ANTIBIOTIC AND CHEMOTHERAPY

LAWRENCE P. GARROD
Emeritus Professor of Bacteriology, University of London
Formerly Bacteriologist, St. Bartholomew's Hospital
and Hon. Consultant in Chemotherapy,
Royal Postgraduate Medical School.

HAROLD P. LAMBERT
Professor of Microbial Diseases, University of London
Consultant Physician, St. George's Hospital.

FRANCIS O'GRADY
Professor of Bacteriology, University of London
Bacteriologist, St. Bartholomew's Hospital.

PAMELA M. WATERWORTH
Senior Microbiologist, Department of Microbiology,
University College Hospital, London.

Antibiotic and Chemotherapy

LAWRENCE P. GARROD
M.D. (Camb.) Hon.LL.D. (Glasgow) F.R.C.P.

HAROLD P. LAMBERT
M.A., M.D. (Camb.) F.R.C.P.

FRANCIS O'GRADY
T.D., M.D. (Lond.) M.Sc. (Lond.) F.R.C. Path.

With a chapter on Laboratory Methods by
PAMELA M. WATERWORTH
M.I.Biol., F.I.L.M.T.

FOURTH EDITION

CHURCHILL LIVINGSTONE
EDINBURGH AND LONDON 1973

ISBN 0 443 01032 3

First Edition	.	.	. 1963
Second Edition	.	.	. 1968
Third Edition	.	.	. 1971
Reprinted	.	.	. 1972
Fourth Edition	.	.	. 1973

Printed in Great Britain

PREFACE TO FIRST EDITION

THIS book is mainly about antibiotics, but embraces sulphonamides and other synthetic drugs employed in the chemotherapy of the microbic infections of temperate climates. That of malaria and most other protozoal infections, helminthiases and malignant disease is excluded. The first part describes the properties of antibiotics and other drugs, with emphasis on their degree of activity against different bacterial species. The large body of detailed information on this presented in a series of tables, some of it hitherto unpublished, provides one essential basis for rational prescribing, since the first requirement of any drug is an adequate and preferably high degree of activity against the species responsible for the infection.

The second part is concerned with chemotherapy in its practical aspects, in infections which are classified by systems. As professional bacteriologists who have had no clinical responsibilities for many years we are fully conscious of our temerity in invading the sphere of therapeutics. Nevertheless each of us has been so frequently consulted by clinical colleagues about the treatment of individual patients that we can claim a knowledge of this subject in its practical as well as theoretical aspects, and feel justified in writing of what we have learned. The treatment we describe is solely that directed against the microbe. We are well aware that other kinds of treatment, quite outside our sphere, are sometimes an important element in success, and moreover that circumstances may exist, again beyond our ken, which can modify the usual indications for chemotherapy. The clinician must be the ultimate judge: our aim has been to provide him with as much factual information as possible, and accounts of the results achieved by previous competent observers. We believe that this information may be found useful at all levels in the profession; to both junior and senior members of hospital staffs and to consultants as well as general practitioners. We trust also that laboratory workers may find the book helpful.

We are indebted to many colleagues for advice, mainly on clinical matters, among whom we would particularly mention Miss J. Allen, F.P.S., Professor J. W. Crofton, Mr. H. G. Dixon, Dr. S. C. Gold, Dr. D. A. Mitchison, Dr. C. S. Nicol, Professor J. G. Scadding, Mr. W. H. Stephenson and Dr. J. P. M. Tizard. They have not actually read our text, and should not be held responsible for the views expressed, or for any errors. Our special thanks are due to Miss Pamela M. Waterworth, who has served both of us as a research assistant. She performed most of the experiments on which our original observations are based: among those hitherto unpublished are numerous data in Tables XI and XXII, and the findings illustrated in Figures 6 and 9. Some of her other contributions to the subject are referred to in the text. We are also indebted to her for advice about Chapter XXVII and for preparing the index.

London, 1963.   M. B.
                                                        L. P. G.

PREFACE TO FOURTH EDITION

As the only author of all four editions of this book, I have the privilege of introducing to its readers a third author of this one, Professor Harold P. Lambert, who brings to it a clinical authority which it could not previously claim.

The success of the Third Edition has been most gratifying; it was sold out in less than twelve months, as was a reprint which followed. The task of revision, despite the short interval which has elapsed, has been heavy. Not only have new drugs to be described—although most are only derivatives of older ones —but basic knowledge has advanced rapidly in several directions. We now devote a separate chapter to modes of action, and much new material will be found in those on synthetic drugs, dosage, penicillins, anti-fungal agents, urinary tract infections and tuberculosis, but every other chapter except the first, which is purely historical, has been revised and brought up to date. The last chapter has been much expanded, and we believe it to be the most complete guide in existence to the provision of those laboratory services without which the clinician prescribing antibiotics can sometimes be ' a navigator without chart or compass '.

Reference lists are longer, and we trust that they will be found useful to the seeker after further information. It may be regrettable that titles are not included, but to have done so would have added about 20 pages to the book and thus perhaps have affected its price.

We are again indebted to many colleagues and friends for advice and information, both proffered and sought. The help of Dr Naomi Datta on the subject of drug resistance has been most valuable. Miss Pamela M. Waterworth's responsibility for Chapter 29 is now acknowledged on the title page. She has also provided some of the new illustrations, made many additions, some based on original observations, to the double-page Table of sensitivities in Chapter 16, checked the reference lists and prepared the index. Lastly, we are grateful to our publishers for allowing us to make numerous alterations and additions in proof, so that it has been possible to notice new work published very few months before this edition itself.

London, 1973   L. P. G.

ACKNOWLEDGMENTS

In addition to the figures acknowledged in the text, we are indebted to the following authors and editors for permission to reproduce original material:

Dr. G. H. Hitchings and *Trans. N.Y. Acad. Sci.* for Fig. 25,

Prof. R. Kilpatrick and *Lancet* for Fig. 2,

Dr. T. D. Brock and *Experimental Chemotherapy* for Fig. 10,

Dr. M. Finland and *Amer. J. med. Sci.* for Fig. 13,

J. med. Lab. Technol. for Fig. 37A,

Dr. I. H. Leopold and *Invest. Ophthal.* for Table 41,

Office of Health Economics for Fig. 30,

J. clin. Path. for Figs. 33 and 34.

Prof. M. H. Richmond for Fig. 3 and Cambridge University Press for Figs. 3 and 20 C and D.

We are indebted for photographs to the Photographic Department of the Royal Postgraduate Medical School, to Mr. P. Crocker of the Department of Pathology, St. Bartholomew's Hospital, and to Mr. P. Luton, Department of Microbiology, University College Hospital.

CONTENTS

PART I

Chapter 1

THE EVOLUTION OF ANTI-MICROBIC DRUGS

No one recently qualified even with the liveliest imagination, can picture the ravages of bacterial infection which continued until rather less than forty years ago. To take only two examples, lobar pneumonia was a common cause of death even in young and vigorous patients, and puerperal septicaemia and other forms of acute streptococcal sepsis had a high mortality, little affected by any treatment then available. One purpose of this chapter is therefore to place the subject of this book in historical perspective.

This subject is chemotherapy, which may be defined as the administration of a substance with a systemic anti-microbic action. Some would confine the term to synthetic drugs, and the distinction is recognized in the title of this book, but since some all-embracing term is needed, this one might with advantage be understood also to include substances of natural origin. Several antibiotics can now be synthesized, and it would be ludicrous if their use should qualify for description as chemotherapy only because they happened to be prepared in this way. The essence of the term is that the effect must be systemic, the substance being absorbed, whether from the alimentary tract or a site of injection, and reaching the infected area by way of the blood stream. 'Local chemotherapy' is in this sense a contradiction in terms: any application to a surface, even of something capable of exerting a systemic effect, is better described as antisepsis.

THE THREE ERAS OF CHEMOTHERAPY

There are three distinct periods in the history of this subject. In the first, which is of great antiquity, the only substances capable of curing an infection by systemic action were natural plant products. The second was the era of synthesis, and in the third we return to natural plant products, although from plants

1

of a much lower order, the moulds and bacteria forming antibiotics.

1. ALKALOIDS. This era may be dated from 1619, since it is
from this year that the first record is derived of the successful
treatment of malaria with an extract of cinchona bark, the
patient being the wife of the Spanish governor of Peru. Another
South American discovery was the efficacy of ipecacuanha root
in amoebic dysentery. Until the early years of this century these
extracts, and in more recent times the alkaloids, quinine and
emetine, derived from them, provided the only curative chemotherapy known.

2. SYNTHETIC COMPOUNDS. Therapeutic progress in this
field, which initially and for many years after was due almost
entirely to research in Germany, dates from the discovery of
salvarsan by Ehrlich in 1909. His successors produced germanin
for trypanosomiasis and other drugs effective in protozoal infections. A common view at that time was that protozoa were
susceptible to chemotherapeutic attack, but that bacteria were
not: the treponemata, which had been shown to be susceptible
to organic arsenicals, are no ordinary bacteria, and were
regarded as a class apart.

The belief that bacteria are by nature insusceptible to any
drug which is not also prohibitively toxic to the human body
was finally destroyed by the discovery of Prontosil. This, the
forerunner of the sulphonamides, was again a product of
German research, and its discovery was publicly announced in
1935. All the work with which this book is concerned is subsequent to this year: it saw the beginning of the effective treatment of bacterial infections.

Progress in the synthesis of anti-microbic drugs has continued
to the present day. Apart from many new sulphonamides,
perhaps the most notable additions have been the synthetic
compounds used in the treatment of tuberculosis.

3. ANTIBIOTICS. The therapeutic revolution produced by the
sulphonamides, which included the conquest of haemolytic
streptococcal and pneumococcal infections and of gonorrhoea
and cerebrospinal fever, was still in progress and even causing
some bewilderment when the first report appeared of a study
which was to have even wider consequences. This was not the
discovery of penicillin—that had been made by Fleming in

1929—but the demonstration by Florey and his colleagues that it was a chemotherapeutic agent of unexampled potency. The first announcement of this, made in 1940, was the beginning of the antibiotic era, and the unimagined developments from it are still in progress. We little knew at the time that penicillin, besides providing a remedy for infections insusceptible to sulphonamide treatment, was also a necessary second line of defence against those fully susceptible to it. During the early 'forties resistance to sulphonamides appeared successively in gonococci, haemolytic streptococci and pneumococci: nearly twenty years later it has appeared also in meningococci. But for the advent of the antibiotics, all the benefits stemming from Domagk's discovery might by now have been lost, and bacterial infections have regained their pre-1935 prevalence and mortality.

The earlier history of two of these discoveries calls for further description.

Sulphonamides

Prontosil, or sulphonamido-chrysoidin, was first synthesized by Klarer and Mietzsch in 1932, and was one of a series of azo dyes examined by Domagk for possible effects on haemolytic streptococcal infection. When a curative effect in mice had been demonstrated, cautious trials in erysipelas and other human infections were undertaken, and not until the evidence afforded by these was conclusive did the discoverers make their announcement. Domagk (1935) published the original claims, and the same information was communicated by Hörlein (1935) to a notable meeting in London.

These claims, which initially concerned only the treatment of haemolytic streptococcal infections, were soon confirmed in other countries, and one of the most notable early studies was that of Colebrook and Kenny (1936) in England, who demonstrated the efficacy of the drug in puerperal fever. This infection had until then been taking a steady toll of about 1,000 young lives per annum in England and Wales, despite every effort to prevent it by hygienic measures and futile efforts to overcome it by serotherapy. The immediate effect of the adoption of this treatment can be seen in Figure 1: a steep fall in mortality began in 1935, and continued, as the treatment became universal and better understood, and as more potent sulphonamides were introduced, until the present-day low level had almost been reached *before penicillin became generally available.* The effect of penicillin between 1945 and 1950 is perhaps more evident on incidence: its widespread use tends completely to

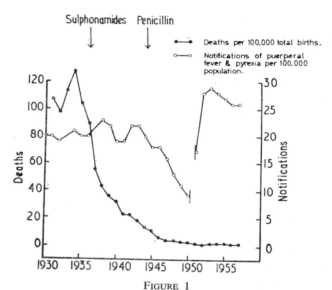

FIGURE 1

Puerperal pyrexia. Deaths per 100,000 total births and incidence per 100,000 population in England and Wales, 1930-1957.

N.B. the apparent rise in incidence in 1950 is due to the fact that the definition of puerperal pyrexia was changed in this year (see text).

(Reproduced from Barber (1960), *J. Obs tet. & Gynaec.* **67,** 727, by kind permission of the editor.)

banish haemolytic streptococci from the environment. The apparent rise in incidence after 1950 is due to the redefinition of puerperal pyrexia as any rise of temperature to 38 °C., whereas previously the term was only applied when the temperature was maintained for 24 hours or recurred. Needless to say, fever so defined is frequently not of uterine origin.

Prontosil had no anti-bacterial action *in vitro,* and it was soon suggested by workers in Paris (Tréfouel *et al.,* 1935) that it owed its activity to the liberation from it in the body of *p*-amino-benzene sulphonamide (sulphanilamide); that this compound is so formed was subsequently proved by Fuller (1937). Sulphanilamide had a demonstrable inhibitory action on streptococci *in vitro,* much dependent on the medium and particularly on the size of the inoculum, facts which are readily understandable in the light of modern knowledge. This explanation of the therapeutic action of prontosil was hotly contested by Domagk. It must be remembered that it relegated the chrysoidin component to an inert role, whereas the affinity of dyes for bacteria had been a basis of German research since the time of Ehrlich, and was the doctrine underlying the choice of this series of compounds for examination. German workers also took the attitude that there must be something mysterious about the action of a true chemotherapeutic agent: an effect easily demonstrable in a test tube by any tyro was too banal altogether to explain it. Finally, they felt justifiable resentment that sulphanilamide, as a compound which had been described many years earlier, could be freely manufactured by anyone.

Every enterprising pharmaceutical house in the world was soon making this drug, and at one time it was on the market under at least 70 different proprietary names. What was more important, chemists were soon busy modifying the molecule to improve its performance. Early advances so secured were of two kinds, the first being higher activity against a wider range of bacteria: sulphapyridine (M and B 693), discovered in 1938, was the greatest single advance, since it was the first drug to be effective in pneumococcal pneumonia. The next stage, the introduction of sulphathiazole and sulphadiazine, while retaining and enhancing anti-bacterial activity, eliminated the frequent nausea and cyanosis caused by earlier drugs. Further developments, mainly in the direction of altered pharmacological properties, have continued to the present day and are described in Chapter 2.

ANTIBIOTICS

' Out of the earth shall come thy salvation.'—S. A. Waksman.

Definition

Of many definitions of the term antibiotic which have been proposed the narrower seem preferable. It is true that the word ' antibiosis ' was coined by Vuillemin in 1889 to denote antagonism between living creatures in general, but the noun ' antibiotic ' was first used by Waksman in 1942 (Waksman and Lechevalier, 1962), which gives him a right to re-define it, and his definition confines it to substances produced by micro-organisms antagonistic to the growth or life of others in high dilution (the last clause being necessary to exclude such metabolic products as organic acids, hydrogen peroxide and alcohol). To define an antibiotic simply as an anti-bacterial substance from a living source would embrace gastric juice, antibodies and lysozyme from man, essential oils and alkaloids from plants, and such oddities as the substance in the faeces of blowfly larvae which exerts an antiseptic effect in wounds. All substances known as antibiotics which are in clinical use and capable of exerting a systemic effect are in fact products of micro-organisms.

Early History

The study of inter-microbic antagonism is almost as old as microbiology itself: several instances of it were described, one by Pasteur himself, in the seventies of the last century. Therapeutic applications followed, some employing actual living cultures, others extracts of bacteria or moulds which had been found active. One of the best known products was an extract of *Ps. aeruginosa,* first used as a local application by Czech workers, Honl and Bukovsky, in 1899: this was commercially available as ' pyocyanase ' on the continent for many years. Other investigators used extracts of species of *Penicillium* and *Aspergillus* which probably or certainly contained antibiotics, but in too low a concentration to exert more than a local and transient effect. Florey (1945) gave a revealing account of these early developments in a lecture with the intriguing title ' The Use of Micro-organisms as Therapeutic Agents ': this was amplified in a later publication (Florey, 1949).

The systematic search, by an ingenious method, for an organism which could attack pyogenic cocci, conducted by Dubos (1939) in New York, led to the discovery of tyrothricin (gramicidin + tyrocidine), formed by *Bacillus brevis,* a substance which although too toxic for systemic use in man, had in fact a systemic curative effect in mice. This work exerted a strong influence in inducing Florey and his colleagues to embark on a study of naturally formed anti-bacterial substances, and penicillin was the second on their list.

Penicillin

The present antibiotic era may be said to date from 1940, when the first account of the properties of an extract of cultures of *Penicillium notatum* appeared from Oxford (Chain *et al.*, 1940): a fuller account followed, with impressive clinical evidence (Abraham *et al.*, 1941). It had been necessary to find means of extracting a very labile substance from culture fluids, to examine its action on a wide range of bacteria, to examine its toxicity by a variety of methods, to establish a unit of its activity, to study its distribution and excretion when administered to animals, and finally to prove its systemic efficacy in mouse infections. There then remained the gigantic task, seemingly impossible except on a factory scale, of producing in the School of Pathology at Oxford enough of a substance, which was known to be excreted with unexampled rapidity, for the treatment of human disease. One means of maintaining supplies was extraction from the patients' urine and re-administration.

It was several years before penicillin was fully purified, its structure ascertained, and its large-scale commercial production achieved. That this was of necessity first entrusted to manufacturers in the United States gave them a lead in a highly profitable industry which was not to be overtaken for many years.

Later Antibiotics

The dates of discovery and sources of the principal antibiotics are given chronologically in Table 1. A few, including penicillin, were chance discoveries, but ' stretching out suppliant Petri dishes ' (Florey, 1945) in the hope of catching a new antibiotic-producing organism was not to lead anywhere. Most further discoveries resulted from soil surveys, a process from which a large annual outlay might or might not be repaid a hundredfold, a gamble against much longer odds than most oil prospecting. Soil contains a profuse and very mixed flora varying with climate, vegetation, mineral content and other factors, and is a medium in which antibiotic formation may well play a part in the competition for nutriment. A soil survey consists of

TABLE 1

Date of Discovery and Source of the More Important Antibiotics

Name	Date of Discovery	Microbe	Source
Penicillin	1929–1940	*Penicillium notatum*	Air, London
Tyrothricin { Gramicidin / Tyrocidine }	1939	*Bacillus brevis*	Soil, New York
Griseofulvin	1939	*Penicillium griseofulvum Dierckx*	Soil, Dorset
	1945	*Penicillium janczewski*	A chicken's throat
Streptomycin	1944	*Streptomyces griseus*	Contaminated wound
Bacitracin	1945	*Bacillus licheniformis*	Mulched field, Venezuela
Chloramphenicol	1947	*Streptomyces venezuelae*	Soil, Britain and U.S.A.
Polymyxin	1947	*Bacillus polymyxa*	Damp patch on wall, Paris
Framycetin	1947–1953	*Streptomyces lavendulae*	Soil
Chlortetracycline	1948	*Streptomyces aureofaciens*	Sewage outfall, Sardinia
Cephalosporin C, N and P	1948	*Cephalosporium sp.*	Soil, New Jersey
Neomycin	1949	*Streptomyces fradiae*	Soil
Oxytetracycline	1950	*Streptomyces rimosus*	Farm soil, Fauquier County, Va.
Nystatin	1950	*Streptomyces noursei*	Soil, Island in Philippines
Erythromycin	1952	*Streptomyces erythreus*	Pastureland, Vermont, U.S.A.
Novobiocin	1955	*Streptomyces spheroides*	
		Streptomyces niveus	
Cycloserine	1955	*Streptomyces orchidaceus*	Soil, Indiana
		Streptomyces gaeryphalus	Soil, Guatemala
Vancomycin	1956	*Streptomyces orientalis*	Soil, Borneo and Indiana
Kanamycin	1957	*Streptomyces kanamyceticus*	Soil, Japan
Paromomycin	1959	*Streptomyces rimosus*	Soil, Colombia
Fusidic acid	1960	*Fusidium coccineum*	Monkey dung, Japan
Lincomycin	1962	*Streptomyces lincolnensis*	Soil, Lincoln, Nebraska
Gentamicin	1963	*Micromonospora purpurea*	Soil, Syracuse, N.Y.

obtaining samples from as many and as varied sources as possible, cultivating them on plates, subcultivating all colonies of promising organisms such as actinomycetes and examining each for anti-bacterial activity. Alternatively the primary plate culture may be inoculated by spraying or by agar layering with suitable bacteria, the growth of which may then be seen to be inhibited in a zone surrounding some of the original colonies. This is only a beginning : many thousands of successive colonies so examined are found to form an antibiotic already known or useless by reason of toxicity.

It will be noticed from Table 1 that antibiotics have been derived from some odd sources other than soil. Although the original strain of *Penicillium notatum* apparently floated in through a window at St. Mary's Hospital, that of *P. chrysogenum* now used for penicillin production was derived from a mouldy Canteloupe melon in a market at Peoria, Illinois. Perhaps the strangest derivation was that of helenine, an antibiotic with some anti-viral activity, isolated by Shope (1953) from *Penicillium funiculosum* growing on ' the isinglass cover of a photograph of my wife, Helen, on Guam, near the end of the war in 1945 '. He proceeds to explain that he chose the name because it was non-descriptive, non-committal and not pre-empted, ' but largely out of recognition of the good taste shown by the mold . . . in locating on the picture of my wife '.

Those antibiotics out of thousands now discovered which have qualified for therapeutic use are described in chapters which follow.

FUTURE PROSPECTS

All successful chemotherapeutic agents have certain properties in common. They must exert an anti-microbic action, whether inhibitory or lethal, in high dilution, and in the complex chemical environment which they encounter in the body. Secondly, since they are brought into contact with every tissue in the body, they must so far as possible be without harmful effect on the function of any organ. To these two essential qualities may be added others which are highly desirable, although sometimes lacking in useful drugs : stability, free solubility, a slow rate of excretion, and diffusibility into remote areas.

If a drug is toxic to bacteria but not to mammalian cells the probability is that it interferes with some structure or function peculiar to bacteria. When the mode of action of sulphanilamide was elucidated by Woods and Fildes, and the theory was put forward of bacterial inhibition by metabolite analogues, the way seemed open for devising further anti-bacterial drugs on a rational basis. Immense subsequent advances in knowledge of the anatomy, chemical composition and metabolism of the bacterial cell should have encouraged such hopes still further. This new knowledge has been helpful in explaining what drugs do to bacteria, but not in devising new ones. Discoveries have continued to result only from random trials, purely empirical in the antibiotic field, although sometimes based on reasonable theoretical expectation in the synthetic.

Not only is the action of any new drug on individual bacteria any drug. It seems unlikely that any totally new antibiotic remains to be discovered, since those of recent origin have similar still unpredictable on a theoretical basis, but so are its effects on the body itself. Most of the toxic effects of antibiotics have come to light only after extensive use, and even now no one can explain their affinity for some of the organs attacked. Some new observations in this field have contributed something to the present climate of suspicion about new drugs generally, which is insisting on far more searching tests of toxicity, and delaying the release of drugs for therapeutic use, particularly in the United States.

The Present Scope of Chemotherapy

Successive discoveries have added to the list of infections amenable to chemotherapy until nothing remains altogether untouched except the smaller viruses. On the other hand, some of the drugs which it is necessary to use are far from ideal, whether because of toxicity or of unsatisfactory pharmacological properties, and some forms of treatment are consequently less often successful than others. Moreover microbic resistance is a constant threat to the future usefulness of almost properties to others already known. It therefore will be wise to husband our resources. and employ them in such a way as to preserve them. The problems of drug resistance and policies for preventing it are discussed in Chapters 15 and 16.

Adaptation of Existing Drugs

A line of advance other than the discovery of new drugs is the adaptation of old ones. An outstanding example of what can be achieved in this way is presented by the sulphonamides. Similar attention has naturally been directed to the antibiotics, with fruitful results of two different kinds. One is simply an alteration for the better in pharmacological properties. Thus procaine penicillin, because less soluble, is longer acting than potassium penicillin: the esterification of macrolides improves absorption: chloramphenicol palmitate is palatable, and other variants so produced are more stable, more soluble and less irritant.

Most of these changes are produced by additions to the drug molecule, but modifications in its essential structure can alter its anti-microbic properties as well—usually for the worse, but sometimes with advantage. The outstanding success here has been achieved by synthetic manipulation of the molecule of penicillin, since new penicillins have thus been obtained with three desirable properties: resistance to acid, resistance to penicillinase, and enhanced action on some Gram-negative species. Derivatives of cephalosporin C and rifamycin now in clinical use have been obtained in the same way. The present complexity of choice among antibiotics for some types of infection is an embarrassment, resulting largely from these efforts, of which it would be ungrateful to complain.

REFERENCES

ABRAHAM, E. P., CHAIN, E., FLETCHER, C. M., FLOREY, H. W., GARDNER, A. D., HEATLEY, N. G. & JENNINGS, M. A. (1941). *Lancet* **2**, 177.
CHAIN, E., FLOREY, H. W., GARDNER, A. D., HEATLEY, N. G., JENNINGS, M. A., ORR-EWING, J. & SANDERS, A. G. (1940). *Lancet* **2**, 226.
COLEBROOK, L. & KENNY, M. (1936). *Lancet* **1**, 1279.
DOMAGK, G. (1935). *Dtsch. med. Wschr.* **61**, 250.
DUBOS, R. J. (1939). *J. exp. Med.* **70**, 1, 11.
FLOREY, H. W. (1945). *Brit. med. J.* **2**, 635.
FLOREY, H. W. (1949). *Antibiotics*, chap. I. London: Oxford University Press.
FULLER, A. T. (1937). *Lancet* **1**, 194.
HONL, J. & BUKOVSKY, J. (1899). *Zbl. Bakt.* Abt. I. **26**, 305. (See Florey, 1949.)
HÖRLEIN, H. (1935). *Proc. R. Soc. Med.* **29**, 313.
SHOPE, R. E. (1953). *J. exp. Med.* **97**, 601, 627, 639.
TRÉFOUEL, J., TRÉFOUEL, J., NITTI, F. & BOVET, D. (1935). *C.R. Soc. Biol. (Paris)* **120**, 756.
WAKSMAN, S. A. & LECHEVALIER, H. A. (1962). *The Actinomycetes*, vol. 3. London: Baillière.

CHAPTER 2

SULPHONAMIDES

THE discovery and early history of the sulphonamides are described in Chapter 1. The introduction of further compounds has now continued for over 30 years; advances have been made in the directions of lower toxicity and better tolerance, and of higher antibacterial activity. Compounds of low solubility, which are little absorbed and so act mainly in the bowel, have been developed, and the most recent additions are long-acting preparations which enable the frequency of doses to be reduced.

It no longer seems necessary to include a full account of all these numerous drugs in a work of this kind, particularly since the scope of their therapeutic use has been much diminished by the substitution of antibiotics.

ANTIBACTERIAL ACTIVITY

Sulphonamides have what in an antibiotic is now called a broad spectrum. Among Gram-positive organisms, group A streptococci and pneumococci are highly sensitive, staphylococci and *Cl. welchii* moderately so (other clostridia are more resistant), but *Str. faecalis* is resistant. The most sensitive Gram-negative species are the *Neisseria,* but the list includes many enterobacteria. Thus in the early days sulphonamide treatment was successful in all forms of streptococcal sepsis, pneumococcal pneumonia and other infections, gas gangrene, gonorrhoea and cerebrospinal fever, and some enterobacterial infections of both gastro-intestinal and urinary tracts. Of these uses only the last is now common.

All sulphonamides act alike, and an organism sensitive to one will be sensitive in some degree to all others. Much has been written about the relative degrees of activity of different sulphonamides against individual species. Such findings are difficult to evaluate, because comparisons have rarely been made with more than a few other drugs. A greater difficulty is the strong dependence of the result of any *in vitro* test on the composition of the culture medium and on the size of the inoculum (see Fig. 35 and p. 503). Because of the magnitude of these effects it is impossible to state the minimum inhibitory concentration (M.I.C.) of a sulphonamide for a given organism with anything approaching the precision such as is possible, for instance, with penicillin, which is little affected by either of these factors.

The results of tests of therapeutic activity in mice are also difficult to interpret in comparative terms, since they also are much affected by the conditions of the experiment. As an example, single doses or doses given only once daily strongly favour long-acting compounds, whereas had they been administered at the usual clinical intervals, a more rapidly eliminated compound might have performed as well or better.

Rather than attempting to review the voluminous and sometimes contradictory literature on the relative *in vitro* activities of different sulphonamides, we have felt it necessary to make our own comparison. The following tests were carried out recently and the results were published for the first time in the third edition of this book.

Determinations of the M.I.C. of Different Sulphonamides for Strains of More Important Susceptible Pathogens

DRUGS. Sulphacetamide was chosen as a representative of the earliest and less potent compounds, since alone among them it is still in use. The remainder include the more widely used short-acting compounds and nearly all the recently introduced long-acting. Compounds of low solubility administered only for their effect on the bowel flora are excluded. The drugs were dissolved by adding the minimum necessary amount of NaOH.

BACTERIA. These were mostly recent clinical isolates with approximately normal sulphonamide sensitivity. Some had been kept at $-70°$C. for varying periods of time.

METHOD. A single batch of Oxoid DST Agar was used throughout. Freshly lysed horse-blood was added in a concentration of 5 per cent, and 14 ml. of medium was mixed in plates with 1 ml. of drug dilution to give final concentrations varying two-fold and based on 1μg./ml., the whole range used for different organisms varying from 128 to 0·12 μg./ml.

The plates were inoculated with a 32-prong replicator from approximately 1 in 200 dilutions of overnight broth or blood broth cultures. Ditches were cut to isolate areas inoculated with swarming *Proteus*. Plates were read for the presence or absence of growth on the following day. Each organism was tested against the whole range of drugs in a single experiment, always controlled by the inclusion of a standard strain of *E. coli* (N.C.T.C. 10418).

The results are given in Table 2. They confirm the low activity of sulphacetamide and of sulphadimidine, and the high activity of sulphadiazine, which is equalled and in a few instances exceeded by that of several other compounds, including sulphafurazole and sulphamethoxazole. They conflict in innumerable particulars with the results of others. As an example Neipp (1964) in tests of which the results were quoted (Table 3, p. 15) in the second edition of this book, credits sulphadiazine with an incredibly low degree of activity against *Str. pneumoniae*, the M.I.C. being forty times greater than that of sulphamethoxazole. This test was done with a single strain: those in Table 2 were done with six. For two of these strains the M.I.C. of sulphadiazine and sulphamethoxazole were the same; for the other four they differed only two-fold. Various claims for the superior activity of individual sulphonamides against particular species are not confirmed. We venture to suggest that the findings reported here are more dependable than some comparisons in the literature, because they relate to a wide range of representative sulphonamides, all of which were tested together in one experiment, they were done with multiple strains of all the more important bacteria, and particularly because they were all carried out in the same way on a single batch of a suitable medium.

The main conclusion to be drawn is that there is very little indeed to choose between the antibacterial activities of the more potent sulphonamides. Choice among them should rather depend on their pharmacological properties, and when these are similar it is almost indifferent.

Acquired Bacterial Resistance

Bacteria can be slowly trained to sulphonamide resistance *in vitro,* and every important pathogenic species has sooner or later been found resistant *in vivo*. This change occurred earliest and most rapidly in gonococci, which nevertheless have reverted to sensitivity during the many years which have elapsed since sulphonamide treatment for gonorrhoea was abandoned. A further quarter-century elapsed before it was seen in the closely related meningococcus (Millar *et al.*, 1963). Resistant strains of *Str. pyogenes* and pneumococci began to appear in the early 'forties, and but for the advent of the antibiotics there might by now be no effective specific treatment for the important infections caused by these organisms. Resistance in all enterobacteria is now common, and in *Sh. sonnei* almost invariable. Needless to say, resistance to any sulphonamide is accompanied by resistance to all others.

Some mutants owe their sulphonamide resistance to the synthesis of a folic acid synthetase with a lowered affinity for sulphonamide. Some other mutants appear to owe their resistance to changes in the feed-back mechanism. Some overproduce *p*-aminobenzoic acid (Pato and Brown, 1963), an effect which could result from 'switching off' the feed-back control, thereby making the organism insusceptible to sulphonamide interference with enzyme production and function (Richmond, 1966).

Combined Action with Other Antibacterial Drugs

Although the effect of sulphonamides is purely bacteristatic, it does not, like that of some similarly acting antibiotics, antagonize the bactericidal effect of penicillin. This is not to say that such a combination is often indicated. With one antibiotic, polymyxin, sulphonamides may act synergically (Herman, 1959; Russell, 1963). By far the most important combination is with trimethoprim, which is so much more effective than a sulphonamide alone that we ventured even in previous editions of this book to say: 'the possibility arises that trimethoprim should also be given whenever sulphonamides are used'. This drug is described in Chapter 3.

PHARMACOKINETICS

Absorption

Most sulphonamides are well absorbed after oral administration, reaching a peak concentration in the blood after 2-4 hours, which after a dose of 2 g. is of the order of 100 μg./ml. Parenteral preparations of some are available, usually sodium salts, which are strongly alkaline and can only be given intravenously or, in the case of sodium sulphadimidine, by deep intramuscular injection.

Conjugation

After absorption a proportion of the drug is conjugated, usually with acetate, this proportion varying considerably with different compounds. The lower this is the better, since the conjugates are inactive therapeutically and the acetyl derivatives are rather more toxic than the free drug. Their solubility in the urine is also a factor to be considered.

Plasma Binding

Of sulphonamide in the blood a proportion, varying considerably with different compounds, is contained in the red cells, some is free in the plasma, and another proportion, again varying greatly, is bound to plasma albumin. This bound drug is usually considered to be antibacterially inactive (Newbould & Kirkpatrick, 1960; Anton, 1960), but the findings of Bøe (1966) suggest that this may be an over-simplified view. He

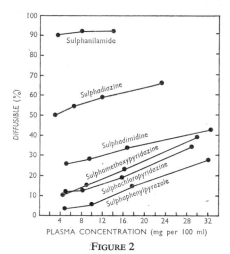

FIGURE 2

Effect of increasing concentration of various sulphonamides on binding of sulphonamide to plasma-proteins at pH 7·4.

Redrawn from Newbould and Kilpatrick (1960).

compared the effects of adding different amounts of protein on the activity of sulphadiazine and of sulphadimethoxine, which at the same concentration in plasma are respectively 45·1 per cent and 98·7 per cent protein-bound, and found discrepancies inexplicable on this basis.

It will be seen from Figure 2 that the percentage bound varies, although not directly, with the total drug concentration in the blood. It is also affected by the albumin concentration: in hypoalbuminaemia the percentage is much decreased (Anton, 1968).

Protein-bound drug is distributed as protein, and binding consequently affects the concentration of drug entering the tissues from the capillaries. Access to the C.S.F. for example, is normally limited to the unbound drug but with increasing capillary permeability and the passage of protein into the C.S.F. in inflammation, protein-bound sulphonamide enters and the total concentration of sulphonamide in the C.S.F. rises.

The concentration of the short-acting sulphonamides achieved in C.S.F. varies between 30 per cent and 80 per cent of the corresponding plasma concentration.

Sulphonamides can be displaced from their protein binding sites by a variety of compounds including phenylbutazone and ethyl-bis-coumarin, and simultaneous administration of these substances produces higher concentrations of diffusible sulphonamide (Anton, 1961). This competition for plasma albumin binding sites is also responsible for the effect of sulphonamide in displacing albumin-bound bilirubin (see p. 21).

PASSAGE THROUGH PLACENTA. Sulphonamides pass readily through the placenta into the foetal circulation and the possible dangers of this to the foetus must be remembered when treating pregnant women with sulphonamides (p. 21).

Excretion

The plasma level of free sulphonamide depends on the rate of absorption, the rate and extent of conjugation, and above all, on the rate of excretion. Sulphonamides are excreted mainly in the urine, the free drug and its conjugates being frequently excreted at different rates and by different mechanisms. As a result, the peak plasma concentrations of free drug and conjugate may occur at different times and the proportion of free drug to conjugate may be very different in the plasma and urine.

As with isoniazid (p. 435), the capacity to inactivate sulphadimidine is bimodally distributed in the population, those who acetylate most (62-90 per cent) of the drug being clearly different from those who acetylate only 40-53 per cent (Evans and White, 1964). Active acetylators of sulphadimidine correspond with rapid inactivators of isoniazid.

Sulphonamides are partly filtered through the glomeruli and partly secreted by the tubules, where some of the excreted drug is reabsorbed. The extent of these processes differs amongst the sulphonamides and may differ markedly for the free drug and its conjugates. As a result, the plasma clearance values vary from <10 to >200 ml./min. Substances with high clearances like sulphafurazole are rapidly eliminated from the plasma and achieve high concentrations in the urine. Substances with low clearances are slowly excreted, plasma levels are maintained for long periods, and low concentrations appear in the urine. If renal function is impaired, excretion may be still further delayed and therapeutic levels may persist for considerably longer. Equally, if such drugs are given repeatedly, high and possibly toxic levels may develop. Naturally no protein-bound drug escapes through the kidney, and therefore highly protein-bound compounds are in general long-acting, but correspondence between the two properties is far from exact because of differences in the degree of tubular re-absorption, which may be a major factor in maintaining the plasma level.

EXCRETION IN BILE. Less than 1 per cent of the dose of the older sulphonamides is excreted in the bile but the proportion is greater (2·4-6·3 per cent) for the new long-acting compounds (Neipp et al., 1964).

TOXICITY

There has been a tendency recently to exaggerate the ill effects produced by these drugs. Proper choice of compound and reasonable dosage can ensure that such effects will be uncommon.

The cyanosis frequently caused by the earliest compounds is now almost never seen, and such effects as nausea and vomiting, headache and dizziness have become very exceptional. Several other distinct types of possible effect require separate consideration.

Renal Blockage

The first edition of this book (Barber & Garrod, 1963) contained a full page table of the solubilities of 17 sulphonamides and of their conjugates in urine at 4 different ranges of pH. It is now perhaps enough to say that all are more soluble in alkaline than acid urine, that long-acting compounds present little danger because of their slow rate of excretion, and that among others only sulphapyridine (no longer used), sulphathiazole, sulphadiazine and sulphamerazine have dangerously low solubilities. The risk of giving even these and even in maximum doses can be much diminished by giving alkali and enough fluid to ensure a good output of urine, although sulphamerazine may be an exception to this. Triple mixtures containing them render the risk almost negligible. Failing such precautions crystals deposited in the urine may block either the renal tubules or the upper orifice of the ureter. Haematuria is a common early sign. Renal damage during sulphonamide therapy may often, however, be due to a hypersensitivity reaction, rather than to tubular blockage. These reactions are discussed below.

Hypersensitivity Reactions

Protein-bound sulphonamide can function as a haptene, and the usual result of antibody formation is moderate fever with an urticarial or maculo-erythematous rash occurring on about the ninth day of a course of treatment. Repetition after an interval will elicit the reaction immediately.

Stevens-Johnson syndrome. This fortunately rare but frequently fatal variety of erythema multiforme has been described as an occasional complication of sulphonamide therapy (Salvaggio and Gonzales, 1959). The relative dangers of different sulphonamides cannot be accurately assessed but those which persist in plasma for prolonged periods present a double hazard. They are extensively bound to plasma proteins—and to this extent are more liable to function as haptenes—and their persistence means that toxic manifestations may continue to develop for days after cessation of therapy. A number of reports have described the condition following treatment with long-acting sulphonamides (Beveridge *et al.*, 1964) and the F.D.A. collected 116 cases in which it was believed these drugs were implicated (Carroll, Bryan and Robinson, 1966). The majority (79) were under the age of 15 and there were 20 deaths. Of the 37 adults, 9 died. The time of onset varied from 2 to 24 days, sometimes as long as 6 days after discontinuing the drug. It was estimated that there had been about 1 or 2 cases per 10 million doses distributed. Toxic epidermal necrolysis (Lyell's syndrome) has also been recorded after administration of long-acting sulphonamides.

EFFECTS OF APPLICATION TO THE SKIN. Local treatment of skin conditions with sulphonamides is now recognized as contra-indicated because a very intractable type of sensitization may result, manifested at first by a local dermatitis, later by extension of this to other areas, and sometimes by fever, and persistence of the reaction long after the treatment has been stopped.

Blood Dyscrasias

AGRANULOCYTOSIS. The commonest effect of sulphonamides on the bone marrow is a depression of leucopoiesis, and this rarely proceeds to agranulocytosis. Modern sulphonamides seem less liable to have this effect than the earlier (Yow, 1953). Before concluding that a sulphonamide is responsible, the prescription sheet should be reviewed. Discombe (1952), having seen necropsies on three patients from one surgical unit within a month where deaths from agranulocytosis were attributed to sulphapyridine, found that each of them had also been given a proprietary sedative which, unknown to the prescriber, contained amidopyrin. It seems possible here that two marrow depressants had acted synergically.

Haemolytic anaemia

Sulphonamides, like a number of other drugs, tend to oxidize haemoglobin to methaemoglobin, and this effect is normally combated through the activity of glucose-6-phosphate dehydrogenase. In patients with inherited deficiency of this enzyme, treatment with sulphonamides may cause denatured haemoglobin to accumulate in the red cells in the form of Heinz bodies, and intravascular haemolysis and haemoglobinuria to occur.

Jaundice

Jaundice resulting from liver damage is a very rare complication of sulphonamide treatment in the adult.

Bilirubin is transported in the blood bound to plasma albumin and a number of drugs, including some sulphonamides (O'Dell, 1959), compete for the binding sites and so interfere with bilirubin excretion. Sulphonamides administered to pregnant women cross the placenta and may circulate in the foetus for several days or even weeks (Sparr and Pritchard, 1958; Lucey and Driscoll, 1961). Interference with bilirubin transport during this period may increase the free plasma bilirubin level and result in kernicterus. For this reason, sulphonamides should not be given to pregnant women where there is a possibility of rhesus incompatibility, premature delivery, or any history of previous neo-natal jaundice. Sulphonamides should not be given to neonates and this is especially important in premature infants in whom bilirubin conjugation is particularly imperfectly developed.

Embryopathy

There have been several reports of teratogenic activity in experimental animals by some long-acting sulphonamides (Paget and Thorpe, 1964), but in a retrospective study, Cahal (1965) found no evidence of embryopathy in man.

CLINICAL APPLICATIONS

Sulphonamides have a wide antibacterial range, yet they do not produce the troublesome disturbances of gut flora which frequently occur with other broad spectrum agents, notably the tetracyclines. They are active not only against staphylococci, haemolytic streptococci and pneumococci, but also against many enterobacteria including some species resistant to common antibiotics. It has also been claimed—though the evidence for this is not particularly good—that sulphonamides may usefully augment the action of antibiotics in the treatment of a variety of infections.

Although severe toxic manifestations have been described and some authors have condemned sulphonamides on this account, severe reactions are uncommon and treatment for 14 days with conventional doses of current sulphonamides rarely gives rise to trouble. From amongst the thousands that have been synthesized a sulphonamide can be chosen which possesses almost any desirable pharmacological attribute: free absorption from the gut with high blood levels, wide distribution in the body, and ready penetration into the C.S.F.; little or no absorption from the gut; rapid excretion with high urinary concentrations; or very slow excretion with prolonged blood levels. In addition to all this, sulphonamides are cheap and very stable.

In short, except for the fact that they are not bactericidal, sulphonamides approximate closely to the ideal antibacterial agent.

Despite this, absolute indications for their use are very few since the same effect can usually be achieved more rapidly with an antibiotic. Their principal use is for the treatment of urinary tract infection. Their applicability to the treatment of respiratory tract infection is more doubtful, and their value in alimentary tract infection has diminished owing to increasingly frequent resistance in enteropathogenic bacteria. The less soluble compounds remain useful in combination with neomycin for pre-operative suppression of the bowel flora. Their value in the treatment of meningococcal meningitis is everywhere threatened and in some countries destroyed by the emergence of resistant strains, and few now regard them as a useful adjunct in treating pneumococcal and *H. influenzae* meningitis. Among more exotic uses, sulphonamides appear currently to be the best treatment for nocardiosis, and, in combination with pyrimethamine, for toxoplasmosis, and perhaps for pyrimethamine-resistant malaria (p. 35).

It is a tenable position that except for a few special purposes, such as pre-operative suppression of the gut flora, sulphonamides should no longer be prescribed alone, but only in combination with trimethoprim, a drug which greatly enhances their effect. Its properties, and the wider indications which exist for this combined treatment, are described in the following chapter.

CHOICE OF A SULPHONAMIDE

There is no present need for the existence of so many different sulphonamides, and in our view there is no longer any need to attempt to balance their individual merits by a consideration of all the properties in which they differ. The following brief account only categorizes them and refers to some of the properties of those in commonest use.

Sulphonamides for General Use

Among the older compounds, sulphanilamide has been discarded because of its low activity, sulphacetamide for the same reason (except for use as eye drops) and sulphapyridine because of its toxicity. The following remain for consideration.

SULPHATHIAZOLE B.P.C. (2-sulphanilamido-thiazole) is highly potent, but peculiarly liable to cause side effects, and is now rarely prescribed alone.

SULPHADIAZINE B.P.C. (2-sulphanilamido-pyrimidine). This compound has the advantages of high potency, a rate of excretion such that adequate blood concentrations are easily maintained, and low protein binding, facilitating diffusion into the tissues and cerebrospinal fluid. Hence it is often regarded as the best choice for treating meningitis. Renal blockage has to be guarded against.

SULPHADIMIDINE B.P. (2-sulphanilamido-4 : 6-methylpyrimidine; sulphamezathine, sulphamethazine). This compound is well absorbed, and excreted moderately slowly. Both the drug and its acetyl derivative are highly soluble, which renders the chance of renal blockage remote, and toxic effects of other kinds and sensitivity reactions are rare. These properties account for its high popularity in this country, but in others this does not obtain : in the United States, for instance, consumption is very small and diminishing (Zbinden, 1964). A good reason for this is its low potency: the concentrations required to inhibit many species according to our findings (Table 2) are up to 8-fold higher than those of sulphadiazine, and according to Neipp (1964) some of these differences are much greater. Similar although less extreme differences have been observed in the curative doses for experimental infections. It also suffers by comparison with sulphadiazine in being acetylated to a greater degree and much more highly protein-bound (Fig. 2).

Sulphadimidine has evidently given satisfaction in clinical use, and it may seem unjustified to detract from its merits on largely theoretical grounds. It must nevertheless be pointed out that advantage can be taken of the higher potency of other compounds, and some of the risks of using them can be reduced by the use of one of the following combinations.

TRIPLE SULPHONAMIDES. The mixture originally advocated by Lehr contained 37 per cent of each of sulphadiazine and sulphathiazole and 26 per cent of sulphamerazine. Sulphamerazine is more highly protein-bound and less slowly excreted than sulphadiazine and is unsuitable for administration alone in full doses. The main advantage of the mixture is that each drug retains its individual solubility in the urine, and since the dose of each is small, so is the risk of renal blockage: indeed if adequate fluids and alkali are given it may well be negligible. Other advantages claimed are a reduced risk of sensitization reactions and the maintenance of a steadier blood level. Several modifications of the original ' sulphatriad ' are now in use.

Highly Soluble Compounds

The following are highly soluble, even in acid urine, in which they attain high concentrations, and have been largely used for treating urinary tract infections.

SULPHAFURAZOLE B.P. (3 : 4-dimethyl - 5 - sulphanilamido-isoxazole, sulfisoxazole, U.S.P., Gantrisin). According to our findings (Table 2) this compound is highly active, and if given in sufficiently frequent doses to compensate for its rapid excretion, should serve for treating infections elsewhere as well as in the urinary tract.

SULPHAMETHIZOLE, B.P. (2-sulphanilamido-5-methyl-1 : 3 : 4-thiodiazole, Urolucosil, Thiosulphil).

SULPHASOMIDINE B.P. (6-sulphanilamido-2:4-dimethylpyrimidine, sulphadimetine, Elkosin). This compound appears rather less active than sulphafurazole. It has also been used as a general purpose sulphonamide.

Compounds of Low Solubility

SUCCINYLSULPHATHIAZOLE, B.P. (2(p-succinyl-sulphanila-mido)-thiazole, sulfasuxidine), and PHTHALYLSULPHATHIAZOLE B.P. (2(p-phthalyl-sulphanilamido)-thiazole, sulphathalidine) are very little absorbed and owe their activity to the slow liberation of sulphathiazole in the bowel. They may be given together with an antibiotic for pre-operative suppression of the bowel flora. (Sulphaguanidine, B.P.C. is less suitable for this purpose because less potent and more absorbed.)

Long-Acting Compounds

These are further divisible into three categories according to their rate of excretion. ' Medium '-long-acting, with half-lives such that two daily doses are given, include the following:

SULPHAMETHOXAZOLE (5-methyl-3-sulphanilamido-isoxazole, Gantanol) has a high potency (Table 2) and is the compound with which trimethoprim is combined in co-trimoxazole.

The best known long-acting compounds, of which only one daily dose need be given, are:

SULPHAMETHOXYPYRIDAZINE B.P. (3-sulphanilamido-6-meth-oxy-pyridazine, Lederkyn, Midicel).

SULPHADIMETHOXINE, B.P.C. (2 : 4-dimethoxy-6-sulphanila-mido-1 : 3-diazine, Madribon).

SULPHAPHENAZOLE B.P.C. (3-sulphanilamido-2-phenylpyra-zole, Orisulf).

SULPHAMETHOXYDIAZINE (2-sulphanilamido-5-methoxypyri-midine, Durenate).

Among these compounds sulphadimethoxine is the most highly protein-bound and sulphamethoxydiazine the least. Various merits have been claimed for each of them and some of these were discussed in previous editions of this book. According to our findings (Table 2) none possesses any outstanding *in vitro* activity, and that of sulphaphenazole is distinctly inferior against all enterobacteria in contrast to the high activity against *Str. pyogenes*. No advantage is clearly discernible in their use except the convenience of a single daily dose, and against this has to be set the possible extra risk referred to on page 19.

Very long acting compounds include sulfametopyrazine (2-sulphanilamido-3-methoxypyrazine, Kelfizine), for which adequate blood levels can be maintained by giving a dose of 2 g. once weekly, and sulfadoxine (formerly sulphormethoxine, 4,*p*-aminobenzenesulphonamido-5, 6-dimethoxypyrimidine, Fanasil), given in a dose of 1 g. once a week. These compounds have been used in single dose treatment of urinary infections (Gruneberg and Brumfitt, 1967; Williams and Smith, 1970), in chronic bronchitis (Pines, 1967), and in malaria (Laing, 1964). Long acting sulphonamides have also been recommended for the prophylaxis of rheumatic fever and of meningococcal meningitis (but see p. 353).

Sulphonamides for Special Uses

MARFANIL. This simple compound, *p*-aminomethylbenzene sulphonamide, now available as the hydrochloride under the name *sulfamylon*, has an interesting history. Synthesized in the U.S.A. where it was soon abandoned as being only feebly active, it was used by the Germans during the war, evidently with great success, as a local application to wounds for the prevention of gas gangrene. It has recently come into its own again as a local preparation for burns (page 338). It is active against *Ps. aeruginosa*. It rapidly diffuses through burned skin and is unusual in that it is not neutralised by *p*-aminobenzoic acid or tissue exudates.

SULPHASALAZINE. This compound of sulphapyridine and salicylic acid (*p*-(benzylsulphonyl-(amino-α-pyridine))-azo-salicylic acid, Salazopyrin, Azopyrin) is used almost exclusively for treating ulcerative colitis. The prolonged courses usually given are liable to cause side effects, including fever and rashes and blood dyscrasias. In a double-blind trial, Baron *et al.* (1962) found sulphasalazine effective in acute attacks of ulcerative colitis, but side effects are common. Truelove, Watkinson and Draper (1962) found corticosteroid therapy to be superior. In a controlled trial of sulphasalazine as maintenance therapy for ulcerative colitis, Misiewicz *et al.* (1965) found that the drug reduced the relapse rate.

PHARMACEUTICAL PREPARATIONS AND DOSAGE

PHTHALYL SULPHATHIAZOLE (Sulphathalidine, *Merck, Sharp and Dohme;* Thalazole, *May and Baker*)
Tablets, B.P., B.N.F.: 500 mg.; Mixture: 500 mg. per 5 ml. Dose: 5-10 g. daily in divided doses.

SUCCINYLSULPHATHIAZOLE (Sulfasuxidine, *Merck, Sharp and Dohme*)
Tablets, B.P., B.N.F.: 500 mg.; Mixture: 500 mg. per 5 ml. Dose: 10-20 g. daily in divided doses.

SULFAMETOPYRAZINE (Kelfizine, Pharmitalia)
Tablets: 200 mg. and 2 g.; Syrup: 20 mg./ml. Dose: Initial 800 mg. subsequent 200 mg. daily, or 2 g. once weekly.

SULPHACETAMIDE
Eye drops B.P.C., B.N.F. 10 per cent w/v, 30 per cent w/v.
Eye ointment B.P., B.N.F., 2·5 per cent, 6 per cent, 10 per cent.

SULPHADIAZINE (Adiazine, *Fr.;* Microsulfon, *U.S.A.*)
Tablets, B.P.: 500 mg. Sodium sulphadiazine injection B.P., B.P.C. 1 g. in 4 ml. for i.v. use. Dose: Initial 3 g.; Subsequent: up to 4 g. daily in divided doses.

SULPHADIMETHOXINE (Madribon, *Roche*)
Tablets, B.P.: 500 mg.; U.S.N.F.: 250 and 500 mg.; Suspension, U.S.N.F.: 250 mg. per 5 ml. Dose: Initial: 1-2 g.; Subsequent: 500 mg. daily.

SULPHADIMIDINE (Sulphamethazine, *U.S.P.;* Sulphamezathine, and S-mez, *I.C.I.*)
Tablets, B.P., B.N.F.: 500 mg. Injection B.P., B.N.F. 1 g. in 3 ml. for i.v. or i.m. Dose: *Systemic infections*: Initial: 3 g.; Subsequent: up to 6 g. daily in divided doses. *Urinary infections*: Initial: 2 g.; Subsequent: up to 4 g. daily in divided doses.

SULPHAFURAZOLE (Sulfisoxazole, *U.S.P.;* Gantrisin, *Roche*)
Tablets, B.P., B.N.F., U.S.P.: 500 mg. Dose: As for sulphadimidine. Sulphafurazole diethanolamine: Equiv. 2 g. sulphafurazole in 5 ml. Dose i/m: Not to exceed oral dose of sulphafurazole. Not more than 5 ml. one site.

SULPHAGUANIDINE
Tablets, B.P.C.: 500 mg. Dose: 10-20 g. daily in divided doses.

SULPHAMETHIZOLE (Urolucosil, *Warner;* Sulfurine, Thiolsulfil, Ultrasul, *U.S.A.*)
Tablets, B.P.,: 100 mg.; U.S.N.F.: 250 mg. Suspension U.S.N.F.: 250 mg. per 5 ml. Dose: 100-200 mg. 4-6 hourly.

SULPHAMETHOXAZOLE (Gantanol, *Roche*)
Tablets, 500 mg. Syrup. 500 mg. per 5 ml. Dose: Initial: 2 g.; Subsequent: 1 g. 12 hourly. Not more than 3 g. per day.

SULPHAMETHOXYDIAZINE (Durenate, *F.B.A.* and Schering, *A.G.*)
Tablets, B.P.: 500 mg. Suspension 500 mg. per 5 ml. Dose: Initial: 1-2 g.; Subsequent: 500 mg. daily.

SULPHAMETHOXYPYRIDAZINE (Lederkyn, *Lederle;* Midicel, *Parke Davis*)
Tablets, B.P. 500 mg.; Suspension: 250 mg. per 5 ml. Dose: Initial: 1 g.; Subsequent: 500 mg. daily.

SULPHAPHENAZOLE (Orisulf, *Ciba*)
Tablets, B.P.: 500 mg.; Suspension: 500 mg. per 5 ml. Dose: Initial: 1 g. 12 hourly for 2 days; Subsequent: 500 mg. 12 hourly.

SULPHASALAZINE (Salazopyrin, Asulfidine, *Pharmacia*)
Tablets, B.N.F.: 500 mg. Dose: 1 g. 4-6 hourly.

SULPHASOMIDINE (formerly Elkosin, *Ciba;* Aristamid, *Ger.*)
Tablets, B.P.: 500 mg. Dose: As for sulphadimidine.

TRISULFAPYRIMIDINES (*equal parts sulphadiazine, sulphadimidine, sulphamerazine;* numerous similar preparations)
Tablets, U.S.P.: 500 mg. Suspension, U.S.P.: 500 mg. per 5 ml. Dose: Initial: 4 g.; Subsequent: 1 g. 4 hourly.

REFERENCES

ANTON, A. H. (1960). *J. Pharmacol. exp. Ther.* **129,** 282.
ANTON, A. H. (1961). *J. Pharmacol. exp. Ther.* **134,** 291.
ANTON, A. H. (1968). *Clin. Pharmacol. Ther.* **9,** 561.
BARBER, M. & GARROD, L. P. (1963). *Antibiotic and Chemotherapy,* p. 26. Edinburgh: Livingstone.
BARON, J. H., CONNELL, A. M., LENNARD-JONES, J. E. & AVERY JONES, F. (1962). *Lancet* **1,** 1094.
BEVERIDGE, J., HARRIS, M., WISE, G. & STEVENS, L. (1964). *Lancet,* **2,** 593.
BØE, O. (1966). *Acta path. microbiol. scand.* **68,** 81.
CAHAL, D. A. (1965). In *Embryopathic Activity of Drugs,* ed. Robson, J. M., Sullivan, F. M. & Smith, R. L. London: Churchill.
CARROLL, O. M., BRYAN, P. A. & ROBINSON, R. J. (1966). *J. Amer. med. Ass.* **195,** 691.
DISCOMBE, G. (1952). *Brit. med. J.* **1,** 1270.
EVANS, D. A. P. & WHITE, T. A. (1964). *J. Lab. clin. Med.* **63,** 394.
GRÜNEBERG, R. N. & BRUMFITT, W. (1967). *Brit. med. J.* **3,** 649.
HERMAN, L. G. (1959). *Antibiotic Ann.* (1958-9) p. 836.
LAING, A. B. G. (1964). *Brit. med. J.* **2,** 1439.
LUCEY, J. F. & DRISCOLL, T. J. (1961). In *Symposium on Kernicterus,* 1959. Toronto: Toronto University Press.
MILLAR, J. W., SIESS, E. E., FELDMAN, H. A., SILVERMAN, C. & FRANK, P. (1963). *J. Amer. med. Ass.* **186,** 139.
MISIEWICZ, J. J., LENNARD-JONES, J. E., CONNELL, A. M., BARON, J. H. & AVERY JONES, F. (1965). *Lancet* **1,** 185.
NEIPP, L. (1964). In *Experimental Chemotherapy,* vol. 2, p. 169, ed. Schnitzer, R. J. & Hawking, F. New York & London: Academic Press.
NEWBOULD, B. B. & KILPATRICK, R. (1960). *Lancet* **1,** 887.
O'DELL, G. B. (1959). *J. Paediat.* **55,** 268.
PAGET, G. E. & THORPE, E. (1964). *Brit. J. Pharmacol.* **23,** 305.
PATO, M. L. & BROWN, G. M. (1963). *Arch. Biochem. Biophys.* **103,** 443.
PINES, A. (1967). *Brit. med. J.* **3,** 202.
RICHMOND, M. H. (1966). *Symp. Soc. gen. Microbiol.* **16,** 301.
RUSSELL, F. E. (1963). *J. clin Path.* **16,** 362.
SALVAGGIO, J. & GONZALEZ, F. (1959). *Ann. intern. Med.* **51,** 60.
SPARR, R. A. & PRITCHARD, J. A. (1958). *Obstet. Gynaec.* **12,** 131.
TRUELOVE, S. C., WATKINSON, G. & DRAPER, G. (1962). *Brit. med. J.* **2,** 1708.
WILLIAMS, J. D. & SMITH, E. K. (1970). *Brit. med. J.* **4,** 651.
YOW, E. M. (1953). *Amer. Practit.* **4,** 521.
ZBINDEN, G. (1964). *Molecular Modification in Drug Design.* Advances in Chemistry Series No. 45, p. 25. Washington D.C.: American Chemical Society.

CHAPTER 3

OTHER SYNTHETIC ANTIMICROBIAL AGENTS

SYNTHETIC agents active against mycobacteria are discussed in Chapter 26, those active against virus infections in Chapter 28, and those used principally or exclusively as topical applications in Chapter 19.

DIAMINOPYRIMIDINES

A group of folate antagonists which owe their importance as antimicrobial agents to an inhibitory effect on the target enzyme in protozoa or bacteria which is enormously greater than that on the corresponding human enzymes.

TRIMETHOPRIM

Trimethoprim (Fig. 3) was synthesized in the Burroughs Wellcome Laboratories, N.Y. (Hitchings and Bushby, 1961) and was released for general therapeutic use as a mixture with

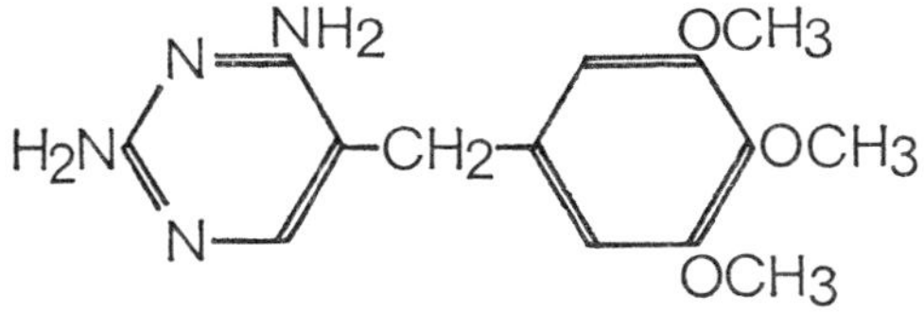

FIGURE 3
Structure of trimethoprim.

sulphamethoxazole, now called *cotrimoxazole,* in 1969. It is a weak base with a pKa of about 7·3 soluble to the extent of 44 μg./ml. water. The lactate is much more soluble: 50 mg./ml. water. It is active in concentrations achievable in the plasma, against all the common pathogenic bacteria except mycobacteria and pseudomonas (Table 3). Its effect is predominantly bacteristatic.

Precautions necessary in sensitivity testing are discussed on page 502. Addition of trimethoprim (8 μg./ml.) to the medium inhibits the overgrowth of *Proteus* without interfering with the recovery of *N. gonorrhoeae* (Seth, 1970).

TABLE 3

Sensitivity of bacteria to trimethoprim

	M.I.C. μg./ml.		M.I.C. μg./ml.
Staph. aureus	0·2-1	N. gonorrhoeae	8-128
Str. pyogenes	0·4-1	N. meningiditis	8
Str. pneumoniae	0·5-2	H. influenzae	0·12-1
Str. viridans	0·25	Bord. pertussis	3
Str. faecalis	0·25-0·5	Esch. coli	0·01-1
C. diphtheriae	0·4	K. pneumoniae	0·5-2
Cl. perfringens	50·0	Ent. aerogenes	1-3
M. tuberculosis	250	Proteus spp.	1-4
		Salmonella spp.	0·01-0·4
		Shigella spp.	0·4
		Ps. aeruginosa	100

Bushby, S. R. M. (1969) *Postgrad. med. J.* **45** (Suppl. Nov) 10; Waterworth, P. M. (1969) *ibid.*, p. 21; Williams *et al.* (1969) *ibid.*, p. 71.

Synergy

A most important feature of trimethoprim is that it is not only a potent antibacterial agent in its own right, but acts on bacteria in the same metabolic sequence as sulphonamides (p. 245) so that the two agents when given together markedly potentiate each other. Maximum potentiation occurs when the drugs are present in the ratio of their M.I.C.s. For example, an organism sensitive to 1 μg./ml. trimethoprim and 20 μg./ml. sulphonamide, will show maximum inhibition when exposed to a 1:20 mixture. This is the optimum ratio for many organisms, but for others proportionately more trimethoprim is required. Some (of which the *Neisseria* are an important example) are more susceptible to sulphonamide than trimethoprim and the ratio must be reversed. An idea of the magnitude of increased susceptibility of various organisms to one drug in the presence of subinhibitory concentrations of the other is given in Table 4. In addition to lowering the concentration required to inhibit growth the mixture may be bactericidal, where either drug alone is bacteristatic.

In some cases, synergy may be so marked that it can be demonstrated with organisms which would be conventionally regarded as resistant to one or other agent (Bushby, 1969; Lexomboon *et al.*, 1972). In other cases, some degree of sensitivity to both agents must be demonstrable. In a study of over 200 strains of *Sh. sonnei*, all of which were inhibited by 0·23 μg. trimethoprim per ml., Jarvis and Scrimgeour (1970) found that only the sulphonamide-sensitive strains showed potentiation.

TABLE 4

Degree of potentiation of trimethoprim by sulphonamide

	M.I.C. (μg./ml.)		Mean Potentiation Factor*
	Sulphafurazole	*Trimethoprim*	
Staph. aureus	4-8	0·12-0·5	5.4
Str. pyogenes	1-16	0·25-0·5	7
Str. pneumoniae	2-128	0·5-2	8·4
N. gonorrhoeae	0.5-8	32-64	25
H. influenzae	0.5-64	0·01-·0125	3·5
Esch. coli	4-32	0·12-0·5	5·7
Klebsiella spp.	8-64	0·5-1	4·6
Pr. mirabilis	4-16	0·5-2	26
Pr. vulgaris	4-16	0·5-2	10
Salmonella spp.	16-128	0·06-0·25	2·4
Shigella spp.	4-16	0·03-0·5	6·2

*Factor by which the M.I.C. of trimethoprim is reduced by presence of 9 parts of sulphafurazole (in the case of *N. gonorrhoeae*, 0·3 parts of sulphafurazole): Darrell *et al.* (1968) *J. clin. Path.*, **21**, 202.

Polymyxin acts synergically both with sulphonamides and trimethoprim against Gram-negative bacilli. Simmons (1970) found that the triple mixture of sulphamethoxazole, trimethoprim and colistin was more active than any pair of these agents against 66 out of 72 enterobacteria. The exceptions were all resistant to sulphamethoxazole.

Resistance

Organisms can be rendered resistant to trimethoprim *in vitro* by serial passage in increasing concentrations of the drug, enterobacteria becoming resistant to 500 μg./ml. or more, after 12-35 passages (Bushby, 1969). Resistance has emerged in the course of treatment of patients infected with klebsiella and haemophilus (May and Davis, 1972). One strain each of *E.*

coli and *Kl. aerogenes,* both isolated from urine, in which high-level trimethoprim resistance was R-factor mediated were described by Fleming *et al.* (1972).

Absorption and Excretion

Trimethoprim is rapidly and near-completely absorbed from the gut, giving peak plasma levels of about 0·9-1·2 μg./ml. 1½-3½ hours after a dose of 100 mg., and 2·2-3·2 μg./ml. after 250 mg. At these concentrations, 42-46 per cent of the drug is protein-bound. The plasma half-life is 6-12 hours (Schwartz and Ziegler, 1969). Excretion of the drug is almost wholly via the urine giving levels of 50-100 μg./ml. of which less than 8 per cent is in conjugated inactive forms. About 70 per cent of the drug is excreted in the first 24 hours, but detectable levels are present in the urine for 4-5 days during which time about 90 per cent of the dose can be recovered.

Sharpstone (1969) found the renal clearance of trimethoprim in the normal subject to be 19-148 ml./min., the wide variation being accounted for to a large extent by the influence of pH. Trimethoprim is a weak base and urinary excretion rises sharply with falling pH as the drug ionises and non-ionic back-diffusion in the tubules decreases. Trimethoprim clearance declines with renal function, but less rapidly than that of creatinine so that at the poorest function levels, trimethoprim clearance exceeds that of creatinine (supporting other evidence that the drug is partly excreted by active tubular secretion) and therapeutic concentrations of the drug are still found in the urine.

CHOICE OF MATCHING SULPHONAMIDE. In order to maintain in treated patients a ratio of trimethoprim to sulphonamide as close as possible to the synergic optimum, it was necessary to choose a sulphonamide with absorption and excretion characteristics as close as possible to those of trimethoprim. Sulphamethoxazole was a particularly happy choice for this purpose, since it combines pharmacokinetic behaviour closely similar to that of trimethoprim with high antibacterial activity (Table 2).

The available preparations contain 5 times as much sulphamethoxazole as trimethoprim and this produces a plasma level of sulphamethoxazole about 20-25 times the simultaneous level of trimethoprim, so achieving the optimum synergic ratio. Against *Neisseria* infections the optimum ratio is markedly different and it may be that for the treatment of infections with these organisms other formulations would be preferable (Garrod, 1969). Similarly, in renal failure differences in handling of the two compounds may disturb the plasma ratio and dosage of the two components may need to be suitably adjusted if treatment of such patients is contemplated (Sharpstone, 1969).

Toxicity and Side Effects

Nausea, vomiting (occasionally severe enough to require withdrawal of treatment) and skin rashes have occurred in some patients. With the drug available only as a mixture with sulphamethoxazole, it is not usually immediately plain which component is responsible for any reactions which occur.

The most serious foreseeable toxic effect of trimethoprim is the induction of folate deficiency. The very low affinity of the drug for the mammalian enzyme and the possibility of by-passing any depressant effect by feeding folate supplements (which cannot be utilized by the parasite—p. 245) makes the likelihood of serious haematological disorder seem relatively remote, but it is nevertheless plain that folate metabolism in man does not entirely escape the attentions of trimethoprim (Kahn *et al.*, 1968). In 10 subjects receiving the large dose of 1 g. per day, Whitman (1969) found bone marrow abnormalities in 8, and FiGlu excretion in 5, but no abnormality on 200 mg. per day. O'Grady *et al.* (1969) found no evidence of folate deficiency in patients treated with small doses (see p. 409) for periods up to six years.

Reversible thrombocytopenia and leucopenia, which may have been due to the sulphonamide component, has been recorded several times (Evans and Tell, 1969; Mohan, 1969; Hammett, 1970). Hulme and Reeves (1971) observed leucopenia in four out of 14 patients who received cotrimazole together with immunosuppressive agents after renal transplantation.

Chanarin and England (1972) describe four patients with megaloblastic anaemia who responded very poorly to haematinics while receiving cotrimazole; and a patient of Jewkes *et al.* (1970), who received 320 mg. trimethoprim and 1·6 g. sulpha-methoxazole daily for a year, is described as having disordered folate metabolism most of the time. By way of convincing confirmation of the site of action of the drug (page 245), folic acid (100 μg./day) was without effect but folinic acid (60 μg./day) restored normoblastic erythropoiesis and banished giant metamyelocytes from the bone marrow. On the other hand, in 10 elderly patients with chronic bronchitis treated for three months, Jenkins *et al.* (1970) found a transient early fall in folate levels with little haematological change except in two patients who were already in poor nutritional state. They were restored to normal by folinic acid supplements.

Review of these and other cases so far described leaves no doubt that disordered folate metabolism with attendant haema-tological changes can occur in patients treated with the drug, but not surprisingly this is most likely when other deficiencies, disorders or drugs have already sapped the patient's haemato-logical resilience.

In the rat, doses greater than 200 mg./kg./day were terato-genic, but complete protection was afforded by folinic acid or dietary folate supplements. No abnormalities were produced in the rabbit (Udall, 1969). Williams *et al.* (1969) treated 120 patients with bacteriuria of pregnancy, half of whom were more than half way towards delivery, but 10 were less than 16 weeks pregnant, and in none of their infants was there any ab-normality.

Ochoa (1971) reports a patient successfully treated for nocar-diasis throughout pregnancy without mishap to mother or baby.

Clinical Use

The range of pathogens against which cotrimoxazole is active opens up a wide field of potentially successful therapeutic ex-ploration (Garrod, 1969). The extent to which such exploration has already been rewarded is indicated by the successful treat-ment of infections as diverse as acne (p. 329), nocardiasis (Beau-mont, 1970; Adams *et al.*, 1971; Evans and Benson, 1971) gonorrhoea (p. 465), brucellosis (p. 322), endocarditis (Fowle and Zorab, 1970; Freeman and Hodgson, 1972) and severe enterobacterial infections including enteric fever (p. 366), cholera and generalised infection of childhood (Roy, 1971).

The principal use of the drug, however, remains in the control, and especially the long term control, of urinary (p. 409 and respiratory (p. 389) infections.

PYRIMETHAMINE

This agent is principally used as a malaria suppressant, but has also been successfully used to treat leishmaniasis and toxoplasmosis. In effective anti-parasitic doses the drug is more active than trimethoprim against mammalian dihydrofolate reductase, and evidence of folate deficiency is more commonly seen during treatment. Its depressant effect on haemopoiesis disappears on withdrawing the drug and can be reversed during treatment by folinic acid.

Combinations of sulphonamide with pyrimethamine are at present the treatment of choice for human toxoplasmosis (Nolan and Rosen, 1968).

PHARMACEUTICAL PREPARATIONS AND DOSAGE

PYRIMETHAMINE (' Daraprim ', *Burroughs Wellcome,* ' Malodice ', *Specia*)
Tablets, B.P., U.S.P., B.N.F. 25 mg.; Elixir 6·25 mg./5 ml. Dose: (leishmaniasis and toxoplasmosis) 25-50 mg. daily.
CO-TRIMOXAZOLE: Drapsules ('Bactrim', *Roche*) Tablets ('Septrin', *Burroughs Wellcome*)
80 mg. trimethoprim + 400 mg. sulphamethoxazole; Paediatric tablets 20 mg. trimethoprim + 100 mg. sulphamethoxazole. Suspension 40 mg. trimethoprim + 200 mg. sulphamethoxazole/5 ml. Adult dose: 1-2 tablets (drapsules) twice daily.
Severe infections 2 tablets (drapsules) 3 times daily.

REFERENCES

ADAMS, A. R., JACKSON, J. M., SCOPA, J., LANE, G. K. & WILSON, R. (1971). *Med. J. Aust.* **1,** 669.
BEAUMONT, R. J. (1970). *Med. J. Aust.* **2,** 1123.
BUSHBY, S. R. M. (1969). *Postgrad. med. J.* **45** (Suppl. Nov.), 10.
CHANARIN, I. & ENGLAND, J. M. (1972). *Brit. med. J.* **1,** 651.
EVANS, D. I. K. & TELL, R. (1969). *Brit. med. J.,* **1,** 578.
EVANS, R. A. & BENSON, R. E. (1971). *Med. J. Aust.* **1,** 684.
FLEMING, M. P., DATTA, N. & GRÜNEBERG, R. N. (1972). *Brit. med. J.* **1,** 726.
FOWLE, A. S. E. & ZORAB, P. A. (1970). *Brit. Heart J.* **32,** 127.
FREEMAN, R. & HODSON, M. E. (1972). *Brit. med. J.* **1,** 419.
GARROD, L. P. (1969). *Postgrad med. J.* **45** (Suppl. Nov.), 52.
HAMMETT, J. F. (1970). *Med. J. Aust.* **2,** 200.
HITCHINGS, G. H. & BUSHBY, S. R. M. (1961). *Proc. 5th int. Cong. Biochem.* (Moscow). Sect. 7. p. 165. London, Pergamon.
HULME, B. & REEVES, D. S. (1971). *Brit. med. J.* **3,** 610.
JARVIS, K. J. & SCRIMGEOUR, G. (1970). *J. med. Microbiol.* **3,** 554.
JENKINS, G. C., HUGHES, D. T. D. & HALL, P. C. (1970). *J. clin. Path.* **23,** 392.

JEWKES, R. F., EDWARDS, M. S. & GRANT, B. J. B. (1970). *Postgrad. med. J.* **46**, 723.
KAHN, S. B., FEIN, S. A. & BRODSKY, I. (1968). *Clin. Pharmacol. Ther.* **9**, 550.
LEXOMBOON, U., MANSUWAN, P., DUANGMANI, C., BENJADOL, P. & McMINN, M. T. (1972). *Brit. med. J.* **3**, 23.
MAY, J. R. & DAVIES, J. (1972). *Brit. med. J.* **3**, 376.
MOHAN, P. (1969). *Practitioner* **202**, 553.
NOLAN, J. & ROSEN, E. S. (1968). *Brit. J. Ophthal.* **52**, 396.
OCHOA, A. G. (1971). *J. Amer. med. Ass.* **217**, 1244.
O'GRADY, F., CHAMBERLAIN, D. A., STARK, J. E., CATTELL, W. R., SARDESON, J. M., FRY, I. K., SPIRO, F. I. & WATERS, A. H. (1969). *Postgrad. med. J.* **45**, (Suppl. Nov.), 61.
ROY, L. P. (1971). *Med. J. Aust.* **1**, 148.
SCHWARTZ, D. E. & ZIEGLER, W. H. (1969). *Postgrad. med. J.* **45**, (*Suppl.* Nov.), 32.
SETH, A. (1970). *Brit. J. vener. Dis.* **46**, 201.
SHARPSTONE, P. (1969). *Postgrad. med. J.* **45** (Suppl. Nov.), 38.
SIMMONS, N. A. (1970). *J. clin. Path.* **23**, 757.
UDALL, V. (1969). *Postgrad. med. J.* **45** (Suppl. Nov.), 42.
WHITMAN, E. N. (1969). *Postgrad. Med. J.* **45** (Suppl. Nov.), 46.
WILLIAMS, J. D., BRUMFITT, W., CONDIE. A. P. & REEVES, D. S. (1969). *Postgrad. med. J.* **45** (Suppl. Nov.), 71.

HEXAMINE

Hexamethylenetetramine was for many years the only drug capable of killing bacteria in the urine. It has no action *per se*, but in an acid medium is slowly decomposed with the liberation of formaldehyde. The odour of sweat is partly due to the action of skin bacteria and hexamine is included in some deodorant preparations where on contact with acid sweat it liberates formalin which inhibits bacterial activity. It is absorbed from the gut and mainly excreted unchanged in the urine. Because of the effect of acid, formalin will be liberated in the stomach unless the drug is given in enteric–coated tablets. To ensure that this reaction shall be adequate in the urine the pH needs reducing to about 5·0. The treatment is therefore inapplicable to infection with any urea-splitting organism. All micro-organisms are susceptible to the action of formaldehyde, and hexamine may still have a place in treating infection by yeasts (*Candida* or *Torula*), which are completely resistant to antibiotics, and by otherwise resistant coliform bacilli. Some patients on the drug complain of frequent and burning micturition and it is still sometimes recommended that these side-effects be controlled by giving alkali— so guaranteeing an absence of any effect. Prolonged administration or high dosage may produce proteinuria, haematuria and bladder changes.

HEXAMINE SALTS

Hexamine is now generally given in the form of its salts with organic acids which may both exert some antibacterial effect in their own right and serve to reduce the urinary pH to the low levels necessary for the liberation of formaldehyde from hexamine. According to Matsumoto *et al.* (1970) 20 per cent of formaldehyde is liberated at pH 5, 6 per cent at pH 6 and none at pH 7·6; but Greenfield *et al.* (1969) detected some formaldehyde even at pH 8. Of the two salts generally available, hexamine mandelate and hexamine hippurate, the hippurate appears to give higher urinary formaldehyde levels. The performance of the mandelate may be impaired by its enteric coating (Greenfield *et al.*, 1969). Mandelic acid is sometimes given alone, usually as the ammonium or calcium salt.

Miller and Phillips (1970) claim that *Pseudomonas* is particularly sensitive to the action of hexamine hippurate although the role of the acid in this effect is obscure. They agree with Katul and Frank (1970) and previous workers that if treatment is to be successful excessive fluid intake must be avoided and that fluid restriction may be more important than rigorous acidification of the urine. Possible benefits of diuresis in the treatment of urinary infection which must be waived if this policy is pursued are discussed on p. 403. Gibson (1970) used no additional acidifying agents in treating bacteriuria of pregnancy with hexamine hippurate. As with hexamine itself, excessive dosage of the salts may produce gastrointestinal upset or haemorrhagic cystitis (Ross and Conway, 1970).

PHARMACEUTICAL PREPARATIONS AND DOSAGE

HEXAMINE (' Methenamine ', *U.S.N.F.*)

Tablets, B.P.C., U.S.N.F. 300 mg. and 500 mg. (should be dissolved in a large volume of water). Mixture, B.P.C. 650 mg. in 15 ml. Dose: 0·6-2 g. after meals.

HEXAMINE, HIPPURATE (' Hiprex ', *Riker*) Tablets 1 g. Dose: 1 g. twice daily.

HEXAMINE MANDELATE (' Methenamine mandelate ', *U.S.P.;* ' Mandelamine ' *Warner* and other proprietary names)

Tablets 250 and 500 mg. Suspensions 250 and 500 mg. in 5 ml. Dose: 1 g. up to 4 times daily.

Other salts are available as proprietary preparations.

MANDELIC ACID usually given as *ammonium mandelate* (Mixture, *N.W.F.* 1 g./5 ml. Dose: 15 ml. in water 3 times daily) or as *calcium mandelate* (granules or suspension). Dose: 3 g. 4 times daily.

REFERENCES

Gibson, G. R. (1970). *Med. J. Aust.* **1,** 167.
Greenfield, W., Berg, R. & Moore, R. (1969). *Clin. Chem.* **15,** 1180.
Katul, M. J. & Frank, I. N. (1970). *J. Urol.* **104,** 320.
Matsumoto, T., Wolferth, C. C. & Hayes, M. F. (1970). *Arch. Surg.* **101,** 71.
Miller, H. & Phillips, E. (1970). *Invest. Urol.* **8,** 21.
Ross, R. R. & Conway, G. F. (1970). *Amer. J. Dis. Child.* **119,** 86.

N-ETHYLPYRIDONE CARBOXYLIC ACIDS

Two compounds which have in common a number of properties presumably based on the substituted pyridone moiety which they share (Fig. 4). One, nalidixic acid, has been widely and successfully used, and the other has been tried, for the treatment of urinary tract infection.

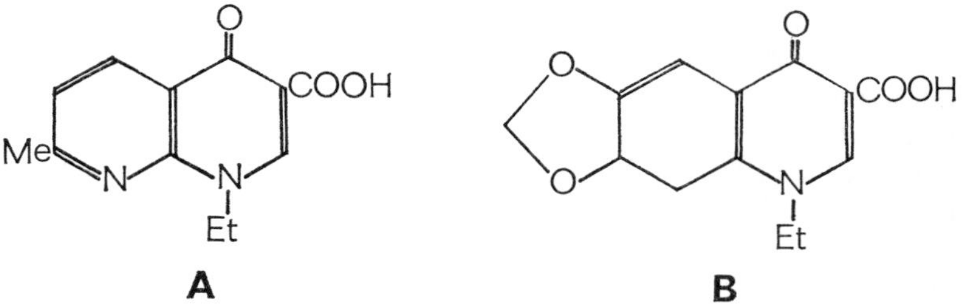

FIGURE 4
Structures of nalidixic acid (A) and oxolinic acid (B).

NALIDIXIC ACID

Pale yellow crystals slightly soluble in water and soluble in dilute alkali (Lesher *et al.,* 1962). Solutions withstand autoclaving.

Antibacterial Activity

It is active principally against Gram-negative organisms, the majority of which, with the exception of *Ps. aeruginosa,* are inhibited by 10 μg. per ml. or less. Gram-positive organisms are relatively resistant (Table 5). Nalidixic acid is bactericidal, although for some organisms concentrations substantially in excess of the M.I.C. are required. The addition of nalidixic acid improves the performance of cetrimide-agar as a selective medium for the isolation of *Ps. aeruginosa* (Lilly and Lowbury, 1972).

Resistance is easily produced by serial passage of organisms in increasing concentrations of the drug and sometimes emerges during the treatment of patients (Atlas *et al.*, 1969).

TABLE 5

Sensitivity of Bacteria to Nalidixic Acid

	M.I.C. μg./ml.		M.I.C. μg./ml.
Staph. aureus	50	N. meningitidis	0·5-5
Str. pyogenes	500	H. influenzae	1-75
Str. pneumoniae	250	Brucella spp	7·5-10
Str. faecalis	500	Esch. coli	3·0-7·5
C. diphtheriae	500	Proteus spp	2·5-20
B. anthracis	75	Klebsiella spp	1·6-50
Clostridium spp	12·5-800	Salmonella spp	2·5-75
M. tuberculosis	250	Shigella spp	2·5-50
		Ps. aeruginosa	4·0-500
		Bacteroides spp	200

Deitz, W. H. *et al.* (1964). *Antimicrob. Agents Chemother.*—1963, p. 584 Feldman, H. A. and Melnyk, C. *ibid*-1964, p. 440; Finegold, S. M. *et al.*, *ibid*-1966, p. 189.

Absorption

The drug is readily absorbed from the gut, giving peak plasma levels in normal subjects of about 25 μg./ml. following a dose of 1 g. but levels may differ greatly from one individual to another (Harrison and Cox, 1970). Administration of the drug with alkali can increase both the plasma and urinary levels partly by increasing dissolution (the drug is much more soluble at higher pH) and absorption in the gut, and partly by decreasing its tubular reabsorption. The plasma half-life is about $1\frac{1}{2}$ hours. Buchbinder *et al.* (1963) found no accumulation of the drug on a 6-hourly regimen of 1-2 g., the blood levels being <3·9-62·5 μg./ml.

A high proportion of the drug is reversibly bound to plasma albumin from which it may displace other compounds. Sellers and Koch-Weser (1970) draw attention to the danger of haemorrhage in patients treated with warfarin and nalidixic acid which can raise the plasma concentration of free anticoagulant by displacing it from its albumin binding sites.

Excretion

About 4 per cent of the drug can be recovered from the faeces and virtually all the administered dose appears in the urine over 24 hours. Only about 2-3 per cent is in the unchanged form. Nalidixic acid is rapidly metabolized, principally to the hydroxy-acid (which is also microbiologically active) and about 13 per cent of the drug in the urine is in this form. The rest is inactive glucuronides of these two compounds apart from about 4 per cent which appears as dicarboxylic derivatives.

Nalidixic acid, like chloramphenicol and nitrofurantoin, is eliminated almost exclusively by the renal route, but before excretion is largely converted to microbiologically inactive metabolites. As a result, in renal failure there is comparatively little accumulation of the active compound since it continues to be metabolized, but the elimination of its inactive derivatives is progressively delayed as renal function declines. This is no doubt why Adam and Dawborn (1971) found that creatinine clearance correlated with clearance of the inactive but not of the active compound.

For the treatment of urinary infection in patients with impaired renal function, therefore, compounds handled in this way have the general disadvantage that breakdown of the drug at a rapid rate relative to its delayed excretion causes accumulation of useless and possibly harmful products and the passage of little active compound into the urine. Plainly such agents should be avoided if possible but if nalidixic acid has to be used justification may be found in the claims that the metabolic products are harmless (Stamey *et al.*, 1969) and adequate concentrations of the active agent still reach the urine. Excretion is impaired in the premature infant.

Excretion products of nalidixic acid interfere with the measurement of urinary 17-ketosteroids and in at least one case have led to mistaken diagnosis of endocrine tumour (Llerena and Pearson, 1968).

Toxicity and side-effects

Nausea, rashes and C.N.S. disturbances, including seizures, have occurred in patients receiving the drug. Amongst 515 reported reactions (Alexander and Forman, 1971) 219 involved visual disturbances, hallucinations or disordered sensory perception. Of 97 skin reactions, 25 were phototoxic (negative lymphocyte transformation tests supported the view that blistered photoreactive eruptions are not of immunological origin), 24 urticarial, 17 ' drug rash ' erythema and 15 maculopapular.

Several examples of intracranial hypertension in children highly reminiscent of the ' bulging fontanelle syndrome ' occasionally seen in infants treated with tetracycline (p. 158—and even less commonly in adults or following other agents (Bhowmick, 1972)—have been reported. In the five-year old child described by Anderson *et al.* (1971)—who had received 53·5 g. of nalidixic acid over 58 days—papilloedema was accompanied by bilateral 6th nerve palsies which rapidly improved on stopping the drug although strabismus remained.

Haemolytic anaemia in babies (one G6PD-deficient) has been described twice (Mandal and Stevenson, 1970).

Clinical Use

Nalidixic acid has been successfully used for the oral treatment of urinary tract infection and also by instillation into the bladder and for the prophylaxis of transurethral operations to cover the period of catheterization.

Although principally used for its effects on the urinary tract, success has also been described in the treatment of brucellosis and of enteric fever (Hassan *et al.*, 1970).

OXOLINIC ACID

Turner *et al.* (1968) described oxolinic acid (Fig. 4) as having greater activity over a similar bacterial range to nalidixic acid, and as being in addition active against *Staph. aureus*. Organisms passaged in the presence of the drug acquire resistance to both oxolinic and nalidixic acids. Oxolinic acid is absorbed by mouth and on a regimen of 240 mg. 4 times daily d'Alessio *et al.* (1968) obtained mean serum and urine levels of 1·8 and 40 μg./ml. In patients treated for urinary tract infection side effects were common; amongst those given 750 mg. of the drug twice daily by Cox (1970) 27 per cent suffered nausea and vomiting or restlessness and insomnia. In both series the emergence of bacterial resistance was a notable cause of failure.

PHARMACEUTICAL PREPARATIONS AND DOSAGE

NALIDIXIC ACID ('Negram', *Winthrop*), B.P.C., B.N.F. Tab. 500 mg.; U.S.N.F. 250, 500 mg. Mixt. B.P.C., B.N.F. 300 mg./5 ml. Dose 1 g. 4 x daily; children 60 mg. per kg. daily in divided doses.

REFERENCES

ADAM, W. R. & DAWBORN, J. K. (1971). *Aust. N.Z. J. Med.* **1**, 126.
ALEXANDER, S. & FORMAN, L. (1971). *Brit. J. Derm.* **84**, 429.
ANDERSON, E. E., ANDERSON, B. & NASHOLD, B. S. (1971). *J. Amer. med. Ass.* **216**, 1023.
ATLAS, E., CLARK, H., SILVERBLATT, F. & TURCK, M. (1969). *Ann. intern. Med.* **70**, 713.
BHOWMICK, B. K. (1972). *Brit. med. J.*, **3**, 30.
BUCHBINDER, M., WEBB, J. C., ANDERSON, L. A. V. & MCCABE, W. R. (1963). *Antimicrob. Agents. Chemother.* 1962. p. 308.
COX, C. E. (1970). *Delaware med. J.* **42**, 327.
D'ALESSIO, D. J., OLEXY, V. M. & JACKSON, G. G. (1968). *Antimicrob. Agents. Chemother.* 1967. p. 490.
HARRISON, L. H. & COX, C. E. (1970). *J. Urol.* **104**, 908.
HASSAN, A., WAHAB, M. F. A., FARID, Z. & EL ROOBY, A. S. (1970). *J. trop. Med. Hyg.* **73**, 145.
LESHER, G. Y., FROELICH, E. J., GRUETT, M. D., BAILEY, J. H. & BRUNDAGE, R. P. (1962). *J. med. pharm. Chem.* **5**, 1063.
LILLY, H. A. & LOWBURY, E. J. L. (1972). *J. med. Microbiol.* **5**, 151.
LLERENA, O. & PEARSON, O. H. (1968). *New Engl. J. Med.* **279**, 983.
MANDAL, B. K. & STEVENSON, J. (1970). *Lancet* **1**, 614.
SELLERS, E. M. & KOCH-WESER, J. (1970). *Clin. Pharmacol. Ther.* **11**, 524.
STAMEY, T. A., NEMOY, N. J. & HIGGINS, M. (1969). *Invest. Urol.*, **6**, 582.
TURNER, F. J., RINGEL, S. M., MARTIN, J. F., STORINO, P. J., DALY, J. M. & SCHWARTZ, B. S. (1968). *Antimicrob. Agents. Chemother.* 1967. p. 475.

NITROFURANS

A group of nitrofurfurane derivatives (Fig. 5) with broad spectrum antimicrobial activity. Many have been synthesised and some of those which are not commercially available, for example *nitrofuratone* (Matsen, 1971) and *niferpipone* (Massarani *et al.*, 1971) are said to compare favourably with those which are. Of the preparations in current therapeutic use, nitrofurazone and nifuroxine are used locally and are available in preparations suitable for application to the skin, ears, eyes and vagina. The other agents are given systemically: furazolidone for intestinal infections, nifuratel for vaginitis and nitrofurantoin for urinary infections. Search continues for compounds which surpass nitrofurantoin in antibacterial spectrum, plasma and urine levels, and patient tolerance. The very closely related nifuradine (also called oxafuradine) has had several clinical trials but according to Ronald and Turck (1968) offers no advantages.

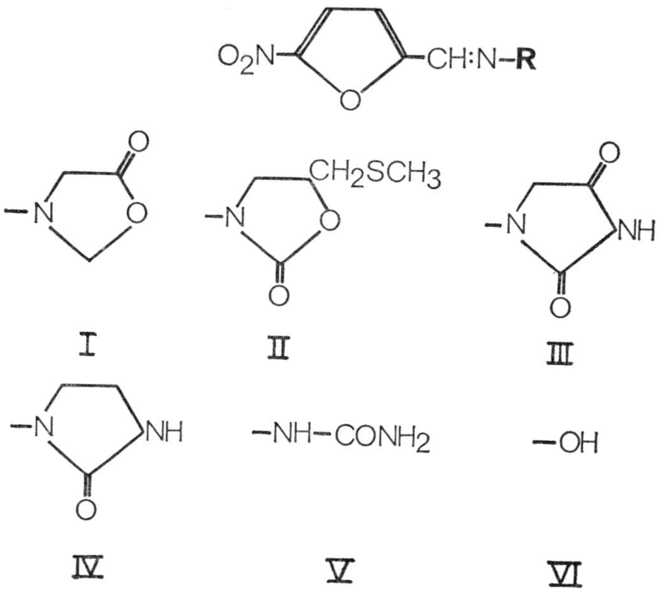

$$O_2N \underset{O}{\overset{}{\diagdown}} CH\!:\!N\!-\!\mathbf{R}$$

I   II   III

IV   V   VI

FIGURE 5

Structures of furazolidone (R = I); nifuratel (R = II); nitrofurantoin (R = III); nifuradene (R = IV); nitrofurazone (R = V) nifuroxime (R = VI).

FURAZOLIDONE

Yellow odourless crystals almost insoluble in water and alcohol, slightly soluble in chloroform. Should be protected from light.

TABLE 6

Antibacterial Activity of Nitrofurans

	M.I.C. Nitrofurazone $\mu g./ml.$	M.I.C. Nitrofurantoin $\mu g./ml.$
Staph. aureus	10	4-30
Str. pyogenes	10	10
Str. viridans	25	8
Str. faecalis	25	4-125
N. gonorrhoeae	10	15
Esch. coli	10	0·4->250
Proteus spp	40	7·5->200
Klebsiella-Aerobacter spp	10-20	25->200
Salmonella spp	5-10	5-15
Shigella spp	5	5
Ps. aeruginosa	>200	>200

Furazolidone is bactericidal to a wide range of Gram-positive and negative organisms. Headache, nausea, diarrhoea, rashes and alcohol intolerance may occur. Furazolidone inhibits mono-amine oxidase, and Aderhold and Muniz (1970) describe acute toxic psychosis in women given the drug together with amitryp-tiline similar to that seen on combined treatment with other monoamine oxidase inhibitors and tricyclic depressants. It has been successfully used for the treatment of a variety of gastro-intestinal infections including entreic fever (p. 365) and other salmonelloses, and shigelloses.

NIFURATEL

This nitrofuran (Fig. 5) was first described by Arnold and Delnon (1965), and on the basis of the broad antimicrobial spectrum claimed for it has been promoted for the combined oral and local treatment of vaginitis of mixed aetiology. It has had some successful trials (Aure and Gjonnaess, 1969; Gjon-naess and Aure, 1969) but the consensus of opinion in Britain is that it compares unfavourably with metronidazole for the treatment of vaginal trichomoniasis (Evans and Catterall, 1970). It has also been suggested that its effect relies heavily on the local application and owes little to the systemically adminis-tered agent. Its broad antimicrobial spectrum has the advantage that treatment is unlikely to be complicated by the emergence of candidiasis as sometimes occurs with metronidazole (Oller, 1969) and the disadvantage that unrecognised gonorrhoea may be masked (Churcher and Evans, 1969).

NITROFURANTOIN

Yellow odourless crystals discoloured by exposure to light, from which it should be protected. Soluble: 50 μg./ml. alcohol; and 60 mg./ml. dimethylformamide. Its solubility in water in-creases markedly with pH (from 220 μg./ml. at pH 4·0 to 2·3 mg./ml. at pH 7·7), but discoloration occurs in strongly alkaline solutions. The sodium salt is much more soluble and is used to prepare solutions for parenteral administration.

Antibacterial Activity

Nitrofurantoin is active against many organisms responsible for urinary infection, particularly *E. coli*, but *Ps. aeruginosa* and some *Klebsiella-Aerobacter* and *Proteus* strains are insensitive (Table 6). The M.I.C. may greatly increase with increasing size of inoculum. It is bactericidal in concentrations not much above the M.I.C. but its activity may be reduced as much as 100-fold at pH 8 as compared with pH 5·5, and a bactericidal effect may be obtained only in an acid medium.

Sensitivity to high concentrations of nitrofurantoin (700 μg/ml.) may be used to divide *Nocardia* into two groups (Tanzil and Linton, 1971).

Resistant variants may be produced by passage in the presence of the drug and have been observed to emerge during the treatment of patients. There is no cross-resistance with other important antibacterial agents but nitrofurantoin antagonises *in vitro* the action of nalidixic acid and the two agents should not be prescribed together (p. 283).

A variety of biochemical abnormalities have been observed in organisms exposed to nitrofurantoin but its precise mode of action is unknown (Waterbury *et al.*, 1966).

Absorption and Excretion

Nitrofurantoin is well absorbed by mouth and rapidly excreted in the urine but very low levels appear in the plasma, partly as the result of rapid tissue breakdown. Only about a third of the dose can be recovered from the urine. The peak plasma level appears 1-2 hours after an oral dose and has been found by many workers not to exceed 2·5 μg./ml. What little drug is present soon disappears, the plasma half-life being about 20 min. (Reckendorf *et al.*, 1963). Urine levels are usually in the range 15-46 μg./ml. and levels above the M.I.C. for the most sensitive organisms are detectable for about 6 hours.

By the intramuscular route 180 mg. of sodium nitrofurantoin gave peak plasma levels of 1·8-6·4 μg./ml. half an hour after injection and peak urine levels of 180-264 μg./ml. after one hour (Cox *et al.*, 1971). Following conventional oral doses, the concentrations in milk and amniotic fluid are insignificant and the concentration in cord blood generally less than the maternal level (Perry and LeBlank, 1967). Since the maternal levels are so low there is little danger of foetal toxicity. Levels in prostatic fluid were only about $\frac{1}{4}$-$\frac{1}{2}$ the plasma level (Dunn and Stamey, 1967).

Nitrofurantoin is excreted by the kidney both in the glomerular filtrate and by tubular secretion. The drug is a weak acid and in alkaline urine about a third is reabsorbed by nonionic back diffusion in the distal tubule. Calculations suggest that this could result in peri-tubular concentrations of the drug of the order of 12-48 μg/ml.—sufficient to exert a useful antibacterial effect (Shirmeister et al., 1966). Direct assays of renal lymph (supposed to reflect the composition of renal interstitial fluid) have shown concentrations about twice those of the plasma. In azotaemic patients too little appears in the urine to inhibit sensitive organisms (Felts et al., 1971). At the same time rapid breakdown of the retained drug may allow toxic metabolites to accumulate. Nitrofurantoin is consequently contraindicated in renal failure (Sachs et al., 1968).

Toxicity and side-effects

In a large series of patients studied by Koch-Weser et al. (1971) reactions sufficiently severe to require withdrawal of therapy were seen in 9·2 per cent of those treated with nitrofurantoin. Most were gastrointestinal upsets but skin rashes, eosinophilia and ' drug fever ' were seen in 4·1 per cent. Serious reactions were very rare. There have been reports of anaphylaxis following nitrofurantoin, none fatal (Satter, 1966). Particularly in elderly patients a few days' therapy has been followed by dramatic onset of chills, cough and breathlessness resembling cardiac failure. In the 10 years from 1959 about 200 cases of such pleuropneumonic reactions to nitrofurantoin were described (Hailey et al., 1969). The chest signs are often followed by eosinophilia or skin rash. On X-ray there is infiltration especially at the bases with consolidation or effusion. The reaction is probably of allergic origin (Ngan et al., 1971). On withdrawal of the drug the condition rapidly clears. In a few patients receiving long-term treatment chronic lung involvement has been described.

Peripheral neuropathy has developed in a number of patients sometimes following excessive treatment, usually in those with impaired renal function. Onset may be sudden with increasing distal sensory disturbances, severe pain, depressed reflexes, and muscular wasting progressing to severe disablement. As the cases described by Craven (1971) clearly show, neuropathy can develop without renal impairment being sufficiently severe to raise the blood urea. Recovery is usually complete some weeks after stopping treatment but it appears from the observations of Felts *et al.* (1971) that normal nerve conduction cannot regularly be restored simply by reducing the dose.

The neurotoxicity is evidently not simply an exaltation of the effects of uraemia since impaired nerve conduction can be demonstrated in normal subjects treated with conventional doses (Toole *et al.*, 1968). A possible role for folic acid deficiency in neuropathy has been considered since megaloblastic anaemia develops in occasional patients (perhaps as a toxic effect of the hydantoin moiety of nitrofurantoin) but Felts *et al.* (1971) were unable to find any changes supporting this aetiology in their patients. As with a number of other drugs, haemolytic episodes may occur in patients with G, 6–PD deficiency (Pritchard *et al.*, 1965).

Clinical use

For practical purposes the use of nitrofurantoin is restricted to the prophylaxis and treatment of urinary tract infection (p. 409). The low plasma levels achieved make oral treatment useless for systemic infections. Some success has been claimed for treatment of peritonitis and Gram-nevative bacteraemia by intravenous infusion of sodium nitrofurantoin (Fadhli and Cross, 1965; Litvak and Melnick, 1966).

PHARMACEUTICAL PREPARATIONS AND DOSAGE

FURAZOLIDONE ('Furoxone', *Smith, Kline and French*)
Tablets B.P.C. 100 mg.; Suspension 100 mg./tablespoon (14 ml.). Dose: 400 mg. daily in divided doses.
NIFURATEL ('Magmilor', *Calmic*; 'Macmiror', *Ital.*). Oral tab. 200 mg.; vaginal pessaries 250 mg. Dose 200 mg. 2—4 x daily plus vaginal pessary nightly x 10.
NITROFURANTOIN ('Berkfurin', *Berk*; 'Furadantin', *Smith, Kline and French*, 'Furan', *Chelsea Drug and Chemical Co.*)
Tablets, B.P., B.N.F. 50 mg.; U.S.P. 50 mg. and 100 mg. Mixture, B.N.F. 25 mg. in 5 ml. Oral suspension, U.S.P. 0·5 per cent w/v. Dose: 50-150 mg. 6 hourly.

REFERENCES

ADERHOLD, R. M. & MUNIZ, C. E. (1970). *J. Amer. med. Ass.* **213**, 2080.
ARNOLD, M. & DELNON, J. (1965). *Ther. Umsch. med. Biblphie* **22**, 490.
AURE. J. C. & GJØNNAESS, H. (1969). *Acta obstet. gynec. Scand.* **48**, 95.
CHURCHER, G. M. & EVANS, A. J. (1969). *Brit. J. vener. Dis.* **45**, 149.
COX, C. E., O'CONNOR, F. J. & LACY, S. S. (1971). *J. Urol.* **105**, 113.
CRAVEN, R. S. (1971). *Aust. N.Z. J. Med.* **1**, 246.
DUNN, B. L. & STAMEY, T. A. (1967). *J. Urol.* **97**, 505.
EVANS, B. A. & CATTERALL, R. D. (1970). *Brit. med. J.* **2**, 335.
FADHLI, H. A. & CROSS, F. S. (1965). *Amer. J. Surg.* **109**, 160.

FELTS, J. H., HAYES, D. M., GERGEN, J. A. & TOOLE, J. F. (1971). *Amer. J. Med.* **51**, 331.
GJØNNAESS, H. & AURE, J. C. (1969). *Acta obstet. gynec. Scand.* **48**, 85.
HAILEY, F. J., GLASCOCK, H. W., JR. & HEWITT, W. F. (1969). *New Engl. J. Med.* **281**, 1087.
KOCH-WESER, J., SIDEL, V. W., DEXTER, M., PARISH, C., FINER, D. C. & KANAREK, P. (1971). *Arch. intern. Med.* **128**, 398.
LITVAK, A. S. & MELNICK, J. (1966). *J. Urol.* **96**, 107.
MASSARANI, E., NARDI, D., DEGEN, L. & SETNIKAR, I. (1971). *Experientia* **27**, 1243.
MATSEN, J. M. (1971). *Antimicrob. Agents Chemother.*—1970, p. 260.
NGAN, H., MILLARD, R. J., LANT, A. F. & TRAPNELL, D. H. (1971). *Brit. J. Radiol.* **44**, 21.
OLLER, L. Z. (1969). *Brit. J. vener. Dis.* **45**, 163.
PERRY, J. E. & LEBLANC, A. L. (1967). *Texas Rep. Biol. Med.* **25**, 265.
PRITCHARD, J. A., SCOTT, D. E. & MASON. R. A. (1965). *J. Amer. med. Ass.* **194**, 457.
RECKENDORF, H. K., CASTRINGIUS, R. G. & SPINGLER, H. K. (1963). *Antimicrob. Agents Chemother.*—1962, p. 531.
RONALD, A. R. & TURCK, M. (1968). *Antimicrob. Agents Chemother.*—1967, p. 506.
SACHS, J., GEER, T., NOELL, P. & KUNIN, C. M. (1968). *New Engl. J. Med.* **278**, 1032.
SATTER, E. J. (1966). *J. Urol.* **96**, 86.
SCHIRMEISTER, J., STEFANI, F., WILLMANN, H. & HALLAUER, W. (1966). *Antimicrob. Agents Chemother.*—1965, p. 223.
TANZIL, H. O. K. & LINTONG, M. (1971). *Amer. Rev. resp. Dis.* **104**, 438.
TOOLE, J. F., HAYES, D. M. & FELTS, J. H. (1968). *Arch. Neurol.* **18**, 680.
WATERBURY, W. F., BOYDSTUN, J., CASTELLANI, A. G.. FREEDMAN, R. & GAVIN, J. J. (1966). *Antimicrob. Agents Chemother.*—1965, p. 339.

NITROIMIDAZOLES

A large group of heterocyclic compounds based on a 5-membered nucleus reminiscent of the nitrofurans (page 43). Between them, the compounds exhibit activity against a wide variety of protozoa and bacteria (Bachman *et al.*, 1969; Miller *et al.*, 1970). Few have come into clinical use. We describe only the best known of the systemic trichomonacides—metronidazole—and its congeners nimorazole and tinidazole (Fig. 6).

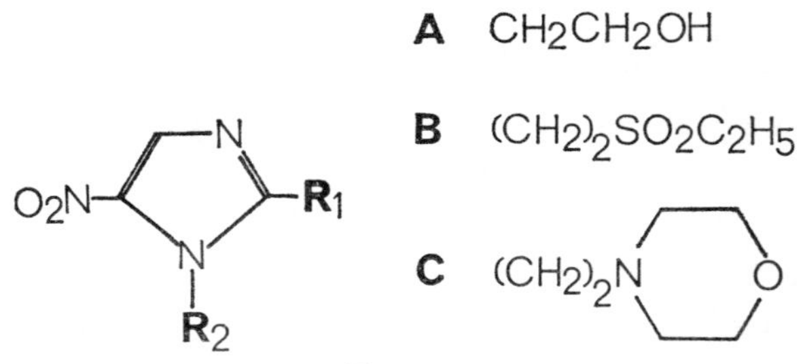

A CH_2CH_2OH

B $(CH_2)_2SO_2C_2H_5$

C $(CH_2)_2N$ — O

FIGURE 6

Structures of metronidazole ($R_1 = CH_3$; $R_2 = A$); tinidazole ($R_1 = CH_3$; $R_2 = B$) and nimorazole ($R_1 = H$; $R_2 = C$).

METRONIDAZOLE

An almost white crystalline powder, soluble 100 mg./ml. water; 5 mg./ml. alcohol; and 4 mg./ml. chloroform. Metronidazole is a potent trichomonacide, active in concentrations of 1·0-2·5 μg./ml. It is inactive against *Candida*. It is a potent inhibitor of obligate anaerobic bacteria and protozoa (*Trichomonas vaginalis*, *Tr. foetus*, and *Entamoeba histolytica*: Table 7) but not of aerobic bacteria or protozoa—such as trypano-

TABLE 7
Inhibitory activity of metronidazole

	MIC μg./ml.
Cl. tetani	0·01
Cl. septicum	0·03
Fusobact. polymorphum	0·03
Veill. alkalescens	0·03
Tr. vaginalis	1·0
Tr. foetus	4·0
Aerobic organisms	>1000

Prince, H. N. *et al.* (1969). *Appl. Microbiol.* **18**, 728.

somes. It is active against Vincent's organisms, and has been shown to inhibit the Nicols strain of *Tr. pallidum* in a concentration of 3·6-9·5 μg./ml. (Wilkinson *et al.*, 1967). It is absorbed by mouth, doses of 200 mg. producing serum levels of 2·5-13 μg./ml. About 60 per cent is excreted in the urine (about 70 per cent in the unchanged form) giving levels of 50-390 μg./ml. It also appears in the saliva, peak levels up to 9·7 μg./ml. being found 3 hours after a 200 mg. dose on the third day of treatment (Stephen *et al.*, 1966).

Toxicity

Nausea, a metallic taste in the mouth, or furry tongue are fairly common. Rashes, central nervous symptoms, dysuria and dark urine have been occasionally reported. Leucopenia has been described but the changes are generally insignificant (Peterson *et al.*, 1967). Disulfiram-like flushing and hypotension are sufficiently common and severe in those taking alcohol while receiving metronidazole for the drug to have been used in the treatment of chronic alcoholism (Merry and Whitehead, 1968).

Clinical Use

The principal use of metronidazole is in the treatment of trichomoniasis in which it has been very successful even as shortened (McLean, 1971) or single dose (Csonka, 1971) courses. Re-treatment, intensive treatment or additional measures are required in some patients (p. 468). Metronidazole is as effective as penicillin in the treatment of Vincent's angina (p. 362). Its anti-spirochaetal effect has led to trials of its use in syphilis but it is considered inferior to penicillin. Its only importance in that connection is that it may lead to misdiagnosis since the serum of patients receiving the drug may immobilize treponemes in the T.P.I. test (Wilkinson *et al.*, 1967). Metronidazole is described as the drug of choice in giardiasis (Bassily *et al.*, 1970) and amoebic liver abscess (Scragg and Powell, 1970), and as remarkably effective in dracunculiasis (Antani *et al.*, 1970).

NIMORAZOLE

This nitroimidazole (Fig. 6), also known as nitrimidazine, and first described by De Carnieri *et al.* (1970) has had a number of successful trials for the oral treatment of vaginal trichomoniasis (p. 469).

TINIDAZOLE

This close congener (Fig. 6) of methonidazole was synthesized by Miller *et al.* (1970). The concentrations in which it inhibits *Tr. vaginalis* and *Tr. foetus* (2·5 μg./ml.) and *Entamoeba histolytica* (40 μg./ml.) are similar to those of metronidazole. Howes *et al.* (1970) comment on the difficulty of interpreting the inhibitory activity of antitrichomonal agents after 24 hours' incubation because of spontaneous death of the parasite. Assessed at 6 hours, the concentration of both agents inhibitory to both trichomonads was 10 μg./ml. Tinidazole appeared to be more actively trichomonacidal in that killing of *Tr. vaginalis* by metronidazole required concentrations 4-8 times the effective concentrations of tinidazole. In a dose of 125 mg., tinidazole produced human plasma levels around 1·5 μg./ml. with a half-life of 9·4 hours (Taylor *et al.*, 1970). They found considerably less metronidazole in its active form in the urine than had previous workers, and concluded from their recovery of almost half the dose of tinidazole (and that exclusively in the active form) that it is more resistant to biotransformation.

PHARMACEUTICAL PREPARATIONS AND OTHER DOSAGE

METRONIDAZOLE (' Flagyl ', *May and Baker*)
 Tablets B.P., B.N.F. 200 mg. Dose: 600 mg. daily in divided doses for 7 days.
NIMORAZOLE (Nitrimidazine; ' Naxogin ', *Carlo Erba*; ' Nulogyl ', *Bristol*)
Tab. 250 mg. Dose 250 mg. 2–3 x daily.

REFERENCES

ANTANI, J., SRINIVAS, H. V., KRISHNAMURTHY, K. R. & JAHAGIRDAR, B. R. (1970). *Amer. J. trop. Med. Hyg.* **19,** 821.
BACHMANN, H. J., SHIRK, R. J., LAYTON, H. W. & KEMP, G. A. (1969). *Antimicrob. Agents Chemother.* 1968, p. 524.
BASSILY, S., FARID, Z., MIKHAIL, J. W., KENT, D. C. & LEHMANN, J. S. JR. (1970). *J. trop. Med. Hyg.* **73,** 15.
COHEN, L. (1971). *Brit. J. vener. Dis.* **47,** 177.
CSONKA, G. W. (1971). *Brit. J. vener. Dis.* **47,** 456.
DE CARNIERI, I., CANTONE, A., GIRALDI, P. N., LOGEMANN, W., MEINARDI, G. & TRANE, F. (1970). *Proc. 6th internat. Cong. Chemother., Tokyo.* (Progress in Antimicrobial and Anticancer chemotherapy: I) p. 149.
HOWES, H. L. JR., LYNCH, J. E. & KIVLIN, J. L. (1970). *Antimicrob. Agents Chemother.*—1969, p. 261.
MCLEAN, A. N. (1971). *Brit. J. vener. Dis.* **47,** 36.
MERRY, J. & WHITEHEAD, A. (1968). *Brit. J. Psychiat.* **114,** 859.
MILLER, M. W., HOWES, H. L. & ENGLISH, A. R. (1970). *Antimicrob. Agents Chemother.*—1969, p. 257.
MOFFETT, M., MCGILL, M. I., SCHOFIELD, C. B. S. & MASTERTON, G. (1971). *Brit. J. vener. Dis.* **47,** 173.
PETERSON, W. F., HANSEN, F. W., STAUCH, J. E. & RYDER, C. D. (1967). *Amer. J. Obstet. Gynec.* **97,** 472.
SCRAGG, J. N. & POWELL, S. J. (1970). *Arch. Dis. Child.* **45,** 193.
STEPHEN, K. W., MCLATCHIE, M. F., MASON, D. K., NOBLE. H. W. & STEVENSON, D. M. (1966). *Brit. dent. J.* **121,** 313.
TAYLOR, J. A. JR., MIGLIARDI, J. R. & VON WITTENAU, M. S. (1970). *Antimicrob. Agents Chemother.*—1969, p. 267.
WILKINSON, A. E., RODIN, P., MCFADZEAN, J. A. & SQUIRES, S. (1967). *Brit. J. vener. Dis.* **43,** 201.

CHAPTER 4

PENICILLINS

1. NATURAL

PENICILLIN, the first of the antibiotics to come into general therapeutic use, is still in many ways the best. Indeed, some of its properties are unique, and it is nothing short of a miracle that so astonishing a substance should have been the first of its kind to be discovered. This is not to say that antibiotics were unknown before that time: many were discovered and used locally for therapeutic purposes much earlier, but this was the first which was suitable for systemic use in man.

The story of the discovery of penicillin by Fleming and of its isolation and systematic study by Florey, Chain and their colleagues in Oxford over ten years later, is now too well known to need re-telling. It took years of hard work to obtain penicillin in the pure state, and the unit of activity by which it had first to be measured, now known to represent 0·6 μg., has persisted to the present day, although all later penicillins are prescribed by weight.

BENZYL PENICILLIN

Physical and Chemical Properties

Penicillin can be prepared in quantity only by the original process of cultivating a mould forming it (a high-yielding mutant of a strain of *P. chrysogenum* is now used) in a suitable liquid medium. In the early stages of large-scale production it was found that four different penicillins were being formed, known as F, G, X and K. Of these G, or benzyl penicillin, had the most desirable properties, and its almost exclusive formation is ensured by adding the appropriate ' precursor ', phenylacetic acid, to the medium.

As formed, penicillin is an unstable acid, and in production it is converted to a salt, that of either potassium or sodium, which is more stable. The structure of benzyl penicillin is shown in the figure below. The potassium salt is what is commonly known as 'soluble' or 'crystalline' penicillin, both unsatisfactory terms, because they apply to any penicillin, but this salt is distinguishable from other forms of benzyl penicillin introduced later by its high degree of solubility in water and by its rapid absorption and excretion.

BENZYLPENICILLIN

a. Site of action of penicillinase
b. Site of action of amidase

STABILITY. Penicillin is stable in the dry state, but deteriorates slowly in solution, this process being accelerated by heat. Among many incompatible chemicals the most important is acid, since the action of gastric acid accounts for the loss of most of a dose of benzyl penicillin if it is swallowed. It is also destroyed by an enzyme, penicillinase, formed by various bacteria, including some staphylococci, various *Bacilli,* some species of *Proteus, Ps. aeruginosa,* other coliforms and the tubercle bacillus. Not all these penicillinases are the same. The resistance of staphylococci to penicillin in clinical practice is largely due to this factor: their intrinsic resistance may be comparatively low, but they appear to withstand high concentrations because in fact they destroy them. This can happen in the body, where further injury may be added to insult by interference with the action of the antibiotic on an accompanying sensitive species.

Anti-bacterial Activity

SPECIES SUSCEPTIBILITY. At one time bacteria were classed simply as sensitive or resistant to penicillin, but they exhibit degrees of sensitivity over an exceedingly wide range, and the fact that if necessary very large doses can be given enables infections by some moderately resistant species to be treated successfully. Table 8 states the concentrations usually required to inhibit the growth of the more sensitive organisms, which include almost all the Gram-positive pathogens and some of the Gram-negative. The least sensitive organisms listed among the latter are included because they can occur in the urine, where high concentrations of penicillin are easily attained.

ABNORMAL RESISTANCE. In some species naturally resistant strains are found: these include *Str. viridans,* resistant strains of which predominate in the mouth of patients undergoing penicillin treatment (Garrod and Waterworth, 1962) and *Staph. aureus,* in which resistance depends on penicillinase formation. Bacteria do not *acquire* resistance to penicillin, unless to a small extent during very prolonged treatment, and the sensitivity of most susceptible pathogens has remained unchanged despite years of extensive therapeutic use. An exception is the gonococcus, moderately resistant strains of which are now being encountered. Another is now the pneumococcus, resistant strains of which have been found by Hansman *et al.* (1971) in an area in New Guinea where monthly injections of procaine penicillin were being given for the prophylaxis of pneumonia. Apart from two other strains isolated in Australia, resistance in this species has not so far been reported, and the peculiar circumstances of its occurrence in New Guinea encourage the belief that it is not likely to be seen often elsewhere. Nevertheless the fact that it can occur at all is disturbing.

TYPE OF ANTI-BACTERIAL ACTION. In a nutrient medium (i.e. when bacterial growth can occur, but not otherwise) penicillin is bactericidal. About four hours is required to produce a high mortality, and this may proceed to extinction, or there may be a few survivors. This effect is best exerted by a concentration 5-10 times greater than the minimum inhibiting growth, and no increase above this level will accelerate it. Against many strains of two species, *Staph. aureus* and *Str. faecalis,* such an increase actually reduces the death rate, the so-called paradoxical zone phenomenon (Eagle, 1951). This behaviour of penicillin is unique, and no certain explanation for it is known, but one hypothesis is proposed by Eagle in his description of the phenomenon.

Spectrum of Activity of Benzyl Penicillin
(Minimum inhibitory concentrations in μg./ml.)

Gram-positive Organisms		Gram-negative Organisms	
Cocci	Streptococcus pyogenes (A)	0·006	
	Streptococcus pneumoniae	0·006	
	Streptococcus viridans	0·012*	
	Streptococcus faecalis	2	
	Staphylococcus aureus	0·012*	
	Staphylococcus albus	0·012*	
	Sarcina lutea	0·0015	
Bacilli	Bacillus anthracis	0·01 –0·04	
	Clostridium tetani	0·007–0·3	
	Clostridium welchii	0·06 –0·25	
	Clostridium oedematiens	0·007–0·015	
	Clostridium septicum	0·03	
	Clostridium histolyticum	0·03	
	Corynebacterium diphtheriae	0·02 –0·6	
	Actinobacillus muris	0·06	
	Erysipelothrix rhusiopathiae	0·04 –0·08	
	Listeria monocytogenes	0·2 –0·6	
Fungi	Actinomyces israeli	0·02 –0·1	

Gram-negative Organisms:

Neisseria gonorrhoeae	0·003*
Neisseria meningitidis	0·012
Neisseria catarrhalis	0·012*
Haemophilus influenzae	0·25 –1
Haemophilus pertussis	0·5 –2
Haemophilus ducreyi	0·045–0·15
Bacteroides fragilis	16*
Bacteroides fusiformis	0·06 –0·5
Bacteroides melaninogenicum	0·007–0·06
Bacteroides necrophorus	0·06 –0·12
Escherichia coli	20*
Klebsiella pneumoniae	2–100
Proteus mirabilis	8*
Salmonella spp.	2–5
Pasteurella septica	0·5

* Denotes that some strains are more resistant.

Other sensitive species, the susceptibility of which cannot be measured in this way, are T. pallidum and other treponemata and a few of the larger viruses. Leptospira spp. are also sensitive to 0·05-0·5 μg./ml.

Resistant species not included in the Table are all organisms of the genera Brucella, Mycobacterium, Pfeifferella, Pseudomonas, Vibrio, Proteus (other than P. mirabilis). Klebsiella aerogenes, all fungi other than A. israeli, most viruses, all rickettsias and mycoplasmas.

The concentrations given for commoner species are the approximate mean of many estimations by various authors. Some of the less familiar are derived as follows: From the present writer's own observations B. anthracis (Antibiot. and Chemother. 1952, 2, 689), A. israeli (Brit. med. J. 1952, i, 1263). Bacteroides (Brit. med. J. 1952, ii, 1529), Clostridia (J. roy. Army med. Corps. 1958, 104, 209). For C. diphtheriae R. Cruickshank et al. (Lancet 1948, ii, 517), E. rhusiopathiae P. H. A. Sneath et al. (Brit. med. J. 1951, ii, 1063), L. monocytogenes I. A. Bakulov (Antibiotics 1959, 4, 575), H. pertussis E. B. Wells et al. (J. Pediat. 1950, 36, 752).

(This table also appears in a contribution by one of the authors (L. P. G.) to 'Experimental Chemotherapy', Ed. F. Hawking & R. J. Schnitzer.)

Pharmacokinetics

The salts of benzyl penicillin are very freely diffusible: after intramuscular injection absorption occurs within a few minutes to produce a high concentration in the blood. Diffusion takes place into the foetal circulation and into serous cavities: lower concentrations are found in glandular secretions, and still lower in the cerebro-spinal fluid, but these are raised in meningitis owing both to the presence of penicillin in the exudate, and to its more ready diffusibility through the walls of dilated capillaries. Concentrations two to five times that in the blood are found in the bile, but excretion is mainly renal, accounting for about 60 per cent of the dose, some of which is apparently destroyed in the body. This excretion is mainly tubular, and exceedingly rapid—much more so than that of any other drug with an anti-microbic action. Some idea of the wasteful nature of this treatment may be gained from the fact that in an adult with anuria an ample dose for the treatment of a fully sensitive infection would be only 2,000 units.

The usual way of overcoming this difficulty is simply to give very large doses: the initially very high concentrations thus produced in the body are no bar to this because penicillin is virtually non-toxic. It is important to recognise that doubling the dose does not double the duration of effect. According to Eagle (1948) the doses required to maintain a blood level in excess of 0·16 unit per ml. for different periods are:

1 hour	20,000	units.
2 hours	50,000	„
3 „	140,000	„
4 „	235,000	„
6 „	600,000	„
8 „	1,400,000	„

These figures give a good idea of the dosage and intervals which must be observed if a *continuous effect* is considered necessary. It may not be: Eagle (1949) has also shown that it takes bacteria damaged but not killed by penicillin three to four hours to recover and resume growth. In some kinds of infection treatment which is intermittent to this degree may be satisfactory.

It has often been said that the blood level is not what matters, but that in the lesion: that penicillin diffuses into this when the blood level is high and persists there much longer. This is true of collections of exudate (Florey, Turton and Duthie, 1946), but not of inflammation in a vascular area without tissue destruction (Eagle, Fleischman and Levy, 1953), and it is to this category that most acute infections belong. It would certainly appear safer to administer doses calculated to maintain an effective concentration in the blood continuously, and by using forms of penicillin to be described later this is easily achieved.

One way of prolonging the action of each dose of penicillin is to administer another substance which interferes with tubular excretion. Probenecid (benemid) (Burnell and Kirby, 1951) serves this purpose well. It is used not so much for extending the intervals between doses as for maintaining higher blood levels between doses given at usual intervals when such levels are considered necessary, as in the treatment of endocarditis due to less sensitive streptococci.

Long-acting Forms of Benzyl Penicillin

The second possible way of prolonging the effect of a dose is to delay absorption. This was first achieved by suspending the calcium salt in a water-immiscible medium containing oil and beeswax. Much more satisfactory results have since been obtained with penicillin compounds of lesser solubility. The first of these was procaine penicillin, an equimolecular compound of penicillin and procaine, which is administered as a suspension of crystals which dissolve slowly at the site of injection. The ' peak ' blood level (which is not a peak but a plateau, and relatively low) is reached in about four hours, and the level falls slowly, being still detectable 24 hours after a moderate dose (Fig. 7).

Still less soluble and therefore longer-acting compounds are benethamine penicillin and benzathine penicillin, a single dose of which will provide a low concentration in the blood for four to five days and several weeks respectively. Various mixtures are available, some including the potassium salt for an immediate high level, and procaine penicillin and one of the least soluble compounds to sustain diminishing levels for a long period.

An orally administered form of benzathine penicillin (Penidural) converts the advantage of this compound when injected
into a drawback, since, owing to its low solubility, little of a
swallowed dose is absorbed. Henry, White and Meynell (1957)

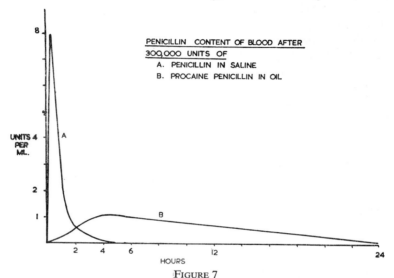

FIGURE 7

Blood levels produced by the administration of penicillin in two different
forms.

(Garrod (1950), reproduced by kind permission of the editor of the *British Medical Journal*.)

recovered only 6·7 per cent of an oral dose from the urine, in
contrast to 30 per cent of an oral dose of phenoxymethyl penicillin, and over 70 per cent of a dose of either penicillin or
procaine penicillin given intramuscularly. These tests were done
in adults: benzathine penicillin appears to be better absorbed
in children, but here account must be taken of the relatively
large dose usually given in proportion to body weight. Even so
the blood concentration most often found three hours after a
dose of 300,000 units given to 101 children by Cathie and
MacFarlane (1953) was only 0·125 units per ml. In neonates a
relatively still larger dose (150,000 units) of either benzathine or
sodium penicillin produced higher and more sustained levels,
with little to choose between the two treatments (Laurence and
Alder, 1954). The only advantage of oral benzathine penicillin
is palatability.

PHENOXYMETHYL PENICILLIN

The existence of several natural penicillins was recognised in early studies, and many more have been obtained by adding various derivatives of acetic acid to the fermentation medium as ' precursors '. None of these is therapeutically important except phenoxymethyl penicillin, or penicillin V. which is obtained when phenoxyacetic acid is the precursor. This substance, originally described in 1948, but without its most important property having been detected, was re-discovered in Austria in 1953, and owes its value to acid stability: it is not destroyed in the stomach, and can therefore be given with confidence by mouth. Absorption is not in fact complete: the proportion of the dose recoverable from the urine is only 25 per cent (Heatley, 1956) but this was a great improvement on the absorption of benzyl penicillin, which is not only on the average much less, but unaccountably variable. Absorption is slower than that after injection, but excretion is equally rapid: hence a moderate dose needs repetition at intervals of four hours. Of different forms of penicillin V, the potassium salt is the best absorbed, the calcium salt next and the free acid least, that being their diminishing order of solubility: absorption is also better from a rapidly disintegrating tablet and after administration in the fasting state (Juncher and Raaschou, 1957).

It was for some time assumed that penicillin V has the same anti-bacterial activity as benzyl penicillin, but this is not so. It is rather *more* active against resistant staphylococci because more slowly destroyed by penicillinase, and slightly *less* active against streptococci, but much less active against Gram-negative species, including the gonococcus, *H. influenzae* and *Proteus* (Garrod, 1960a, b). These differences are exaggerated in the synthetic acid-resistant penicillins described later. Penicillin V therefore affords a very convenient means of treating Gram-positive infections, but is not indicated for gonorrhoea or for Gram-negative infections involving the respiratory or urinary tract.

THERAPEUTIC APPLICATIONS

These are dealt with individually in the second part of this book, and need only be briefly reviewed here. In the first place, penicillin is almost wholly responsible for the fact that fatal haemolytic streptococcal infection is now almost unheard of: in all serious forms of this infection, whether involving wounds, the air passages or the uterus, it is usually the treatment of choice. The pneumococcus is also invariably susceptible to it (with a hitherto geographically limited exception mentioned on p. 54), and its efficacy can therefore be depended on in lobar pneumonia. In staphylococcal infections its value has been reduced by the increasing prevalence of resistant strains, but if the strain is sensitive natural penicillins are preferable to the synthetic.

Among its other principal uses may be mentioned the treatment of both syphilis and gonorrhoea, bacterial endocarditis and actinomycosis. Rarer indications for which it is highly effective are gas gangrene, anthrax and erysipeloid.

Dosage

Because both of the variety of its uses and of its lack of toxicity, the dosage of penicillin is remarkably elastic, certainly more so than that of any other drug. The factors determining the necessary dose are, first and foremost, the concentration required to inhibit the growth of the infecting organism, and the accessibility and gravity of the infection. If the inhibitory concentration is known or can be deduced, the aim should be to maintain one exceeding this, preferably several-fold, in the affected tissues. If these are intact and fully vascularized, the concentration in them will be much the same as that in the blood. If there are foci of suppuration or of necrosis, or fibrotic areas with a poor blood supply as in such a condition as actinomycosis, penetration is more difficult. A special indication for high dosage owing to inaccessibility is the attainment of an adequate concentration in the cerebro-spinal fluid in meningitis.

To translate these principles into practical terms, a fully sensitive infection in an area well supplied with blood should respond to 0·5 or even 0·25 g. of penicillin V given orally at intervals of four hours or to procaine penicillin given by injection in doses of 300,000 units (180 mg.) at intervals of 12 hours. Somewhat higher concentrations can be attained by increasing the dose of either of these preparations, but for maximum effects ' soluble ' (i.e. potassium) penicillin must be given either by intramuscular injection at intervals not exceeding six hours or by continuous intravenous infusion: the amount so administered may be anything from four to 20 million units daily or even more.

TOXICITY

Penicillin has no toxicity in the ordinary sense except when administered intrathecally: the dose by this route should never exceed 20,000 units, if indeed the route need be used at all, which is doubtful. It is almost impossible to poison a patient with penicillin if he has properly functioning kidneys, but if there is gross renal impairment the antibiotic may accumulate in the blood, in which the level should be estimated, the dose being reduced accordingly. Doses of 25 to 40 mega units of potassium penicillin daily given for presumed or known Gram-negative infections to 4 elderly patients, all with raised blood ureas, caused partial or complete loss of consciousness with myoclonic movements and sometimes generalized seizures (Bloomer, Barton and Maddock, 1967). From a study of 15 patients similarly treated (some with doses of up to 120 mega units daily) in whom the penicillin was assayed in the blood and cerebrospinal fluid, Smith, Lerner and Weinstein (1967) conclude that this ' neurotoxicity ' results only when a concentration of 10 units per ml. is exceeded in the c.s.f. These patients received either the Na or the K salt, the effects of which are not distinguished. An effect from the cation must be considered whenever large doses of a single salt are given, and it is now usually thought desirable in these circumstances to use a mixture of the Na and K salts. The disturbances which may follow massive doses of the Na salt are described by Brunner and Frick (1968).

The unique toxicity of penicillin for guinea-pigs, in which a single intramuscular dose is often fatal within a few days, seems finally to have been explained by the work of Farrar and Kent (1965). The two following effects in man may be classified as sensitivity reactions, but it is convenient to refer to them here.

NEPHRITIS. Very rarely patients receiving long courses of large doses of penicillin develop fever, eosinophilia, proteinuria and haematuria with a raised blood urea. Baldwin *et al.* (1968) describe 3 cases, in one of which persistence with the treatment ended in oliguria and death. The kidneys showed tubular necrosis and dense interstitial infiltration with mononuclears and eosinophiles.

HAEMOLYTIC ANAEMIA. This complication occurs only in patients who have been treated with penicillin before and again receive a prolonged course of large doses (commonly 20 mega units daily) usually for bacterial endocarditis. The haemolysis is due to the action of 1gG antibody on cells which have adsorbed the antibiotic. Rapid recovery ensues when administration is stopped. White *et al.* (1968) describe 2 cases and review the findings in 12 others.

SENSITIZATION REACTIONS

These present a more serious problem with penicillin than with any other antibiotic. Previous treatment is probably the usual cause of sensitization: various ' hidded contacts ' (Siegel, 1959), such as consumption in milk, are possible causes; the idea that fungus infections may be responsible is less well founded. Reactions are of two kinds, the ' serum sickness ' type, characterized by urticaria and fever; and immediate profound shock. which may be fatal within a few minutes. This condition, first recorded about 1952, has since been frequently described, some authors having knowledge of numerous cases (Cheng and Chiang, 1956; Rosenthal, 1958): penicillin is even described as having ' replaced foreign sera as the commonest cause of anaphylactic shock ' (Kern and Wimberley, 1953). It usually follows a therapeutic injection, but has also been caused by oral administration, by local application, and by the injection of a minute dose as a test for sensitivity. The condition is one of profound vasomotor collapse, with an impalpable pulse, usually loss of consciousness, with or without facial or laryngeal oedema or a generalized rash.

Several authors (Hoigné and Schoch, 1959; Lewis, 1957;

Tompsett, 1967) distinguish from this another kind of immediate reaction attributed to the accidental intravenous injection of a suspension of procaine penicillin, characterized by vertigo, disturbances of sensation (one of Tompsett's patients saw a green giraffe jump over her bed) and a sense of impending death: this can occur in individuals not sensitized to penicillin, as has sometimes been proved by giving a further dose without ill effects. Some other features, including tachycardia and cyanosis, may occur in either kind of reaction, and the two are not always easily distinguishable (Hoigné, 1962). Although sometimes regarded as manifestations of procaine poisoning, these reactions are undoubtedly due to blockage of pulmonary capillaries by the crystals, as demonstrated experimentally by Bell, Rannie and Wynne (1954). Bredt (1965) observed 7 cases after injections of Megacillin, a depot preparation containing no procaine, and prevented further cases by having the crystals in this milled to a smaller size.

Tests for sensitivity. Dermal tests, by the ' patch ', ' scratch ' or intradermal methods, are far from infallible, and seem better able to predict reactions of the serum sickness type than that of shock. Thus in a study in Taiwan (Idsöe and Wang, 1958), in which such tests were performed before therapeutic injection, the results were negative in each of five cases subsequently suffering from fatal shock and six having severe shock; they were positive only in a proportion of those later developing less severe shock or urticaria.

Further study of this problem has been pursued on three lines, and has produced an extensive recent literature which will not be fully reviewed here. One is the use of *penicilloyl-polylysine* for tests of sensitivity, based on the work of de Weck and Eisen (1961) and de Weck (1962). According to these authors, penicillin itself does not combine firmly enough with protein to produce an antigen: the actual haptene is penicillenic acid or a penicillenate or penicilloyl derivative of it. This substance is slowly formed from penicillin in solution. The result of a test with a solution of penicillin may thus depend on whether degradation products have formed in it. Penicillenic acid itself cannot be used for fear of producing sensitization, but the penicilloyl-polypeptide compound penicilloyl-polylysine is a suitable antigen and is said not to sensitize. (But

Resnik and Shelley (1966) report shock following a repeat test with it.) The reliability claimed for this test by Parker *et al.* (1962) and in particular the claim that it gives no false negatives, have not always been confirmed by others (Rytel *et al.*, 1963; Finke *et al.*, 1965; Smith, Johnson and Cluff, 1966). On the other hand, much more dependable findings are claimed by Levine and Zolov (1969) from tests with both penicilloyl-poly-lysine and a Minor Determinant Mixture (containing benzyl penicillin, penicilloate, penilloate and α-benzyl penicilloyl amine, a preparation apparently not available commercially). Scratch tests with each of these were followed if negative by intradermal tests. In 185 patients negative to both and treated with penicillin only one atypical reaction occurred. Of 32 patients positive to one or both, 21 were not treated, and among 11 who were there were 7 accelerated and one immediate urti-carial reactions. Similar findings are reported by Adkinson *et al.* (1971), who claim that the application of these tests has much reduced the frequency of penicillin reactions in their unit at the Johns Hopkins Hospital.

Another method, the *basophil degranulation test* proposed by Shelley (1963) appears from a further study (Katz, *et al.*, 1964) to be a somewhat chancy procedure, and though others have used it in parallel with tests of different kinds, the results are unimpressive.

Impurities in penicillins as antigens. All work until very recently has been based on the belief that the sensitizing antigen is a combination of a penicillin derivative with body protein. The subject has now been much complicated by the discovery that a highly reactive pre-formed antigen may exist in penicillin itself (Batchelor *et al.*, 1967; Stewart, 1967). That found by these authors in 6-aminopenicillanic acid, and hence liable to be present in any semi-synthetic penicillin, is believed to be derived from the enzyme used in production, and that in benzyl penicillin from *P. chrysogenum* itself, each existing as a peni-cilloyl conjugate. These authors also recognized that a reactive substance can be formed in a solution of pure benzyl penicillin by polymerization. Dewdney, Smith and Wheeler (1971) have since shown that such polymers, to which sensitized animals react, are formed on standing for 8-14 days in solutions not only of benzylpenicillin, but of ampicillin, hetacillin, carbenicillin and cephaloridine. The use of freshly prepared solutions for injection should be a safeguard against the possible effects of this change.

The effects of removing protein impurities have been studied. Penicillin freed from the penicilloyl protein impurity (BRL 3000, ' Purapen G ') produced no reaction in 11 sensitive volunteers who reacted to ordinary penicillin, but 9 reacted to both and 1 to the purified material only (Knudsen *et al.*, 1967). Similar treatment of ampicillin reduced the incidence of rashes by about one half (Knudsen, Dewdney and Trafford, 1970). de Weck and Schneider (1969) contest the view that these impurities are responsible for reactions, at least to benzyl penicillin, on two grounds: that in animals they have found purified benzyl penicillin to retain its full immunogenicity, and that hydrolysed crude benzyl penicillin, which owing to the opening of the β-lactam ring cannot form penicilloyl conjugates, does not induce the formation of anti-penicilloyl antibodies.

ANTI-PENICILLIN ANTIBODIES. An agglutination test with penicillin-treated red cells is often positive, even in normal subjects or patients actually under treatment without ill effects. Positive results were obtained by Ascari and Gorman (1969) in 22·2 per cent of subjects with a history of reactions to penicillin and 37·8 per cent of treated syphilitics; Epp (1962) obtained them in over 50 per cent of all subjects and in a higher proportion of those with a history of a reaction. Levine *et al.* (1966) using an antigen prepared by coupling penicilloyl groups to red cells in a special suspending medium, obtained enormous titres, and demonstrated agglutinin in almost all of 76 ' consecutive ' patients, only one of whom had a history of a reaction to penicillin.

It seems that the method of preparing the cell suspension affects the frequency of positive results. These agglutinins can be either 1gM or 1gG, and the latter can function as ' blocking antibodies ', preventing the reaction between administered penicillin and the antibodies responsible for reactions.

These, the so-called ' skin-sensitizing ' antibodies, are certainly of two kinds, respectively responsible for urticarial and shock-like reactions. The former can be detected with penicilloyl-polylysine and the latter with benzyl penicillin itself, applied in a scratch test.

The expert application of these tests, if necessary employing different amounts of penicilloyl-polylysine, is recommended by de Weck and Schneider (1969) when penicillin treatment is strongly indicated in a supposedly sensitized patient, in a general review of this very complex subject, which should be consulted for further details. Apart from this only common sense precautions can be advocated, including regular inquiry about previous reactions whenever penicillin is to be given, extreme caution and preferably the substitution of other antibiotics in asthmatics and patients with other known sensitivities, and the immediate availability of adrenaline.

PHARMACEUTICAL PREPARATIONS

Benzyl penicillin (Na or K salt: ' crystalline ' or ' soluble ' penicillin. Vials containing 100,000 units and much more for solution for intramuscular injection. Dosage widely variable according to nature of condition treated: see text. Tablets containing 200,000 or 400,000 units or other amounts for oral administration. Also ointment, lozenges and other preparations.

Procaine benzyl penicillin. Available under numerous proprietary names as a suspension, usually containing 300,000 units per ml., or as a powder for preparing such a suspension, for intramuscular injection. Some preparations (e.g. Fortified Procaine Penicillin Injection, B.P.) also contain benzylpenicillin. Dose 300,000 to 1,200,000 units; need usually be given only once daily.

Benzathine penicillin. Suspension usually containing 600,000 units per ml. for intramuscular injection: long interval dosage (one dose of 1,200,000 units monthly for rheumatic fever prophylaxis). Also available as tablets or suspension (' Penidural ', Wyeth) for oral administration.

Phenoxymethyl penicillin (Penicillin V). Usually phenoxymethyl penicillin potassium (' Compocillin VK ', Abbott; ' Crystapen V ', Glaxo; ' Distaquaine V ', Dista Products, and many others). Tablets containing 125 or 250 mg.: also as capsules and suspensions. Usual dose 250 mg. at 4- or 6-hourly intervals; this may be considerably exceeded, but gastric intolerance may result from larger doses.

REFERENCES

ADKINSON, N. F., THOMPSON, W. L., MADDREY, W. C. & LICHTENSTEIN, L. M. (1971). *New England J. Med.* **285**, 22.
ASCARI, W. Q. & GORMAN, J. G. (1969). *Transfusion,* **9**, 35.
BALDWIN, D. S., LEVINE, B. B., McCLUSKEY, R. T. & GALLO, G. R. (1968). *New Engl. J. Med.* **279**, 1245.
BATCHELOR, F. R., DEWDNEY, J., FEINBERG, J. G. & WESTON, R. D. (1967). *Lancet* **2**, 1175.
BELL, R. C., RANNIE, I. & WYNNE, N. A. (1954). *Lancet*, **2**, 62.
BLOOMER, H. A., BARTON, L. J. & MADDOCK, R. K., Jr. (1967). *J. Amer. med. Ass.* **200**, 121.
BREDT, J. (1965). *Dtsch. med. Wschr.* **90**, 1602.
BRUNNER, F. P. & FRICK, P. G. (1968). *Brit. med. J.* **4**, 550.
BURNELL, J. M. & KIRBY, W. M. M. (1951). *J. clin. Invest.* **30**, 697.
CATHIE, I. A. B. & MACFARLANE, J. C. W. (1953). *Brit. med. J.* **1**, 805.
CHENG, C. L. & CHIANG, C-T. (1956). *Chinese med. J.* **74**, 513.
DEWDNEY, J. M., SMITH, H. & WHEELER, A. W. (1971). *Immunology* **21**, 517.

EAGLE, H. (1948). *Ann. intern. Med.* **28**, 260.
EAGLE, H. (1949). *J. clin. Invest.* **28**, 832.
EAGLE, H. (1951). *J. Bact.* **62**, 663
EAGLE, H., FLEISCHMAN, R. & LEVI, MINA (1953). *J. Lab. clin. Med.* **41**, 122.
EPP, M. (1962). *Canad. J. pub. Hlth.* **53**, 79.
FARRAR, W. E. JR. & KENT, T. H. (1965). *Amer. J. Path.* **47**, 629.
FINKE, S. R., GRIECO, M. H., CONNELL, J. T., SMITH, M. C. & SHERMAN, W. B (1965). *Amer. J. Med.* **38**, 71.
FLOREY, M. E., TURTON, E. C. & DUTHIE, E. S. (1946). *Lancet* **2**, 405.
GARROD, L. P. (1950). *Brit. med. J.* **2**, 453.
GARROD, L. P. (1960a). *Brit. med. J.* **1**, 527.
GARROD, L. P. (1960b). *Brit. med. J.* **2**, 1695.
GARROD, L. P. & WATERWORTH. P. M. (1962). *Brit. Heart J.* **24**, 39.
HANSMAN, D., GLASGOW, H., STURT, J., DEVITT, L. & DOUGLAS, R. (1971). *New England J. Med.* **284**, 175.
HEATLEY, N. G. (1956). *Antibiot. Med.* **2**, 33.
HENRY, L., WHITE, G. & MEYNELL, M. J. (1957). *Brit. med. J.* **1**, 17.
HOIGNÉ, R. (1962). *Acta med. scand.* **171**, 201.
HOIGNÉ, R. & SCHOCH, K. (1959). *Schweiz. med. Wschr.* **89**, 1350.
IDSÖE, O. & WANG, K. Y. (1958). *Bull. Wrld Hlth Org.* **18**, 323.
JUNCHER, H. & RAASCHOU, F. (1957). *Antibiot. Med.* **4**, 497.
KATZ, H. I., GILL, K. A., BAXTER, D. L. & MOSCHELLA, S. L. (1964). *J. Amer. med. Ass.* **188**, 351.
KERN, R. A. & WIMBERLEY, N. A. JR. (1953). *Amer. J. med. Sci.* **226**, 357.
KNUDSEN, E. T., DEWDNEY, J. M. & TRAFFORD, J. A. P. (1970). *Brit. med. J.* **1**, 469.
KNUDSEN, E. T., ROBINSON, O. P. W., CROYDON, E. A. P. & TEES, E. C. (1967). *Lancet* **2**, 1184.
LAURANCE, B. & ALDER, V. G. (1954). *Brit. med. J.* **2**, 1392.
LEVINE, B. B., FELLNER, M. J., LEVYTSKA, V., FRANKLIN, E. C. & ALISBERG, N. (1966). *J. Immunol.* **96**, 707, 719.
LEVINE, B. B. & ZOLOV, D. M. (1969). *J. Allergy* **43**, 231.
LEWIS, G. W. (1957). *Brit. med. J.* **1**, 1153.
PARKER, C. W., SHAPIRO, J., KERN, M. & EISEN, H. N. (1962). *J. exp. Med.* **115**, 821.
RESNIK, S. S. & SHELLEY, W. B. (1966). *J. Amer. Med. Ass.* **196**, 740.
ROSENTHAL, A. (1958). *J. Amer. med. Ass.* **167**, 1118.
RYTEL, M. W., KLION, F. M., ARLANDER, T. R. & MILLER, L. F. (1963). *J. Amer. med. Ass.* **186**, 894.
SHELLEY, W. B. (1963). *J. Amer. Med. Ass.* **184**, 171.
SIEGEL, B. B. (1959). *Bull. Wrld. Hlth. Org.* **21**, 703.
SMITH, H., LERNER, P. I. & WEINSTEIN, L. (1967). *Arch. intern. Med.* **120**, 47.
SMITH, J. W., JOHNSON, J. E. III & CLUFF, L. E. (1966). *New Engl. J. Med.* **274**, 998.
STEWART, G. T. (1967). *Lancet* **2**, 1177.
TOMPSETT, R. (1967). *Arch. intern. Med.* **120**, 565.
WECK, A. L. DE (1962). *Schweiz. med. Wschr.* **92**, 1155.
WECK, A. L. DE & SCHNEIDER, C. H. (1969). *Minnesota Med.* **52**, 137.
WECK, A. L. DE & EISEN, H. N. (1960). *J. exp. Med.* **112**, 1227.
WHITE, J. M., BROWN, D. L., HEPNER, G. W. & WORLLEDGE, S. M. (1968). *Brit. med. J.* **3**, 26.

CHAPTER 5

PENICILLINS

2. SEMI-SYNTHETIC PENICILLINS AND CEPHALOSPORINS

THE existence of the penicillin ' nucleus ', 6-aminopenicillanic acid, in *Penicillium chrysogenum* fermentations was first detected by discrepancies between the results of chemical and microbiological assays, and more was found to be formed in the absence of added precursor (Batchelor *et al.*, 1959). The second discovery made at this time was that this substance

6 − amino − penicillanic acid   7 − amino − cephalosporanic acid

could also be prepared in quantity from benzyl or phenoxymethyl penicillin by the action of an enzyme derived from other micro-organisms : the effect of this amidase is to separate the side chain (for site of action see p. 53). The amidase acting on benzyl penicillin is obtainable from numerous enterobacteria (*Escherichia, Klebsiella,* etc.) and that attacking phenoxymethyl penicillin is derived from moulds (e.g. *Streptomyces lavendulae* (Batchelor *et al.*, 1961).

Until this discovery different penicillins could only be obtained by adding precursors to the medium, among which only derivatives of acetic acid were effective. The availability of the nucleus itself enabled side chains in a great variety to be attached by a semi-synthetic process. In the Beecham Research Laboratories, where these discoveries were made, over 2,000 new penicillins have been prepared by this process, and those which have come into therapeutic use possess one or more of the following advantages: (1) resistance to acid, (2) resistance

TABLE 9

CLINICALLY USEFUL PENICILLINS

Side Chain	Approved Name and Full Chemical Name	Trade Names	Important Properties
⬡—CH_2–CO–	**Benzyl penicillin** 6-phenylacetamido penicillanic acid		
⬡—O–CH_2–CO–	**Phenoxymethyl penicillin** Penicillin V 6-phenoxyacetamido penicillanic acid		Acid-resistant
⬡—O–CH–CO– $\quad$ CH_3	**Phenethicillin** DL-6-(α-phenoxypropionamido) penicillanic acid	Broxil	Acid-resistant
⬡—O–CH–CO– $\quad$ CH_2 $\quad$ CH_3	**Propicillin** DL-6-(α-phenoxy-n-butyramido) penicillanic acid	Brocillin Ultrapen	Acid-resistant
⬡—CH–CO– $\quad$ NH_2	**Ampicillin** 6-(D(-)-α-aminophenylacetamido) penicillanic acid	Penbritin	Active against Gram-negative bacilli Acid-resistant
⬡—CH–CO– $\quad$ COONa	**Carbenicillin** Disodium α-carboxy-benzyl-penicillin	Pyopen	Active against Gram-negative bacilli
⬡ (OCH_3)(OCH_3)—CO–	**Methicillin** 6-(2,6 dimethoxybenzamido) penicillanic acid	Celbenin	Penicillinase-resistant
⬡(Cl)—C–C–CO– $\quad$ N C O CH_3	**Cloxacillin** 6-(5-Methyl-3-orthochlorophenyl-isoxazole-4-carboxyamido) penicillanic acid	Orbenin	Penicillinase-resistant Acid-resistant

to penicillinase, (3) broader spectrum. The names, structures, and important properties of those in established use in Great Britain are stated in Table 9. More recent additions are amoxycillin p. 84) and flucloxacillin (p. 76).

ACID-RESISTANT PENICILLINS (PHENOXYPENICILLINS)

The property of acid resistance, permitting a reliable effect from oral administration, was not new, since it already existed

TABLE 10

Sensitivity of Bacteria to the Penicillins

Usual Minimum Concentration (μg./ml.) causing Complete Bacteristasis with a Moderate Inoculum

	Benzyl Penicillin	Phenoxy-methyl Penicillin	Phenethi-cillin	Propicillin	Ampicillin	Methi-cillin	Cloxa-cillin
1. Highly Sensitive Species							
Staph. aureus*	0·03	0·03	0·03	0·06	0·06	2	0·125
Str. pyogenes	0·015	0·015	0·03	0·03	0·03	0·125	0·06
Str. pneumoniae	0·015	0·015	0·06	0·03	0·06	0·25	0·25
B. anthracis	0·008	0·015	0·06		0·06	0·125	0·5
Cl. welchii	0·06						
N. gonorrhoeae	0·015	0·03	0·125	0·125	0·125	0·06	0·5
N. meningitidis	0·03	0·125	1		0·06	0·25	0·5
N. catarrhalis	0·03	0·125			0·015	0·25	1
2. Less Sensitive Species							
Str. faecalis	2	4	4		2	32	32
H. influenzae	1	4	4		0·25	2	16
Salmonella spp.	8	128	>250		2	>250	250
Salm. typhi	4	64	250		1	>250	250
Shigella spp.	16	64			4	>250	128
Esch. coli	64	128	>250		8	250	250
Proteus mirabilis*	32	128	>250		4	4	250
Proteus mirabilis†	>250	>250	>250	>250	>250	>250	>250
Proteus vulgaris	>250	>250	>250	>250	64	>250	>250
Proteus rettgeri	4 - >250	>250	>250	>250	2 - >250	>250	>250
Proteus morgani	>250	>250	>250	>250	128 - >256	>250	>250
Klebsiella aerogenes	>250	>250	>250	>250	16 - >250	>250	>250

* Non-penicillinase-forming.   † Penicillinase-forming.

in phenoxymethyl penicillin (p. 59). Despite this property, only about 25 per cent of the dose is absorbed, and better absorption is the main advantage of the semi-synthetic penicillins in this class, phenethicillin (Knudsen and Rolinson, 1959) and propicillin (Williamson, Morrison and Stevens, 1961). Details of their anti-bacterial activity are given in Table 10. Like phenoxymethyl penicillin they are almost as active as benzyl penicillin against sensitive Gram-positive bacteria, but they share and in some instances exaggerate the deficiencies of phenoxymethyl penicillin in dealing with various Gram-negative species. Their clinical application should be restricted accordingly.

The therapeutic efficacy of these penicillins is the product of three factors, anti-bacterial activity, efficiency of absorption, and extent of protein binding in the blood. The only adequate study taking all these factors into account is that of Bond, Lightbown, Barber and Waterworth (1963) who assayed not only total but free antibiotic in the blood of volunteers at intervals after a dose, as well as studying the anti-bacterial activity *in vitro* in the presence and absence of serum. This study included phenbenicillin, another such compound, no longer manufactured, which is better absorbed but also much more highly protein-bound than the others. Taking all these factors into account, phenoxymethylpenicillin was judged the most active of the three for streptococcal infections and phenethicillin for staphylococcal.

A sufficient dose of any of these drugs given at 4-hour intervals should serve any ordinary suitable purpose. If any of them is to be used for a serious and unusual purpose, notably for bacterial endocarditis, its suitability should be verified by an accurate test of the sensitivity of the organism *to the penicillin which it is proposed to use*. It cannot be assumed that the result will be the same as that to be obtained with benzylpenicillin.

PENICILLINASE-RESISTANT PENICILLINS

Of far greater practical importance than the discovery of the acid-resistant penicillins was the discovery that changes in the side-chain of penicillin can protect the central β-lactam ring from the action of penicillinase without removing anti-bacterial activity. Several such penicillins are now available for clinical use. They comprise a single compound, methicillin, which is acid-labile and has therefore to be injected, and a group, the isoxazolyl penicillins, which are also acid-stable and can hence be given orally.

Methicillin

CHEMISTRY. Methicillin is 2 : 6 dimethyloxybenzyl penicillin (Table 10) and is supplied as the sodium salt. It is readily soluble in water, but solutions are very unstable. Neutral solutions lose 50 per cent of their activity in five days at room temperature and 20 per cent when stored at 5°C. Acid solutions are much more unstable and at pH 2·0 half the activity is lost in 20 minutes at room temperature (Rolinson *et al.*, 1960).

ANTI-BACTERIAL ACTIVITY. Methicillin is highly resistant to staphylococcal penicillinase, although less so to the penicillinase of many other species (Rolinson *et al.*, 1960). It is, therefore, equally active against penicillin-sensitive and penicillinase-producing strains of *Staph. aureus*. On the other hand, its activity is much less than that of benzyl penicillin against most other penicillin-sensitive species (Table 10). Methicillin, like benzyl penicillin, is actively bactericidal in optimum concentrations, but, at least against staphylococci, may be less so in higher concentrations. In view of its lack of activity against other species there is no indication for its use except a severe penicillin-resistant staphylococcal infection.

RESISTANCE IN STAPHYLOCOCCI. Strains of *Staph. aureus* resistant to methicillin, thought at first not to exist and then to be exceedingly rare, are now being encountered more frequently: the percentage resistant among many thousands of strains tested at the Central Public Health Laboratory rose from 0·06 in 1960 to 0·97 in 1964 (Dyke, Jevons and Parker, 1966) and to 4·11 per cent in 1969 (Parker and Hewitt, 1970). Much higher frequencies of resistance in strains isolated from infections in hospitals have been reported from France (Chabbert *et al.*, 1965), Switzerland (Benner and Kayser, 1968; Kayser and Hollinger, 1968) and Denmark (Siboni and Poulsen, 1968). It is now clear that such infections may not respond to treatment with methicillin alone, and the strains concerned are usually resistant to many other antibiotics. An appropriate treatment for serious infections of this nature may be a combination of methicillin or cephalothin with kanamycin, which exerts a synergic bactericidal effect (Bulger, 1967; see also p. 314).

Although these strains form large amounts of penicillinase, they do not destroy methicillin, as has been asserted: their resistance is intrinsic. Only a small minority of the cells in these cultures appears resistant (Sutherland and Rolinson, 1964a)—except on a medium containing an excess of electrolytes, such as 5 per cent NaCl (Barber, 1964)—with the result that a diffusion test of sensitivity with a light inoculum may give a misleading result. Methods for detecting methicillin resistance are discussed in Chapter 29.

Resistance to methicillin is much commoner in *Staph. albus*: Kjellander and Finland (1963) found 10 per cent of clinical isolates resistant. They formed penicillinase, but also possessed intrinsic resistance.

PHARMACOKINETICS. Methicillin is not acid-resistant and has, therefore, to be administered by intramuscular (or intravenous) injection. Like benzyl penicillin it is rapidly excreted and injections must, therefore, be frequent. The usual regime is 1 g. every four hours for the first 24 hours and every six hours thereafter but much larger doses can and may have to be given, and their effect can be reinforced with probenecid. Only about 40 per cent of the drug in the blood is protein-bound, an important fact in assessing its relative merits.

TOXICITY. Methicillin has in general the same low toxicity as benzyl penicillin, but has apparently caused bone marrow depression, mainly affecting leucocytes, in a few patients (McElfresh and Huang, 1962; Levitt *et al.*, 1964). Nephritis has also been described (Brauninger and Remington, 1968) and its occurrence has been advanced in the United States as a reason for preferring isoxazolyl penicillins to methicillin. Condemnation because of this very rare complication seems unjustifiable when it is remembered that benzyl penicillin can have the same effect: among patients with penicillin nephritis described by Baldwin *et al.* (1968), 3 had been treated with methicillin, 3 with benzyl penicillin, and one with both (see p. 62). Patients sensitized to benzyl penicillin will usually, although not always, react to methicillin.

Isoxazolyl Penicillins

These compounds combine resistance to penicillinase with resistance to acid. The series of 3 : 5-disubstituted 4-isoxazolyl penicillins was originally described by Doyle *et al.* (1961), and among them cloxacillin was first brought into use in this country and oxacillin in the United States. Their sodium salts are readily soluble in water and neutral solutions are stable at room temperature for 24 hours. They also show a similar degree of resistance to acid to that of phenoxymethyl penicillin.

CLOXACILLIN is 3-chlorophenyl-5-methyl-4 isoxazolyl penicillin. The usual inhibitory concentration for all staphylococci is about $0.12-0.25$ μg. per ml. : i.e. cloxacillin has fully eight times the *in vitro* activity of methicillin, although still considerably less than that of benzyl penicillin against sensitive strains. It is slightly less resistant than methicillin to staphylococcal penicillinase, with the result that a 2-4 fold higher concentration may be required to inhibit a large inoculum. Activity is diminished even more by protein: in 95 per cent serum this reduction is 8-fold (Barber and Waterworth, 1964). The susceptibility of all other species is less than that to benzyl penicillin (Table 10), but that of *Str. pyogenes* is noteworthy, since cloxacillin—or oxacillin (Simon and Sakai, 1963)—will eliminate a streptococcal infection complicated by the presence of penicillinase-forming staphylococci when benzyl penicillin has failed because of local inactivation.

Cloxacillin and methicillin exhibit cross-resistance : the position with regard to staphylococci is thus the same for both antibiotics.

PHARMACOKINETICS. Cloxacillin should be administered before meals, since food interferes with absorption. Even so this is incomplete : higher blood levels are produced by intramuscular injection, when 30 per cent of the dose is excreted in the urine, compared with 20 per cent after an oral dose (Kislak, Eickhoff and Finland, 1965). About 10 per cent of an oral dose is excreted in the bile ((Nayler *et al.*, 1962). It is clear from excretion studies that much of the drug is unaccounted for, evidently owing to inactivation in the body.

The usual dose recommended is 500 mg. orally or 250 mg. intramuscularly at 6-hour intervals: this can be increased if necessary and reinforced with probenecid. Absorption is better than that of oxacillin: differences of up to 2-fold in favour of cloxacillin have been reported in the blood levels attained (Report, 1962; Turck, Ronald and Petersdorf, 1965). The degree of protein binding is very high, as would be expected from the effect of serum on activity *in vitro*. Toxicity is low, and no special effects have been reported.

OXACILLIN. This compound, 3-methyl-5-phenyl-4-isoxazolyl penicillin, has been extensively used and studied in the United States while similar studies of cloxacillin have been pursued in this country. As would be expected from the fact that only a single chlorine atom distinguishes them, their properties are closely similar and call for no separate description. As already stated, oxacillin is less well absorbed and this difficulty has been overcome in some clinical studies by intramuscular injection for the early stages of severe infections. Its activity against penicillinase-forming staphylococci is also slightly less, and these differences have led some American authors (Sidell *et al.*, 1964) to compare it unfavourably with cloxacillin. It also seems that oxacillin may be more rapidly destroyed in the body (Gravenkemper *et al.*, 1965): in patients with ' end-stage kidney disease ' having regular renal dialysis, the oxacillin level in the blood fell to *nil* in eight hours after a 1 g. dose (Bulger *et al.*, 1964).

DICLOXACILLIN. This more recently introduced compound, which is 3(2,6-dichlorphenyl)-5-methyl-4-isoxazolyl penicillin, furnished as the sodium monohydrate, has interesting properties, well described in comparison with those of cloxacillin and oxacillin by Gravenkemper *et al.* (1965). Its inhibitory concentration for both sensitive and resistant staphylococci is somewhat lower than that of the other two compounds, and it is also highly active against streptococci and pneumococci. The concentrations attained in the blood exceed those of cloxacillin by 2-fold, just as those of cloxacillin exceed those of oxacillin to the same degree, and these concentrations are better sustained.

This difference is due not only to better absorption, but to slower excretion: Rosenblatt *et al.* (1968) found the renal clearances of oxacillin, cloxacillin and dicloxacillin to be 226·8, 162·2 and 113·7 ml./min. respectively. These authors and Naumann and Kempf (1965) have also shown that >70 per cent of a dose of dicloxacillin is excreted in the urine, the figures for both other compounds being lower (oxacillin 55·5 and cloxacillin 62, according to Rosenblatt *et al.*, 1968). The main defect of dicloxacillin is its very high degree of protein binding: according to these authors the percentages bound are oxacillin 94-96, cloxacillin 93-95 and dicloxacillin 95-97.

FLUCLOXACILLIN. This new compound, now in general clinical use, is 3-(2-chloro-6-fluorophenyl)-5-methyl-4-isoxazolyl penicillin. Its anti-bacterial activity is almost identical with that of cloxacillin, but it is much better absorbed after oral administration, the blood levels attained being about double those produced by the same dose of cloxacillin at all times up to 4 hours. Protein binding has been determined as 94·7 per cent, in a test showing oxacillin 93·1 and dicloxacillin as 96·9 per cent. The usual dose proposed, which may be exceeded if necessary, is 250 mg. either orally or intramuscularly at intervals of 4-6 hours (Sutherland *et al.*, 1970). Clinical trials in various infections, such as those reported by Harding and Knudsen (1970) and Leigh and Spencer (1971) afford evidence of therapeutic efficacy, but naturally not of any distinct superiority, to demonstrate which a comparative trial on an enormous scale would be needed.

Other Penicillinase-Resistant Penicillins

Of several other such compounds only one appears to have been retained in clinical use.

NAFCILLIN is 6-(2-ethoxy-1-naphthamido) penicillanic acid. Its anti-bacterial activity was studied by Lane (1964) and by Klein and Finland (1963) who also studied absorption, which was irregular and incomplete, although no specific reason for this is adduced. Hence in an extensive clinical trial in severe staphylococcal infections Eickhoff, Kislak and Finland (1965a) used mainly the parenteral route in a dose of usually 6 but up to 18 g. daily, sometimes with probenecid. Results compared favourably with those obtained with methicillin, oxacillin, etc. According to Kind *et al.* (1970) the relatively low blood levels attained by nafcillin are due, not to defective absorption, but to inactivation in the liver.

Others are DIPHENICILLIN (ANCILLIN), which is 2-biphenylyl penicillin, similar to oxacillin, but less acid-stable and thus poorly absorbed, and even when given parenterally yielding inferior clinical results (Klein *et al.*, 1963), and QUINACILLIN, which is 3-carboxy-2-quinoxalinyl penicillin, described by Richards, Housley and Spooner (1963), which has a low activity against organisms other than staphylococci and is very poorly absorbed.

General Therapeutic Efficacy

All these penicillinase-resistant penicillins have been used mainly for treating severe staphylococcal infections. These are notoriously varied in nature, and many occur in patients with a still greater variety of predisposing conditions, some of these being of the gravest nature in themselves. Hence all extensive clinical studies embrace a mixture of patients with pneumonia, septicaemia, wound infections, etc., with sometimes a few of endocarditis or meningitis, many occurring as a complication of malignant disease, or serious cardiac, hepatic or renal lesions, often in elderly subjects. Such miscellaneous clinical material does not lend itself to an assessment of the relative value of antibiotics which are themselves closely related, and no attempt at such an analysis will be made here.

The main choice lies between methicillin, which has much the lowest intrinsic anti-staphylococcal activity, but of which 60 per cent in the blood is free, and one of the isoxazolyl or other acid-resistant compounds, with higher anti-bacterial activity, but of which perhaps only 5 per cent is free. These contrasting properties are largely self-cancelling, and the probability is that adequate doses of almost any of these penicillins will achieve very similar effects. The possibilities of reducing protein binding by displacement with other drugs which have been explored by Kunin (1966) do not seem hopeful. Initial treatment of a severe staphylococcal infection should always be with one of these penicillins unless or until the strain has been shown to be sensitive to benzylpenicillin.

BROAD SPECTRUM PENICILLINS

Adicillin

This is the name now given to cephalosporin N, one of three distinct antibiotics formed by the Sardinian *Cephalosporium* referred to in the succeeding section. It is identical with synnematin B, an antibiotic isolated by Gottshal *et al.* in 1951 from a mould of the *Tilachlidium* genus. It is a penicillin with a side-chain derived from D-α-aminoadipic acid, which, although much less active than benzyl penicillin against Gram-positive cocci, is rather more so against various Gram-negative species, including *Salm. typhi.* Although it gave promising results in the treatment of typhoid fever (Benavides *et al.*, 1955) it has never been manufactured in quantity: this is understood to be due to difficulties in purification.

Ampicillin

This semi-synthetic compound, α-aminobenzyl penicillin, was first described by Rolinson and Stevens (1961). It is administered orally as the free acid, which unlike most other penicillins is soluble only to the extent of about 10 per cent in water.

ANTI-BACTERIAL ACTIVITY. Ampicillin is slightly less active than benzyl penicillin against most Gram-positive bacteria, but slightly more so against *Str. faecalis.* It is destroyed by staphylococcal penicillinase, and is therefore not indicated for resistant staphylococcal infections. *Listeria monocytogenes* is highly sensitive (Seeliger, Laymann and Finger, 1967) and several recent papers (Weingartner and Ortel, 1967; MacNair, White and Graham, 1968; Seeliger and Matheis, 1969) commend ampicillin for the treatment of listeriosis.

The outstanding property of ampicillin is an activity four to eight times greater than that of benzyl penicillin against various Gram-negative bacilli (Table 10), including *H influenzae, Salmonella* and *Shigella* spp., non-penicillinase-forming *Proteus mirabilis*, and most strains of *E. coli* (Sutherland and Rolinson, 1964b; Anderson *et al.*, 1964). *Kl. pneumoniae* may be sensitive, but *Kl. aerogenes,* penicillinase-forming *Proteus,* and *Pseudomonas* spp. are resistant, as are other coliform bacilli forming a penicillinase. *Kl. aerogenes* possesses a high degree of intrinsic resistance, apart from its capacity to destroy ampicillin enzymically (Hamilton-Miller, 1965). The effect of ampicillin, like that of benzyl penicillin, is bactericidal.

PHARMACOKINETICS. Ampicillin is resistant to acid, and is well absorbed when administered orally, but not completely: 30 per cent of an oral dose is recoverable from the urine, but 60-70 per cent of an intramuscular (Naumann, 1965), for which reason the parenteral route may be preferred for maximal effect. This can also be enhanced with probenecid. When different oral doses are compared, plotting the dose against the blood concentration gives a straight line (Knudsen, Rolinson and Stevens, 1961): i.e. the same proportion of a large dose is absorbed as of a small, whereas the larger the dose of a tetracycline, the less the proportion absorbed. The peak concentration is reached in about 2 hours, and the subsequent fall is gradual, a detectable amount persisting for 6 hours after a moderate dose (250 mg.).

Although excretion is mainly renal, fairly high concentrations are attained in the bile. The report by Brown and Acred (1961) of a level in the bile of dogs 300 times that in the blood, does not seem to represent conditions in the human biliary tract, since Ayliffe and Davies (1965) found a mean difference of only 9-fold (extremes 3- 48-fold) in a series of patients. There were wide variations in the content among patients with normal biliary tracts: in those with obstructive lesions it was very low or nil. These observations have been confirmed and extended by Mortimer, Mackie and Haynes (1969). Blecher *et al.* (1966) have shown that ampicillin accumulates and persists in the amniotic fluid, evidently in consequence of renal excretion by the foetus: in most specimens the level exceeded 2·5 μg. per ml. after 3 maternal doses of 500 mg.

Ampicillin can also be administered intramuscularly or intravenously, the sodium salt, which behaves identically (Eickhoff, Kislak and Finland, 1965b) being more suitable by the latter route. High concentrations are attained in the cerebrospinal fluid in patients with purulent meningitis when 150-200 mg. per kg. are given intravenously daily (Naumann, 1965) although ampicillin, like benzyl penicillin, traverses the normal blood-brain barrier in very small amounts. Impairment of renal function reduces the rate of excretion, and the dose can be reduced accordingly: renal dialysis will reduce the blood level (Höffler, Stegemann and Scheler, 1966).

TOXIC EFFECTS. Ampicillin appears to be as free from toxicity as benzyl penicillin. Apart from occasional gastric intolerance, the only significant side effects seen have been rashes, which are decidedly commoner than with other penicillins. A large-scale survey by Shapiro *et al.* (1969) showed that 9·5 per cent of patients treated with ampicillin developed rashes and only 4·5 per cent of those given other penicillins. The route of administration was not a factor, but the effect of dosage was not analysed: it may be significant that a series of patients of whom 20 per cent had rashes were given 6 g. daily (Sleet, Sangster and Murdoch, 1964). A rash almost invariably results when ampicillin is given to a patient with glandular fever.

An ampicillin rash is almost always maculo-papular and not urticarial, like that produced by benzylpenicillin. This fact, its much greater frequency, and the usual delay in its inset, strongly suggest that a different mechanism is responsible. Geddes (1972), who confirms that purified ampicillin less often causes it, believes it to be due to impurities and not to true sensitization to the penicillin nucleus. A prospective study on a large scale (Report, 1973) in which a rash occurred in 7·3 per cent of 933 patients, and was more frequent in those suffering from viral infections and in females, confirms the distinct nature of this exanthem.This is important, since an ampicillin rash is then not a contraindication to later penicillin treatment.

CLINICAL APPLICATIONS. Early reports dealt largely with the treatment of urinary tract infections. Ampicillin is unquestionably the best penicillin for this purpose when the organism is sensitive: it is not only more active than benzyl penicillin (although the same species are moderately sensitive to this) but has the great practical advantage of oral administrability. The phenoxy penicillins, although also administrable by mouth, are insufficiently active against Gram-negative species.

The high hopes originally entertained of efficacy in enteric fever have not altogether been fulfilled. This and other important uses are discussed in the later chapters on the treatment of alimentary tract and respiratory tract infections and meningitis.

Hetacillin

This derivative of 6-aminopenicillanic acid ('Versapen', Bristol) was said to be a new chemical entity, 'the first penicinate': It is described as 6-(2,2-dimethyl-5-oxo-4-phenyl-1-imidazolidinyl)-3,3-dimethyl-7-oxo-4-thia-1-azabicyclo (3.2.0) heptane-2-carboxylic acid (Hardcastle *et al.*, 1966). Its range and degree of antibacterial activity are said in earlier papers to be very similar to those of ampicillin. According to Bunn, Milicich and Lunn (1965) and Tuano *et al.* (1966) it is more slowly excreted than ampicillin, each dose therefore having a more prolonged effect. On the other hand, the levels attained by ampicillin earlier in the inter-dose period are considerably higher than those of hetacillin. It is acknowledged that hetacillin undergoes hydrolysis with the formation of ampicillin, both *in vitro* and in the body, but the first descriptions of this change do not specify its rate or extent. According to Sutherland and Robinson (1967) this hydrolysis is rapid and complete, both *in vitro* and in the blood : these authors even suggest that hetacillin may itself have no anti-bacterial activity and the studies by two methods of Smith and Hamilton-Miller (1970) go far to confirm this. The *in vitro* activities of hetacillin and ampicillin against 15 species of bacteria were identical, as would be expected. Comparative studies of absorption showed lower initial blood levels from hetacillin, and only such prolongation of effect in some experiments as would be accounted for by the time required for conversion to ampicillin. It seems from these findings that hetacillin is only another form in which to administer ampicillin and possesses no advantages over it. Most subsequent clinical trials of hetacillin have been non-comparative, but in the few in which hetacillin and ampicillin have been compared their effects were indistinguishable.

Carbenicillin

This compound, numbered 2064 in the Beecham Research Laboratories series, is disodium α-carboxybenzyl penicillin (Knudsen, Rolinson and Sutherland, 1967). It is distinguished from all other penicillins by its degree of activity against *Ps. aeruginosa*. most strains of which are inhibited *in vitro* by 25 or 50 μg./ml. (Table 11). It is olso active against all species of *Proteus* and some other enterobacteria, but inferior to benzyl penicillin against Gram-positive species. Its action is bactericidal.

It must be administered by injection and gives a peak level at 1 hour with some persistence to 6 hours (about 25 and 4 μg./ml. respectively after a dose of 1 g.). Probenecid enhances these levels and excretion is renal. Usual dosage is 1 g. at 4-hour intervals, but larger doses, if necessary by intravenous drip, are safe. The results of treating 74 patients are reported by Brumfitt, Percival and Leigh (1967), including 54 with urinary tract infections and 14 with Gram-negative bacteriaemia. Among the latter only 2 out of 7 with *Ps. aeruginosa* infection responded, but all of those with *E. coli* or *Proteus* infections: success was also less frequent in *Ps. aeruginosa* urinary infections. Jones and Lowbury (1967) obtained encouraging results in *Ps. aeruginosa* infection of experimental burns, with some verification in the clinical field.

TABLE 11

Minimum Inhibitory Concentrations of Carbenicillin (μg./ml.)

Escherichia coli	5
Proteus mirabilis*	2·5
„ morganii	5
„ rettgeri	2·5
„ vulgaris	5
Pseudomonas aeruginosa	50
Klebsiella aerogenes	250
Staphylococcus aureus*	0·5
Streptococcus pyogenes	0·25
„ pneumoniae	0·5
„ faecalis	25

* non-penicillinase-forming
(From Knudsen, Rolinson & Sutherland, 1967.)

Massive dosage was highly successful in the hands of Van Rooyen *et al.* (1967) in treating this infection in a series of very extensive burns, but the impression is gaining ground that whenever a systemic effect is necessary it may be unwise to rely on carbenicillin alone. Several authors, among whose observations those of Sonne and Jawetz (1969) are perhaps the most convincing, have demonstrated synergy between carbenicillin and gentamicin, and it is now a common practice to administer both. In our own experience this combination was effective even in a case of *Pseudomonas* endocarditis, although in a patient whose greatly impaired renal function enabled very high carbenicillin blood levels to be maintained. Cooper, Rice and Penfold (1969) used this combination successfully in four very severe *Ps. aeruginosa* infections in children, two having septicaemia and two, including one of these, leukaemia.

An added reason for using this combination is that during treatment with carbenicillin alone *Ps. aeruginosa* may become resistant. Such strains were recovered from 17 patients by Darrell and Waterworth (1969), 5 of whom had been treated with carbenicillin and 10 with other penicillins. Lowbury *et al.* (1969) report the appearance and rapid predominance of highly resistant strains in the Burns Unit at Birmingham. Subsequent study in the Unit by Roe, Jones and Lowbury (1971) showed that such resistance was transferable to and from other species, both *in vitro* and in experimental burns in mice. These organisms produced a carbenicillinase. Further interesting observations made by Ayliffe, Lowbury and Roe (1972) suggest that

TABLE 12

Antibiotic Sensitivities of Proteus Species

	Ampicillin	Carbenicillin	Cephaloridine	Kanamycin
P. mirabilis	+	+	+	+
„ (penicillinase-forming)	0	0	+	+
P. morganii	0	+	0	+
P. rettgeri	0	+	0	+
P. vulgaris	0	+	0	+

+ = sensitive
0 = resistant

resistance transferred to *Ps. aeruginosa* in a burn from a *Klebsiella* or *Proteus* may be latent, only manifesting itself when carbenicillin is administered.

The possible usefulness of carbenicillin in *Proteus* infections should not be forgotten. *P. mirabilis*, if penicillinase-forming, is resistant, as it is to ampicillin, but the other three species which are resistant to ampicillin and in general also to the cephalosporin antibiotics, are sensitive, and for infections of the urinary tract or elsewhere caused by these less common species carbenicillin may be the antibiotic of choice. The sensitivities of these organisms to four antibiotics are stated in simplified form in Table 12.

NEW BROAD SPECTRUM PENICILLINS

Recently several new penicillin derivatives have been produced, improving in some way on the properties of either ampicillin or carbenicillin. Most of these are not yet in general use, and information about them is incomplete; they will therefore be only briefly described. They may be classified according to the new properties which commend them.

Better Absorbed Derivatives of Ampicillin

Oral ampicillin is incompletely absorbed, about twice the dose having to be given to achieve the same effect as that from intra-muscular injection. Two new derivatives overcome this defect. One of these is pivampicillin (pivaloyloxymethyl D-α-aminobenzyl penicillinate), evolved by Leo Pharmaceutical Products from a study of ampicillin esters. This substance is believed to be completely absorbed, and is then rapidly hydrolysed in the blood and tissues with liberation of ampicillin. This process is 99 per cent complete in blood within 15 minutes. The blood levels attained in animals and man are 2-3 times higher than those produced by the same oral dose of ampicillin, and 73 per cent of the dose is excreted in the urine in 6 hours (von Daehne et al., 1970). These findings with regard to blood and urine levels are confirmed by Jordan, de Maine and Kirby (1971) and by Foltz et al. (1971), who add that administration with food actually improves total absorption although slightly slowing it, whereas it impairs that of ampicillin.

The second and more recent of these derivatives, prepared by Beecham Research Laboratories, is BRL 2333 (amoxycillin: 6[D(-)α-amino-p-hydroxyphenylacetamido] penicillanic acid). This is not an ester, but a compound absorbed and acting as such. Its anti-bacterial spectrum is almost identical with that of ampicillin, with which it also shares the properties of acid

resistance, low protein binding and susceptibility to penicillinase (Sutherland and Rolinson, 1971). Absorption and excretion were studied by Croydon and Sutherland (1971) and Neu
and Winshell (1971a) with very similar results to those reported
for pivampicillin, i.e. peak levels in the blood twice those given
by ampicillin, and corresponding differences in the amount
excreted in the urine. Food does not interfere with absorption.
These findings are assembled in a more up-to-date paper by
Sutherland, Croydon and Rolinson (1972). In therapeutic tests
in mice Acred et al. (1971a) found it superior to ampicillin in
almost all of 14 infections, in some considerably so, and to
some extent after subcutaneous as well as oral administration,
a finding which appears to indicate an intrinsically greater
activity in addition to its superiority in pharmacological
behaviour. In view of these findings it would seem advisable to
define any indications for which ampicillin is still to be preferred.

An Orally Absorbed Derivative of Carbenicillin

An ester of carbenicillin, 6-[2-phenyl-2-(5-indanyloxycar-
bonyl)acetamido] penicillanic acid, has been the subject of two
papers (Wallace et al., 1971; Bran, Karl and Kaye, 1971). After
absorption, it is said to be rapidly hydrolysed to carbenicillin.
The peak blood level after a dose of 1 g. is only about 10
μg./ml., but about one third of the dose is excreted in the urine
in 6 hours, thus giving high concentrations. These authors
treated 26 and 28 patients with 2 g. (for Ps. aeruginosa 4 g.) and
1 g. daily respectively for urinary tract infections, the majority
due to E. coli, with success in the majority. A bitter after-
taste was much complained of, and vomiting compelled dis-
continuance in 3 patients in each series. Such unpleasant
treatment seems unlikely to find favour except for otherwise
resistant infections due to Ps. aeruginosa or indole-forming
Proteus.

Derivatives with Improved Anti pseudomonad Activity

BL-P1654 is 6-[R-α-(guanylureido) phenylacetamido]-peni-
cillanic acid. According to van Scoy, Warren and Washington
(1971) it has a low solubility which may prove a drawback. Its
main advantage is a higher activity than that of carbenicillin

against *Ps. aeruginosa,* but the difference varied with the medium used, and results were much affected by inoculum size. Its activity is also higher against *Enterobacter, Serratia* and *H. influenzae.* Price *et al.* (1971) find its superiority against *Ps. aeruginosa* greater; 75 per cent of 82 strains were inhibited by 8 μg./ml. or less, giving it an activity exceeding that of carbenicillin by 8–fold. Moreover its CD_{50} for this infection in mice is about one tenth of that of carbenicillin, and it attains higher concentrations in the blood. On the other hand, resistance to it in this organism is acquired more quickly than to carbenicillin.

BRL 2288 is 6[D(-)-α-carboxyl-3-thienylacetamido] penicillanic acid. It closely resembles carbenicillin, having a poor activity against Gram-positive species, but activity against indole-forming *Proteus;* that against *Ps. aeruginosa* exceeds that of carbenicillin by 2– to 4– fold (Sutherland, Burnett and Rolinson, 1971; Neu and Winshell 1971). Its CD_{50} for this infection in mice is about half that of carbenicillin (Acred *et al.,* 1971b), and it acts synergically with both gentamicin and polymyxin. A pharmacological study by Sutherland and Wise (1971) shows behaviour apparently identical with that of carbenicillin, including prolongation of effect by probenecid. The possible dosage of carbenicillin is so elastic that another product with only moderately higher activity may not prove a serious rival to it.

Epicillin (Squibb) is 6-[D-2-amino-2-(1,4-cyclohexadienyl) acetamido]-penicillanic acid, and according to Basch, Erickson and Gadebusch (1971) and Gadebusch *et al.* (1971) closely resembles ampicillin in many properties, but is somewhat more active against *Ps. aeruginosa.* Therapeutic studies in mice are reported, and degrees of sensitivity to epicillin are plotted in a complex scatter diagram in relation to clinical results, but no details of these are given. Urinary tract infections were treated with epicillin by Woodruff *et al.* (1971), 11 out of 14 *E. coli* infections responding and 4 out of 7 due to *P. mirabilis,* but only 1 out of 4 due to *Ps. aeruginosa,* a discouraging result in view of the activity claimed for it against this species.

A Derivative with Enhanced Activity Against Enterobacteria

Lund and Tybring (1972) of Leo Pharmaceutical Products report a study of 6-β-amidinopenicillanic acids, a new group of substances among which a series of analogues was examined for activity against *E. coli.* The maximum was attained by 6-β [(hexahydro-1 H-azepin-1-yl) methyleneamino] - penicillanic acid, designated FL1060. The activity of this substance, compared with that of benzylpenicillin and ampicillin, is low against all Gram-positive species, but remarkably high against *E. coli,* the IC_{50} for 4 strains varying from 0·016 to 0·1 μg./ml. It is also much greater than that of ampicillin against some strains of *Klebsiella* spp. and of *P. mirabilis* and various other Gram-negative organisms including *Serratia marcescens.* Like other β-lactam antibiotics, FL1060 has bactericidal activity, mitigated by increased osmolality, and induces cell wall changes which lead to the production of spherical osmotically fragile forms. These differ from spheroplasts, however, in that a proportion of them not only survive but actively grow in the presence of the agent without osmotic protection. Such phenotypically resistant variants revert to bacillary form on subculture but retain their resistance to FL1060 for several generations. Greenwood and O'Grady (1973) suggest that FL1060 is a ' half penicillin ' which inhibits surface cell-wall mucopeptide synthesis, but lacks the cell division-inhibiting property which causes Gram-negative rods to grow into long filaments in the presence of low concentrations of other β-lactam antibiotics.

CEPHALOSPORINS

This group of antibiotics, the early studies of which at Oxford are described by Florey (1955) and then later by Abraham (1962) is formed by a species of *Cephalosporium* cultivated from the sea near a sewage outfall off Sardinia by Brotzu, who used the crude products of its growth with some success for treating typhoid fever and brucellosis. When the culture was examined at Oxford it was found to produce three quite distinct antibiotics, cephalosporin N, a penicillin (adicillin : p. 78), cephalosporin P, an antibiotic of steroid structure similar to fucidin (p. 199) and cephalosporin C.

Cephalosporin C

The existence of this substance among the products of the mould was not even detected for several years, and the yield

4

was at first so small that great difficulty was experienced in obtaining enough for essential laboratory tests. It has the same side chain as cephalosporin N, attached to a nucleus now known as 7-aminocephalosporanic acid (p. 68). The degree of anti-bacterial activity of cephalosporin C is only moderate, but the property which attracted most attention, at that time unique among antibiotics of this general structure, was a high degree of resistance to staphylococcal penicillinase: moreover it competitively inhibited the action of penicillinase on benzyl penicillin (Abraham and Newton, 1956). It was shown to be therapeutically active in mice and to have a very low toxicity.

Thanks to the prophetic foresight of its discoverers, determined and prolonged attempts were made to obtain an adequate yield, and when this had been achieved, chemical manipulations, similar to those being applied at the same time to the penicillin nucleus, were undertaken to improve its performance. The substitution of other side chains greatly enhanced anti-bacterial activity and three valuable derivatives so produced are now in therapeutic use. These are cephalothin, the first to come into use, cephaloridine and cephalexin.

Cephalothin

This derivative is 7-(thiophene-2-acetamido)-cephalosporanic acid, supplied as the sodium salt. The range of its anti-bacterial activity, and that of cephaloridine, may be seen from Table 13, condensed from the findings of Barber and Waterworth (1964) in whose paper cephaloridine is referred to as Ceph 87/4. All staphylococci, whether penicillinase-forming or not, and streptococci (except *S. faecalis*) are highly sensitive. *Neisseria* spp. are sensitive and *H. influenzae* less so. Among enterobacteria *E. coli*, *Salmonella* and *Shigella* spp. are inhibited by concentrations not exceeding 8 μg per ml., as is *Proteus mirabilis*, whether penicillinase-forming or not. This is a point of distinction from ampicillin, which is destroyed by the penicillinase of this species. The three other species of *Proteus* (not in the Table) are variable but in general resistant. *Kl. edwardsii* (*pneumoniae*) is sensitive, as to a rather lesser degree is *Kl. aerogenes*, but *Enterobacter aerogenes* is much more resistant. This difference is evidently that referred to by Benner *et al.* (1965b) employing different nomenclature. They distinguish the species by motility, and contrast *Aerobacter,* which is motile, and highly resistant to cephalothin and cephaloridine, but sensitive to various other drugs including tetracycline, chloramphenicol, streptomycin and sulphonamides, with the non-motile *Klebsiella* which is frequently resistant to these other drugs, but consistently sensitive to the cephalosporins. *Pseudomonas* spp. are all highly resistant.

TABLE 13

Minimum Inhibitory Concentrations (μg. per ml.)

	Cephalothin	Cephaloridine
Staph. pyogenes pen. sens.	0·25	0·12
„ pen. res.	0·25-0·5	0·12-0·25
Strep. pyogenes	0·06	0·007
„ *pneumoniae*	0·06-0·12	0·015-0·03
faecalis	32	8-16
N. gonorrhoeae	0·25-0·5	4
N. meningitidis	0·12-0·5	0·5-1
H. influenzae	2-8	4-16
E. coli	2-8	2-4
Salm. typhi	0·5-2	2
Sh. flexneri	1-2	1-2
Pr. mirabilis	4-8	8
Kl. edwardsii	1-4	1-4
Kl. aerogenes	2-32	2-8
Ent. aerogenes	128-256	128-256

(Condensed from Barber and Waterworth, 1964)

Serum somewhat reduces the activity of cephalothin, but the inoculum effect with penicillinase-producing staphylococci is small. On the other hand methicillin-resistant staphylococci are also more resistant to cephalothin, and here the inoculum effect is large.

The cephalosporin antibiotics, like penicillins, are bactericidal, and like them, they inhibit the synthesis of staphylococcal cell walls (Abraham, 1959).

PHARMACOKINETICS. Absorption after oral administration is quite inadequate, and administration is by intramuscular injection; adequate blood levels can be maintained by giving 1 g. at intervals of 4 to 6 hours. Excretion is mainly renal, and tubular. According to Kunin and Atuk (1966) cephalothin loses activity in the body, its half-life in ' severely oliguric ' patients being comparatively short whereas that of cephaloridine is much prolonged. Perkins, Smith and Saslaw (1969) found much less difference in their behaviour: both are removed by peritoneal dialysis. Penetration into the cerebrospinal fluid is poor (Vianna and Kaye, 1967; Lerner, 1969). Unlike cephalothin, cephaloridine is excreted via the glomeruli.

CLINICAL APPLICATIONS. Patients sensitized to penicillin do not usually react to cephalosporins; hence they may be indicated on this account for a variety of infections susceptible to both, and several clinical studies report successful use for pneumococcal and Group A streptococcal infections (Turck *et al.*, 1965; Perkins and Saslaw, 1966). The second important property of cephalothin is its activity against penicillin-resistant staphylococci, and many patients with severe staphylococcal infections including pneumonia, septicaemia and endocarditis have been treated with a high proportion of successes (Walters, Romansky and Johnson, 1963; Merrill *et al.*, 1966). Doses of up to 12 g. daily have been used. Superinfections with *Pseudomonas* or resistant *Klebsiella* are liable to occur and may be fatal. The third principal use is for Gram-negative infections, mainly of the urinary tract, caused by sensitive enterobacteria : it is noteworthy in this connection that cephalothin has a rather broader spectrum than ampicillin.

SIDE EFFECTS. Injections may be painful, and rashes are sometimes produced : thus cephalothin, although usually without effect on a penicillin-sensitive patient, may itself sensitize. It is claimed that cephalothin does not cause the renal damage which may be produced by cephaloridine, and although there are at least two cases in the literature in which it seems that this may have occurred, it can be accepted that the relative degree of risk is much smaller.

Cephaloridine

This derivative, resulting from the addition of not one but two side chains to the nucleus, is described chemically as 7-[(2-thienyl) acetamido]-3-(1-pyridylmethyl)-3-cephem-4-carboxylic acid betaine. It was made available at the end of 1964, its properties being described by Muggleton, O'Callaghan and Stevens (1969). These authors give particulars of its *in vitro* activity and the results of therapeutic tests in mice in which its CD_{50} was shown to be lower than that of four other appropriate antibiotics for infections by *Staph. aureus, E. coli* and *Pr. mirabilis.* After an intramuscular dose of 500 mg. in man the blood content was >12 μg. per ml. at 1 hour and still nearly 2 μg. per ml. at 6 and 8 hours. About 80 per cent of the dose was excreted in the urine.

This paper was accompanied by an account of clinical results (Murdoch *et al.*, 1964) in 6 cases of septicaemia, 4 of pneumococcal meningitis, for which intrathecal injections were also given, and 24 of pyelonephritis. Among later clinical reports are those of Apicella, Perkins and Saslaw (1966a) on 92 patients with a variety of infections and by the same authors (1966b) on the treatment of endocarditis.

The properties of cephaloridine and the indications for its use are very similar to those of cephalothin, and it seems necessary only to point out the differences between them. Cephaloridine has three advantages: rather greater activity against some bacteria, better stability in the body, and indifference to protein effect. Another is that injections are less painful than those of cephalothin. It also attains better concentrations than cephalothin in the cerebrospinal fluid in the presence of meningitis: Oppenheimer, Beaty and Petersdorf (1969) in an experimental study found peak c.s.f. levels as percentages of those in the blood to be for cephaloridine 10·9, cephalothin 5·6 and methicillin 2·9.

On the other hand it has one serious disadvantage which was not at first appreciated. The large inoculum effect in tests with penicillinase-forming staphylococci first noted by Barber and Waterworth (1964) and found to be still larger by Kislak, Steinhauer and Finland (1966), suggests that cephaloridine is more susceptible than had been supposed to the action of penicillinase. Ridley and Phillips (1965) have shown that when a heavy inoculum is used, the minimum inhibitory concentration of cephaloridine for different strains of staphylococci varies widely, those possessing multiple antibiotic resistance and particularly those resistant to methicillin being inhibited only by much higher concentrations than those at first reported. Benner *et al.* (1965a) have also shown that some strains destroy cephaloridine rapidly, but not cephalothin, and suggest that the latter is preferable for treating infections due to such organisms. Burgess and Evans (1966) report the failure of cephaloridine to control a staphylococcal endocarditis, blood cultures remaining positive despite the demonstrated presence of high concentrations of the antibiotic in the same specimens of blood.

It must be concluded that cephaloridine cannot always be relied on for treating one of the principal infections for which it was first recommended. It is in fact doubtful whether any single antibiotic can regularly be depended on to control staphylococcal endocarditis: a combination with another antibiotic which has been shown to be totally bactericidal *in vitro* may be necessary (Chap. 18).

SIDE EFFECTS. Rashes due to sensitization may occur as with cephalothin. A much more serious possible effect is that on the kidney. That large doses of cephaloridine cause necrosis of the proximal convoluted tubules has been amply demonstrated in animals. There is a wide variation in species susceptibility, a single dose of only 90 mg./kg. producing this change in the rabbit, the doses required in the monkey, guinea-pig and mouse being 300, 400 and 3100 mg./kg. (Atkinson *et al.*, 1966). In the mouse and hen the effect can be prevented by giving probenecid (Child and Dodds, 1967). It is well recognized that only moderate doses may cause the appearance of large numbers of hyaline casts in the urine. Larger doses—8 g. daily or more—have unquestionably sometimes caused increasing proteinuria with a raised blood urea, going on in some cases to oliguria and renal failure, the lesion responsible being a tubular necrosis. We ourselves know of several patients in whom in retrospect it seems that this must have occurred, although the reason for it was unsuspected at the time. In severely ill patients renal failure is not uncommon and may be produced in other ways, but careful observers with extensive experience of the use of this drug have satisfied themselves that it has sometimes been responsible for renal damage. Kaplan, Reisberg and Weinstein (1968) observed it in 4 out of 7 patients given 12 g. daily, and Steigbigel *et al.* (1968) attributed renal failure in 2 out of 7 patients in whom it occurred out of a total of 122 treated directly to cephaloridine. In one case in each of these series it was fatal. It is now recognized that diuretics, which may also be indicated in such patients, enhance the renal toxicity of cephaloridine; this was demonstrated experimentally for both frusemide and ethacrynic acid by Dodds and Foord (1970). This is therefore a drug combination to be avoided.

Cephapirin

This substance, 7-[D-(pyridylthio)-acetamido]-cephalosporanic acid, prepared by Bristol Laboratories, is the subject of two papers, that by Axelrod, Meyers and Hirschman (1971) describing *in vitro* findings, and Bodner and Koenig (1972) also reporting results of a small clinical trial, in which administration was either intramuscular or by continuous intravenous infusion. Both papers compare *in vitro* activity with that of cephalothin, showing only small differences. Apparently the only distinct advantage claimed for cephapirin is that it is less liable than cephalothin to cause phlebitis when given intravenously; intramuscular injection is also less painful.

The synthesis of several further cephalosporin derivatives was announced at a recent meeting in the United States of America, but is otherwise hitherto unpublished.

Cefazolin. This is 3 - (5 - methyl - 1,3,4 - thiadiazol - 2 -ylthiomethyl) -7- [2 - (1H - tetrazol-1- 61)acetamido] - 3- cephem - 4 - carboxylic acid. It was first prepared by the Fujisawa Pharmaceutical Co., Japan, and is being manufactured in the United States by Smith, Kline and French. The main advantage claimed for it is that the blood concentrations attained after intramuscular injection are about twice those produced by the same dose of cephaloridine and better prolonged, and a larger proportion of the dose is excreted unchanged in the urine. It also appears to be free of nephrotoxicity. Its anti-bacterial activity is similar to that of cephaloridine. Therapeutic tests in mice gave expected results, and clinical application in pneumococcal pneumonia and urinary tract infections has been successful.

Cefoxitin. This derivative, synthesized by Merck, is 3-(hydroxymethyl) -7-α-methoxy-7-[2-thienyl) acetamido]-3-cephem-4-carboxylic acid carbamate, monosodium salt. Its only advantage is higher activity than that of other derivatives against *E. coli* and other enterobacteria, which also embraces indolforming *Proteus* and *Serratia*. Against Gram-positive organisms it is comparatively less active. Blood levels attained are intermediate between those of cephalothin and cephaloridine; probenecid prolongs the effect, indicating tubular excretion. Therapeutic results have not yet been reported.

Cephamycins may be mentioned in this connection, although they are not cephalosporins. They have a very similar basic structure, and three have been identified as products of 27 strains of 8 species of *Streptomyces* (Stapley *et al.*, 1972). It is not yet clear whether they are likely to prove therapeutically useful. They possess one advantage in being resistant to enzymes derived from enterobacteria which inactivate cephalothin and cephaloridine. According to Miller *et al.* (1972) cephamycins A and B have no useful activity except against two species of *Proteus*, but the activity of C compares favourably with that of cephalothin and cephaloridine against not only *Proteus* spp. but *E. coli* and several other enterobacteria. *P. morganii* and *Providencia* are also sensitive, although cephalosporin-resistant. C is non-toxic in mice and effective against experimental enterobacterial infections, notably those due to cephalosporin-resistant species or strains.

ORAL CEPHALOSPORINS

Neither cephalothin nor cephaloridine is absorbed from the alimentary tract in sufficient amount to exert a therapeutic effect, and much effort has evidently been devoted to finding a derivative which is. Several are now available.

Cephaloglycin

This derivative, which is 7-(D-α-aminophenyl acetamido)-cephalosporanic acid, was first described by Wick and Boniece (1965) eight years ago. It is absorbed from the alimentary tract only to a limited extent: Kunin and Brandt (1968) could detect none in the blood after a 500 mg. dose, and Applestein *et al.* (1968) observed a peak level of 1·5 μg./ml. after a dose of 1 g. Fairly high concentrations are found in the urine, and some success has been obtained in treating urinary tract infections (Ronald and Turck, 1967). According to Wick, Wright and Kuder (1971) urinary excretion is almost entirely in the form of desacetylcephaloglycin, but this derivative retains most of the anti-bacterial activity of the parent substance.

Perkins, Glontz and Saslaw (1969) used it not only for this purpose but even for treating pneumonia, the pneumococcus being a highly sensitive organism. Despite some success they conclude that cephaloglycin should be reserved for the continuation of successful treatment begun with an injectable cephalosporin. Cephaloglycin is unstable in an alkaline medium, and it is suggested that sensitivity tests by a dilution method in broth should be read after 12 hours. In view of this instability it is difficult to trace the fate of this substance in the body, but it is clear that not more than about 10 per cent of a dose is excreted in the urine. Cephaloglycin is commercially available in the United States but not in Great Britain, and is used for treating urinary tract infections.

Cephalexin

Cephalexin, which is 7-(D-α-amino-α-phenylacetamido)-3-methyl-3-cephem-4-carboxylic acid, has like cephaloglycin a closely similar anti-bacterial spectrum to that of cephalothin, but with a somewhat lower degree of activity against most species (Thornhill *et al.,* 1969). Its action is particularly weak on *H. influenzae,* and the only Gram-negative organisms out of 23 varieties examined against which its activity exceeds that of cephalothin and cephaloridine are ampicillin-resistant strains of *E. coli* (Waterworth, 1971). Unlike cephaloglycin it is stable, and very well absorbed: mean 1-hour blood levels after doses of 250, 500 and 1,000 mg. were 6·8, 17·6 and 25 μg./ml., falling to 0·6, 1·5 and 3·1 μg./ml. at 4 hours. Urinary recovery in 6 hours was from 85 to 96 per cent of the dose given (Perkins, Carlisle and Saslaw, 1968). Similar findings are reported by Braun *et al.* (1968). In experimental streptococcal infection in monkeys oral cephalexin had an efficacy equal to that of cephalothin but inferior to that of cephaloridine, each of these being of course administered by injection (Saslaw and Carlisle, 1969). In a further similar study by these authors (1970) it is suggested that cephalexin is relatively more active *in vivo* than *in vitro* because of its low degree of protein binding, said in monkey serum to be only 11 per cent.

Cephalexin has now been fairly extensively used, mainly for urinary tract and respiratory infections (Symposium, 1970; Symposium, 1971) but it is still difficult to assess its merits, apart from that of convenience of administration, in comparison with those of the injectable cephalosporins. A pointer to one valuable use may be the study of Stillerman, Isenberg and Moody (1972) of the treatment of acute streptococcal sore throat in children; cephalexin was more successful than the same dose of either phenoxymethyl penicillin or ampicillin in eliminating the organism from the throat.

Cephradine. This derivative ('Eskasef', Smith, Kline and French; 'Velosef', Squibb) has a structure almost identical with that of cephalexin, and is also administered orally. At the time of writing there is not enough information on which to assess its merits.

Bacterial Resistance to the Cephalosporins

It is important to recognize that staphylococci resistant to methicillin are also abnormally resistant to both cephalothin and cephaloridine. How effective the latter are in the treatment of infections caused by such strains cannot yet be judged. These fortunately exceptional organisms are thus not fully susceptible to any of this general group of antibiotics. Appropriate sensitivity tests for assessing the behaviour of individual strains are discussed in Chapter 29.

The natural resistance of some Gram-negative species is in part intrinsic, and in part dependent on enzymic destruction of the antibiotic. The distribution of 'cephalosporinase' the enzyme responsible, as described by Fleming, Goldner and Glass (1963), corresponds to that of resistance among enterobacteria. Although also a β-lactamase, this enzyme has little action on benzyl penicillin. Hamilton-Miller, Smith and Knox (1965) determined the action of cell-free extracts of various Gram-negative species on benzyl penicillin, ampicillin and cephaloridine, and observed several patterns of activity, some extracts destroying ampicillin more rapidly than cephaloridine or vice versa. Jack and Richmond (1970) classify β-lactamases from Gram-negative bacteria in eight distinct types on the basis both of their patterns of relative activity and of other characters.

PHARMACEUTICAL PREPARATIONS

PHENETHICILLIN POTASSIUM ('Broxil', Beecham). Tablets of 125 or 250 mg., and syrup. Dosage of this and the two following as for phenoxymethyl penicillin.

PROPICILLIN POTASSIUM ('Brocillin', Beecham; 'Ultrapen', Pfizer). Tablets of 125 or 250 mg., and syrup.

METHICILLIN (Sodium methicillin, 'Celbenin', Beecham). Vials of 1 g. for solution for intramuscular injection: the solution should be freshly prepared (particularly unstable if the distilled water is acid from dissolved CO_2). Usual adult dose 1 g. at 4-hour intervals, but this may be increased if necessary to a total of 12 or 18 g. daily.

CLOXACILLIN (Sodium cloxacillin, 'Orbenin', Beecham). Capsules of 250 mg. (oral) and vials containing 250 mg. for solution in 1·5 ml. water for intramuscular injection. Usual adult oral dose 500 mg. at 6-hour intervals, administered 1 hour *before* meals: admixture with food in bulk greatly reduces absorption. Half this dose intramuscularly produces similar blood levels, but larger amounts, up to 8 g. daily, have been given by this route for severe infections.

FLUCLOXACILLIN ('Floxapen', Beecham). Capsules of 250 mg. (oral) and vials containing 250 mg. for intramuscular injection. Usual adult dose 250 mg. at 6-hour intervals, administered 1 hour *before* meals. Similar or larger doses up to 8 g. daily by injection.

OXACILLIN (Sodium Oxacillin, 'Prostaphlin', Bristol Laboratories). Preparations and dosage as for cloxacillin.

AMPICILLIN ('Penbritin', Beecham). Capsules of 250 and 500 mg.; vials of 100, 250 and 500 mg. for solution for intramuscular injection; also tablets and syrup. Adult dose from 250 mg. orally at 6-hour intervals to a total of up to 12 g. daily given at the same intervals intramuscularly.

AMOXICILLIN ('Amoxil', Bencard). Capsules of 250 mg. (oral). Usual dose 250 mg. 8-hourly, but may be increased to 12 g. daily.

CARBENICILLIN ('Pyopen', Beecham). Vials of 1 g. and 5 g. for solution for intramuscular or intravenous injection. Dosage: urinary tract infections 1-2 g. 6-hourly. Systemic infections 2 g. 6-hourly. (*Pseudomonas* 20-30 g. intravenously daily).

CEPHALORIDINE ('Ceporin', Glaxo). Vials of 250, 500 and 1,000 mg. for solution for intramuscular injection. Dose 250 mg. or more (up to 1·5 g.) at 6-hour intervals.

CEPHALOTHIN ('Keflin', Lilly). Preparations and doses as for cephaloridine.

CEPHALEXIN ('Ceporex', Glaxo, 'Keflex', Lilly). Tablets 250 mg. and syrup: dosage 250 mg. or more 6-hourly up to 4 g. daily.

REFERENCES

ABRAHAM, E. P. (1959). *Endeavour* **18**, 212.
ABRAHAM, E. P. (1962). *Pharmacol. Rev.* **14**, 473.
ABRAHAM, E. P., & NEWTON, G. G. F. (1956). *Biochem. J.* **63**, 628.
ACRED, P., HUNTER, P. A., MIZEN, L. & ROLINSON, G. N. (1971a). *Antimicrobial Agents and Chemotherapy*—1970, p. 416.
ACRED, P., HUNTER, P. A., MIZEN, L. & ROLINSON, G. N. (1971b). *Antimicrobial Agents and Chemotherapy*—1970, p. 396.
ANDERSON, K. N., KENNEDY, R. P., PLORDE, J. J., SHULMAN, J. A. & PETERSDORF, R. G. (1964). *J. Amer. med. Ass.* **187**, 555.
APICELLA, M. A., PERKINS, R. L. & SASLAW, S. (1966a). *Amer. J. med. Sci.* **251**, 266.
APICELLA, M. A., PERKINS, R. L. & SASLAW, S. (1966b). *New Engl. J. Med.* **274**, 1002.
APPLESTEIN, J. M., CROSBY, E. B., JOHNSON, W. D. & KAYE, D. (1968). *Appl. Microbiol.* **16**, 1006.
ATKINSON, R. M., CURRIE, J. P., DAVIS, B., PRATT, D. A. H., SHARPE, H. M. & TOMICH, E. G. (1966). *Toxicol. appl. Pharmacol.* **8**, 398.

AXELROD, J., MEYERS, B. R. & HIRSCHMAN, S. Z. (1971). *Appl. Microbiol.* 22, 904.
AYLIFFE, G. A. J. & DAVIES, A. (1965). *Brit. J. Pharmacol.* 24, 189.
AYLIFFE, G. A. J., LOWBURY, E. J. L. & ROE, E. (1972). *Nature (New Biol.)* 235, 141.
BALDWIN, D. S., LEVINE, B. B., McCLUSKEY, R. T. & GALLO, G. R. (1968). *New Engl. J. Med.* 279, 1245.
BARBER, M. (1964). *J. gen. Microbiol.* 35, 183.
BARBER, M. & WATERWORTH, P. M. (1964). *Brit. med. J.* 2, 344.
BASCH, H., ERICKSON, R. & GADEBUSCH, H. (1971). *Infection Immunity* 4, 44.
BATCHELOR, F. R., CHAIN, E. B., RICHARDS, M. & ROLINSON, G. N. (1961). *Proc. roy. Soc. B.* 154, 522.
BATCHELOR, F. R., DOYLE, F. P., NAYLER, J. H. C. & ROLINSON, G. N. (1959). *Nature (Lond.)* 183, 257.
BENAVIDES, V. L., OLSON, B. H., VARELGA, G. & HOLT, S. H. (1955). *J. Amer. med. Ass.* 157, 989.
BENNER, E. J., BENNET, J. V., BRODIE, J. L. & KIRBY, W. M. M. (1965a). *J. Bact.* 90, 1599.
BENNER, E. J. & KAYSER, F. H. (1968). *Lancet* 2, 741.
BENNER, E. J., MICKLEWAIT, J. S., BRODIE, J. L. & KIRBY, W. M. M. (1965b). *Proc. Soc. exp. Biol. (N.Y.)* 119, 536.
BLECHER, T. E., EDGAR, W. M., MELVILLE, H. A. H. & PEEL, K. R. (1966). *Brit. med. J.* 1, 137.
BODNER, S. J. & KOENIG, M. G. (1972). *Amer. J. med. Sci.* 263, 43.
BOND, J. M., LIGHTBOWN, J. W., BARBER, M. & WATERWORTH, P. M. (1963). *Brit. med. J.* 2, 956.
BRAN, J. L., KARL, D. M. & KAYE, D. (1971). *Clin. Pharmacol. Ther.* 12, 525.
BRAUN, P., TILLOTSON, J. R., WILCOX, C. & FINLAND, M. (1968). *Appl. Microbiol.* 16, 1684.
BRAUNINGER, G. E. & REMINGTON, J. S. (1968). *J. Amer. med. Ass.* 203, 103.
BROWN, D. M. & ACRED, P. (1961). *Brit. med. J.* 2, 197.
BRUMFITT, W., PERCIVAL, A. & LEIGH, D. A. (1967). *Lancet* 1, 1289.
BULGER, R. J. (1967). *Lancet* 1, 17.
BULGER, R. J., LINDHOLM, D. D., MURRAY, J. S. & KIRBY, W. M. M. (1964). *J. Amer. med. Ass.* 187, 319.
BUNN, P. A., MILICICH, C. & LUNN, J. S. (1966). *Antimicrobial Agents and Chemotherapy* 1965: p. 947.
BURGESS, H. A. & EVANS, R. J. (1966). *Brit. med. J.* 2, 1244.
CHABBERT, Y. A., BAUDENS, J. G., ACAR, J. F. & GERBAUD, G. R. (1965). *Rev. franc. clin. biol.* 10, 495.
CHILD, K. J. & DODDS, M. G. (1967). *Brit. J. Pharmacol.*, 30, 354.
COOPER, R. G., RICE, J. C. & PENFOLD, J. L. (1969). *Med. J. Aust.* 1, 517.
CROYDON, E. A. P. & SUTHERLAND, R. (1971). *Antimicrobial Agents and Chemotherapy*—1970, p. 427.
v.DAEHNE, W., FREDERIKSEN, E., GUNDERSEN, E., LUND, F., MORCH, P., PETERSEN, H. J., ROHOLT, K., TYBRING, L. & GODTFREDSEN, W. O. (1970). *J. med. Chem.* 13, 607.
DARRELL, J. H. & WATERWORTH, P. M. (1969). *Brit. med. J.* 3, 141.
DODDS, M. G. & FOORD, R. D. (1970). *Brit. J. Pharmacol.* 40, 227.
DOYLE, F. P., LONG, A. A. W., NAYLER, J. H. C. & STOVE, E. R. (1961). *Nature (Lond.)* 192, 1183.
DYKE, K. G. H., JEVONS, M. P. & PARKER, M. T. (1966). *Lancet* 1, 835.
EICKHOFF, T. C., KISLAK, J. W. & FINLAND, M. (1965a). *New Engl. J. Med.* 272, 699.
EICKHOFF, T. C., KISLAK, J. W. & FINLAND, M. (1965b). *Amer. J. med. Sci.* 249, 163.
FLEMING, P. C., GOLDNER, M. & GLASS, D. G. (1963). *Lancet* 1, 1399.
FLOREY, H. W. (1955). *Ann. intern. Med.* 43, 480.

FOLTZ, E. L., WEST, J. W., BRESLOW, I. H. & WALLIK, H. (1971). *Antimicrobial Agents and Chemotherapy*—1970, p. 442.

GADEBUSCH, H., MIRAGLIA, G., PANSY, F. & RENZ, K. (1971). *Infection Immunity* 4, 50.

GALBRAITH, H. J. B. (1967). *Brit. J. clin. Pract.* 21, 331.

GEDDES, A. M. (1973). *Current Antibiotic Therapy*. Ed. A. M. Geddes & J. D. Williams. Edinburgh. Churchill Livingstone. p. 231.

GOTTSHALL, R. Y., ROBERTS, J. M., PORTWOOD, L. M. & JENNINGS, J. C. (1951). *Proc. Soc. exp. Biol. (N.Y.)* 76, 307.

GRAVENKEMPER, C. F., BENNETT, J. V., BRODIE, J. L. & KIRBY, W. M. M. (1965). *Arch. intern Med.* 116, 340.

GREENWOOD, D. & O'GRADY, F. (1973). *J. clin. Path.* 26, 1.

HAMILTON-MILLER, J. M. T. (1965). *J. gen. Microbiol.* 41, 175.

HAMILTON-MILLER, J. M. T., SMITH, J. T. & KNOX, R. (1965). *Nature (Lond.)* 208, 235.

HARDCASTLE, G. A. JR., JOHNSON, D. A., PANETTA, C. A., SCOTT, A. I. & SUTHERLAND, S. A. (1966). *J. organic Chem.* 31, 897.

HARDING, J. W. & KNUDSEN, E. T. (1970). *Practitioner* 205, 801.

HÖFFLER, D., STEGEMANN, I. & SCHELER, F. (1966). *Dtsch. med. Wschr.* 91, 206.

JACK, G. W. & RICHMOND, M. H. (1970). *J. gen. Microbiol.* 61, 43.

JONES, R. J. & LOWBURY, E. J. L. (1967). *Brit. med. J.* 3, 79.

JORDAN, M. C., DE MAINE, J. B. & KIRBY, W. M. M. (1971). *Antimicrobial Agents and Chemotherapy*—1970, p. 438.

KAPLAN, K., REISBERG, B. & WEINSTEIN, L. (1968). *Arch. intern. Med.* 121, 17.

KAYSER, F. H. & HOLLINGER, A. (1968). *Dtsch. med. Wschr.* 93, 1933.

KIND, A. C., TUPASI, T. E., STANDIFORD, H. C. & KIRBY, W. M. M. (1970). *Arch intern Med.* 125, 685.

KISLAK, J. W., EICKHOFF, T. C. & FINLAND, M. (1965). *Amer. J. med. Sci.* 249, 636.

KISLAK, J. W., STEINHAUER, B. W. & FINLAND, M. (1966). *Amer. J. med. Sci.* 251, 433.

KJELLANDER, J. O. & FINLAND, M. (1963). *Proc. Soc. exp. Biol. (N.Y.)* 113, 1031.

KLEIN, J. O. & FINLAND, M. (1963). *Amer. J. med. Sci.* 246, 10.

KLEIN, J. O., SABATH, L. D., STEINHAUER, B. W. & FINLAND, M. (1963). *Amer. J. med. Sci.* 246, 385.

KNUDSEN, E. T. & ROLINSON, G. N.(1959). *Lancet* 2, 1105.

KNUDSEN, E. T., ROLINSON, G. N. & STEVENS, S. (1961). *Brit. med. J.* 2, 198.

KNUDSEN, E. T., ROLINSON, G. N. & SUTHERLAND, R. (1967). *Brit. med. J.* 3, 75.

KUNIN, C. M. (1966). *Clin. Pharmacol. Ther.* 7, 166.

KUNIN, C. M. & ATUK, N. (1966). *New Engl. J. Med.* 274, 654.

KUNIN, C. M. & BRANDT, D. (1968). *Amer. J. med. Sci.* 255, 196.

LANE, W. R. (1964). *Med. J. Aust.* 2, 499.

LEIGH, D. A. & SPENCER, R. (1971). *Brit. J. clin. Pract.* 25, 371.

LERNER, P. I. (1969). *Amer. J. med. Sci.* 257, 125.

LEVITT, B. H., GOTTLIEB, A. J., ROSENBERG, I. R. & KLEIN, J. J. (1964). *Clin. Pharmacol. Ther.* 5, 301.

LOWBURY, E. J. L., KIDSON, A., LILLY, H. A., AYLIFFE, G. A. J. & JONES, R. J. (1969). *Lancet* 2, 448.

LUND, F. & TYBRING, L. (1972). *Nature (New Biol.)* 236, 135.

McELFRESH, A. E. & HUANG, N. N. (1962). *New Engl. J. Med.* 266, 246.

MacNAIR, D. R., WHITE, J. E. & GRAHAM, J. M. (1968). *Lancet* 1, 16.

MERRILL, S. L., DAVIS, A., SMOLENS, B. & FINEGOLD, S. M. (1966). *Ann. intern. Med.* 64, 1.

MILLER, A. K., CELOZZI, E., PELAK, B. A., STAPLEY, E. O. & HENDLIN, D. (1972). *Antimicrobial Agents & Chemotherapy*, 2, 281, 287.

MORTIMER, P. R., MACKIE, D. B. & HAYNES, S. (1969). *Brit. med. J.* 3, 88.

MUGGLETON, P. W., O'CALLAGHAN, C. H. & STEVENS, W. K. (1964). *Brit. med. J.* **2**, 1234.
MURDOCH, J. McC., SPIERS, C. F., GEDDES, A. M. & WALLACE, E. T. (1964). *Brit. med. J.* **2**, 1238.
NAUMANN, P. (1965). *Dtsch. med. Wschr.* **90**, 1085.
NAUMANN, P. & KEMPF, B. (1965). *Arzneimittel Forsch.* **15**, 139.
NAYLER, J. H. C., LONG, A. A. W., BROWN, D. M., ACRED, P., ROLINSON, G. N., BATCHELOR, F. R., STEVENS, S. & SUTHERLAND, R. (1962). *Nature (Lond.)* **195**, 1264.
NEU, H. C. & WINSHELL, E. B. (1971a). *Antimicrobial Agents and Chemotherapy*—1970, p. 385.
NEU, H. C. & WINSHELL, E. B. (1971b). *Antimicrobial Agents and Chemotherapy*—1970, p. 423.
OPPENHEIMER, S., BEATY, H. N. & PETERSDORF, R. G. (1969). *J. Lab. clin. Med.* **73**, 535.
PARKER, M. T. & HEWITT, J. H. (1970). *Lancet* **1**, 800.
PERKINS, R. L., CARLISLE, H. N. & SASLAW, S. (1968). *Amer. J. med. Sci.* **256**, 122.
PERKINS, R. L., GLONTZ, G. E. & SASLAW, S. (1969). *Clin. Pharmacol. Ther.* **10**, 244.
PERKINS, R. L. & SASLAW, S. (1966). *Ann. intern. Med.* **64**, 13.
PERKINS, R. L., SMITH, E. J. & SASLAW, S. (1969). *Amer. J. med. Sci.* **257**, 116.
PRICE, K. E., LEITNER, F., MISIEK, M., CHISHOLM, D. R. & PURSIANO, T. A. (1971). *Antimicrobial Agents and Chemotherapy*—1970, p. 17.
REPORT FROM SIX HOSPITALS (1962). *Lancet* **2**, 634.
REPORT (1973). CROYDON, E.A.P. & 13 others. *Brit. med. J.*, **1**, 7.
RICHARDS, H. C., HOUSLEY, J. R. & SPOONER, D. F. (1963). *Nature (Lond.)* **199**, 354.
RIDLEY, M. & PHILLIPS, I. (1965). *Nature (Lond.)* **208**, 1076.
ROE, E., JONES, R. J. & LOWBURY, E. J. L. (1971). *Lancet* **1**, 149.
ROLINSON, G. N. & STEVENS, S. (1961). *Brit. med. J.* **2**, 191.
ROLINSON, G. N., STEVENS, S., BATCHELOR, F. R., WOOD, J. C. & CHAIN, E. B. (1960). *Lancet* **2**, 564.
ROLLO, I. M., SOMERS, G. F. & BURLEY, D. M. (1962). *Brit. med. J.* **i**, 76.
RONALD, A. R. & TURCK, M. (1967). *Antimicrobial Agents & Chemotherapy*—1966, p. 83.
ROSENBLATT, J. E., KIND, A. C., BRODIE, J. L. & KIRBY, W. M. M. (1968). *Arch. intern. Med.* **121**, 345.
SASLAW, S. & CARLISLE, H. N. (1969). *Amer. J. med. Sci.* **257**, 395.
SASLAW, S. & CARLISLE, H. N. (1970). *Amer. J. med. Sci.* **259**, 383.
SEELIGER, H. P. R., LAYMANN, V. & FINGER, H. (1967). *Dtsch. med. Wschr.* **92**, 1095.
SEELIGER, H. & MATHEIS, H. (1969). *Dtsch. med. Wschr.* **94**, 853.
SHAPIRO, S., SLONE, D., SISKIND, V., LEWIS, G. P. & JICK, H. (1969). *Lancet* **2**, 969.
SIBONI, K. & POULSEN, E. D. (1968). *Dan. med. Bull.* **15**, 161.
SIDELL, S., BULGER, R. J., BRODIE, J. L. & KIRBY, W. M. M. (1964). *Clin. Pharmacol. Ther.* **5**, 26.
SIMON, H. J. & SAKAI, W. (1963). *Pediatrics* **31**, 463.
SMITH, J. T. & HAMILTON-MILLER, J. M. T. (1970). *Chemotherapy* **15**, 365.
SLEET, R. A., SANGSTER, G. & MURDOCH, J. McC. (1964). *Brit. med. J.* **1**. 148.
SONNE, M. & JAWETZ, E. (1969). *Appl. Microbiol.* **17**, 893.
STAPLEY, E. O. & 8 others (1972). *Antimicrobial Agents &Chemotherapy* **2**, 122.
STEIGBIGEL, N. H., KISLAK, J. W., TILLES, J. G. & FINLAND, M. (1968.) *Arch. intern. Med.* **121**, 24.
STILLERMAN, M., ISENBERG, H. D. & MOODY, M. (1972). *Amer. J. Dis. Child.* **123**, 457.

SUTHERLAND, R., CROYDON, E. A. P. & ROLINSON, G. N. (1970). *Brit. med. J.* **4**, 455.

SUTHERLAND, R., BURNETT, J. & ROLINSON, G. (1971). *Antimicrobial Agents & Chemotherapy*—1970, p. 390.

SUTHERLAND, R., CROYDON, E. A. P. & ROLINSON, G. N. (1972). *Brit. med. J.* **3**, 13.

SUTHERLAND, R. & ROBINSON, O. P. W. (1967). *Brit. med. J.* **2**, 804.

SUTHERLAND, R. & ROLINSON, G. N. (1964a). *J. Bact.* **87**, 887.

SUTHERLAND, R. & ROLINSON, G. N. (1964b). *J. clin. Path.* **17**, 461.

SUTHERLAND, R. & ROLINSON, G. N. (1971). *Antimicrobial Agents and Chemotherapy*—1970, p. 411.

SUTHERLAND, R. & WISE, P. J. (1971). *Antimicrobial Agents and Chemotherapy*—1970, p. 402.

SYMPOSIUM (1970). *Postgrad. med J.* **46**, Suppl. Oct.

SYMPOSIUM (1971). *Postgrad. med. J.* **47**, Suppl. Feb.

THORNHILL, T. S., LEVISON, M. E., JOHNSON, W. W. & KAYE, D. (1969). *Appl. Microbiol.* **17**, 457.

TUANO, S. B., JOHNSON, L. D., BRODIE, J. L. & KIRBY, W. M. M. (1966). *New Engl. J. Med.* **275**, 635.

TURCK, M., ANDERSON, K. N., SMITH, R. H., WALLACE, J. F. & PETERSDORF, R. G. (1965). *Ann. intern. Med.* **63**, 199.

TURCK, M., RONALD, A. & PETERSDORF, R. G. (1965). *J. Amer. med. Ass.* **192**, 961.

VAN ROOYEN, C. E., ROSS, J. F., BETHUNE, G. W. & MACDONALD, A. C. (1967). *Canad. med. Ass. J.* **97**, 1227.

VAN SCOY, R. E., WARREN, E. & WASHINGTON, J. A. (1971). *Antimicrobial Agents and Chemotherapy*—1970, p. 12.

VIANNA, N. J. & KAYE, D. (1967). *Amer. J. med. Sci.* **254**, 216.

WALLACE, J. F., ATLAS, E., BEAR, D. M., BROWN, N. K., CLARK, H. & TURCK, M. (1971). *Antimicrobial Agents and Chemotherapy*—1970, p. 223.

WALTERS, E. W., ROMANSKY, M. J. & JOHNSON, A. C. (1963). *Antimicrobial Agents and Chemotherapy*—1962, 706.

WATERWORTH, P. M. (1971). *Postgrad. med. J.* February Suppl., 25.

WEINGARTNER, L. & ORTEL, S. (1967). *Dtsch. med. Wschr.* **92**, 1098.

WICK, W. E. & BONIECE, W. S. (1965). *Appl. Microbiol.* **13**, 248

WICK, W. E., WRIGHT, W. E. & KUDER, H. V. (1971). *Appl. Microbiol.* **21**, 426.

WILLIAMSON, G. M., MORRISON. J. K & STEVENS. K. J. (1961). *Lancet* **1**. 847.

WOODRUFF, M. W., COVERT, S. V., LITINSKY, S. M. & VANNEMAN, W. M. (1971). *New York State med. J.* **71**, 1087.

CHAPTER 6

AMINOGLYCOSIDES

1. STREPTOMYCIN

UNLIKE penicillin, streptomycin was discovered as the result of a deliberate search for antibiotics. Starting in 1939, Waksman and his colleagues examined a large series of microorganisms, particularly soil bacteria, for activity against Gram-negative bacilli. The first antibiotic of any value resulting from this investigation was streptothricin, which was isolated in 1942 by Waksman and Woodruff from a strain of *Streptomyces lavendulae*, but was subsequently found to be too toxic for clinical use. In 1944, after more than ten thousand microorganisms had been examined, Schatz, Bugie and Waksman recorded the isolation of streptomycin from a strain of *Streptomyces griseus*, found in a diagnostic culture from a chicken's throat.

Different strains of *Streptomyces griseus* vary very much in antibiotic production. Some strains appear to produce no antibiotics, others produce streptomycin; and yet others produce grisein or the antifungal agent, candicidin. The species was first isolated by Krainsky in Russia in 1914 and soon after by Waksman and Curtis (1916). When this original strain was tested in 1946 it produced no antibiotics, but after irradiation, a streptomycin-producing variant was obtained (Waksman and Lechevalier, 1953).

CHEMICAL PROPERTIES

Streptomycin (Fig. 8) is readily soluble in water and is a strong base. Many organic and inorganic salts have been prepared, of which the sulphate is the most important preparation since it causes the least pain and irritation at the site of injection.

Streptomycin sulphate is a white almost colourless substance with a slightly bitter taste. It is very soluble in water and almost insoluble in alcohol. Watery solutions are acid, those

containing 250 mg./ml. having a pH as low as 4·5. Solutions
are stable for long periods at a pH between 3 and 7 and a
temperature below 28° C.; solutions kept in the cold retain their
potency for at least a year.

Catalytic reduction of streptomycin yields dihydrostreptomycin (also isolated from *Streptomyces humidus*: Imamura
et al., 1956). Its structure is shown in Fig. 8 and its properties
are described in earlier editions of this book. It closely resembles
streptomycin in most respects but as it is much more liable to
produce deafness (Table 16, p. 111), it should no longer be used
therapeutically.

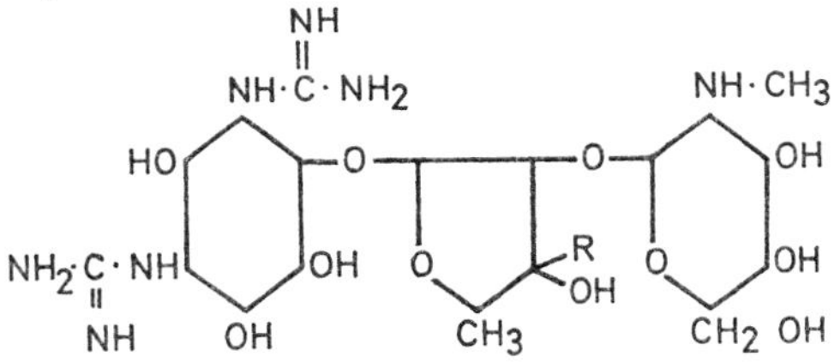

FIGURE 8
Structure of Streptomycin (R = CHO) and Dihydrostreptomycin
(R = CH$_2$OH).

ANTI-BACTERIAL ACTIVITY

Streptomycin is a bactericidal antibiotic particularly active
against *Mycobacteria*, Gram-negative bacilli and some strains
of staphylococci. Streptococci and pneumococci are relatively

TABLE 14
Sensitivity of Bacteria to Streptomycin
N.B.—Resistant variants are common with all species

Gram-negative Bacteria	M.I.C. µg./ml.	Gram-positive Bacteria	M.I.C. µg./ml.
E. coli	2 - 4	Staph. aureus	2
Kl. aerogenes	2	Str. pyogenes	32
Kl. pneumoniae	1	Str. pneumoniae	64
Proteus spp.	4 - >256	Str. faecalis	64 - >256
Ps. aeruginosa	16 - 64	Clostridium spp.	> 128
Salm. typhi	8 - 16		
Salm. paratyphi	4 - 8		
Salm. spp.	4 - 16	Myco. tuberculosis	0·5
Sh. sonnei	2 - 4		
Sh. flexneri	2 - 8		
N. gonorrhoeae	4		

resistant, and anaerobic sporing bacilli and fungi almost completely insensitive (Table 14).

The anti-bacterial activity of streptomycin is greatest in a slightly alkaline medium (pH 7·8) and is considerably reduced in media with a pH of 6·0 or less. Streptomycin is so sensitive to the effect of pH that the natural acidity of a solution of streptomycin sulphate may be sufficient to depress its anti-bacterial activity. Krauss *et al.* (1968) found that 20 μg./ml. streptomycin sulphate (pH 7·1) inhibited a strain of pneumococci, while 50 μg./ml. (pH 6·8) failed to do so. It is less active under anaerobic conditions, but some strains of anaerobic cocci are inhibited by from 2·0 to 10·0 μg./ml.

Mode of Action

Streptomycin is actively bactericidal to sensitive organisms, including *Myco. tuberculosis,* in concentrations which can be attained in the blood-stream. Thus a population of 10^7 staphylococci per ml. is completely extinguished in eight hours by 20 μg. streptomycin per ml.; 50 and 200 μg./ml. extinguishes it in four and two hours respectively and 2,000 μg./ml. produces a 99·8 per cent mortality in 10 minutes. Thus, unlike penicillin, which has a quite low optimum concentration for bactericidal effect, above which no enhancement is obtainable, streptomycin behaves like an ordinary germicide, the velocity of its bactericidal action increasing progressively with rise in concentration. Parallel with this the uptake of streptomycin by bacteria increases with exposure time and is directly related to the concentration of the drug. Uptake involves two processes which may or may not be separated by a lag (Beggs and Williams, 1971). The first rapid phase probably represents simple binding to the cell surface. The second phase is inhibited by chloramphenicol, low temperature and anaerobiosis, and is presumably dependent on biosynthetic processes. It is probably through this effect that anaerobic conditions inhibit the action of streptomycin.

Acquired Resistance

Large populations of nearly all species of bacteria, including the tubercle bacillus, are liable to contain a few cells resistant to 1,000 μg. per ml. streptomycin which are readily selected by the antibiotic. Increase in resistance to streptomycin after only a few passages in the presence of the antibiotic *in vitro* or within a few days (for the tubercle bacillus a few weeks) of the beginning of streptomycin treatment is common. Streptomycin-resistant strains sometimes have a reduced growth-rate and virulence, but many appear to be as virulent as their sensitive parents.

Resistance appears to arise from several distinct mechanisms. High level resistance results from a single step mutation which alters one of the 20 or so proteins which go to make up the ribosomes (p. 247) so that binding of streptomycin to the ribosome is reduced (Chang and Flaks, 1970). Low level resistance is due to decreased uptake of the antibiotic (Gundersen, 1967). An important therapeutic consequence of this is seen in enterococci, wild strains of which show two distinct levels of resistance (Standiford *et al.*, 1970). Moderate resistance (M.I.C. 62-500 μg./ml.) is due to impermeability of the bacterial cell which prevents the drug reaching its sensitive ribosome. This impermeability can be overcome by simultaneous exposure to agents, such as penicillin, which interfere with synthesis of the bacterial cell wall (p. 252) where the permeability barrier is presumably located. As a result strains showing moderate resistance to streptomycin exhibit synergy with penicillin (p. 312). In contrast, strains showing high levels of resistance (M.I.C. 1000 μg./ml.) have ribosomes which are resistant to streptomycin and hence simultaneous treatment with penicillin is without effect (Zimmermann *et al.*, 1971). R-factor mediated resistance (p. 264) is different in that genetic material transferred during conjugation confers on the recipient cell the capacity to synthesize a specific enzyme which destroys streptomycin. All 54 streptomycin-resistant wild strains of *E. coli* examined by Rassekh and Pitton (1971) inactivated streptomycin—even the four strains which did not transfer their resistance. They conclude that resistance in wild strains is generally R-factor mediated even when not transferable (Yamada *et al.*, 1968).

It is not infrequent to find strains of meningococci, *Staph. aureus, E. coli, Ps. aeruginosa, Proteus* and *Myco. tuberculosis* which are actually favoured by the presence of the antibiotic or completely dependent on it. Isolated ribosomes from streptomycin-dependent *Escherichia* will synthesize peptides only in the presence of the drug (Dixon and Polglase, 1969). The antigenicity and virulence of streptomycin-dependent variants of *Salm. typhi* is unchanged (Reitman, 1967).

Cross-Resistance

There is complete cross-resistance between streptomycin and dihydrostreptomycin, and partial cross resistance between streptomycin and neomycin, kanamycin and paromomycin. This is usually one–way: strains that have developed resistance to neomycin and kanamycin nearly always show a significant increase in resistance to streptomycin (Table 18, p. 118) while streptomycin-resistant bacteria are frequently still sensitive to neomycin and kanamycin (Brock, 1964). These cross-resistances probably arise from differences in the ribosomal sites of action of the antibiotics (Tanaka *et al.*, 1964).

PHARMACOKINETICS

Absorption

Streptomycin is not absorbed in any quantity from the intestinal tract. Its activity in the gut is retained and it is excreted unchanged in the faeces. It may, therefore, be used orally for its action on bacteria in the lumen of the intestine. For systemic treatment streptomycin is usually administered by intramus-

TABLE 15

Plasma Levels of Streptomycin

	Dose	Peak Plasma Level		Plasma Half-life Hours
		Hour	$\mu g./ml.$	
Adult	0·5G	$\frac{1}{2}$-1$\frac{1}{2}$	16-42	2·4-2·7
	1·0G		25-50	
Adult over 40 yrs	0·75G		26-58	up to 9·0
Premature Infant	10 mg. per kg.	2	17-42	7·0

Adcock, J. D. & Hettig, R. A. (1946). *Arch. intern. Med.* **77,** 179.
Buggs, C. W., *et al.* (1946). *J. clin. Invest.* **25,** 94.
Axline, S. G. & Simon, H. J. (1965). *Antimicrob. Agents Chemother.* 1964. p. 135.
Line, D. H. *et al.* (1970).

cular injections which are liable to be painful. The levels obtained are shown in Table 15. In patients treated for tuberculosis, Line *et al.* (1970) found considerable variation in the same patient on repeat testing, the peak levels following a dose of 0·75 g. sometimes differing by as much as 50 μg./ml. In premature infants the ability to excrete streptomycin is impaired (Table 15) and therapeutic levels (10 μg./ml. or more) are still present 4-5 hours after 5 mg./kg. (half the adult dose). As renal function declines with age too, so in patients over the age of 40 streptomycin tends to persist longer in the blood and in older adults excretion is commonly incomplete at 24 hours (Line *et al.*, 1970).

Distribution

Streptomycin diffuses fairly rapidly into most body tissues but is distributed as if it were present in extracellular fluid only. Little or no streptomycin can be demonstrated inside macrophages in the presence of therapeutic blood levels, even when the cells are actively phagocytic (Bonventre *et al.*, 1967). It appears in the peritoneal fluid in concentrations of about one-quarter to one-half those present in the blood, and in pleural fluid the concentrations may equal those in the blood.

It does not penetrate into the C.S.F. or thick-walled abscesses but significant amounts are usually present in tuberculous cavities. Levels in cord blood are similar to those in maternal blood.

Excretion

URINE. Streptomycin is rapidly excreted in the urine, when the kidneys are normal, but the amount excreted in 24 hours differs very much in different individuals. Excretion is by glomerular filtration and is unaffected by agents which block tubular secretion. The renal clearance is 30-70 ml./min. and between 30 and 90 per cent of the dose is usually excreted in the first 24 hours, some being destroyed or retained in the body. The concentrations of streptomycin in the urine are often very high: 300-400 μg. per ml. after doses of 0·5 g. and 1,000 μg. per ml. or more after doses of 1 g. In oliguria, the plasma half life is prolonged to 50-100 hours and dosage must be reduced if toxic levels are to be avoided (p. 299).

Small amounts of streptomycin, probably less than one per cent, are excreted in the bile and levels of from 3 to 12·5 μg./ml. have been recorded.

TOXICITY AND SIDE-EFFECTS

Pain and irritation at the site of injection of streptomycin are common, but pain can be relieved by giving the antibiotic with procaine.

Many patients experience unpleasant symptoms within a few hours of an intramuscular injection of streptomycin, such as paraesthesiae in and round the mouth, vertigo and ataxia, headaches and lassitude and ' muzziness in the head '. These are often trivial, but in ambulant patients in whom blood levels are appreciably higher than in those at rest, they are sometimes sufficient to render the patient unable to work. Occasional cases of aplastic anaemia and agranulocytosis have been recorded but the most common serious toxic effect of streptomycin is vestibular disturbance.

Effects on Eighth Nerve

In early clinical trials of streptomycin in tuberculosis the drug was given in a daily dose of 2 g. and in the first American series the incidence of vertigo was 96 per cent, and in the first British report it was 66 per cent. If the daily dose was only 1 g. the incidence of vertigo was greatly reduced and with half this dose rarely occurred earlier than the forty-fifth day of treatment. Although there are considerable species differences, animal experiments confirm that the principal toxic effect of streptomycin is on the sensory epithelia of the labyrinth. Cats treated with a daily dose of 100-200 mg. per kg. became incoordinated after 16-19 days and with continuation of treatment lost their righting reflexes and eventually had difficulty in standing. Some recovery occurred after cessation of treatment but they were still unable to jump without falling and some showed the circling movement characteristic of chronic vestibular damage. Lindeman (1969), who reviews the various claims and conclusions of those who have examined the histological manifestations of experimental streptomycin ototoxicity, found the sensory epithelia of the cristae ampullares to be the most severely affected. It has been suggested that the damage results from an inhibitory effect on the ribosomes of these cells analogous to that which is responsible for the antibacterial action of the drug. The vestibular end-organs are essential to the development of the typical symptoms of motion sickness, and even partial impairment of vestibular function will afford some protection. This has led to the treatment of patients suffering from Menière's disease with just enough streptomycin to produce unsteadiness.

Deafness

On prolonged follow-up of patients treated with streptomycin for Menière's disease there was no recurrence and none had developed deafness (Graybiel et al., 1967). Nevertheless there is no doubt that both in man and animals, damage to hearing can occur. Robinson and Cambon (1964) described two cases of congenital hearing loss in children born to mothers treated with streptomycin in pregnancy, and amongst 17 children whose mothers had received the drug, Conway and Birt (1965) found abnormalities in the caloric test in 6 and in the audiogram in 4. In all 8 monkeys treated with streptomycin, Igarashi et al. (1966) found pathological changes in the organ of Corti in addition to vestibular damage.

There is a good deal of evidence that the incidence of vestibular disturbance is related to total dosage and also to excessive blood levels maintained for shorter periods. There is also some evidence that streptomycin is actively secreted into the endolymph and such local concentration may play an important part in its specific ototoxicity. It has also been postulated that it is through interference with this secretory mechanism that streptomycin exerts its beneficial effect in Menière's disease by reducing the endolymph hydrops which supposedly underlies the disease (Fairbanks et al., 1971). Two other factors are important: the age of the patient and the state of renal function. In the older patient the risk of damage is higher and when it does occur compensation is less good than in younger patients. In the cases reported by Erlanson and Lundgren (1964) two thirds of the patients had received a total dose of only

4-10 g. over 5-14 days, but in some the daily dose was high, and two thirds had impaired renal function. Line *et al.* (1970) studied 27 patients treated with 0·75 g. streptomycin daily for tuberculosis, 8 of whom became dizzy within 6 weeks of starting treatment. There was no significant relation between incidence of dizziness and peak streptomycin level, but a highly significant relation with the 24-hour level. Serum levels exceeding 3 μg./ml. at 24 hours were found in 5 out of 8 dizzy patients but only 2 out of 18 unaffected patients, and both of these had had their dosage reduced when it was found that their renal function was impaired.

While there is no doubt of the importance of excessive dosage, there is also considerable individual variation in susceptibility to the drug. In their studies in monkeys, Igarashi *et al.* (1966) found damage to the cristae which varied from very slight to very severe and which bore no relation to the amount of drug given. Prazic *et al.* (1964), who emphasize the possibility of damage to hearing after only a few doses of streptomycin, describe a family of 7 in which 4 sisters all became deaf after receiving 5-30 g. streptomycin. The hearing of the remaining members of the family was normal and there was no history of familial deafness. It may be that such familial susceptibility to streptomycin was implicated in the case of a mother treated in pregnancy and her child both of whose audiograms were abnormal (Conway and Birt, 1965).

The possibility of toxic effects needs taking into account, therefore, not only in connection with a long course given for tuberculosis, but when streptomycin is prescribed for shorter periods for other purposes. Among 22 patients with eighth nerve damage, affecting vestibular function in 21 and hearing in three, seen by Cawthorne and Ranger (1957), only four had been treated for tuberculosis: none had received more than 20 g., and 12 had had only 10 g. or less. Some of their diagnoses imply renal insufficiency, and most of them were middle aged or elderly. In some cases the antibiotic had been given only as ' cover ' for what should have been a clean operation. It is quite unjustifiable to use streptomycin for such a purpose in anyone in whom there is any possibility of impaired renal function, including that which naturally accompanies the advance of age. When such impairment exists, and alternative treatment cannot be adopted, the dose should be carefully regulated by the results of blood assays (p. 518). Table 16 shows that there is no foundation for the claim that streptomycin pantothenate is less ototoxic than other preparations.

TABLE 16

Relative Ototoxicity of Streptomycin Preparations

	Average dose g.	Number of patients	Ototoxic %
Streptomycin	105	91	12
Streptomycin pantothenate	106	104	11·5
Streptomycin plus dihydro-streptomycin	79	100	22·7
Dihydrostreptomycin pantothenate	67	47	44·7

WILLEMOT, J. J. et al. (1962). Acta tuberc. Belg. 53, 128.

Hypersensitivity

Skin rashes and drug-fever occur in about 5 per cent of treated patients. They are usually trivial and respond to antihistamine treatment so that in most cases streptomycin therapy can be continued, although this should be done with caution, since occasionally severe and even fatal exfoliative dermatitis may develop.

Skin sensitization is also common in nurses and dispensers who handle streptomycin and may lead to severe dermatitis, sometimes associated with periorbital swelling and conjunctivitis. This can be avoided by exercising care in giving injections, and wearing gloves and, where solution may be ejected, goggles.

Desensitization of those who handle streptomycin is usually possible, but may take several months and quite severe reactions may occur even with the minute doses used. Cover with antihistamines or corticosteroids, together with the use of repeated minute doses, instead of steadily increasing ones, may help to reduce the reactions but will not necessarily eliminate them.

Patients showing hypersensitivity during therapy are generally much more readily desensitized. Reactions most frequently develop between 4 and 6 weeks, but may appear after the first dose or after 6 months' treatment. Desensitization may be achieved by giving 20 mg. prednisolone daily plus 10 daily increments from 10-100 mg. streptomycin followed by 10 daily increments from 0·1-1·0 g. (Hutfield, 1965). Alternatively, Lal and Ferguson (1963) gave increasing doses of streptomycin every six hours. By the ninth day, the whole dose was tolerated in a single injection and the patients were able to continue treatment without reaction.

Neuromuscular Blockade

Several antibiotics have attracted attention because of their capacity to produce neuromuscular blockade (pp. 120 and 192). According to Hokkanen (1964) streptomycin and its relatives function as membrane stabilizers in the same way as curare, reducing the sensitivity of the post-junctional end-plate membrane to the depolarizing effect of acetyl-choline. To give some idea of the potency of these compounds, it has been estimated that if D-tubocurarine has a blocking value of 1,000, that of polymyxin B is 5, neomycin 2·5, streptomycin 0·7, and kanamycin 0·5. Their effect is, therefore, relatively feeble and it is rare for streptomycin to show any neuromuscular blocking effects in those whose neuromuscular mechanisms are normal. However, as Hokkanen points out, antibiotics are customarily given in much larger amounts than curare and it is relatively common to see blocking effects in patients who are also receiving muscle relaxants or anaesthetics or in those suffering from myasthenia gravis (Toivakka and Hokkanen, 1965).

A similar depressant effect on cardiac muscle has been demonstrated in several experimental systems by Cohen *et al.* (1970) who thought that streptomycin toxicity was responsible for persistent hypotension in one of their patients.

CLINICAL APPLICATIONS

The most important use of streptomycin is in the treatment of tuberculosis (Chap. 26).

Apart from this streptomycin is the most effective antibiotic for the treatment of plague and tularaemia and sometimes, also, for infections due to otherwise resistant coliform bacilli. In the treatment of such infections, particularly of the urinary tract, large doses should be given for a short period, and combined therapy should be considered, since unless the infection is sterilized within a day or two of the onset of treatment drug-resistant strains are almost certain to appear.

Streptomycin is a good drug to give in combination with penicillin, since both are bactericidal antibiotics (Chap. 16) and this combination is often useful in the treatment of bacterial endocarditis. Streptomycin in combination with tetracycline has been considered to be the most effective antibiotic treatment for brucellosis (p. 321).

Since streptomycin is not absorbed from the intestinal tract, oral administration may be used for its effect on the intestinal flora.

PHARMACEUTICAL PREPARATIONS AND DOSAGE

STREPTOMYCIN SULPHATE (Streptolin. *Glaxo;* Streptoquaine, *Dista*)
INJECTION: B.P., B.N.F., equiv. 330 mg. in 1 ml; U.S.P., equiv. 500 mg. in 1 and 1·25 ml.; equiv. 1 g. in 2 ml. and 2·5 ml.; equiv. 5 g. in 10 ml. and 12·5 ml. Proprietary: 250, 330 and 500 mg. per ml. Sterile powder in vials 100 mg. and 1 g. Dose: i.m. 0·5-1·0 g. daily; intrathecal: 100 mg.
ORAL: tablets (Dista) equiv. 250 mg. Dose: 2 tab. 4 times daily. Paediatric mixture, B.P.C., A.P.F.: equiv. 125 mg. per ml.

REFERENCES

BEGGS, W. H. & WILLIAMS, N. E. (1971). *Appl. Bacteriol.* 21, 751.
BONVENTRE, P. F., HAYES, R. & IMHOFF, J. (1967). *J. Bact.* 93, 445.
BROCK, T. D. (1964). *Fed. Proc.* 23, 965.
CAWTHORNE, T. & RANGER, D. (1957). *Brit. med. J.* 1, 1444.
CHANG, F. N. & FLAKS, J. G. (1970). *Proc. Nat. Acad. Sci. U.S.* 67, 1321.
COHEN, L. S., WECHSLER, A. S., MITCHELL, J. H. & GLICK, G. (1970). *Amer. J. Cardiol.* 26, 505.
CONWAY, N. & BIRT, B. D. (1965). *Brit. med. J.* 2, 260.
DIXON, H. & POLGLASE, W. J. (1969). *J. Bact.* 100, 247.
ERLANSON, P. & LUNDGREN, A. (1964). *Acta med. scand.* 176, 147.
FAIRBANKS, D. N. F., SHIMIZU, H. & WARFIELD, D. (1971). *Arch. Otolaryngol.* 93, 590.
GRAYBIEL, A., SCHUKNECHT, H. F., FREGLY, A. R., MILLER, E. F. & McLEOD. M. E. (1967). *Arch. Otolaryng.* 85, 156.
GUNDERSEN, W. B. (1967). *Acta path. microbiol. scand.* 69, 214.
HOKKANEN, E. (1964). *Acta neurol. scand.* 40, 346.
HUTFIELD, D. C. (1965). *Brit. J. vener. dis.* 41, 210.
IGARASHI, M., McLEOD, M. E. & GRAYBIEL, A. (1966). *Acta Oto-laryng. Suppl.* 214, 1.
IMAMURA, A., HORI, M., NAKAZAWA, K., SHIBATA, M., TATSUOKA, S. & MIYAKE, A. (1956). *Proc. imp. Acad. (Japan)* 32, 648.
KRAINSKY, A. (1914). *Zbl. Bakt. 2. Abt.* 41, 649.
KRAUSS, M. R., KING, J. C. & COX, R. P. (1968). *J. Bact.* 95, 2413.
LAL, S. & FERGUSON, A. D. (1963). *Tubercle (Edin.)* 44, 360.
LINDEMAN, H. H. (1969). *Acta Otolaryngol. (Stockh.)* 67, 177.
LINE, D. H., POOLE, G. W. & WATERWORTH, P. M. (1970). *Tubercle (Lond.)* 51, 76.

PRAZIC, M., SALAJ, B. & SUBOTIC, R. (1964). *J. Laryngol.* **78,** 1037.
RASSEKH, M. & PITTON, J. S. (1971). *Chemotherapy* **16,** 239.
REITMAN, M. (1967). *J. infect. Dis.* **117,** 101.
ROBINSON, G. C. & CAMBON, K. G. (1964). *New Engl. J. Med.* **271,** 949.
SCHATZ, A., BUGIE, E. & WAKSMAN, S. A. (1944). *Proc. Soc. exp. Biol.* (*N.Y.*) **55,** 66.
STANDIFORD, H. D., DE MAINE, J. B. & KIRBY, W. M. M. (1970). *Arch. int. Med.,* **126,** 255.
TANAKA, N., SASHIKATA, K., NISHIMURA, T. & UMEZAWA, H. (1964). *Biochem. biophys. Res. Commun.* **16,** 216.
TOIVAKKA, E. & HOKKANEN, E. (1965). *Acta neurol. Scand.* **41,** Suppl. **13,** 275.
WAKSMAN, S. A. & CURTIS, R. E. (1916). *Soil Sci.* **1,** 99.
WAKSMAN, S. A. & LECHEVALIER, H. (1953). *Guide to the Classification and Identification of the Actinomycetes and their Antibiotics.* Baltimore: The Williams and Wilkins Co.
WAKSMAN, S. A. & WOODRUFF, H. B. (1942). *Proc. Soc. exp. Biol.* (*N.Y.*) **49,** 207.
YAMADA, T., TIPPER, D. & DAVIES, J. (1968). *Nature (Lond.)* **219,** 288.
ZIMMERMANN, R. A.. MOELLERING, R. C. Jr. & WEINBERG, A. N. (1971). *J. Bact.* **105,** 873.

CHAPTER 7

OTHER AMINOGLYCOSIDES

A series of further antibiotics has been discovered, now totalling six, sharing with streptomycin a similar chemical structure, the same general range of anti-bacterial activity, the same pharmacological behaviour, and a tendency to damage one or other branch of the eighth nerve. There is also some tendency to cause renal damage, or at least to impair further the function of an already damaged kidney. The degree of toxicity varies; in some it is such as to preclude systemic use.

All are bases, of which the sulphates are usually employed in therapeutics. They will be described in the order of their discovery.

NEOMYCIN

NEOMYCIN, or more accurately the neomycin complex, was first isolated by Waksman and Lechevalier in 1949 from a strain of *Streptomyces fradiae*. The crude material has been shown to contain two chemically similar, biologically active components, neomycins B and C, of which commercial preparations are a mixture.

Anti-bacterial Activity

A general conspectus of the range of activity not only of neomycin but of the whole of this group of antibiotics may be obtained from the original observations detailed in Table 17. It will be seen that that of neomycin differs very little from that of streptomycin. An important omission from this Table is *Myco. tuberculosis*. This species is sensitive to all the aminoglycosides, and three of them other than streptomycin have been used for the treatment of tuberculosis, although not always with happy results.

The effect exerted is rapidly bactericidal like that of streptomycin, and activity is greater on the alkaline side of neutrality. but the degree of pH effect differs. The -fold differences in activity (against *Staph. aureus*) between media of pH 5·5 and

TABLE 17

Mean* Minimum Inhibitory Concentrations (µg. per ml.) of Aminoglycoside Antibiotics

	No. of Strains	Strepto-mycin	Neomycin	Kanamycin	Framycetin	Paromo-mycin	Genta-micin
Staph. aureus	29	2	0·5	1	0·5	1	0·125
Str. faecalis	32	64	64	32	64	64	8
Esch. coli	22	8	8	4	8	8	1
Klebsiella spp.	20	4	2	2	2	2	1
Aerobacter spp.	10	4	2	2	2	2	0·5
P. mirabilis	6	8	8	4	8	8	2
P. vulgaris	6	4	4	4	4	4	1
P. morgani	10	8	8	4	8	4	1
P. rettgeri	7	4	8	2	8	4	1
Ps. aeruginosa	31	32	32	128	32	512	4
Salmonella spp.	14	16	2	2	2	2	1
Shigella spp.	17	8	8	4	8	8	2

* Tests mainly of recent isolates at Hammersmith Hospital by plate dilution method with 2-fold differences. Means are of log₂ of M.I.C. to the nearest log₂. In the series tested strains showing a clearly abnormal degree of resistance (sometimes following treatment with the antibiotic) were omitted from these calculations.

8·5 found by Garrod (1959) were for streptomycin 512, neomycin 64, framycetin 32, kanamycin 16 and paromomycin 8. Gentamicin and tobramycin are similarly affected by pH.

Acquired Resistance

This may also be considered for the group as a whole. The single step mutation to high resistance to streptomycin is not seen with other aminoglycosides; resistance is acquired slowly, although some change may be seen during the treatment of an individual patient. Frequent and long-continued use for a particular purpose certainly seems liable eventually to generate resistance in the pathogen at which it is aimed. The treatment of nasal staphylococcus carriers has had this effect (Harrison, Beavon and Griffin, 1959; Quie, Collin and Cardle, 1960), and in some hospitals resistance in staphylococci is now not uncommon. The use of Polybactrin spray (neomycin-bacitracin-polymyxin) may well have contributed largely to this: a majority of the numerous strains resistant to neomycin and kanamycin examined by Barber and Waterworth (1966) were also resistant to bacitracin. An epidemic of infection by a resistant strain in a Burns Unit where neomycin was being used locally and kanamycin systemically is described by Lowbury et al. (1964): this was a single organism described as ' an atypical 83A', and colonized burns in a majority of patients treated with these antibiotics, but was found in few patients not so treated, and disappeared when their use was given up. This is by no means the only instance in which the administration of an antibiotic has apparently favoured colonization or infection by staphylococci resistant to it: other examples are described by Knight and Holzer (1954) and Simon (1963).

Among enterobacteria, strains of *E. coli* from infants, and of this and other organisms from patients with urinary tract infections, treated with kanamycin, are now not uncommonly resistant. Resistance has also been seen in enterobacteria from the faeces of patients treated orally: we ourselves have found resistant strains of *Proteus* in patients given neomycin for preoperative bowel preparation. The time may come, if liberal oral use for this and other purposes continues, when this group, and kanamycin in particular, can no longer be relied on for treating *Proteus* infections. It is now becoming recognized that

the indiscriminate use of gentamicin, to which most strains of
E. coli and other organisms are still sensitive, may alter this
situation for the worse.

Cross-resistance

Most naturally occurring resistant strains, and all those
trained to resistance *in vitro*, are almost equally resistant to all
four earlier members of this group (Kunin *et al.*, 1958; Andrieu
et al., 1959). On the other hand we have seen strains of enterobacteria which have become resistant, particularly after oral
treatment, only to the antibiotic used and not to other members
of this group. Resistant strains of *Staph. aureus* are usually
more resistant to kanamycin than to neomycin: the converse
has not been seen (Barber and Waterworth, 1966). There is a
less close relationship with streptomycin, which tends to be
one-way: i.e. training to resistance to any of the neomycin group
produces a substantial increase in resistance to streptomycin,

TABLE 18

Cross Resistance among Antibiotics of the Neomycin Group
Index* of Increase in Resistance to

Antibiotic to which habituated	Streptomycin	Neomycin	Framycetin	Kanamycin	Paromomycin
Streptomycin	10	5	4	5	5
Neomycin	6	8	8	8	8
Framycetin	6	8	8	9	10
Kanamycin	6	9	9	10	9
Paromomycin	6	8	8	8	9

* e.g. $8 =$ Increased 2^8 fold (i.e. 256-fold).

but when streptomycin resistance is induced, the increase in
resistance to the neomycin group is much less. Naturally occurring resistance is even less closely related, or not at all, in that
streptomycin-resistant bacteria may be fully sensitive to neomycin. Resistance to gentamicin and tobramycin is distinct
from that to the earlier aminoglycosides.

A typical example of the results of training may be seen in Table 18. A 1,024-fold increase in resistance to streptomycin resulted in no more than a 32-fold increase in resistance to the other four antibiotics, but training to each of these raised streptomycin resistance to a relatively greater degree, as well as producing approximately the same level of resistance in all four.

Pharmacokinetics

Neomycin behaves like streptomycin and other aminoglycosides. Very little absorption occurs after oral administration; the antibiotic retains its activity in the gut and is eliminated unchanged in the faeces. Distribution and excretion after intramuscular injection are as for streptomycin, but systemic administration has now been almost entirely abandoned.

Toxicity

Neomycin is the most liable of all this group to damage the auditory branch of the eighth nerve. It was originally welcomed as a second line drug for treating tuberculosis, but deafness so often resulted that this treatment soon fell into disrepute. Since then a remarkable number of uses have been found for it which entail little or no risk of toxic effects.

Clinical Applications

It should be understood that for many of the purposes here described, other members of this group are alternatives.

TOPICAL APPLICATION. Neomycin is a valuable agent for the local treatment of superficial infections with staphylococci and many Gram-negative bacilli. To avoid the development of resistant strains it is best used in combination with another agent, such as bacitracin, chlorhexidine or, for infection due to *Ps. aeruginosa*, polymyxin. Neomycin in combination with chlorhexidine or bacitracin is also useful in the treatment of staphylococcal nasal carriers. The recent appearance of neomycin-resistant strains has reduced the value of this proceeding.

Prolonged application to skin lesions of either neomycin or framycetin may cause sensitization, usually to both antibiotics (Kirton and Munro-Ashman, 1965).

5

ORAL ADMINISTRATION. This has three distinct objects, one being the treatment of an acute intestinal infection. There is dispute about the efficacy of neomycin or kanamycin in infantile gastro-enteritis due to pathogenic *E. coli* and in any case resistant strains are now common. It is doubtful whether benefit can be expected in *Salmonella* or mild *Shigella* infections, and results as regards elimination of the subsequent carrier state have been disappointing. The supposedly synergic combination of neomycin with ampicillin also failed in this task in the hands of Pettersson, Klemola and Wager (1964).

Neomycin is also useful as an intestinal antiseptic prior to abdominal surgery, for which purpose it may be administered with sulphathalidine or bacitracin (p. 372). Finally oral neomycin has been extensively used for suppressing the intestinal flora in hepatic failure. Large doses so administered for long periods are not without risk of causing deafness (see p. 373). In connection with any long-continued administration, it should be recognized that atrophic changes in the intestinal mucosa may result, with malabsorption of fats and carbohydrates (Jacobson and Faloon, 1961). According to Cheng and White (1962) there is also interference with the absorption of phenoxymethyl penicillin.

INHALATION. Neomycin aerosol is strongly commended by some authors for the treatment of bronchial infections, particularly bronchiectasis. The antibiotic is absorbed from the lung, and if this treatment is overdone, deafness may result.

INTRAPERITONEAL APPLICATION. Neomycin has been introduced into the peritoneal cavity at operation for the prevention or treatment of peritonitis, sometimes in what appear to be excessive amounts (2-3 g. or even more): respiratory depression or apnoea may result. Craig *et al.* (1966) review reports of this effect and describe experiments in dogs showing that neomycin potentiates the action of muscle relaxants.

INTRAVESICAL APPLICATION. Neomycin solution may be introduced into the urinary bladder after cystoscopy etc. to kill any bacteria accidentally introduced. Thornton, Lytton and Andriole (1966) commend irrigation with a solution containing 40 mg. neomycin and 20 mg. polymyxin B per l. for preventing the establishment of infection during catheter drainage prolonged up to 10 days.

FRAMYCETIN

FRAMYCETIN. In 1947 Decaris noticed a pink mould growing on a damp patch on the wall of his home in Paris. He cultivated the mould and identified it as a strain of *Streptomyces lavendulae* and found that culture filtrates were bactericidal for many species of Gram-positive and Gram-negative bacteria. These findings were not published until 1953 (Decaris, 1953). Further extraction and purification of the antibiotic were carried out in the research laboratories of Roussel. According to Rinehart *et al.* (1960) framycetin is identical with neomycin B, but this is disputed by the manufacturers. Framycetin differs in any case from neomycin, since the latter is a mixture of B and C.

In France framycetin is sometimes injected intrathecally as part of the treatment of acute meningitis. Otherwise administration has been topical or oral. Skin infections and nasal carriers of staphylococci have been treated as with neomycin, and *E. coli* enteritis has been successfully treated.

Framycetin has also been recommended for suppression of the intestinal flora prior to operation (Shidlovsky, Marmell and Prigot, 1956). It was compared for this purpose by Stratford and Dixson (1964) with a larger dose of neomycin and found nevertheless to be superior to it: *E. coli, Str. faecalis* and even *Cl. welchii* totally disappeared from the faeces of 10 out of 12 patients given framycetin, but from only 8 out of 17 of those given neomycin. Results in the treatment of post-operative infection were also better in a small series.

KANAMYCIN

This antibiotic was isolated in Japan from a strain of *Streptomyces kanamyceticus* (Umezawa *et al.*, 1957). It differs little from neomycin in anti-bacterial activity (Table 17), but that against all species of *Proteus* is noteworthy, and like neomycin can cause deafness, but its liability to produce this effect is so considerably less that carefully controlled parenteral administration is justifiable. An interesting contrast is afforded by two cases of enterococcal endocarditis described by Garrod and Waterworth (1962) for whom the usual combination of penicillin and streptomycin was unsuitable owing to very high bacterial resistance to the latter. Neomycin was substituted in one and kanamycin in the other, each given in a dose of 1 g. daily for six weeks. The patients were of approximately the same age, and both recovered, but whereas the neomycin caused total deafness, the hearing of the patient given kanamycin was unaffected.

Oral and Topical Applications

The uses which kanamycin shares with others of this group are the treatment of infantile gastro-enteritis and the suppression of the bowel flora, whether pre-operatively or in patients with hepatic disease.

Like neomycin it has been introduced into the peritoneal cavity, but with a more limited object and in more reasonable amounts. Cohn, Cotlar and Richard (1963) treated 360 patients, most with established peritonitis, by local instillation (1 g. in 50 ml. for an adult) with what are claimed to be excellent results: the treatment is specially commended for young children with peritonitis complicating appendicitis.

Parenteral Administration

In patients with good renal function kanamycin can safely be given intramuscularly in a total dose of 1 g. daily for 7 to 10 days, or longer with precautions. The main indication for it is an infection of the urinary tract or elsewhere with coliform organisms, particularly *Proteus* spp., resistant to other drugs. Murdoch, Geddes and Syme (1962) recorded complete cure in 50 out of 55 patients with such infections, including 5 with septicaemia. Murdoch *et al.* (1966) bring this series up to 228, including 49 clinically septicaemic cases (21 confirmed by blood culture), many with shock, among whom the mortality was only 9·5 per cent. A dose of 1 g. daily was not exceeded, and sometimes reduced, and given for not more than 14 days. No toxic effects were seen.

On the other hand, if renal function is sufficiently impaired deafness can be caused by a total dose of less than 10 g. (Erlanson and Lundgren, 1964). Renal insufficiency is unfortunately common in the intractable urinary infections for which this antibiotic is indicated, and the utmost care is necessary both in assessing renal efficiency and controlling dosage accordingly, verifying that it is not excessive by blood assays. Atuk, Mosca and Kunin (1964) treated 10 uraemic patients in this way without toxic effects. A scheme for prolonging the interval between doses in accordance with the serum creatinine level is proposed by Sørensen et al. (1967). Mawer et al. (1972) advocate the use of a computer to calculate the dose on a similar basis.

Kanamycin is also a recognized second line drug for the treatment of tuberculosis; here administration at longer intervals diminishes the risk of toxic effects.

PAROMOMYCIN

This antibiotic was first described by Haskell, French and Bartz (1959). The following differently named substances are identical with it (Schillings and Schaffner, 1962); aminosidine (marketed in Italy as Gabbromycina), catenulin and hydroxymycin.

Clinical reports on the use of this antibiotic refer mainly to oral administration. Good results in various forms of enteritis are claimed by Mössner (1962). A convincing account of effects in acute infantile enteritis by Kahn, Stein and Wayburne (1963) is referred to in Chapter 21. According to Weinstein, Samet and Meade (1961) paromomycin is superior to neomycin in suppressing the bowel flora, but they made no direct comparison of the two, and their bacterial counts in faeces before administering paromomycin (up to 10^{18} aerobes per g.) are impossibly high. Like neomycin, it can cause intestinal malabsorption (Keusch, Troncale and Buchanan, 1970).

The main difference between paromomycin and other aminoglycosides is its activity against E. histolytica. Excellent results were reported with paromomycin in an extensive study involving treatment of 432 patients with amoebic dysentery in 12 different countries in Asia, Africa and the Americas (Courtney et al., 1960). Another peculiar use is as an anthelmintic. In the hands of Wittner and Tanowitz (1971) a single oral dose of 4 g. regularly eliminated T. saginata, T. solium and D. latum; repeated doses were often necessary for H. nana.

Since paromomycin is not recommended for systemic use, it is presumably regarded as too toxic for this purpose, but it is interesting that Teik and Siew (1964) treated 7 severe staphylococcal infections with intramuscular aminosidine (paromomycin) without causing deafness, possibly because the total dose given never exceeded 15 g.

GENTAMICIN

This antibiotic was discovered in 1963 as the product of a strain of *Micromonospora purpurea*. (Its name is so spelt because the termination ' mycin ' should be considered to denote derivation from a *Streptomyces*). It is the most active of the entire group, and is now being used for a great variety of purposes, sometimes in place of other aminoglycosides. As naturally formed gentamicin contains several components, of which those designated C1, C1a and C2 are required by U.S.A. regulations to be present in the commercial product in certain flexible proportions. Gentamycin A (referred to on p. 264) is unimportant, and the product contains little or none of it.

Anti-bacterial Activity

It will be evident from Table 17 that gentamicin is more active than other aminoglycosides against all species listed. According to Weinstein *et al.* (1964) the inhibitory concentration of gentamicin is lower than that of neomycin or kanamycin for all enterobacteria tested, including species of *Aerobacter, Escherichia, Klebsiella* and *Salmonella. Proteus* spp. are also sensitive, but *P. vulgaris* least so.

Serratia spp. are also more sensitive to gentamicin than to other antibiotics, and according to Denis and Brisou (1971) are even more so to the combined action of gentamicin and carbenicillin. The most significant activity is against *Ps. aeruginosa,* shown by these authors to be 5-10 times greater than that of neomycin or kanamycin. This is fully confirmed by Barber and Waterworth (1966), who examined 25 recently isolated strains and found them decidedly more sensitive to gentamicin than to either kanamycin or streptomycin.

The actual M.I.C. of gentamicin for sensitive strains of *Ps. aeruginosa* found by different workers varies considerably. The probable explanation for this has been proposed by Garrod and Waterworth (1969) who found that the result of any such test can vary as much as 32-fold with the magnesium content of the medium: Mg, which is essential for the growth of this species and enhances its pigment production, also with increasing concentration reduces its apparent sensitivity to this antibiotic. Since this is a factor very difficult to control, the test is better conducted by direct comparison with another strain of the same organism having a known normal sensitivity.

Activity against streptococci is only moderate, although again claimed to exceed that of neomycin or kanamycin. Watanakunakorn (1971) examined 100 strains of enterococci, and not only were all inhibited by 50 μg./ml. gentamicin or less, but all were subject to synergic bactericidal action by gentamicin + penicillin, whereas some, resistant to streptomycin, were not so affected by the combination of this antibiotic with penicillin, an observation to be borne in mind in connection with the treatment of enterococcal endocarditis. The main Gram-positive species of therapeutic interest is *Staph. aureus,* in connection with which the findings of Barber and Waterworth (1966) are both extensive and decisive. They tested 102 strains with normal sensitivity to kanamycin (M.I.C. most often 1 μg. per ml.) and found gentamicin four times more active (M.I.C. of majority 0·25 μg. per ml.). They also tested 57 strains resistant to both kanamycin and neomycin (the majority also to bacitracin) and found that with two minor exceptions their sensitivity to gentamicin was normal. Naturally acquired resistance to neomycin and kanamycin may therefore be unaccompanied by resistance to gentamicin. It was shown by these authors in training experiments that a considerable degree of crossing results when resistance is artificially produced.

The action of gentamicin is bactericidal, and influenced in the usual way by pH, but to different degrees according to bacterial species (Rubenis, Kozij and Jackson, 1964); these authors also showed that high concentrations of NaCl greatly depress its activity.

Resistance to gentamicin in normally sensitive species is still uncommon, but may be transmissible. The R factor responsible inactivates the antibiotic (Davies, 1971).

Pharmacokinetics. Like the rest of this group gentamicin is almost unabsorbed from the alimentary tract, and is administered by intramuscular injection. Absorption, distribution and excretion also do not materially differ, but owing to the relatively small dose usually given the duration of an effective blood level may be less. Excretion is mainly renal, over 80 per cent being recoverable from the urine. Gentamicin traverses the placenta, attaining a concentration in the foetal blood about one third of that in the maternal (Yoshioka, Monma and Matsuda, 1972). In the newborn infant, like many other antibiotics, it is excreted slowly, and dosage should be adjusted accordingly (Rohwedder and Goll, 1970; McCracken, West and Horton, 1971).

Carbenicillin is now often given with gentamicin, and McLaughlin and Reeves (1971) have shown that when the two are mixed in an intravenous fluid and the concentration of carbenicillin is much the higher, the gentamicin is progressively inactivated. This is a somewhat unexpected finding, since in another mixture, that of methicillin and kanamycin, it is the penicillin and not the aminoglycoside which suffers. These authors also claim to have obtained evidence of similar inactivation *in vivo*. Further work has amply confirmed the first of these observations but not the second. Noone and Pattison (1971) found that when the antibiotics were diluted in serum instead of saline the rate of inactivation was so slow as to be immaterial, and Winters *et al.* (1971) in an elaborate study in both animals and patients have shown that a large dose of carbenicillin given during gentamicin therapy does not affect the blood levels of the latter.

The dose originally recommended was 0·5 mg. per kg. (i.e. about 40 mg. for an adult of average weight) at 8-hour intervals. This may suffice for some purposes, but as shown by Darrell and Waterworth (1967) the blood concentration produced by this does not for long exceed the M.I.C. for *Ps. aeruginosa*, and if a systemic effect is required it must clearly be increased. These authors also report that three strains of *Ps. aeruginosa* isolated after unsuccessful treatment on this low scale of dosage had become more resistant. It is now usually considered that a dose of 80 mg. three times a day is safe if renal function is normal.

Toxicity

Gentamicin is ototoxic, vestibular function being that usually affected. To what extent it is also nephrotoxic is disputed, but at least this effect is rare. It seems originally to have been assumed that the enhanced anti-bacterial activity of gentamicin in comparison with other aminoglycosides is paralleled by an equal enhancement of ototoxicity, and a lower scale of dosage was decided on accordingly. The original scale suggested carried caution too far. In our experience the present normal dosage has never proved ototoxic in patients with good renal function, and in the series of 57 patients reported by Jao and Jackson (1964), of 5 who suffered various degrees of loss of labyrinthine function, 4 had raised blood ureas, and the fifth had had to be given large doses to overcome *Pseudomonas* septicaemia. Nevertheless it must be recognized that gentamicin is more ototoxic than, say, kanamycin, if it be accepted that the safe upper limit for the blood level is 10 μg./ml., and this is frequently stated and generally believed.

This subject is placed in proper perspective by the extensive study of Jackson and Arcieri (1971). They found the overall incidence of ototoxicity to have been 2 per cent; vestibular damage occurred in 66 per cent of these, auditory in 16 per cent and both in 18 per cent. Analysis of 913 courses of treatment, in 70 of which damage occurred, showed its main determinant to be impaired renal function. A very important conclusion is that duration of treatment was without effect. A dose of 2·6 mg./kg. daily, but not one of 3·4 mg./kg., is safe if renal function is normal; this limitation is rather surprising, and it may be doubted whether some of the patients on whose records it is based had in fact normal renal function.

In patients at risk, the blood level can be kept within safe limits by lengthening the interval between doses of 80 mg. from 8 hours to as long as 48 hours in accordance with the degree of impairment of renal function (Gingell and Waterworth, 1968). During such treatment it should be verified by blood assays that the expected levels are not being exceeded. Although such assays are sometimes essential, they need not be done either as frequently or in so large a proportion of patients as is suggested by Stratford and Dixson (1971).

Clinical Applications

These are referred to elsewhere in this book, but may be briefly summarized here. The principal field for gentamicin treatment, which has clearly increased in scope and popularity in the past few years, is serious coliform infections in various sites. In the urinary tract it is particularly indicated for *Ps. aeruginosa* infection. In Gram-negative septicaemia many workers now regard gentamicin as the antibiotic of choice; Cox and Harrison (1971) and Holloway and Taylor (1971) obtained results with it as good as those with kanamycin, usually combined with polymyxin B. Martin *et al.* (1969) commend for this purpose a combination of gentamicin and cephaloridine. In systemic *Ps. aeruginosa* infections it is advisable to combine gentamicin with large doses of carbenicillin. Among rather diverse findings on the behaviour of this combination, the majority point to a synergic action on most strains, not only *in vitro* (Yuce and van Rooyen, 1971) but *in vivo* (Andriole, 1971).

A noteworthy feature of recent therapeutic studies has been success in treating these infections in neonates. In three of the cases of septicaemia reported by McCracken and Jones (1970) the condition had developed during treatment with kanamycin and penicillin; gentamicin was successful in two of them. Klein *et al.* (1971), reporting similar experience, advocate a dose of 3 mg./kg every 12 hours; no toxic effects have been seen by these or other authors. The conditions successfully treated in infants include meningitis, for which intrathecal injection may be necessary. Two cases of *Ps. aeruginosa* meningitis in adults were successfully treated with gentamicin and other antibiotics by Helm and Stille (1971). Gatmaitan, Carruthers and Lerner (1970) reduced the usual mortality of Gram-negative pneumonia from 49 to 31 per cent by treatment with gentamicin. It should be remembered that another organism highly sensitive to gentamicin is *Staph. aureus,* and Richards, McCall and Cox (1971) report success with it in various staphylococcal infections, some severe.

Various forms of local application have been successful, the effect evidently being mainly or wholly on the highly sensitive staphylococcus. A 0·1 per cent cream has been used for burns, bedsores, various forms of dermatitis and for the nasal staphylococcus carrier state. Oral administration for pre-operative suppression of the bowel flora is said to be successful with much smaller doses than those of neomycin used for this purpose.

Tobramycin

The history of this antibiotic goes back six years, to the description by Wick and Welles (1968) of nebramycin, the product of a strain of *Streptomyces tenebrarius*, so named because of its sensitivity to light. At least seven factors were identified in this, of which that numbered 6 had the most desirable properties, and it is this which is now known as tobramycin. The outsanding property of this antibiotic is an activity against *Ps. aeruginosa* exceeding that of gentamicin by about two-fold, and retained against some gentamicin-resistant strains (Meyer, Young and Armstrong, 1971; Traub and Raymond, 1972). The first of these papers also reports synergy with carbenicillin against a few of the strains examined. This superiority applies to no other species; staphylococci are about equally sensitive to both, various enterobacteria generally rather more sensitive to gentamicin, and *S. marcescens* more so by four-fold.

The fullest information about the anti-bacterial activity of tobramycin under different conditions and in comparison with other aminoglycosides is in a recent paper by Waterworth (1972). These studies include one of the combined bactericidal action of tobramycin and carbenicillin on *Ps. aeruginosa* by means of serial viable counts, showing that each antibiotic alone and lower concentrations of the combination caused a steep initial fall followed by re-growth. The M.I.C. of survivors in these tests was re-determined and found to have increased. Carbenicillin 100 μg./ml. + tobramycin 0·5 μg./ml. was totally bactericidal, and it is concluded that in these concentrations each antibiotic is able to kill the small minority of mutants resistant to the other.

Black and Griffith (1971) report a pharmacological study in which single doses of 25, 50 and 75 mg. were given intramuscularly to volunteers. The curve of blood levels follows the same pattern as that of other aminoglycosides, but urinary recovery in

24 hours amounted only to 16-36 per cent of the dose. At the time of writing there is no other published information on which to base an assessment of possible clinical utility.

PHARMACEUTICAL PREPARATIONS

NEOMYCIN SULPHATE (' Mycifradin ', *Upjohn;* 'Neomycin ', *Glaxo;* 'Nivemycin ', *Boots).* Supplied as tablets containing 500 mg. for oral administration: usual dose 4-6 g. daily, and in vials of 500 mg. sterile powder for parenteral administration, the dose not normally exceeding 1 g. daily: also in numerous creams, powders, etc. for local application, often combined with other antibacterial substances. In future, doses are to be stated in units. The minimum acceptable potency of a preparation is 650 units per mg.

KANAMYCIN SULPHATE ('Kannasyn ', *Bayer;* 'Kantrex ', *Bristol Laboratories,.* Available for parenteral administration in vials containing 1·43 g. (= 1 g. kanamycin base) (Kannasyn), or in vials of a stable aqueous solution containing 500 mg. in 2 ml. or 1 g. in 3 ml. (Kantrex Injection). Usual dose 1 g. daily. Also in capsules or suspension for oral administration: usual dose up to 2 g. daily for intestinal infections and up to 6 g. daily for a short period for pre-operative bowel preparation.

FRAMYCETIN SULPHATE ('Soframycin ', *Roussel).* Tablets of 250 mg. for oral administration: dosage as for kanamycin. Also as ointment, nasal spray solution, etc.

PAROMOMYCIN SULPHATE ('Humatin ', *Parke Davis).* Capsules of 250 mg. and syrup for oral administration: dosage similar to the foregoing.

GENTAMICIN SULPHATE ('Garamycin ', *Schering Corporation;* 'Genticin ', *British Schering;* 'Cidomycin ', *Roussel).* Genticin and Cidomycin are supplied for intramuscular injection in vials containing a solution of 80 mg. of the base in 2 ml. with certain excipients.

REFERENCES

ANDRIEU, G., MONNIER, J. & BOURSE, R. (1959). *Pr. méd.* **67**. 718.
ANDRIOLE, V. T. (1971). *J. infect. Dis.* **124,** Dec. Suppl. 46.
ATUK, N. O., MOSCA, A. & KUNIN, C. (1964). *Ann. intern. Med.* **60,** 28.
BARBER, M. & WATERWORTH. P. M. (1966). *Brit. med. J.* **1,** 203.
BLACK, H. R. & GRIFFITH, R. S. (1971). *Antimicrobiotic Agents and Chemotherapy*—1970, 314
CHENG, S. H. & WHITE, A. (1962). *New Engl. J. Med.* **267,** 1296
COHN, I., COTLAR, A. M. & RICHARD, L. (1963). *Amer. Surg.* **29,** 756.
COURTNEY, K. O., THOMPSON. P. E., HODGKINSON, R. & FITZSIMMONS, J. R. (1960). *Antibiot. Ann.* 1959-60, p. 304.
COX, C. E. & HARRISON, L. H. (1971). *J. infect. Dis.* **124,** Suppl., Dec. 156.
CRAIG, H. V., GUILLET, G. G., WALKER, J. A. & ARTZ. C. P. (1966). *Amer. Surg.* **32,** 27.
DARRELL. J. H. & WATERWORTH, P. M. (1967). *Brit. med. J.* **2,** 535.
DAVIES, J. (1971). *J. infect. Dis.* **124,** Dec. Suppl., 7.
DECARIS. L. J. (1953). *Ann. Pharmacol. franç.* **2,** 44.
DENIS, F. & BRISOU, J. (1971). *Arch. Roum. Path. exp. Microbiol.* **30,** 209.
ERLANSON, P. & LUNDGREN, A. (1964). *Acta med. scand.* **176,** 147.
GARROD, L. P. (1959). *Royal College of Physicians of Edinburgh,* Publication No. 11.
GARROD, L. P. & WATERWORTH, P. M. (1962). *J. clin. Path.* **15,** 328.
GARROD, L. P. & WATERWORTH, P. M. (1969). *J. clin. Path.* **22,** 534.
GATMAITAN, B. G., CARRUTHERS, M. M. & LERNER, A. M. (1970). *Amer. J. med. Sci.* **260,** 90.
GINGELL, J. C. & WATERWORTH, P. M. (1968). *Brit. med. J.* **2,** 19.

HARRISON, K. J., BEAVON, J. & GRIFFIN, E. (1959). *Lancet* 1, 908.
HASKELL, T. H., FRENCH, J. C. & BARTZ, Q. R. (1959). *J. Amer. chem. Soc.* 81, 3480, 3481, 3482.
HELM, E. & STILLE, W. (1971). *Dtsch. med. Wschr.* 96, 1435.
HOLLOWAY, W. J. & TAYLOR, W. A. (1971). *J. infect. Dis.* Dec. Suppl., 180, JACKSON, G. G. & ARCIERI, G. (1971). *J. infect Dis.* Suppl., Dec. 130.
JACOBSON, E. D. & FALOON, W. W. (1961). *J. Amer. med. Ass.* 175, 187.
JAO, R. L. & JACKSON, G. G. (1964). *J. Amer. med Ass.* 189, 817.
KAHN, E., STEIN, H. & WAYBURNE, S. (1963). *Lancet* 2, 703.
KEUSCH, G. T., TRONCALE, F. J. & BUCHANAN, R. D. (1970). *Arch. intern. Med.* 125, 273.
KIRTON, V. & MUNRO-ASHMAN, D. (1965). *Lancet* 1, 138.
KLEIN, J. O., HERSCHEL, M., THERAKAN, R. M. & INGALL, D. (1971). *J. infect. Dis.* 124, Dec. Suppl., 224.
KNIGHT, V. & HOLZER, A. R. (1954). *J. clin. Invest.* 33, 1190.
KUNIN, C. M., WILCOX, C., NAJARIAN, A. & FINLAND, M. (1958). *Proc. Soc. exp. Biol. (N.Y.)* 99, 312.
LOWBURY, E. J. L., BABB, J. R., BROWN, V. I. & COLLINS, B. J. (1964). *J. Hyg. (Lond.)* 62, 221.
MARTIN, C. M., CUOMO, A. J., GERAGHTY, M. J., ZAGER, J. R. & MANDES, T. C. (1969). *J. infect. Dis.*, 119, 506.
MAWER, G. E., KNOWLES, B. R., LUCAS, S. B., STIRLAND, R. M. & TOOTH, J. A. (1972). *Lancet* 1, 12.
MCCRACKEN, G. H. JR. & JONES, L. G. (1970). *Amer. J. Dis. Child.* 120, 524.
MCCRACKEN, G. H., WEST, N. R. & HORTON, L. J. (1971). *J. infect. Dis.* 123, 257.
MCLAUGHLIN, J. E. & REEVES, D. S. (1971). *Lancet* 1, 261.
MEYER, R. D., YOUNG, L. S. & ARMSTRONG, D. (1971). *Appl. Microbiol.* 22, 1147.
MÖSSNER, G. (1962). *Dtsch. med. Wschr.* 87, 185.
MURDOCH, J. McC., GEDDES, A. M. & SYME, J. (1962). *Lancet* 1, 457.
MURDOCH, J. McC., GRAY, J. A., GEDDES, A. M. & WALLACE, E. T. (1966). *Annal. New York Acad. Sci.* 132, 842.
NOONE, P. & PATTISON, J. R. (1971). *Lancet* 2, 575.
PETTERSSON, T., KLEMOLA, E. & WAGER, O. (1964). *Acta med. scand.* 175, 185.
QUIE, P. G., COLLIN, M. & CARDLE, J. B. (1960). *Lancet* 2, 124.
RICHARDS, F., MCCALL, C. & COX, C. (1971). *J. Amer. med. Ass.* 215, 1297.
RINEHART, K. L. JR., ARGOUDELIS, A. D., GOSS, W. A., SOHLER, A. & SCHAFFNER, C. P. (1960). *J. Amer. chem. Soc.* 82, 3938.
ROGERS, K. B., BENSON, R. P., FOSTER, W. P., JONES, L. E., BUTLER, E. B. & WILLIAMS, T. C. (1956). *Lancet* 2, 599.
ROHWEDDER, H.-J. & GOLL, U. (1970). *Dtsch. med. Wschr.* 95, 1171.
RUBENIS, M., KOZIJ, V. M. & JACKSON, G. G. (1964). *Antimicrob. Agents and Chemother.*—1963, p. 153.
SCHILLINGS, R. T. & SCHAFFNER, C. P. (1962). *Antimicrob. Agents and Chemother.*—1961, p. 274.
SHIDLOVSKY, B. A., MARMELL, M. & PRIGOT, A. (1956). *Antibiot. Ann.* 1955-6, p. 118.
SIMON, H. J. (1963). *Proc. Soc. exp. Biol. (N.Y.)* 113, 518.
SØRENEN, A. W. S., SZABO, L., PEDERSEN, A. & SCHARFF, A. (1967). *Postgrad. med. J.*, 1967 Suppl. ' The Clinical Aspects of Kanamycin ', p. 37.
STRATFORD, B. C. & DIXSON, S. (1964). *Med. J. Aust.* 1, 74.
STRATFORD, B. C. & DIXSON, S. (1971). *Med. J. Aust.* 1, 1107.
TEIK, K. O. & SIEW, L. G. (1964). *Med. J. Malaya* 19, 8.
THORNTON, G. F., LYTTON, B. & ANDRIOLE, V. T. (1966). *J. Amer. med. Ass.* 195, 179.
TRAUB, W. H. & RAYMOND, E. A. (1972). *Appl. Microbiol.* 23, 4.

132 ANTIBIOTIC AND CHEMOTHERAPY

UMEZAWA, H., UEDA, M., MAEDA, K., YAGISHITA, K., KONDÖ, S., OKAMI, Y., UTAHARA, R., ÖSATO, Y., NITTA, K. & TAKEUCHI, T. (1957). *J. Antibiot. (Tokyo). Series A.* **10**, 181.
WAKSMAN, S. A. & LECHEVALIER, H. A. (1949). *Science* **109**, 305.
WATANAKUNAKORN, C. (1971). *J. infect. Dis.* **124**, 581.
WATERWORTH, P. M. (1972). *J. clin. Path.* **25**, 979.
WEINSTEIN, M. J., LUEDEMANN, G. M., ODEN, E. M. & WAGMAN, G. H. (1964). *Antimicrob. Agents and Chemother.*—1963, p. 1.
WEINSTEIN, L., SAMET, C. A. & MEADE, R. H. (1961). *J. Amer. med. Ass.* **178**, 891.
WICK, W. E. & WELLES, J. S. (1968). *Antimicrobial Agents & Chemotherapy—* 1967, p. 341.
WINTERS, R. E., CHOW, A. W., HECHT, R. H. & HEWITT, W. L. (1971). *Ann. intern. Med.* **75**, 925.
WITTNER, M. & TANOWITZ, H. (1971). *Amer. J. trop. Med. Hyg.* **20**, 433.
YOSHIOKA, H., MONMA, T. & MATSUDA, S. (1972). *J. Pediat.* **80**, 121.
YUCE, K. & van ROOYEN, C. E. (1971). *Canad. med. Ass. J.* **105**, 919.

CHAPTER 8

CHLORAMPHENICOL

CHLORAMPHENICOL was the first broad spectrum antibiotic to be discovered. It was isolated independently by Ehrlich *et al.* (1947) from a streptomycete (*S. venezuelae*) from soil in Venezuela and by Carter *et al.* (1948) from a similar organism found in a sample of soil from a compost heap in Illinois. A method of synthesizing chloramphenicol from *p*-nitroacetphenone has proved practicable on a large scale, and alone among clinically important antibiotics chloramphenicol is manufactured synthetically.

Chemical Properties

Chloramphenicol consists of yellowish-white crystals with an intensely bitter taste. Its solubility is about 2·5 mg./ml. water and about 400 mg./ml. alcohol. Aqueous solutions have a pH of about 5·5 and are extremely stable. They keep indefinitely at ordinary room temperature if protected from light, and will withstand boiling. Some hydrolysis occurs on autoclaving.

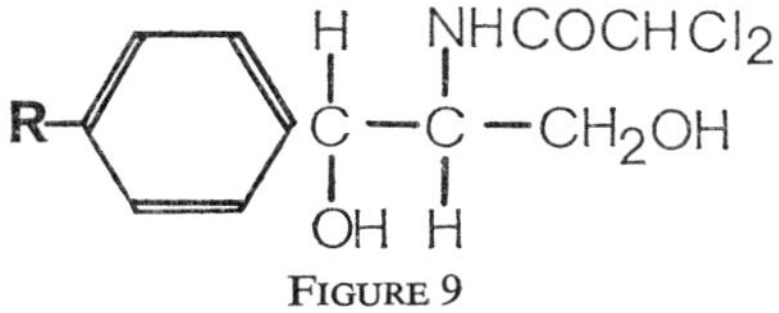

FIGURE 9

Structures of chloramphenicol ($R = NO_2$) and thiamphenicol ($R = CH_2SO_2$)

There are four isomers of chloramphenicol, all of which have been synthesized, but neither its isomers nor the many structurally related compounds which have been synthesized have greater activity than natural chloramphenicol. The side chain is critical to antibacterial activity but contrary to the original view the precise nature of the aromatic ring is of little importance (von Strandtmann *et al.*, 1967).

One antibacterially active derivative, thiamphenicol (Fig. 9: Dextrosulphenicol, Thiomycetin), in which the nitro group of chloramphenicol is replaced by a sulphomethyl group

(Cutler *et al.*, 1952) has received intermittent attention over the years because of potentially advantageous pharmacokinetic behaviour (p. 138) and also because it was originally thought

TABLE 19

Sensitivity of Bacteria to Chloramphenicol

	M.I.C. μg./ml.		M.I.C. μg./ml.
C. diphtheriae	0·5-3·0	H. influenzae	0·2-0·5
Str. pneumoniae	1·0-4·0	Pasteurella spp.	0·2-10
Actino. israeli	1·0-4·0	B. pertussis	0·2-12·5
Clostridium spp.	1·5->500	N. meningitidis	0·5-1·5
Str. pyogenes	2·0-4·0	N. gonorrhoeae	0·5-1·5
B. anthracis	2·5-5·0	Kl. pneumoniae	0·5-2·0
Str. faecalis	4·0-12	Salmonella spp.	0·5-10
Staph. aureus	4·0-12	Kl. aerogenes	0·5-30
Myco. tuberculosis	12-25	Brucella spp.	0·8-2·5
		Esch. coli	0·8-8·0
		Bacteroides spp.	1·0-8·0
		Salm. typhi.	2·0-4·0
		Sh. sonnei.	2·5-6·0
		Proteus spp.	2·5-64
		Ps. aeruginosa	50-125

McLean, I. W. *et al.* (1949). *J. clin. Invest.* **28**, 953.
Chen, C. H. *et al.* (1949). *South. med. J.* **42**, 986.
Garrod, L. P. (1952). *Antibiot. Chemother.* **2**, 689.
Garrod, L. P. (1952). *Brit. med. J.* **1**, 1263.
Garrod, L. P. (1955). *Brit. med. J.* **2**, 1529.
Welch, H. *et al.* (1952). *Antibiot. Chemother.* **2**, 693.

that the toxicity of chloramphenicol hinged on the presence of the nitro group. In fact, thiamphenicol is more, not less, liable than chloramphenicol to depress haemopoiesis although it has been optimistically asserted that this is of the reversible benign variety (p. 142) and not a precursor of potentially fatal aplasia.

Antimicrobial Activity

Chloramphenicol is active against a wide range of Gram-positive and Gram-negative bacteria (Table 19), and chlamydia (p. 486). *Salm. typhi, H. influenzae* and *B. pertussis* are more susceptible to chloramphenicol than to almost any other antibiotic, a fact to be remembered in considering indications for clinical use. Chloramphenicol is strictly bacteristatic against almost all bacterial species including *Brucella, Escherichia,* streptococci, staphylococci and *Salmonella* (Fig. 10).

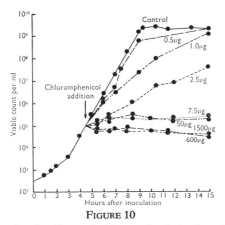

FIGURE 10

The purely bacteristatic effect of chloramphenicol. Growth is slowed or halted but there is no significant decline in the number of viable organisms. (From Brock, 1964.)

The same bacteristatic effect is seen *in vivo*. *Salm typhi* grows rapidly intracellularly and although it can be inhibited within a few minutes of exposure to chloramphenicol, the organism remains viable for long periods and will regrow on removal from the drug. Similar reappearance of the organism when chloramphenicol is withdrawn is seen in the treatment of human typhoid carriers (Woodward and Smadel, 1964).

Acquired Resistance

Resistant strains of various bacterial species have been isolated by serial passage *in vitro* (Reeve and Suttie, 1968). As the concentration of chloramphenicol is increased, mutants resistant at successive genetic loci emerge, and resistance increases in a step-wise fashion. Resistant mutants commonly grow less rapidly than the sensitive parent strain and show antigenic and morphological changes including loss of flagella. Low-order cross-resistance between chloramphenicol and tetracyclines or erythromycin has been described.

Resistance has been seen in many wild strains of both Gram-positive and Gram-negative organisms and the prevalence of resistant strains has often followed faithfully the frequency of usage of the drug.

The chloramphenicol molecule can be attacked at a number of different points by bacteria, and the degradation products have no antibacterial activity. Naturally occurring chloramphenicol-resistant *Staph. aureus* evidently owe their resistance to inactivation of the agent by an inducible acetylase (Shaw and Brodsky, 1968). Such resistance can be spontaneously lost, or ' cured ' by acridines, suggesting a plasmid location for the responsible gene (p. 263). An analogous situation exists in many enterobacteria. In *Escherichia,* where the capacity to acetylate chloramphenicol accounts for the resistance of many clinical isolates, the enzyme is constitutive, that is to say maximum synthesis occurs without prior exposure to the drug, but in this species too the location of the gene controlling synthesis of the enzyme is extrachromosomal, and it may be transferred in conjugation accounting for R factor-mediated resistance (p. 263). Spontaneous chromosomal mutation to high resistance in *Proteus mirabilis* is similarly accompanied by enzyme synthesis. Transfer to such strains of an R factor conferring resistance to chloramphenicol results in additional synthesis of the same enzyme (Shaw, 1971).

The outstandingly important example of transferable chloramphenicol resistance is in the *Salm. typhi* responsible for an outbreak in Mexico and subsequently imported both into Britain and into the U.S.A. (Anderson and Smith, 1972). Chloramphenicol resistance in *Pseudomonas aeruginosa* is apparently not dependent on enzymic destruction of the drug, and the situation in resistant strains of *Proteus, Klebsiella* and *Aerobacter* is variable (Okamoto *et al.,* 1967; Sompolinsky *et al.,* 1968).

Dependent strains which will not grow, or grow very poorly, in the absence of chloramphenicol have also been described.

PHARMACOKINETICS

Absorption and Distribution

The usual route of administration is oral, and the peak blood levels obtained are shown in Table 20. The dissolution and absorption of poorly soluble compounds like chloramphenicol depends to an important extent on size and aggregation of the primary particles. Direct comparisons show that preparations containing large particles may give blood levels

TABLE 20

Serum Levels of Chloramphenicol after Oral Adminstration in Patients of Different Ages

Age	Dose mg./kg.	Peak		Half-life Hours
		Hour	μg./ml.	
Adult	7(0·5 g.)	2-3	8-13	2-5
	30(2 g.)		15-25	
1-2 days	50	6-12	30-40	24-28

Glazko *et al.* (1968) *Clin. Pharmacol. Therap.* **9**, 472.
Weiss *et al.* (1960) *New Engl. J. Med.*, **262**, 787.

only $\frac{1}{4}$-$\frac{1}{2}$ those arising from small particles (Glazko *et al.*, 1968). Reducing or increasing the dose has a proportionate effect on the level attained. This falls comparatively slowly and since there is some cumulative effect, a level of 4-6 μg per ml can be maintained by giving 0·5 g at six-hour intervals, or a correspondingly higher one by raising the dose.

Children can neither swallow the capsules given to adults nor tolerate the exceedingly bitter taste of the free drug. The alternative for them is a suspension of chloramphenicol palmitate, a tasteless compound which is itself inert, and is not absorbed until it is hydrolysed in the gut, liberating chloramphenicol. Chloramphenicol palmitate (and the same is true of the stearate) exists in two distinct crystalline and an amorphous form. Hydrolysis time in the gut is a major determinant of the efficacy of absorption and as one crystalline form is substantially more rapidly hydrolysed than the other, the blood levels obtained are directly related to the proportion of that form which is present in the preparation (Aguiar *et al.*, 1967). Better plasma levels may be obtained if the drug is dispersed in a freely soluble matrix such as urea (Chiou, 1971).

PARENTERAL ADMINISTRATION. Simple suspensions of finely ground chloramphenicol are available which are suitable only for intramuscular injection. Chloramphenicol sodium succinate, on the other hand, which is freely soluble and undergoes hydrolysis in the tissues with the liberation of chloramphenicol, can be injected in a small volume intramuscularly, intravenously or subcutaneously.

The levels of the drug after administration by these routes differ little from those following the same dose by the oral route. The peak level is of course attained immediately after intravenous injection. In contrast to this, the absorption of an intramuscularly injected suspension appears to be slower (peak at 4-5 hours) than that from the bowel, detectable blood levels persisting longer (half-life 4-6 hours).

Distribution

About 60 per cent of the chloramphenicol in the blood is bound to protein. Studies of organ distribution have shown the diminishing order of concentration to be kidney, liver, lung, heart, spleen, muscle and brain. Free diffusion occurs into serous effusions, and into the foetal circulation. Penetration into all parts of the eye has also been demonstrated. Perhaps most important of all, the concentrations attained in the cerebro-spinal fluid are higher than those of any other antibiotic: they amount to 30-50 per cent of those in the blood even in the absence of meningitis. Glandular secretions also contain some of the antibiotic: its presence in the saliva occasions a bitter taste and accounts for changes in the oral flora. Thiamphenicol (p. 133) is said to penetrate particularly well not only into purulent but also into mucoid sputum where it achieves levels bactericidal to *H. influenzae* (Cambieri *et al.*, 1970).

Excretion

Before excretion, most of the chloramphenicol in the body is inactivated either by conjugation with glucuronic acid or by reduction to inactive aryl amines, and the main site of these processes is the liver.

Pre-treatment with phenobarbitone, a potent inducer of the liver microsomal enzymes concerned with glucuronide conjugation, results in diminished blood levels of chloramphenicol and increased urinary excretion of the glucuronide. Blood levels of thiamphenicol which is normally much less conjugated, are correspondingly less affected (Bella *et al.*, 1968). Conversely, it appears that chloramphenicol (in common with other drugs including sulphaphenazole, phenylbutazone and dicoumarol) depresses microsomal enzyme activity so that the levels of some unrelated drugs metabolized by the same pathway may be raised. Toxicity from diphenylhydantoin and hypoglycaemic collapse from tolbutamide in patients also receiving chloramphenicol have been ascribed to this cause (Christensen and Skousted, 1969). Similarly, pre-treatment with chloramphenicol delayed the recovery of experimental animals anaesthetized with pentobarbitone (or other barbiturates eliminated by metabolism) but not of those anaesthetized with barbitone which is largely excreted unchanged in the urine (Adams, 1970).

Excretion is mainly renal: 90 per cent of the dose can be detected in the urine by chemical methods, but only about 10 per cent of this amount is unaltered antibiotic. In experimental animals, the microbiologically active drug (but not its conjugates) exerts a potent relaxant effect on the ureter (Benzi *et al.*, 1970). Chloramphenicol itself is excreted by the glomeruli, but excretion of its inactive derivatives is also by active tubular secretion. Excretion diminishes linearly with renal function. At a creatinine clearance of less than 20 ml/min, maximum concentrations of 10-20 μg/ml in urine are found in contrast to 150-200 μg/ml in the normal. Despite this, blood levels of active chloramphenicol are only marginally elevated but microbiologically inactive metabolites accumulate. This may explain both the poor results of treatment of urinary infection plus exalted toxicity found in some (especially elderly) patients (Lindberg *et al.*, 1966).

Very young infants are deficient in the ability to form glucuronides and their glomerular and tubular excretion capabilities are low. The rate of disappearance of chloramphenicol from the blood is consequently greatly prolonged (Table 20) and in the new-born the dose and frequency of administration must be reduced (p. 291) if toxic quantities of the drug are not to accumulate.

About 3 per cent of the administered dose is excreted in the bile but only about 1 per cent appears in the faeces and that mostly in inactive forms. The idea that high concentrations of chloramphenicol can be demonstrated in the bile appears to have come from studies in the rat, in which, in contrast to man, the bile is a principal route of excretion.

Side Effects and Toxicity

Chloramphenicol passed the usual toxicity tests in animals, and had been in world-wide use for several years before it was recognized as a potentially highly dangerous bone marrow depressant. More years passed before it was observed to be the cause of the ' grey syndrome ' in infants, another usually fatal condition. It thus has the unenviable distinction of exerting lethal toxic effects of two different kinds. Other effects are of only minor importance.

ALIMENTARY TRACT. Soreness of the mouth is fairly common if a course of treatment exceeds one week. It is attributable to depression of the normal flora by the antibiotic in the saliva and consequent overgrowth of *Candida albicans*. Mild cases show little change, but in the more severe there is a frank stomatitis: it is possible that vitamin B deficiency or even a direct action of the antibiotic on the epithelium, which in the tongue shows atrophic changes, may also play some part. Nausea, vomiting and diarrhoea, although they may occur, are much less common and less severe than those capable of being caused by tetracyclines.

Contrary to the claim that chloramphenicol intensifies the destruction of G-6-PD-deficient erythrocytes, Chan *et al.* (1971) found that treatment reduced the rate of red cell destruction in Chinese patients with typhoid fever.

MARROW APLASIA. A few isolated reports of granulocytopenia and aplastic anaemia following chloramphenicol therapy appearing about 1950 attracted little attention. The storm burst in 1952, when a succession of papers described such effects, not merely in single cases but in series. By the end of 1963 the Registry of Blood Dyscrasias of the American Medical Association had collected 674 cases of drug-induced marrow aplasia (Erslev, 1964). Chloramphenicol was implicated in 299 of these and had been the sole drug administered in 151—more cases than all the rest of the listed drugs put together. Despite the publicity given to the relationship between aplasia and chloramphenicol over the years and the reports which regularly appear (Wallerstein *et al.*, 1969; Report, 1971) the drug continues to be given for trivial reasons and in extravagant doses.

Simple granulocytopenia is uncommon: the usual effect is a total aplasia of the marrow. The first signs are purpura and pallor, and a blood count reveals a deficiency of all blood cells including platelets. Most patients die despite repeated transfusions. Survival is most likely in those with early onset of dyscrasia in which few cell types are depressed (Best, 1967). A few patients survive with protracted aplasia and in them myeloblastic leukaemia may ultimately supervene (Brauer and Dameshek, 1967). In over 400 cases reviewed by Best (1967) manifestations appeared *during* treatment in only 22 per cent. In 10 per cent there was an interval between the cessation of treatment and onset of dyscrasia of 130 days or more. Cause and effect may thus never be connected.

The frequency of marrow aplasia in treated patients is difficult to compute with any accuracy because of the problem of establishing the size of the population at risk. The value of overall figures is also doubtful because some physicians have given very large doses or treated thousands of patients (Lietman *et al.*, 1964; Woodward and Smadel, 1964) without encountering haematological abnormalities, while others have seen several cases of aplastic anaemia over a limited period. One of us saw three cases, two of them fatal, among an estimated number of 1,200 patients treated with chloramphenicol at St. Bartholomew's Hospital up to 1952. Apparently the profession is divided into those who, perhaps having seen chloramphenicol cause marrow aplasia, fear this effect and rarely use the drug, and a larger number who ignore this possibility because it seems too remote and prescribe chloramphenicol freely.

It has been claimed (though contested: Letters, 1970) that marrow aplasia is peculiar to patients of Northern European or even those of English stock and that free use of the drug in other populations, for example in Italy, Israel and South America has not resulted in this complication. From a State-wide survey in California Wallerstein *et al.* (1969) calculated that the overall risk of fatal aplastic anaemia was 2 cases per million population per annum. In patients treated with an average of 4 g. of chloramphenicol the risk was 13 times greater. By comparison, the risk in patients treated with oxyphenylbuta-zone was increased 4-fold and that in patients treated with mepacrine was increased 10-fold.

It has several times been suggested (though there is no direct evidence for this) that the toxic agent is not chloramphenicol itself but some metabolite, and that marked differences in the incidence of aplasia may be explained by some genetic pre-disposition. This idea is attractive, but as Best (1967) points out, difficult to reconcile with the extreme rarity of aplasia in more than one member of treated families. The mechanism by which chloramphenicol produces marrow aplasia has natur-ally received a great deal of attention but has yet to be elucidated. It is now established that chloramphenicol exerts a regular dose-related but reversible depressant effect on the marrows of all those treated with the drug, resulting in vacuolization of erythroid and myeloid cells, reticulocytopenia and ferrokinetic changes (increase in serum iron, increased saturation of iron-binding globulin, and reduced plasma-iron clearance and utilization) indicative of decreased erythropoiesis (Manyan and Yunis, 1970). Despite the highly suggestive nature of these changes, there is no evidence that this common marrow depression is the precursor of potentially fatal aplasia which differs in being (fortunately) rare, late in onset, irrever-sible and unrelated to dose. The suggestion has been made that aplasia is not primarily a defect of the stem cell at all, but a disorder of the bone marrow sinusoidal micro-circulation (Knospe and Crosby, 1971). At the present time it can only be said by way of both explanation and warning that chloram-phenicol aplasia is an idiosyncratic response and patients who exhibit it may do so on exposure to the smallest dose. The idiosyncratic nature of the response, and the fact that patients who develop aplasia have frequently received more than one course of therapy has suggested that marrow toxicity has an immunological basis. Chloramphenicol is not ordinarily anti-genic for man but some treated patients develop antibodies which might conceivably exalt the drug's toxicity or diminish its antibacterial effect (Orgel and Hamburger, 1971).

Chloramphenicol is a phenylalanine analogue, and diverse observations link chloramphenicol with phenylalanine metabolism. Chloramphenicol inhibits the intestinal uptake of phenylalanine, and the morphological abnormalities of red cells which regularly follow administration of the antibiotic resemble those seen in phenylalanine deficiency. There is at present, however, no undisputed evidence to support the unifying hypothesis that chloramphenicol toxicity in some way operates through phenylalanine metabolism (Weksler *et al.*, 1968).

ENCEPHALOPATHY. Another toxic effect ascribed to chloramphenicol—encephalopathy—has also been linked to phenylalanine metabolism. Delirium in patients treated with chloramphenicol has usually been explained as an effect of toxic bacterial products liberated spontaneously or in response to treatment. Levine *et al.* (1970) challenge this explanation because they observed episodes of asterexis and delirium in three chloramphenicol-treated patients who had no infection (two were treated in an attempt to depress the synthesis of myeloma protein). Interestingly, doses of the drug which were toxic by mouth were innocuous when given intravenously. It is suggested that chloramphenicol which reaches the liver via the portal vein interferes with hepatic function in such a way as to produce a state of phenylalanine deprivation.

THE 'GREY SYNDROME' IN INFANTS. The practice of giving large doses of chloramphenicol by injection to new-born infants prophylactically seems to have arisen about 1957. Indications mentioned by various authors were prematurity, premature rupture of the membranes, and among post-natal factors such conditions as lethargy and abdominal distension. It is remarkable that in none of these reports was there the slightest evidence that this treatment served any useful purpose. The infants remained well for two or three days, when vomiting, refusal to suck and abdominal distension were succeeded by flaccidity, an ashen colour and hypothermia (the 'grey syndrome'), this circulatory collapse being followed by death within a few hours. In what was described as an 'outbreak' of neonatal deaths among full term infants in Los Angeles, the condition was at first thought to be some obscure infection, and the dose of chloramphenicol was actually increased in an endeavour to overcome it: nine infants died from this cause in only two months. The doses given were from 100 to 160 mg./ kg. daily by intramuscular injection and in infants so treated, because of the deficient capacity of the infant to conjugate and excrete chloramphenicol, blood levels climb as high as 170 μg. per ml.

OPTIC NEURITIS. A number of cases have been described of optic neuritis in children with cystic fibrosis of the pancreas, receiving prolonged chloramphenicol treatment for pulmonary infection. Partial restoration of sight has followed stopping the drug and treatment with large doses of B complex vitamins (Cocke et al., 1966). Harley et al. (1970) describe the development of optic neuritis in 13 out of 98 patients suffering from cystic fibrosis treated for 80-1500 days with 10-100 mg. chloramphenicol/kg./day. The usual presenting ocular symptom was severe bilateral deterioration of visual acuity with dense central scotoma. Of the 13, 11 promptly improved when the drug was discontinued whether or not Vitamin B was given. The central visual acuity in 3 of 6 patients who again received the drug was permanently impaired. It is recommended that if prolonged therapy is thought to be necessary, parents should be taught to test the vision frequently with a small chart, and to note particularly any development of numbness or cramps in the feet which frequently precede the onset of ocular signs. A different form of optic neuritis (resembling that of tobacco amblyopia and possibly associated with abnormal propionate metabolism) is described by Begg et al. (1968) in a woman who had received 386 g. of chloramphenicol over 8 months.

EFFECTS ON MAMMALIAN PROTEIN SYNTHESIS. The ribosomes of mitochondria differ from other mammalian ribosomes and resemble those of bacteria in their structure and susceptibility to inhibition (Freeman, 1970). It appears that the reversible dose-related depressant effect of chloramphenicol on haemopoiesis is one result of this inhibition of mitochondrial protein synthesis (Yunis et al., 1970). Evidence of a quite different and exotic kind for a suppressive effect on mammalian mitochondria is provided by the clinical improvement on chloramphenicol treatment of the patient recognized by Haydar et al. (1971) as suffering from the excessively rare Luft's syndrome in which severe hypermetabolism is associated with pseudoneoplastic overgrowth of abnormal mitochondria in skeletal muscle.

The ability of chloramphenicol to inhibit protein synthesis has naturally produced concern about possible detrimental effects on various host responses, notably antibody synthesis and wound healing. Robertson and Warhab (1970) treated 89 patients suffering from typhoid or paratyphoid fever with chloramphenicol or ampicillin and were unable to find any evidence of consistently low antibody titres in those receiving chloramphenicol, or of any complications likely to have resulted from suppressed antibody synthesis. They concluded that if chloramphenicol treatment affects the antibody response in enteric fever it evidently does not do so to a greater extent than ampicillin. Nevertheless, chloramphenicol can be shown to impair immunological responses in certain experimental circumstances, and Linehan et al. (1969) found the chloramphenicol analogue, thiamphenicol to be a potent immunosuppressant in preventing the rejection of renal homografts in the dog.

Neither Bloom and Grillo (1970) nor Donati (1971) found any evidence that treatment with chloramphenicol (or tetracycline) impaired the healing of experimental wounds in the guinea-pig or rat. Caulfield and Burke (1971) agreed with this as far as oral treatment was concerned, but found that wound healing was greatly delayed in rats treated with intravenous chloramphenicol sodium succinate which presumably produced higher peak plasma levels. Ultramicroscopically, the participating fibroblasts showed changes analogous with those seen in bacteria: fewer fully assembled membrane-bound ribosomes and more free ribosomes in the cytoplasm.

Clinical Applications

There is great diversity of opinion on this subject, depending on the degree of importance to be attached to the possibility of toxic effects. We believe that this possibility should not be disregarded, and the following principles, which have frequently been enunciated, should therefore be not only assented to but observed.

1. Chloramphenicol should never be prescribed for minor

infections. There have been many tragic fatalities following its use for trivial conditions such as respiratory catarrh.

2. It is currently still the drug of choice in typhoid fever and other severe salmonella infections. Some authorities take the view that these are the *only* indications. The least contested of other indications are meningitis or severe respiratory infection due to *H. influenzae*. Pertussis may be an indication in severe cases at an early age and if treatment can be begun early enough. It should be prescribed for other serious infections only when these are resistant, or much less sensitive, to other antibiotics.

3. Both the daily dose (usually not exceeding 2 g.) and the duration of the course (e.g. 10 days) should be limited. Although patients may show toxic manifestations after receiving very little of the drug, the danger is almost certainly increased by excessive or repeated dosage or by treatment of patients with impaired hepatic or renal function—including those at the extremes of life.

Chloramphenicol has a very similar antibacterial spectrum to the tetracyclines which are often antibacterially more active and, although not free from toxicity, are innocent of the production of fatal aplastic anaemia. It is therefore pertinent to consider in what circumstances chloramphenicol is to be preferred. Brock (1964) has assembled extensive direct comparisons of the efficacy of chloramphenicol and tetracyclines in a number of experimental infections. As he comments, there must be reservations about the transfer of these findings to man but they are sufficiently in accord with human therapeutic experience, where that is available, to form a useful guide.

It appears that in the treatment of the majority of experimental infections chloramphenicol fails to show any special advantages.

Nevertheless, many clinicians, guided by their own experience, believe it to be a most valuable drug, preferring it in many situations to agents which on other evidence might be expected to be superior. There is no doubt that chloramphenicol can be, and frequently has been, life-saving in the treatment of severe infections. It is also unique amongst readily available antibiotics in producing a condition which is commonly irreversible and fatal. The onus is on anyone who prescribes it to show that he has excellent reasons for doing so.

PHARMACEUTICAL PREPARATIONS AND DOSAGE

CHLORAMPHENICOL (Alficetyn, *Allen and Hanburys;* Chloromycetin, *Parke Davis;* Kemicetine, *Carlo Erba;* numerous other proprietary names). Capsules, B.P., B.N.F.: 250 mg. U.S.P., 50, 100, 250 mg. Injections: Suspension, U.S.N.F.: 1 and 2 g.; Chloramphenicol sodium succinate, U.S.P.: equiv. 1 g. Mixture, B.N.F., U.S.P.: Chloramphenicol palmitate, equiv. 125 mg. per 4 ml. Dose: 1·5-3 g. daily in divided doses. Children 25-50 mg. per kg. per day in divided doses. Premature infant: not more than 25 mg. per kg. per day.

REFERENCES

ADAMS, H. H. (1970). *J. Amer. vet. med. Ass.* **157,** 1908.
AGUIAR, A. J., KRC, J. JR., KINKEL, A. W. & SAMYN, J. C. (1967). *J. pharm. Sci.,* **56,** 847.
ANDERSON, E. S. & SMITH, H. R. (1972). *Brit. med. J.* **3,** 329.
BEGG, I. S., SMALL, M. & WHITE, A. M. (1968). *Lancet* **2,** 686.
BELLA, D. D., FERRARI, V., MARCA, G. & BONAMOMI, L. (1968). *Biochem. Pharmacol.* **17,** 2381.
BENZI, G., ARRIGONI, E. & SANGUIETTI, L. (1970). *Archs. int. Pharmacodyn. Thér.* **185,** 329.
BEST, W. R. (1967). *J. Amer. med. Ass.* **201,** 181.
BLOOM, G. P. & GRILLO, H. C. (1970). *J. surg. Res.* **10,** 1.
BRAUER, M. J. & DAMESHEK, W. (1967). *New Engl. J. Med.* **277,** 1003.
BROCK, T. D. (1964). In *Experimental Chemotherapy,* vol. 3, p. 119, ed. Schnitzer, R. J. & Hawking, F. New York: Academic Press.
CAMBIERI, F., GAMBINI, A. & LODOLA, E. (1970). *Chemotherapy* **15,** 356.
CARTER, H. E., GOTTLIEB, D. & ANDERSON, H. W. (1948). *Science* **107,** 113.
CAULFIELD, J. B. & BURKE, J. F. (1971). *Arch. Path.* **92,** 119.
CHAN, T. K., CHESTERMAN, C. N., McFADZEAN, A. J. S. & TODD, D. (1971). *J. lab. clin. Med.* **77,** 177.
CHIOU, W. L. (1971). *J. pharm. Sci.* **60,** 1406.
CHRISTENSEN, L. K. & SKOVSTED, L. (1969). *Lancet* **2,** 1397.
COCKE, J. G., BROWN, R. E. & GEPPERT, L. J. (1966). *J. Pediat.* **68,** 27.
CUTLER, R. A., STENGER, R. J. & SUTER, C. M. (1952). *J. Amer. chem. Soc.* **74,** 5475.
DONATI, R. M. (1971). *Arch. Surg.* **102,** 132.
EHRLICH, J., BARTZ, Q. R., SMITH, R. M., JOSLYN, D. A. & BURKHOLDER, P. R. (1947). *Science* **106,** 417.
ERSLEV, A. J. (1964). *J. Amer. med. Ass.* **188,** 531.
FREEMAN, K. B. (1970). *Canad. J. Biochem.* **48,** 479.
GLAZKO, A. J., KINKEL, A. W., ALEGNANI, W. C. & HOLMES, E. L. (1968). *Clin. Pharmacol. Ther.* **9,** 472.
HARLEY, R. D., HUANG, N. N., MACRI, C. H. & GREEN, W. R. (1970). *Trans. Amer. Acad. Ophthalmol. Otol.* **74,** 1011.
HAYDAR, N. A., CONN, H. L., AFIFI, A., WAKID, N., BALLAS, S. & FAWAZ, K. (1971). *Ann. intern. Med.* **74,** 548.
KNOSPE, W. H. & CROSBY, W. H. (1971). *Lancet* **1,** 20.
LETTERS (1970). *New Engl. J. Med.* **282,** 343; 813; 1047.
LEVINE, P. H., REGELSON, W. & HOLLAND, J. F. (1970). *Clin. Pharmacol. Ther.* **11,** 194.
LIETMAN, P. S., DI SANT' AGNESE, P. A. & WONG, V. (1964). *J. Amer. med. Ass.* **189,** 924.

LINDBERG. A. A., son NILSSON, L. H., BUCHT, H. & KALLINGS, L. O. (1966). *Brit. med. J.* **2**, 724.
LINEHAN, J. D., LEE, H. M., ROBERTSHAW, G. E. & HUME, D. M. (1969). *Surg. Forum* **20**, 270.
MANYAN, D. R. & YUNIS, A. A. (1970). *Biochem. Biophys. Res. Comm.* **41**, 926.
OKAMOTO, S., SUZUKI, Y., MISE, K. & NAKAYA, R. (1967). *J. Bact.* **94**, 1616.
ORGEL, H. A. & HAMBURGER, R. N. (1971). *Immunology* **20**, 233.
REEVE, E. C. R. & SUTTIE, D. R. (1968). *Genet. Res.* **11**, 97.
REPORT (1971). *Med. J. Aust* **1**, 928.
ROBERTSON, R. P. & WAHAB, M. F. A. (1970). *Ann. intern. Med.* **72**, 219.
SHAW, W. V. (1971). *Ann. N.Y. Acad. Sci.* **182**, 234.
SHAW, W. V. & BRODSKY, R. F. (1968). *J. Bact.* **95**, 28.
SOMPOLINSKY, D., ZIEGLER-SCHLOMOWITZ, R. & HERCZOG, D. (1968). *Canad. J. Microbiol.* **14**, 891.
VON STRANDTMANN, M., BOBOWSKI, G. & SHAVEL, J. Jr. (1967). *J. med. Chem.* **10**, 888.
WALLERSTEIN, R. O., CONDIT, P. K., KASPER, C. K., BROWN, J. W. & MORRISON, F. R. (1969). *J. Amer. med. Ass.* **208**, 2045.
WEKSLER, M. E., BOURKE, E. & SCHREINER, G. E. (1968). *Clin. Pharmacol. Ther.* **9**, 647.
WOODWARD, T. E. & SMADEL, J. E. (1964). *Ann. intern. Med.* **60**, 144.
YUNIS, A. A., SMITH, U. S. & RESTREPO, A. (1970). *Arch intern. Med.* **126**, 272.

Chapter 9

TETRACYCLINES

In 1948, when aureomycin, the first of the tetracyclines, was discovered, the only other antibiotics in general use were penicillin and streptomycin. Each of these had a limited range of activity, and each had to be given by injection. Aureomycin differed from them in having a wide range of activity, including most organisms susceptible to either and some to neither of them, and a second advantage, shared with chloramphenicol, which was discovered at about the same time, of being administrable by the mouth.

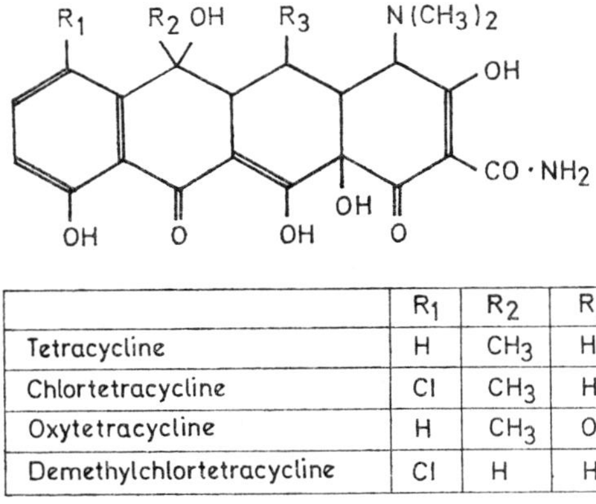

	R_1	R_2	R_3
Tetracycline	H	CH_3	H
Chlortetracycline	Cl	CH_3	H
Oxytetracycline	H	CH_3	OH
Demethylchlortetracycline	Cl	H	H

FIGURE 11
Structure of tetracyclines.

The tetracyclines are a family of closely related antibiotics, to which additions are still being made after over 20 years. The first, aureomycin, was so called from the golden yellow colour of the colony of *Streptomyces aureofaciens,* the organism forming it. Two years later (1950) ' Terramycin ' derived from *Streptomyces rimosus,* was introduced, and within a further two years their structure was ascertained, which differs only in the presence of a Cl atom in one and an OH

group in the other. The names chlortetracycline and oxytetracycline were then proposed for them, and in 1953 tetracycline
was introduced, which has neither of these attachments: this
can be obtained either by catalytic dehalogenation of chlortetracycline or directly from another *Streptomyces*. The properties
of these three will be described before those of several more
recently introduced.

The three earlier tetracyclines are all yellow crystalline
substances, amphoteric in nature and of low solubility (about
0·05 per cent): their hydrochlorides are much more soluble
(that of tetracycline about 10 per cent) and are chiefly used in
therapeutics. Their solutions are acid, and those of tetracycline
and oxytetracycline are reasonably stable, but that of chlortetracycline is the most unstable of any major antibiotic,
particularly in neutral and still more in alkaline solution: in
nutrient broth with pH of 7·4 it loses the greater part of its
activity during overnight incubation.

Anti-microbic Activity

The term 'broad spectrum', denoting a wide range of
activity, was coined in connection with this group of antibiotics, and in fact their spectrum is the broadest known
(Table 31, p. 280). Susceptible species include not only
those, mainly Gram-positive, which are also sensitive to penicillin, but many Gram-negative species which are not, and in
addition mycoplasmas, rickettsias and *Chlamydia* (p. 477). Like
penicillin the tetracyclines are active against *T. pallidum* and
other treponemata: unlike it, they also have some action on
the tubercle bacillus. The only large group of fully resistant
pathogenic organisms are the fungi (not including that of actinomycosis, which is highly sensitive). The possible indications for
administering tetracyclines, to be considered later, are therefore
very numerous.

INDIVIDUAL DIFFERENCES IN ACTIVITY. These are only of
the order of two-fold, and may therefore not be of much
consequence. Chlortetracycline, provided that the test is read
after about 18 hours (further incubation alters the results,
owing to its instability) can be shown to be the most active
against all the pathogenic Gram-positive cocci, particularly

staphylococci and pneumococci. Oxytetracycline is the most active against *Ps. aeruginosa* and tetracycline against *Proteus,* although the inhibitory concentrations for these species are considerably higher. There are no consistent differences among numerous other susceptible species.

ACQUIRED RESISTANCE. The acquisition of resistance to tetracyclines is a slow process, and is not often observed during the treatment of an individual patient, Nevertheless resistant strains of various coliform bacilli and of staphylococci have gradually become fairly common; indeed, tetracycline resistance has come to be regarded as the hall-mark of a virulent and troublesome staphylococcus. Resistance in haemolytic streptococci, first observed as long ago as 1952 in the special environment of a Burns Unit where tetracyclines had been extensively used (Lowbury and Hurst, 1956), has since been reported in strains isolated from the throat: Kuharic *et al.* (1960) found 20 per cent of strains in Seattle resistant, and Mitchell and Baber (1965) 32 per cent of a large number isolated in Bristol from throat swabs and other sources. The frequency of resistance over a number of years in London has been well documented. The proportion of resistant strains rose from 0·7 per cent. in 1958 to 41 per cent in 1965 (Dadswell, 1967), remained at this high level for several years and has since decreased somewhat to 27 per cent in early 1971 (Rees, 1971). Anyone who formerly regarded tetracyclines as suitable for treating acute sore throats and other possibly streptococcal infections should be warned.

Even more discouraging, since it comprises much the largest field of present use of tetracyclines, is the appearance of resistance in pneumococci Earlier reports of this, reviewed in the last edition of this book, refer to small numbers of patients or to isolated outbreaks of infection due to a single serological type in elderly chronic bronchitics in institutions. It was not to be expected that such strains would indefinitely remain rarities and the recent studies of Percival, Armstrong and Turner (1969) show that at least in Liverpool they have not. The frequency of resistance in strains from in-patients at the Royal Infirmary rose from 6 per cent in 1967 to 23 per cent in 1968, and at least half of these infections were judged to have been acquired outside hospital. Among patients attending general

6

practitioners and chest clinics the corresponding figures were 7 and 12 per cent. The degree of resistance (M.I.C. of the order of 50 μg./ml.) is such as to preclude any possibility of successful treatment. No such steep increase in resistance has been observed in *H. influenzae*, although strains with some diminution in sensitivity have been seen.

Another organism now showing resistance is *Cl. welchii*. Johnstone and Cockcroft (1968) of Vancouver report that tetracycline given to a road casualty ' known to be allergic to penicillin ' failed to prevent gas gangrene, and his arm had to be amputated. The strain of *Cl. welchii* responsible was tetracycline-resistant, as were 11 out of 102 further strains from human sources subsequently tested. Another objection to the emergency use of tetracycline for this purpose is that shock delays its absorption (Owen-Smith, 1969).

An organism resistant to one tetracycline is equally or almost equally resistant to any other.

MODE OF ACTION. Antibiotics are classified as bactericidal and bacteristatic, and the tetracyclines decidedly belong in the second category. There may be no such thing as pure bacteristasis, and there is some evidence that high concentrations of tetracyclines cause a steeper fall in the viable count than low ones, but the process is very gradual, with numerous survivors after as long as 24 hours. It is now known that tetracyclines belong to the group of antibiotics acting by interference with protein synthesis, the stage affected being probably the formation of peptide linkages. Resistance may be due to decreased permeability to the antibiotic.

Pharmacokinetics

Although it is possible to prepare solutions suitable for intravenous or even intramuscular injection, the usual route of administration is oral, in capsules containing the hydrochloride.

ABSORPTION. This takes place from all levels of the alimentary tract from the stomach onwards (Gray *et al.*, 1953). but is never complete, and the larger the dose the lower is the proportion of it absorbed. Both because defective absorption militates against effective treatment and because the principal side effects are due to retention of the antibiotic in the bowel, much attention has been devoted to this problem, which has eluded complete solution so far as the earlier tetracyclines are concerned. Two factors appear to be involved. One is simply solubility: the hydrochlorides are reasonably soluble in water, giving a highly acid solution, but in a neutral or alkaline medium they tend to be precipitated, or (as when liberated in the intestine) not to dissolve. Secondly, tetracyclines combine with divalent metals, of which calcium is likely to be present in the largest amount. This was not appreciated for some years, and it is interesting in retrospect that calcium phosphate was actually used as a filler in capsules (Dearborn *et al.*, 1957) long after it had been shown that aluminium hydroxide, which must act in a similar way, interferes with absorption (Waisbren and Hueckel, 1950): this substance had been added to chlortetracycline to allay the gastric disturbance sometimes produced.

When the general significance of this reaction was grasped studies were made of the effect of appropriate additions to the contents of tetracycline capsules on the blood levels attained, and it was shown that calcium phosphate reduced absorption, whereas citric acid or sodium metaphosphate, which combine with calcium and thus render it unavailable for combination with the antibiotic, increased it substantially (Welch *et al.*, 1957; Sweeney *et al.*, 1957). Phosphate is now commonly included in the capsule to enhance absorption either as an addition or in combination with the antibiotic as a tetracycline phosphate complex, but it must not be supposed that this solves the problem: a variable and sometimes large proportion of the dose remains unabsorbed. Neuvonen *et al.* (1970). showed that the concurrent administration of 200 mg. of ferrous sulphate significantly reduced the peak serum concentrations of several tetracyclines.

DISTRIBUTION. The blood level curve is a plateau, having a slow rise and a still slower fall. Factors contributing to this persistence are (1) continued absorption, (2) biliary excretion and reabsorption, (3) protein binding, the extent of which has been determined as 47, 20 and 24 per cent for chlor- and oxytetracycline and tetracycline respectively (Kunin, Dornbush and Finland, 1959). Tetracycline attains the highest level and chlortetracycline the lowest, but the differences are not large: maxima on ordinary doses (e.g. 250 mg. six-hourly) are of the order of 2-4 μg./ml. with a small cumulative increase. Tetracyclines behave much like penicillin in their diffusion into serous cavities, the foetal circulation and glandular secretions. They enter the cerebro-spinal fluid somewhat more freely, concentrations of tetracycline found there being about 10 per cent of those in the blood: those of chlor- and oxytetracycline are somewhat lower (Wood and Kipnis, 1953). A unique feature of their behaviour is deposition in bone in areas where bone is being laid down: here they remain detectable for long periods. Similar deposition in teeth is referred to in the next section.

EXCRETION. Tetracyclines are freely excreted in both bile and urine. In the former the concentrations attained are 10-20 times those in the blood: much of the antibiotic so excreted must be re-absorbed. Urinary excretion accounts for rather over 20 per cent of an oral dose and 50 per cent of an intravenous: the difference between these figures is explained by incomplete absorption from the bowel, and the balance unaccounted for even after injection denotes degradation in the body. Variable but often very large amounts (>1,000 μg./g.) are found in the faeces when administration is oral.

PARENTERAL ADMINISTRATION. Suitable solutions can be administered by slow intravenous infusion, a usual dose being 0·5 g. twice daily. Advantages of this route are the immediate effect and the certainty of attaining an adequate blood level, the factor of variable absorption from the alimentary tract being eliminated. The level is also well maintained, doubtless owing largely to biliary excretion and reabsorption.

Side Effects

At the time when the first edition of this book was in preparation, alimentary tract superinfections were almost the only side-effects recognized from the use of these drugs. After years of worldwide use, a number of new unwanted effects began to be described. There is little foundation for the claim that tetracyclines are teratogenic, but some other side-effects are now well documented and, although uncommon, are potentially important.

GASTRO-INTESTINAL DISTURBANCES. The incidence of these symptoms is dose-dependent, and they are much more common when daily doses of 2 g. or more are given than when the dose is limited to 1g. daily. Nausea and vomiting are presumably due to a direct irritant effect of the drug on the gastric mucosa. Possibly diarrhoea can also be so caused, but this and other effects are more often the result of superinfection, i.e. the replacement of the suppressed normal flora by antibiotic-resistant organisms. It is here that the broad spectrum effect operates to the patient's disadvantage: most of the flora of the mouth, and even of the more complex flora of the lower bowel, including lactobacilli and clostridia as well as streptococci and the normal coliforms, are sensitive, and their suppression leaves a vacuum liable to be filled by less well-disposed inhabitants. The three main varieties of superinfection are by *Candida albicans*, by *Proteus* and *Pseudomonas* species resistant to tetracyclines, and by resistant staphylococci. Any of these may become clinically significant and the dangerous condition of staphylococcal enterocolitis has been especially well described. First recognized as a complication of treatment with oxytetracycline (Jackson *et al.*, 1951), it can in fact be produced by any tetracycline, even one given by the intravenous route (Lundsgaard-Hansen *et al.*, 1960), when its direct action on the bowel must result from biliary excretion; it has also often been caused by treatment with penicillin and streptomycin together, and less often by other antibiotics. The epidemic at the Radcliffe Infirmary, Oxford, embracing 31 cases with 14 deaths (Cook *et al.*, 1957) suggests that cross-infection with an endemic strain is the usual source of the infection. The condition is seen almost exclusively in surgical patients post-operatively, and the operation most commonly followed by it (14 of the Oxford series) is gastrectomy. The emptiness of the bowel in such patients is probably an important factor. The lesion is a superficial necrosis of large areas of small intestinal mucosa, and the clinical manifestations are a profuse watery diarrhoea, with stools swarming with staphylococci, leading to dehydration and circulatory collapse. Treatment includes stopping the offending antibiotic, administering another to which the staphylococcus is or is likely to be sensitive (methicillin or perhaps vancomycin: see p. 369) and fluid replacement. Detection at an early stage by staining films of faeces from all patients with post-operative diarrhoea may enable the development of the full syndrome to be prevented. Staphylococcal enterocolitis has now become less common with the diminished threat from hospital staphylococci in many centres, and the growing tendency to avoid antibiotic regimens which seriously alter the bowel flora.

Although these serious consequences of superinfection are well documented, the relationship between the common minor gastro-intestinal symptoms and the undoubted changes in bowel flora is much less certain. For example, in a double-blind trial of two treatments of bronchitis, although the incidence of *Candida albicans* in the stools was significantly higher in the patients receiving tetracycline alone (37·1 per cent) than in those receiving tetracycline with nystatin (9·1 per cent), the incidence of gastro-intestinal symptoms was identical in the two groups (British Tuberculosis Association, 1968).

STAINING OF TEETH. Tetracyclines are deposited in teeth during the early stages of calcification, just as they are in calcifying bone. This may occur *in utero* if the mother is treated after the fifth month, when calcification of the deciduous teeth begins (Kline, Blattner and Lunin, 1964) or be produced by treatment of the child after birth. For the effect to be visible as yellow staining a certain total dose must be exceeded: the relationship between dosage and effect was well studied by Wallman and Hilton (1962). Different tetracyclines produce different degrees and shades of pigmentation (Owen, 1963) and varying degrees of hypoplasia may accompany it. The main objection to this change is cosmetic, and this applies particularly to the second dentition: it is thus important to remember when the permanent teeth begin to be formed, and it would also be useful to know for how long after this pigmentation can still be produced. The permanent incisors begin to be formed six months after birth, the canines and premolars after two years, and the molars after three to four years (Witkop and Wolf, 1963). There seems to have been no thorough study of the relationship between age at the time of tetracycline treatment and dental staining, but an effect on the anterior teeth seems likely to be small after the third year. Tetracycline treatment is therefore to be avoided in early childhood except for imperative indications or unless a short course will suffice. Doxycycline, which binds less with calcium than other tetracyclines, is said to cause dental changes less frequently (Forti and Benincori, 1969) and should perhaps be preferred if a tetracycline must be given to a child.

RENAL DAMAGE. Recent publications (Edwards *et al.*, 1970) and correspondence have drawn attention again to the risks of tetracyclines in renal failure. This action is probably attributable to the anti-anabolic action of these agents. Shils (1963) pointed out that clinical and biochemical deterioration may occur in patients with impaired renal function, that the changes are proportional to the degree of renal failure and to the dose and duration of tetracycline administration, and that the maximal effects are often reached some days after the course of tetracycline has finished. Tetracyclines should not be given to patients with impaired renal function. An exception may be possible in the case of doxycycline. Several authors have found that the half-life of this drug is unchanged in renal failure, that a progressive rise in plasma levels is not found and that blood urea and creatinine levels do not rise in patients receiving doxycycline (Merier *et al.*, 1969; Little and Bailey, 1970; Ribush and Morgan, 1972). The reason for this difference from other tetracyclines is still uncertain, and since occasional patients with renal failure do show dangerous prolongation of drug action (Morgan and Ribush, 1972), it would be advisable to monitor plasma levels in any patient with impaired renal function for whom any tetracycline has to be prescribed.

LIVER DAMAGE. It has been known since the work of Lepper *et al.* (1951) that tetracyclines given in excessive doses parenterally as well as orally can damage the liver. Since then a number of deaths have been reported in pregnant women given tetracycline in large intravenous doses, usually for the treatment of pyelonephritis (Schulz, 1963; Whalley *et al.*, 1964; Kunelis *et al.*, 1965). The main lesion found at autopsy was diffuse fatty degeneration of the liver.

A total daily dose of tetracycline by the intravenous route of 1 g. is adequate for most purposes, and should rarely be exceeded. Whether pyelonephritis, for which the treatment has usually been given in pregnancy, plays an important part by delaying elimination of the antibiotic has not been actually determined. The alternative possibility is that the liver itself is specially liable to damage in pregnancy : Kunelis *et al.* (1965) make the specific suggestion that it may be more sensitive to agents which depress protein anabolism. Tetracyclines should not be given in late pregnancy, in the interests of both mother and foetus.

BENIGN INTRACRANIAL HYPERTENSION. A number of infants treated with tetracycline have developed bulging of the anterior fontanelle (Fields, 1961). More recently a similar syndrome has been described in older children (Maroon and Mealy, 1971) and even in adults, with headache, photophobia and papilloedema. The signs and symptoms clear when administration of the drug is stopped, but several patients developed the same illness when tetracycline was given again. The mechanism is quite unknown.

OTHER TETRACYCLINES

Several more tetracyclines have now been introduced. They possess the same general properties as the foregoing, and only those in which they differ need be described.

Demethylchlortetracycline

This substance, of which a general account is given by Finland and Garrod (1960) is formed by a mutant strain of *Streptomyces aureofaciens,* and is chlortetracycline without the methyl group in the R_1 position (p. 149). It is astonishing that subtracting this one attachment should have such profound effects. One of these is to confer a high degree of stability, in contrast to the remarkable instability of chlortetracycline. Anti-bacterial activity exceeds that of tetracycline against most species by a factor of about two. Absorption is better than that of tetracycline, and excretion is considerably slower, the rate of renal clearance being 43 per cent of that of tetracycline. This may be due, at least in part, to a higher degree of protein binding than that of the older tetracyclines. The result of these differences in behaviour is that a smaller dose will give at least an equal blood level for a longer time, and indeed the usual daily dose is four 150 mg. capsules when that of tetracycline would be four of 250 mg. It is believed that larger doses than this of demethylchlortetracycline are more liable than those of other tetracyclines to cause gastro-intestinal disturbance, although statistical proof of this is unavailable on a convincing scale.

These findings with regard to absorption and excretion have been confirmed by several groups of workers, but in consequence of one conflicting report (Roberts *et al.*, 1961) a further cross-over test on an impressive scale was carried out, which not only confirmed that the average blood levels produced by 300 mg. demethylchlortetracycline given twice a day equal those produced by 250 mg. tetracycline given four times a day, but showed further that if the former is given in doses of 150 mg. four times a day the levels produced are substantially higher (Sweeney, Dornbush and Hardy, 1962).

Demethylchlortetracycline has the minor drawback of causing photo-sensitization: patients taking it should avoid prolonged exposure to sunlight.

Rolitetracycline

This tetracycline compound (pyrrolidinomethyl tetracycline), known as Reverin in Germany, the country of its origin, unlike any of the foregoing is highly soluble in water (>1 g./ml.), giving a neutral solution. It is thus easily administered intravenously in full doses, and by this means exceptionally high blood and tissue levels can be attained (Otte, 1960; Knothe and Mahler, 1959). There are enthusiastic reports of its clinical use, mainly from the Continent. Its toxicity somewhat exceeds that of tetracycline, and there would appear to be some possibility of the kind of liver damage observed when chlortetracycline was given in large doses parenterally. Although administered only by injection, its use in surgical cases can result in staphylococcal enterocolitis: six cases with two deaths are reported by authors from Berne (Lundsgaard-Hansen *et al.*, 1960).

Lymecycline

This compound (tetracycline-L-methylenelysine), produced in Italy and known as Tetralysal, is formed by a reaction between tetracycline, formaldehyde and L-lysine (Cassano *et al.*, 1961). Like the foregoing it is highly soluble (1 g. in 0·4 ml.), and is said to be particularly well absorbed when given orally, permitting lower dosage and reducing (or according to some statements eliminating) alimentary tract side effects. It can also be administered by intramuscular or intravenous injection. Its *in vitro* activity is stated as identical with that of tetracycline.

Most of the publications on this product are Italian, and those dealing with absorption and excretion include none reporting estimations in the faeces: these should afford the best evidence of good absorption, particularly in subjects shown to be poor absorbers of tetracycline. The finding of de Carneri and Manfredi (1962) that doubling the dose increases the blood level by 82 per cent is suggestive: an increase so nearly corresponding to the increase in the dose is not to be expected with other tetracyclines. In this country Whitby and Black (1964) obtained conflicting results: lymecycline gave higher blood levels than tetracycline in volunteers, but lower ones in treated patients. The 24-hour urinary excretions of tetracycline and lymecycline in volunteers were 21 and 28 per cent of the dose respectively: this figure for lymecycline is less than half that reported in some Italian studies. In their clinical study these authors observed no difference in the frequency of side effects: diarrhoea, sore mouth, etc. occurred in 13 out of 58 patients given lymecycline and in 10 out of 44 given tetracycline. Unwanted effects may be less frequent with lymecycline than with other tetracyclines when it is necessary to give a large dose of a tetracycline, as is sometimes necessary in patients with severe purulent bronchitis (Pines *et al.*, 1968).

Clomocycline

('Megaclor'), described as N-methylolchlortetracycline, is another Italian product for which similar advantages are claimed. It has a solubility in water of over 1:1 over a wide range of pH, and because of this is said to be much better absorbed than less soluble tetracyclines. Its instability is claimed to be an advantage as accountable for minimal deposition in bone (Tubaro, 1964). There is less published evidence about this product than about lymecycline, and some of the same questions call for an independent and authoritative answer in connection with both. It is supplied in capsules containing 170 mg. of which one four times a day is said usually to be an adequate dose.

Methacycline

It is claimed for this compound (6-methylene oxytetracycline: Rondomycin) that its anti-bacterial activity *in vitro* somewhat exceeds that of demethylchlortetracycline, that this difference in its favour is greater *in vivo* (mouse infections) and that it is better absorbed (English *et al.*, 1962). Remington and Finland (1962), on the other hand, found the blood levels produced by methacycline and demethylchlortetracycline to be very similar, except that the latter diminished more slowly. There was little difference between the two in activity against the organisms used for assay. No notable information about this drug has become available, possibly because its manufacturers have concentrated more attention on the newer derivative, doxycycline.

Doxycycline

This compound, which is a α-6-deoxytetracycline, is described by English (1966) as possessing similar *in vitro* activity to that of methacycline and demethylchlortetracycline, and similar therapeutic activity against streptococcal, staphylococcal and *P. multocida* infections in mice when administered subcutaneously: on the other hand the curative dose by oral administration was less, a difference attributed to better absorption. From a further study (English, 1967) using different methods it was calculated that the percentage of an oral dose of doxycycline absorbed exceeded that of several other tetracyclines (including methacycline) by a factor of over 3. The observations of Rosenblatt *et al.* (1967) suggest a different or additional explanation: they found that doses of 100 mg. doxycycline and 300 mg. demethylchlortetracycline gave similar blood levels, but showed that this was due, not to better absorption (about the same proportion of the dose of each being excreted in the urine), but to slower excretion, the renal clearances of the two drugs being respectively 15·95 and 36·49 ml. per min.

An advantage of this drug is that owing to its slow excretion only one daily dose need be given. According to Fabre *et al.* (1967) an initial dose of 200 mg. followed by 100 mg. daily serves to maintain a blood level of between 1·5 and 3 μg./ml. Favourable clinical results are reported by Rennau and Schmiedel (1968) in infections of the lungs and bronchi and of the urinary and biliary tracts.

Minocycline

This derivative was first described by Redin (1967). It is 7-dimethylamino-6-demethyl-6-deoxytetracycline. It appears to be exceptionally well absorbed after oral administration, about one quarter of the dose of demethylchlortetracycline being required to produce the same blood level, and has a long half-life in serum of 13·7 hours (Bernard *et al.*, 1971). Its most interesting property is its activity both *in vitro* and *in vivo* against staphylococci resistant to tetracycline: effective doses against mouse infections by 12 such strains varied from 0·3 to 14 mg. per kg., whereas tetracycline was ineffective at 1 g. per kg. We have had the opportunity of examining this compound and found that its *in vitro* activity greatly exceeds that of tetracycline against tetracycline-resistant strains, not only of staphylococci, but of *Str. pyogenes, Str. faecalis,* and *E. coli.* This difference does not extend to resistant pneumococci or to any other enterobacteria (*Proteus, Pseudomonas, Klebsiella, Salmonella* or *Shigella*). An explanation of why minocycline retains activity against tetracycline-resistant strains of some species but not of others would be of great interest.

In a later *in vitro* study Fedorko, Katz and Allnoch (1968) emphasize the activity of minocycline against strains of staphylococci resistant to other tetracyclines. This is also confirmed by Steigbigel, Reed and Finland (1968) in one of the largest series of determinations of M.I.C. ever published. It embraces 7 tetracyclines and 421 strains of 21 varieties of bacteria. From a vast mass of data they calculate an order of merit based on the percentage of total strains inhibited by each tetracycline either in a lower concentration than by any other or in one not bettered by any other. These percentages, with the organisms most sensitive to each tetracycline are minocycline 67 (staphylococci and streptococci), doxycycline 38 (enterococci), methacycline 32 (*H. influenzae*), chlortetracycline and demethylchlortetracycline each 20 and tetracycline and oxytetracycline each 4. Some clinical results with minocycline are reported by Frisk and Tunevall (1969).

CLINICAL APPLICATIONS

Thanks to their exceptionally broad spectrum, tetracyclines are indicated for a greater variety of infections than any other antibiotic. This fact encourages their choice, particularly by the general practitioner, when a bacteriological diagnosis is unavailable.

Much of their prescription in this country is for infections of the respiratory tract. It used to be said that all organisms capable of causing pneumonia were susceptible, but as resistant strains of pneumococci have become more prevalent this ceases to be true of the most important of them. It holds good for most Gram-negative infections, for psittacosis and infections with *Rickettsia burneti* and *Mycoplasma pneumoniae*. Resistance in haemolytic streptococci is now common, and the prescription of tetracyclines for acute throat infections is therefore inadvisable. Much the largest consumption is in the treatment of chronic bronchitis, for which the tetracyclines, ampicillin and, more recently, cotrimoxazole are the most commonly prescribed antimicrobial drugs.

Tetracyclines are now established as a moderately effective treatment for acne vulgaris (Lane and Williamson, 1969), used in a dose of 250-500 mg. daily, and as somewhat more effective in rosacea (Sneddon, 1966).

Other indications for the use of tetracyclines are diverse but uncommon. They are used for susceptible urinary infections, and in brucellosis, although cotrimoxazole is now a competitor in this disease. Tetracyclines also offer an alternative to penicillin in the treatment of actinomycosis, anthrax and syphilis. Other possible or definite uses are in granuloma venereum, lymphogranuloma inguinale, leptospirosis, relapsing fever, trachoma, tularaemia and typhus. In cholera, tetracyclines reduce the requirement for intravenous fluids by about half, and have also been successfully used for prophylaxis of the disease in infected families (McCormack *et al.,* 1968). Another and surprising use, arising from the spread of drug-resistant malaria in the Far East, is as an adjunct in the eradicative treatment of *P. falciparum* infection (Rieckmann *et al.,* 1971, Clyde *et al.,* 1971).

Tetracyclines were formerly regarded as indicated in mixed infections, notably peritonitis (see p. 373) but acquired resistance in several species has diminished their value. Prophylactic administration to surgical patients should be avoided if possible. A general contra-indication to the use of tetracyclines is any condition in which a bactericidal effect is essential: thus they have no place in the treatment of infective endocarditis, except that caused by *Coxiella burneti.*

PHARMACEUTICAL PREPARATIONS

TETRACYCLINE HYDROCHLORIDE ('Achromycin', *Lederle;* 'Tetracyn', *Pfizer,* and other names).
    Capsules and Tablets B.P., B.N.F. 200 mg., Proprietary 50 mg., U.S.P. 50, 100 and 250 mg., Elixir B.N.F. 125 mg./5 ml., Oral Suspension 250 mg./5 ml., Injection B.P., B.N.F. (i.m.) 200, 400 mg. Proprietary and U.S.P. 100, 250 and 500 mg. Usual adult dose 250 mg. 4 times a day, which may be doubled for severe infections. Intramuscular injection, 100 mg. dose 2-300 mg. daily. Intravenous injection, 250 mg. dose 500 mg.—1 g. daily.

CHLORTETRACYCLINE HYDROCHLORIDE ('Aureomycin', *Lederle*).
    Capsules B.P. 250 mg., Proprietary 50 mg., U.S.N.F. 50, 100 and 250 mg., Injection B.P., B.N.F., U.S.N.F. 100, 250, 500 mg. Dosage: See Tetracycline hydrochloride.

OXYTETRACYCLINE HYDROCHLORIDE ('Terramycin', *Pfizer;* 'Imperacin' *I.C.I.*).
    Capsules and Tablets B.N.F. 250 mg., U.S.N.F. 50, 100 and 250 mg. Syrup 125 mg./5 ml., Oral Suspension 250 mg./5 ml. Intramuscular injection 100 mg. dose 2-300 mg. daily. Intravenous injection 250 mg. dose 500 mg.—1 g. daily.

DEMETHYLCHLORTETRACYCLINE HYDROCHLORIDE('Ledermycin', 'Declomycin' *Lederle*).
    Capsules B.P., B.N.F. 150 mg., U.S.N.F. 75 and 150 mg., Tablets 300 mg., Syrup, B.N.F., U.S.N.F. 75 mg./5 ml., Oral Suspension U.S.N.F. 15 mg./ml.: usual dose 150 mg. 4 times a day, but may be increased. No parenteral preparation. Also ointment and syrup.

ROLITETRACYCLINE ('Reverin', *Hoechst,* Synetrin, Velocycline *U.S.A.*).
    Available as vials of the pure substance for solution for intramuscular or (preferably) intravenous injection. Intramuscular or intravenous injection, 350 mg. Usual dose 350 mg. daily.

LYMECYCLINE ('Tetralysal', *Carlo Erba*).
    Capsules containing equivalent of 150 mg. tetracycline base. Injection (i.m.) 100 mg. Usual dose one capsule 4 times a day.

METHACYCLINE HYDROCHLORIDE (' Rondomycin ', *Pfizer*).
Capsules of 150 mg. Syrup 75 mg./5 ml.: usual dose one capsule 4 times a day.

CLOMOCYCLINE (' Megaclor ', *Pharmax*).
Capsules of 170 mg. Syrup 85 mg./5ml.: usual dose one capsule 4 times a day.

DOXYCYCLINE (' Vibramycin ', *Pfizer*).
Capsules 100 mg.: dosage 100 to 200 mg. once a day.

REFERENCES

BERNARD, B., JONG YIN, E. & SIMON, H. J. (1971). *J. Clin. Pharmacol.* **11**, 332.
BRITISH TUBERCULOSIS ASSOCIATION (1968). *Brit. med. J.* **4**, 411.
CASSANO, A., FILICE, A., COSTA, C. & TRIMARCO, C. (1961). *Rif. med.* **75**, 1383.
COOK, J., ELLIOTT, C., ELLIOT-SMITH, A., FRISBY, B. R. & GARDNER, A. M. N. (1957). *Brit. med. J.* **1**, 542.
CLYDE, D. F., MILLER, R. M., DUPONT, H. L. & HORNICK, R. B. (1971). *J. Trop. Med. Hyg.* **74**, 238.
DADSWELL, J. V. (1967). *J. clin. Path.* **20**, 641.
DEARBORN, E. H., LITCHFIELD, J. T. JR., EISNER, H. J., CORBETT, J. J. & DUNNETT, C. W. (1957). *Antibiot. Med.* **4**, 627.
DE CARNERI, I. & MANFREDI, N. (1962). *Arzneimittal-Forsch.* **12**, 1174.
DOWLING, H. F. & LEPPER, M. H. (1964). *J. Amer. med. Ass.* **188**, 307.
EDWARDS, O. M., HUSKISSON, E. C. & TAYLOR, R. T. (1970). *Brit. Med. J.* **1**, 26.
ENGLISH, A. R. (1966). *Proc. Soc. exp. Biol. (N.Y.)* **122**, 1107.
ENGLISH, A. R. (1967). *Proc. Soc. exp. Biol. (N.Y.).* **126**, 487.
ENGLISH, A. R., MCBRIDE, T. J. & RIGGIO, R. (1962). *Antimicrob. Agents and Chemotherapy*—1961, p. 462. Detroit.
FABRE, J., PITTON, J. S., VIRIEUX, C., LAURENCET, F. L., BERNHARDT, J. P. & GODEL, J. C. (1967). *Schweiz. med. Wschr.* **97**, 915.
FEDORKO, J., KATZ, S. & ALLNOCH, H. (1968). *Amer. J. med. Sci.* **255**, 252.
FIELDS, J. P. (1961). *J. Pediat.* **58**, 74.
FINLAND, M., & GARROD, L. P. (1960). *Brit. med. J.* **2**, 959.
FORTI, G. & BENINCORI, C. (1969). *Lancet* **1**, 782.
FRISK, A. R. & TUNEVALL, G. (1969). *Antimicrob. Agents Chemother.*, 1968, p. 335.
GRAY, W. D., HILL, R. T., WINNE, R. & CUNNINGHAM, R. W. (1953). *J. Pharmacol. exp. Ther.* **109**, 223.
JACKSON, G. G., HAIGHT, T. H., KASS, E. H., WOMACK, C. R., GOCKE, T. M. & FINLAND, M. (1951). *Ann. intern. Med.* **35**, 1175.
JOHNSTONE, F. R. C. & COCKCROFT, W. H. (1968). *Lancet* **1**, 660.
KLINE, A. H., BLATTNER, R. J. & LUNIN, M. (1964). *J. Amer. med. Ass.* **188**, 178.
KNOTHE, H. & MAHLER, J. (1959). *Dtsch. med. Wschr.* **84**, 1687.
KUHARIC, H. A., ROBERTS, C. E. JR., & KIRBY, W. M. M. (1960). *J. Amer. med. Ass.* **174**, 1779.
KUNELIS, C. T., PETERS, J. L. & EDMONDSON, H. A. (1965). *Amer. J. Med.* **38**, 359.
KUNIN, C. M., DORNBUSH, A. C. & FINLAND, M. (1959). *J. clin. Invest.* **38**, 1950.
LANE, P. & WILLIAMSON, D. M. (1969). *Brit. med. J.* **2**, 76.
LEPPER, M. H., WOLFE, C. K., ZIMMERMAN, H. J., CALDWELL, E. R. JR., SPIES, H. W. & DOWLING, H. F. (1951). *Arch. intern. Med.* **88**, 271.
LITTLE, P. J. & BAILEY, R. R. (1970). *N.Z. Med. J.* **72**, 183.
LOWBURY, E. J. L. & HURST, L. (1956). *J. clin. Path.* **9**, 59.
LUNDSGAARD-HANSEN, P., SENN, A., ROOS, B. & WALLER, U. (1960). *J. Amer. med. Ass.* **173**, 1008.

McCORMACK, W. M., CHOWDHURY, A. M., JAHANGIR, N., FARIDUDDIN, A. & MOSLEY, W. H. (1968). *Bull. W.H.O.* **38,** 787.
MAROON, J. C. & MEALY, J. (1971). *J. Amer. Med. Ass.* **216,** 1479.
MÉRIER, G., LAURENCET, F. L., RUDHARDT, M., CHUIT, A. & FABRE, J. (1969). *Helv. Med. Acta* **35,** 124.
MITCHELL, R. G. & BABER, K. G. (1965). *Lancet* **1,** 25.
MORGAN, T. & RIBUSH, N. (1972). *Med. J. Austral.* **1,** 55.
NEUVONEN, P. J., GOTHONI, G., HACKMAN, R. & A. F. BJORKSTEN, K. (1970). *Brit. med. J.* **4,** 532.
OTTE, H. J. (1960). *Zbl. Bakt.* 1, Abt. Orig. **180,** 569.
OWEN, L. N. (1963). *Arch. oral Biol.* **8,** 715.
OWEN-SMITH, M. S. (1969). *J. roy. Army med. Corps* **115,** 23.
PERCIVAL, A., ARMSTRONG, E. C. & TURNER, G. C. (1969). *Lancet* **1,** 998.
PINES, A., RAAFAT, H., PLUCINSKI, K., GREENFIELD, J. S. B., LINSELL, W. D. & SOLARI, M. E. (1968). *Brit. J. Dis. Chest* **62,** 19.
REDIN, G. A. (1967). *Antimicrob. Agents and Chemother.*—1966, p. 371.
REES, T. A. (1971). *Lancet* **1,** 938.
REMINGTON, J. S. & FINLAND, M. (1962). *Clin. Pharmacol. & Ther.* **3,** 284.
RENNAU, H. & SCHMIEDEL, A. (1968). *Münch. med. Wschr.* **110,** 1136.
RIBUSH, N. & MORGAN. T. (1972). *Med. J. Austral.* **1,** 53.
RIECKMANN, K. H., POWELL, R. D., McNAMARA, J. V., WILLERSON, D., KASS, L., FRISCHER, H. & CARSON, P. E. (1971). *Amer. J. Trop. Med. Hyg.* **20,** 811.
ROBERTS, C. E. JR., PERRY, D. M., KUHARIC, H. A. & KIRBY, W. M. M. (1961). *Arch. intern. Med.* **107,** 204.
ROSENBLATT, J. E., BARRETT, J. E., BRODIE, J. L. & KIRBY, W. M. M. (1967). *Antimicrob. Agents and Chemother.*—1966, p. 134.
SCHULZ, J. C., ADAMSON, J. S., WORKMAN, W. W. & NORMAN, T. D. (1963). *New Engl. J. Med.* **269,** 999.
SHILS, M. E. (1963). *Ann. Int. Med.* **58,** 389.
SNEDDON, I. B. (1966). *Brit. J. Dermatol.* **78,** 649.
STEIGBIGEL, N. H., REED, C. W. & FINLAND, M. (1968). *Amer. J. med. Sci.* **255,** 179.
SWEENEY, W. M., HARDY, S. M., DORNBUSH, A. C. & RUEGSEGGER, J. M. (1957). *Antibiot. Med.* **4,** 642.
SWEENEY, W. M., DORNBUSH, A. C., & HARDY, S. M. (1962). *Amer. J. med. Sci.* **243,** 296.
TUBARO, E. (1964). *Brit. J. Pharmacol.* **23,** 445.
WAISBREN, B. A. & HUECKEL, J. S. (1950). *Proc. Soc. exp. Biol. (N.Y.)* **73,** 73.
WALLMAN, I. S. & HILTON, H. B. (1962). *Lancet* **1,** 827.
WELCH, H., LEWIS, C. N., STAFFA, A. W. & WRIGHT, W. W. (1957). *Antibiot. Med.* **4,** 215.
WHALLEY, P. J., ADAMS, R. H. & COMBES, B. (1964). *J. Amer. med. Ass.* **189,** 357.
WHITBY, J. L. & BLACK, H. J. (1964). *Brit. med. J.* **2,** 1491.
WITKOP, C. J. & WOLF, R. O. (1963). *J. Amer. med. Ass.* **185,** 1008.
WOOD, W. S. & KIPNIS, G. P. (1953). *Antibiot. Ann.* 1953-54, p. 98.

CHAPTER 10

MACROLIDES

THIS is a large group of closely similar antibiotics, the more widely used of which were discovered in 1952-4. They all consist of a macrocyclic lactone ring—to which they owe the generic name macrolide—to which sugars are attached. Their chemical inter-relationships are reviewed by Celmer (1966). Erythromycin, the first to be discovered, has the highest activity, at least *in vitro,* and has been used more extensively and studied more thoroughly than either oleandomycin or spiramycin, which rank next in importance and are commercially available.

ERYTHROMYCIN

This antibiotic was obtained in 1952 in the Lilly Research Laboratories, Indianapolis, from a strain of *Streptomyces erythreus* derived from soil from the Philippines. Its structure

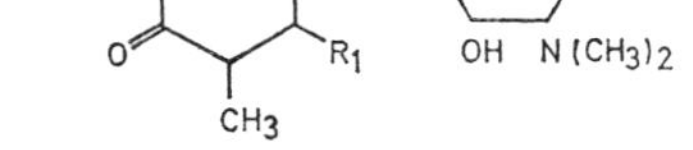

	Erythromycin A	Oleandomycin
R_1	L – cladinose	L – oleandrose
R_2	$CH_2 \cdot CH_3$	CH_3
R_3	$< \begin{array}{l} CH_3 \\ OH \end{array}$	CH_3
R_4	CH_3	$< \begin{array}{l} CH_2 \\ O \end{array}$
R_5	$< \begin{array}{l} CH_3 \\ OH \end{array}$	CH_3

FIGURE 12
Structure of macrolides.

is shown in Fig. 12. There are three erythromycins, of which B and C possess lesser activity. Erythromycin is a faintly yellow crystalline weak base, soluble only to the extent of about 0·1 per cent in water, but readily so in ethanol and other organic solvents. Neutral solutions are stable for many weeks at 5°C, but at room temperature there is some loss after a few days; at a pH below 5 loss of activity is rapid.

Antibacterial Activity

The sensitivity of pathogenic bacteria to erythromycin is shown in Table 21. Inoculum size or presence of serum has only a small effect on the M.I.C. but pH is an important factor, activity increasing with increase in pH up to 8·5.

TABLE 21

Sensitivity of Bacteria to Erythromycin

Gram-positive Bacteria	MIC μg./ml.	Gram-negative Bacteria	MIC μg./ml.
Str. pneumoniae	0·01 - 0·2	N. gonorrhoeae	0·04 - 0·4
Str. pyogenes	0·02 - 0·2	N. meningitidis	0·2 - 1·6
Str. viridans	0·02 - 3·1	H. influenzae	0·4 - 3·1
Str. faecalis	0·6 - 3·1	B. pertussis	0.2
Staph. aureus	0·01 - 1·6	Brucella abortus	10
Staph. albus	0·2 - 3·1	Brucella melitensis	0·3
C. diphtheriae	0·2 - 3·1	E. coli	8 - 300
Cl. tetani	0·2 - 0·6	Shigella spp.	100 - 200
Cl. welchii	0·1 - 0·2	Salmonella spp.	100 - 200
Myco. kansasii	0·5 -2·0	Kl. aerogenes	>100
Myco. scrofulaceum	0·5-16·0	Kl. pneumoniae	>100
Myco. fortuitum	R	Proteus spp.	>100
		Ps. aeruginosa	>100

Noteworthy features of the spectrum are uniformly high activity against pneumococci and haemolytic streptococci of group A and rather less activity against *Staph. aureus*. The more vulnerable Gram-negative genera *Neisseria* and *Haemophilus* are also sensitive, and the hardier enterobacteria generally resistant although some strains of *Escherichia* are inhibited (and killed) by as little as 8 μg./ml. *Mycoplasma pneumoniae* is sensitive to 0·004-0·016 μg erythromycin per ml. (Niitu *et al.*, 1970). Differential sensitivity to erythromycin and lincomycin separates *Mycoplasma hominis*, which is sensitive to lincomycin and resistant to erythromycin, from T-strains (Csonka and Corse, 1970) which are sensitive to erythromycin and resistant to lincomycin. Erythromycin also exerts anti-rickettsial (*R. prowazeki*) activity in the embryonated egg, and an action inferior to that of chlortetracycline on the *Chlamydia* of lymphogranuloma venereum.

Although the action of erythromycin is predominantly bacteristatic in low concentrations, somewhat higher ones are distinctly if slowly bactericidal, there being few survivors after 24 hours' exposure.

Figure 13 shows that erythromycin is the most active agent *in vitro* against *Str. pneumoniae.*

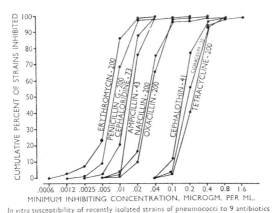

In vitro susceptibility of recently isolated strains of pneumococci to 9 antibiotics

FIGURE 13

Redrawn from Kislak *et al.* (1965). *Amer. J. med. Sci.* 250, 261.

Acquired Resistance

Strains of *Staph. aureus,* enterococcus and *Str. pneumoniae* develop 500-fold increases in resistance after 3-12 subcultures in the presence of the antibiotic, and strains of *Str. pyogenes* and *Str. viridans* 20-fold increases in resistance after 20 subcultures. The resistance is only moderately stable and resistant variants often consist of a mixed population, the individual cells of which have a wide variation in sensitivity to erythromycin. Resistant mutants of *Staph. aureus* produced *in vitro* frequently give rise to small colonies with relatively little pigment production and produce little or no coagulase. Similar changes may also be seen when erythromycin resistance occurs *in vivo.*

Increased resistance is not often observed to develop during successful short-term treatment, but during more prolonged treatment of infections more difficult to eradicate, such as endocarditis, it is common. Where such resistant staphylococci emerge, they may spread rapidly in a hospital where the use of erythromycin is extensive.

Resistant strains of pneumococci (Cooper *et al.*, 1968) and of haemolytic streptococci which spread to several contacts have been reported (Sanders *et al.*, 1968).

Cross-resistance

Staphylococci passaged in the presence of one of the major macrolides (or such minor ones as have been examined) develop resistance not only to the agent to which they were exposed but uniformly to all the macrolides tested. When haemolytic streptococci are passaged *in vitro* (Malke, 1970) or when macrolide-resistant Gram-positive cocci emerge in the course of treatment, they commonly show different degrees of cross resistance with other macrolides and with the chemically unrelated lincomycin. This is well illustrated by the outbreak of haemolytic streptococcal infection described by Lowbury and Kidson (1968) in which streptococci first appeared which were resistant to erythromycin but sensitive to lincomycin, and were then succeeded by strains which were resistant to both agents or resistant to lincomycin but sensitive to erythromycin. The degree of resistance to the two agents varied considerably from strain to strain and resistant Gram-positive cocci have generally exhibited a spectrum of unstable shared resistances with extreme strains resistant to only one agent. At least two kinds of mutants are involved in these resistance patterns (Malke, 1970; Weisblum *et al.*, 1971) and in some, such resistance is probably plasmid-borne.

Dissociated Resistance

There also occurs in some strains of staphylococci which emerge in treated patients a most intriguing form of cross resistance described by Garrod (1957) as *dissociated resistance*.

These strains consist of cells the majority of which are sensitive to erythromycin, but growth on a medium containing the antibiotic produces a uniformly and highly resistant population. A unique feature of the behaviour of such organisms is that in the presence of erythromycin they are also resistant to oleandomycin, spiramycin, lincomycin and group B depsipeptides (p. 81) although in its absence they are fully sensitive (Figs.

14 and 15). Weaver and Pattee (1964) showed that erythromycin is the specific inducer of this resistance which is due to the production by the bacterial cell of a second type of ribosome (Weisblum *et al.*, 1971). Within 40 minutes of exposure (about one generation) more than 90 per cent of the population becomes resistant. Reversion to sensitivity is complete after 90 minutes of growth in the absence of erythromycin.

PHARMACOKINETICS

Absorption

The acid lability of erythromycin base necessitates administration in a form giving protection from gastric acid. Delayed and incomplete absorption is obtained from enteric-coated tablets and there is a good deal of individual variation, adequate levels not being attained at all in a few subjects. Alternatives are to give capsules of erythromycin stearate (which is resistant to gastric acid, and broken down in the intestine liberating the base) or the propionyl ester of erythromycin in the form of its lauryl sulphate (erythromycin estolate), which possesses the two advantages of tastelessness and resistance to gastric acid. The estolate is absorbed as the propionyl ester which is microbiologically inactive and must be hydrolysed in the body to the active base. Initial rapid hydrolysis affects relatively little of the drug and is followed by a period of slow breakdown during which the ratio of active to inactive compound remains fairly constant (Stevens *et al.*, 1969). As with other compounds which depend on *in vivo* liberation of active compound from inactive precursors (see p. 185) there has been some disagreement over the true concentrations of circulating active agent in patients treated with the estolate (Tardrew *et al.*, 1969). In a crossover study in 30 subjects Bell (1971) found peak levels of $1\cdot1$-$2\cdot9$ μg./ml. (nil in one subject) 2-4 hours after 250 mg. of the estolate and $0\cdot05$-$0\cdot37$ μg./ml. ($0\cdot57$ μg./ml. in 1 subject and nil in 3) 2-6 hours after 250 mg. of the stearate. The serum levels obtained after single doses of various preparations are given in Table 22. Other salts of erythromycin sometimes administered are the propionate and the succinate.

PARENTERAL INJECTION. The gluceptate (glucoheptonate) and lactobionate of erythromycin are suitable for intravenous injection and are useful for attaining an immediate effect and higher blood levels (Table 22). Peak values of 3·5-10·7 μg. per ml. were obtained after a dose of 250 mg. of the gluceptate by Lake and Bell (1969). Intramuscular injection is also possible but causes pain, and the dose should not exceed 100 mg.

Distribution

Erythromycin is at first distributed throughout the body water (Lake and Bell, 1969) and tends to be retained longer in the liver and spleen than in the blood (Table 23). Only very

TABLE 22

Erythromycin Serum Levels in Man

Preparation	Dose mg.	Route	Peak Hrs.	Peak μg./ml.	Half life hrs.
Base	250 500 1,000	oral	3-4 2-4 4	0·25-0·5 0·9-1·4 1·3-1·5	2-4
Stearate fasting	250 500	oral	2 2-4	1·3 0·4-1·8	
after food	500		2-4	0·1-0·4	2-4
Propionate fasting	500		2-4	0·4-1·9	3-5
after food	500	oral	4	0·3-0·5	3-4
Estolate fasting	250 500	oral	2-4 1-2	0·36-3·0 1·4-5·0	2-4
after food	250 500		2-4	1·1-2·9 1·8-5·2	
Lactobionate *Gluceptate*	500 300	I/V I/V	0 0	11·5-30·0 20·0-80·0	1-2

Bell, S. M. (1971). *Med. J. Aust.* **2,** 1280.
Davis, D. S. & Romansky, M. J. (1955). *Antibiot. Ann.* 1954-5, p. 286.
Griffith, R. S. (1955). *Antibiot. Ann.* 1954-5, p. 269.
Griffith, R. S. & Black, H. R. (1962). *Antibiot. Chemother.* **12,** 398.
Griffith, R. S. & Black, H. R. (1964). *Amer. J. med. Sci.* **247,** 69.
Hirsch, H. A. & Finland, M. (1959). *Amer. J. med. Sci.* **237,** 693.
Lake, B. & Bell, S. M. (1969). *Med. J. Aust.* **i,** 449.
Lopez-Belio, M. & Takimura, Y. (1955). *Antibiot. Ann.* 1954-5, p. 295.
Reichelderfer, T. E. *et al.* (1960). *Antibiot. Ann.* 1959-60, p. 899.

low levels are attained in the cerebro-spinal fluid. Furgiuele (1964) found good penetration into the aqueous humour after oral erythromycin. Levels of 0·1 μg. per ml. occurred when the serum level was 0·36 μg. per ml. There was no demonstrable penetration into the vitreous. Bass *et al.* (1971) gave 12·5 mg./kg. of two erythromycin preparations 6-hourly to children with otitis media and measured the concentrations of drug in the serum level was 0·36 μg. per ml. There was no demonstrable In those given the succinate the concentrations in serum and exudate were 0·45-2·6 and 0·24-1·02 μg./ml. respectively; in those given the estolate : 3·9-12·3 and 1·7->8 μg. per ml.

Excretion

Erythromycin is excreted both in the urine and in the bile but only a fraction of the dose can be accounted for in this way. Urinary concentrations on 1 g. a day of propionyl erythromycin have been reported to be 13-46 μg. per ml. and on similar doses of erythromycin base 11-24 μg. per ml. Lake and Bell (1969) found peak concentrations of 7·4-15·2 μg. per ml. 3-4 hours after 250 mg. of the estolate. Studies in the dog suggest that what little is excreted in the glomerular filtrate is partially re-absorbed by the tubules.

Fairly high concentrations are found in the bile in man: 10 μg. per ml. in subjects receiving the propionyl ester, and 64 μg. per ml. in those receiving the base, the bile-serum concentration ratio being about 4 for the propionyl ester, and 30 for the base. It is possible that the smaller excretion of the propionyl ester into the bile accounts in part for its better maintained serum levels. Even so, only about 1·5 per cent of the dose of the base (0·2 per cent of the ester) appears in the bile in the first eight hours. Much of the rest is presumably demethylated (Mao and Tardrew, 1965) or otherwise degraded.

Toxicity and Side Effects

No toxic effects of any consequence have ever been recorded from the administration of erythromycin base. This unfortunately cannot be said of erythromycin estolate which, like the similar ester of oleandomycin (p. 175) may give rise in patients treated for more than 14 days to signs of liver damage.

These consist of upper abdominal pain, fever, hepatic enlargement, a raised serum bilirubin, with or without actual jaundice, pale stools and dark urine and eosinophilia. The condition may mimic viral hepatitis, cholecystitis, pancreatitis or cardiac infarction. At least 56 such episodes have been described in detail (11 patients receiving triacetyloleandomycin and the rest in patients receiving erythromycin estolate) according to Braun (1969), who discusses the difficulty of reconciling widely divergent views in the literature about the incidence and origin of this complication.

There have been no deaths and on stopping the drug recovery has been complete (McKenzie and Doyle, 1966). Nevertheless, the relation to the estolate appears to be well founded. Once patients have recovered, recurrence of symptoms can be produced by giving the estolate but not by giving the base or stearate (Brown, 1963). This together with the relative frequency of the reaction after second courses of the drug, peripheral eosinophilia and other evidence of sensitivity, and the histological appearances (Popper *et al.*, 1965) suggest that the reaction results from a mixture of intra-hepatic cholestasis of hypersensitive origin and liver cell necrosis. An element of direct hepatoxicity (which might trigger more severe reactions in hypersensitive individuals) is suggested by the greater damage produced in mouse liver tissue cultures by the estolate than by the base or stearate (Dujovne *et al.*, 1970), and by the common development of abnormal liver function tests in patients receiving the estolate. However, increase in SGOT often occurs as the sole abnormality and this must be interpreted with caution since some metabolite of the estolate interferes with the measurement commonly used (Sabath *et al.*, 1968).

Gastro-intestinal disturbances have been found in 5-6 per cent of those patients treated with the propionate and 2 per cent of those treated with the estolate. Nausea and vomiting are said to be more common with the propionate and diarrhoea with the estolate. Allergic effects occur in about 0·5 per cent of patients.

It would be wrong to give the impression, by reviewing the side effects which have been reported, that erythromycin is a toxic substance. Leaving aside the special problem of the hepatotoxicity of the estolate, there is no doubt that erythromycin is one of the most innocuous antibiotics in current use.

OLEANDOMYCIN

This antibiotic was isolated in 1954 in the laboratories of Charles Pfizer & Co. from a strain of *Streptomyces antibioticus*. Its *in vitro* activity is less than that of erythromycin but greater than that of spiramycin: the factor by which that of erythromycin exceeds it was found to be two to four for *Staph. aureus* and about 10 for *Str. pyogenes*. Like erythromycin it is incompletely absorbed, and an ester, triacetyloleandomycin, gives improved blood levels, but this, like erythromycin estolate, can cause liver damage.

Oleandomycin has been extensively used as a 1:2 mixture with tetracycline (Sigmamycin) a combination for which synergic properties were claimed, but this has not been confirmed either *in vitro* or in assays of the anti-bacterial activity of the serum of subjects to whom tetracycline was given alone and in combination with oleandomycin, erythromycin or spiramycin. There is a good deal of French and a great deal of Russian literature on oleandomycin which we have not attempted to review. As far as clinical utility and safety are concerned, those who admire the drug take much the same view of it as we have taken of erythromycin.

SPIRAMYCIN

Spiramycin (Rovamycin) was obtained in 1954 in the Rhone-Poulenc Research Laboratories from a strain of *Streptomyces ambofaciens* derived from a sample of soil collected near Paris (Pinnert-Sindico *et al.*, 1955). This organism forms three closely related antibiotics, of which spiramycin A is used therapeutically.

Spiramycin has a substantially lower *in vitro* activity than erythromycin: 16-32-fold against *Staph. aureus,* 8-16-fold against *Str. pyogenes,* and 4-8-fold against *Str. pneumoniae.*

If spiramycin had no other property tending to compensate for its lesser anti-bacterial activity, the clinical results claimed for it would be difficult to understand. It seems that this property may be exceptional persistence in the tissues. Macfar-

lane *et al.* (1968) who successfully used the drug for the prevention of post-prostatectomy staphylococcal sepsis, found levels
12 hours after a dose of 1 g. in man of 0·25 μg./ml. in serum,
5·3 μg./ml. in bone, 6·9 μg./ml. in pus, and 4 hours after the
dose, 10·6 μg./ml. in saliva. As with erythromycin, high levels
were found in the prostate (27 μg./ml.) after repeated dosage.
It is evident from comparative studies of different macrolides
that at a time when the spiramycin content of the blood has
fallen to a low level, high concentrations persist in the organs,
whereas the organ content of erythromycin, oleandomycin or
carbomycin declines much more rapidly (Table 23).

TABLE 23

Concentrations of Antibiotic in Organs (μg./g.) and Blood (μg./ml.) of Mice
6 and 24 hrs. after Single Oral Dose of 500 mg. per kg.

	Spiramycin		Erythromycin		Oleandomycin		Carbomycin	
	6 hrs.	24 hrs.	6 hrs.	24 hrs.	6 hrs.	24 hrs.	6 hrs.	24 hrs.
Spleen	122	164	80	6	114	4	97	22
Kidney	107	108	5	<1	5	<1	7	<1
Lung	87	103	43	<1	42	<1	18	>1
Heart	56	46	2·5	2	22	3	6	<3
Liver	150	32	37	<1	170	<1	3	<1
Blood	11.2	3·9	16	5	8·6	1.8	16	7·2

Benazet and Dubost (1959). *Antibiot. Ann.* 1958-9, p. 211.

Spiramycin has been used in the treatment of ocular toxoplasmosis, but is inferior to pyrimethamine (Nolan and Rosen,
1968). It inhibits the growth of some experimental tumours, but
the claim that it might be useful in the treatment of skin cancer
has not been substantiated (Klein *et al.*, 1965).

CLINICAL APPLICATIONS

Since erythromycin was acclaimed as a new barrier to the
onslaught of the staphylococcus our resources have multiplied
remarkably and one of the the newer agents will almost always
be preferred for a resistant staphylococcal infection. This still
leaves a large field of usefulness in pneumococcal and streptococcal infection in which there is ample evidence of its efficacy,

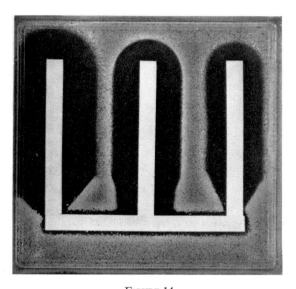

FIGURE 14

Effect of erythromycin on the sensitivity of erythromycin-resistant *Staph.
aureus* to clindamycin, pristinamycin and spiramycin. Strips contain: (hori-
zontal) erythromycin, (left) clindamycin, (centre) pristinamycin, (right)
spiramycin.

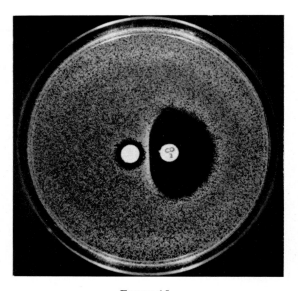

FIGURE 15

Culture of *Staph aureus* showing dissociated resistance to erythromycin.
Discs contain: (left) erythromycin 10 μg., (right) clindamycin 2 μg. Although
the organism appears sensitive to clindamycin (because resistance is induced
only by erythromycin: page 170), treatment with this drug usually produces
full resistance.

and in clostridial infections (p. 334), for which erythromycin is a natural second choice in patients sensitive to penicillin. Erythromycin appears to be as effective as penicillin in the treatment of diphtheria and some authors regard it as the drug of choice in the treatment of carriers. Because of the common cross-resistance between them, erythromycin and lincomycin should not be used together or sequentially (p. 170). Bass *et al.* (1971) point out that while the levels found in middle-ear exudate are more than sufficient to inhibit *Strep. pyogenes* and the pneumococcus they are unlikely to be inhibitory to many strains of *H. influenzae* which is a common cause of otitis media in the very young child. The advisability of using erythromycin in severe infections depends in part on the ultimate view taken of the hepatic toxicity of erythromycin estolate since the absorption of other forms is sometimes inadequate. Some authors have found that despite the higher serum levels achieved by erythromycin estolate, the clinical response is no better than to the stearate or succinate (Billow *et al.*, 1964), and it has been argued that this shows that (despite the results of assays) in treated patients the levels of microbiologically active drug do not markedly differ. Since it appears to take 10 days or more to produce liver changes and these are reversible, our own feeling at present is that if erythromycin must be given by mouth for severe infection—and perfectly satisfactory parenteral preparations are available—the estolate should be used unless the patient is known to have been treated with it before. It should not be given for more than 10 days. Above all, those using the drug should be alert to the significance of any indication of hepatic derangement.

PHARMACEUTICAL PREPARATIONS AND DOSAGE

ERYTHROMYCIN (Erythrocin, *Abbott* (stearate); Ilotycin, *Lilly* (base). Numerous other proprietary names and preparations of various salts). Tablets 100 mg.; B.P., B.N.F.: (base) 250 mg.; B.P. (Stearate) equiv. 250 mg.; U.S.P. (base or various salts or esters): equiv. 100 and 200 mg. Mixture, B.N.F.. equiv. 80 mg. per 4 ml.; Oral suspension, U.S.P.: equiv. 200 mg. per 5 ml. Injection, U.S.P. (Gluceptate, lactobionate, ethylsuccinate, etc.) 250 mg.; 500 mg. and 1 g. Dose: 1-2 g. daily in divided doses.

ERYTHROMYCIN ESTOLATE (Propionyl erythromycin lauryl sulphate; Ilosone. *Lilly*).
Capsules: Equiv. 125 and 250 mg. erythromycin base; Suspension: equiv. 125 mg. erythromycin base per 5 ml. Dose: 1-2 g. daily in divided doses for not more than 10 days.

OLEANDOMYCIN (Oleandomycin phosphate).
Capsules containing equivalent of 250 mg. of base: sterile powder for solution for intramuscular injection. Usual oral dose 250-500 mg. 4 times daily.

SPIRAMYCIN (Rovamycin, *May & Baker*).
Tablets and capsules of 250 mg., and syrup. Usual dose 0·5-1 g. 4 times daily.

REFERENCES

BASS, J. W., STEELE, R. W., WIEBE, R. A. & DIERDORFF, E. P. (1971). *Pediatrics* **48.** 417.
BELL, S. M. (1971).*Med. J. Aust.* **2,** 1280.
BILLOW, B. W., THOMPSON, E. A., STERN, A. & FLORIO, A. (1964). *Curr. ther. Res.* **6,** 381.
BRAUN, P. (1969). *J. infect. Dis.* **119,** 300.
BROWN, A. R. (1963). *Brit. med. J.* **2,** 913.
CELMER, W. D. (1966). *Antimicrob. Agents Chemother.* 1965, p. 144.
COOPER, R. G., RISCHBIETH, H. G. & VESEY, B. (1968). *Med. J. Aust.* **1,** 1131.
CSONKA, G. & CORSE, J. (1970). *Brit. J. vener. Dis.* **46,** 203.
DUJOVNE, C. A., LAVELLE, G., WEISS, P., BIANCHINE, J. R. & LASAGNA, L. (1970). *Arch. int. Pharmacodyn.* **186.** 84.
FURGIUELE, F. P. (1964). *Amer. J. Ophthal.* **58,** 443.
GARROD, L. P. (1957). *Brit. med. J.* **2,** 57.
KLEIN, E., STOLL, H. L., MILGROM, H., CASE, R. W., TRAENKLE, H. L., GRAHAM, S., LAOR, Y. & HELM, F. (1965). *J. invest. Derm.* **44,** 351.
LAKE, B. & BELL, S. M. (1969). *Med. J. Aust.* **1,** 449.
LOWBURY, E. J. L. & KIDSON, A. (1968). *Brit. med. J.* **2,** 490.
MACFARLANE, J. A., MITCHELL, A. A. B., WALSH, J. M. & ROBERTSON, J. J. (1968). *Lancet* **1,** 1.
MALKE, H. (1970). *J. gen. Microbiol.* **64,** 353.
MAO, J. C.-H. & TARDREW, P. L. (1965). *Biochem. Pharmacol.* **14,** 1049.
MCKENZIE, I. & DOYLE, A. (1966). *Med. J. Aust.* **1,** 349.
NIITU, Y., HASEGAWA, S., SUETAKE, T., KUBOTA. H., KOMATSU, S. & HORI-KAWA, M. (1970). *J. Pediat.* **76,** 438.
NOLAN, J. & ROSEN, E. S. (1968). *Brit. J. Ophthal.* **52**, 396.
PINNERT-SINDICO, S., NINET, L., PREUD'HOMME, J. & COSAR, C. (1955). *Antibiot. Ann.* 1954-5, p. 724.
POPPER, H., RUBIN, E., GARDIOL, D., SCHAFFNER, F. & PARONETTO, F. (1965). *Arch. intern. Med.* **115.** 128.
SABATH, L. D., GERSTEIN, D. A. & FINLAND, M. (1968). *New Engl. J. Med.* **279,** 1137.
SANDERS. E., FOSTER, M. T. & SCOTT, D. (1968). *New. Engl. J. Med.* **278**, 538.
STEPHENS, V. C., PUGH, C. T., DAVIS, N. E., HOEHN, M. M., RALSTON, S., SPARKS, M. C. & THOMPKINS, L. (1969). *J. Antibiot.* **22,** 551.
TARDREW, P. L., MAO, J. C. H. & KENNEY, D. (1969) *Appl. Microbiol.* **18,** 159.
WEAVER. J. R. & PATTEE, P. A. (1964).*J. Bact.* **88,** 574.
WEISBLUM, B., SIDDHIKOL, C., LAI, C. J. & DEMOHN, V. (1971). *J. Bact.* **106,** 835.

CHAPTER 11

PEPTIDES

THE peptide antibiotics form a large group of which very few have found any therapeutic application. They are composed of peptide-linked amino acids which commonly include both D- and L-forms and some unusual compounds. Perlman and Bodanszky (1966) list the amino acid composition of 18 families of antibiotic peptides and 37 others. Characteristic non-amino acid moieties, like the long chain fatty acids of the polymyxins (p. 184), also occur. Ring formation is common.

Antibiotic peptides are commonly produced in families of closely related compounds which sometimes differ only in one amino acid residue. The separation of these close relatives may be so difficult that there is doubt about the homogeneity of some of the compounds and hence doubt about the number of members of the family. There are also strong resemblances between some of the members of different families. This kind of inter-relationship is illustrated in Fig. 17, which shows that the tyrocidines not only closely resemble one another but that half the tyrocidine molecule is made up of the amino acid sequence of gramicidin S.

There is a connection between antibacterial range and the number of basic groups in the molecule. Bacitracin and gramicidin are most active against Gram-positive organisms and each has two basic groups. The compounds of greatest therapeutic importance, colistin and polymyxin B, are more active against Gram-negative organisms and have 5 and 6 basic groups respectively (Herr, 1963).

It is of interest that almost all peptide antibiotics have been isolated from the genus *Bacillus,* and that no other type of antibiotic has emerged from this genus. Those that have found a place in clinical medicine are gramicidin, bacitracin, isolated in the United States in 1945, and the polymyxins, discovered independently in Britain and America in 1947.

179

BACITRACIN

Bacitracin was the outcome of a study of the bacterial flora of contaminated civilian wounds in the Presbyterian Hospital, Columbia University (Johnson, Anker and Meleney, 1945). It was observed that following direct plating of material from the injured tissue, bacteria sometimes appeared on blood agar plates that were not subsequently recovered from broth cultures made at the same time from the same material. This occurred most frequently when the broth cultures contained a large number of aerobic Gram-positive sporing bacilli. The cell-free filtrate of one such bacillus was found to have strong antibiotic activity. Further extraction and purification led to the isolation of a group of closely related polypeptide anti- biotics, designated bacitracin A, B and C after Tracy, the patient from whom the bacillus was originally isolated.

Anti-bacterial Activity

Bacitracin is highly active against many species of Gram- positive bacteria and the pathogenic *Neisseriae*. Although strains of *Staph. aureus* are usually sensitive, they are rather less so than most other Gram-positive bacteria. Haemolytic streptococci of Lancefield's Group A are so much more sensi- tive than streptococci of other groups (to discs containing 0·1 unit) that bacitracin sensitivity is used as a screening test for the identification of Group A streptococci.

Toxicity and Clinical Use

The bacitracins are not absorbed by the oral route. All are nephrotoxic when given parenterally, and depression of renal function may persist for weeks.

With the steady accumulation of less toxic antibiotics it has been recommended that it be removed from human use (Re- port, 1969). It is still included in some preparations for local application (p. 326); absorption may occur from application to ulcerated areas and resulting anaphylaxis has been described (Roupe and Strannegard, 1969).

DEPSIPEPTIDES

This large group of natural cyclic peptides is of great general biological interest. They occur, like their relatives, in families of compounds some of which are antibiotics, some powerful poisons and others devoid of biological effect. They were given the name *peptolides*—which expresses well their kinship (Figure 16) with the peptides on the one hand and the macrolides on the other—but the name was withdrawn when it was found that *depsipeptides* had priority (Russell, 1960). Many

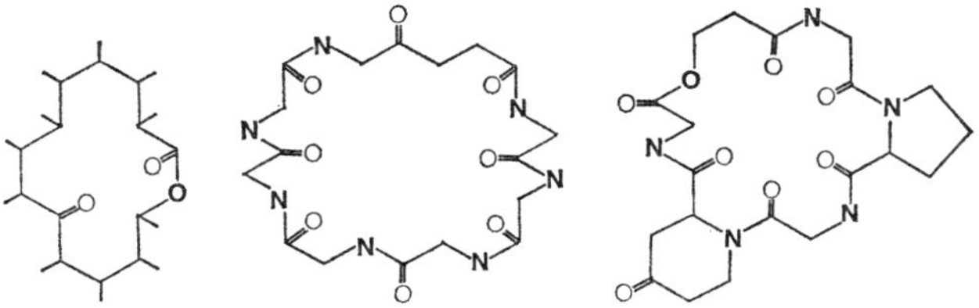

FIGURE 16

Skeleton structures of a typical macrolide (I) peptide (II) and depsipeptide (III) to show the general similarity of their large cyclic molecules, closed in the case of the macrolide through oxygen (O), in the case of the peptide through nitrogens (N) and in the case of the depsipeptide through both.

antibiotic members of the group have been isolated and characterized but few have been pursued with any vigour into the therapeutic field. They are particularly active against streptococci and staphylococci, but include *H. influenzae* and the pathogenic *Neisseria* in their spectrum. Vazquez (1967) reviews the whole group of which the better studied are ostreogrycin, virginiamycin, streptogramin, mikamycin and pristinamycin. With the exception of viridogrisein, which is intrinsically the most active member of the group, they each consist of two components, which act synergically. The group A components of the differently named agents are very closely related if not identical.

Organisms which show ' dissociated resistance ' (p. 170) to the macrolides show cross-resistance with group B depsipeptides. The Group A and B components are separately bacteristatic but in combination not only inhibit staphylococci at much reduced concentrations but kill them. Some have been used in the treatment of staphylococcal septicaemia with ' spectacular' results. Two have been developed commercially: virginiamycin (Staphylomycine, *R.I.T.*, Belgium) which has been fairly extensively studied (Van Dijck, 1969), and pristinamycin (Pyostacine, *Rhone Poulenc*) which has been used a good deal in France almost exclusively for the treatment of infections by staphylococci, most strains of which are inhibited by less than 1 μg./ml. Administration is oral, 2-3 g. being given daily in divided doses.

GRAMICIDIN

This was the first in the field and came from the pioneer work of Dubos (1939) which preceded the extraction and purification of penicillin. It is produced by an aerobic sporing bacillus, *B. brevis*, originally isolated from soil. Crude extracts

Tyrocidine	R_1	R_2
A	L-Phe	D-Phe
B	L-Try	D-Phe
C	L-Try	D-Try

GRAMICIDIN S

$$\begin{bmatrix} \text{L-Val} - \text{L-Orn} - \text{L-Leu} - \text{D-Phe} - \text{L-Pro} \\ \text{L-Pro} - \text{D-Phe} - \text{L-Leu} - \text{L-Orn} - \text{L-Val} \end{bmatrix}$$

TYROCIDINES

$$\begin{bmatrix} \text{L-Val} - \text{L-Orn} - \text{L-Leu} - \text{D-Phe} - \text{L-Pro} \\ \text{L-Tyr} - \text{L-Glu-NH}_2 - \text{L-Asp-NH}_2 - R_1 - R_2 \end{bmatrix}$$

FIGURE 17
Structure of gramicidin S and tyrocidines (Ruttenberg *et al.*, 1965).

of cultures of this bacillus yielded an alcohol-soluble bactericidal substance, tyrothricin, from which two antibiotics, gramicidin and tyrocidine, were separated (Dubos and Hotchkiss, 1941). There are at least four gramicidins in the substance isolated by Dubos and a further compound designated gramicidin S (Soviet), the structure of which is indicated in Fig. 17, was obtained from a strain of *B. brevis* by Gause and Brazhnikova (1944).

Anti-bacterial Activity

Gramicidin is active against most species of aerobic and anaerobic Gram-positive bacteria, including mycobacteria.

Gram-negative bacilli are completely insensitive probably due to the presence of surface phospholipids which inhibit the acton of gramicidin.

Tyrothricin, which contains only 15 to 20 per cent gramicidin, is about as active against pneumococcal infection in mice as gramicidin itself, although the other component of tyrothricin, tyrocidine, is inactive *in vivo*. It has been suggested therefore, that there is a synergic action between tyrocidine and gramicidin, a situation reminiscent of the more recently discovered depsipeptides (p. 181).

Toxicity and Use

By intravenous injection gramicidin is highly toxic to erythrocytes, liver and kidney and therapeutically is of historical interest only. It should never be given systemically and has no special properties to justify its inclusion in mixtures for local application (p. 326).

POLYMYXINS

The polymyxins are a group of basic polypeptide antibiotics derived from a spore-bearing soil bacillus and with a selective action against Gram-negative bacilli. They were first isolated in 1947 independently in one laboratory in Britain (Ainsworth, Brown and Brownlee, 1947) and two in the United States (Stansly, Shepherd and White, 1947; Benedict and Langlykke, 1947). The British investigators called the antibiotic ' aerosporin ' since they identified the bacillus as *B. aerosporus*. The American investigators identified the bacillus as *B. polymyxa* and called the antibiotic polymyxin. Comparative studies in the two laboratories proved the identity of the two bacilli and the name polymyxin was accepted (Symposium, 1949).

Chemical Properties

Five polymyxins, A, B, C, D and E were originally isolated and characterized and others have since been added 'Vogler

7

and Studer, 1966; Kimura *et al.*, 1969). Polymyxin A is the antibiotic originally named aerosporin and polymyxin D is the polymyxin isolated by Stansly, Shepherd and White in 1947. Interestingly, neither has come into therapeutic use for which the less toxic polymyxin B and colistin (Koyama *et al.*, 1950) —shown to be identical with polymyxin E by Suzuki *et al.* (1964)—have been commercially developed. Polymyxins are composed of amino acids linked in the form of a ring with a tail adorned at its end by a characteristic fatty acid. The close relationship of the two components of polymyxin B, B1 and B2, and one of the two components of colistin (colistin *A*, which is identical with polymyxin E1) is shown in Fig. 18. Both polymyxin B and colistin are supplied as the sulphate or the sulpho-methyl derivative.

The sulphates are highly soluble in water and methanol; solutions are fairly stable and withstand heating to 60°C. for one hour. If solutions are sterilized by filtration, there is some loss in either Seitz or sintered glass filters.

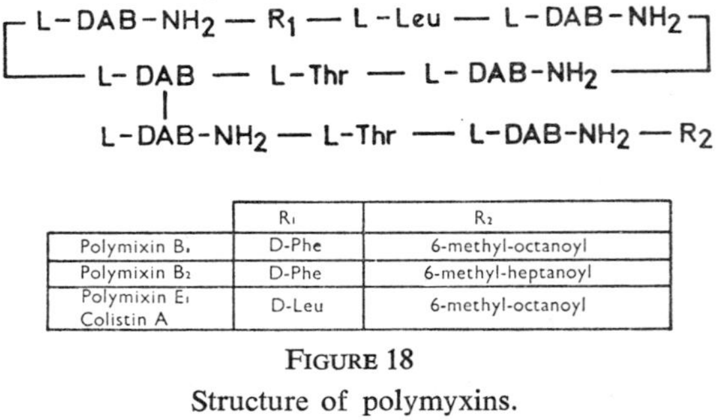

$$L-DAB-NH_2 — R_1 — L-Leu — L-DAB-NH_2$$
$$L-DAB — L-Thr — L-DAB-NH_2$$
$$L-DAB-NH_2 — L-Thr — L-DAB-NH_2 — R_2$$

	R_1	R_2
Polymixin B₁	D-Phe	6-methyl-octanoyl
Polymixin B₂	D-Phe	6-methyl-heptanoyl
Polymixin E₁ Colistin A	D-Leu	6-methyl-octanoyl

FIGURE 18
Structure of polymyxins.
Leu=leucine; Thr=threonine; Phe=phenylalanine; DAB=di-amino-butyric acid.
Suzuki, T. *et al.* (1963). *J. Biochem. (Japan)* **54**, 173, 412, 555.
Suzuki, T. *et al.* (1964). *J. Biochem. (Japan)* **56**, 335.
Wilkinson, S. & Lowe, L. A. (1964). *Nature (Lond.)* **204**, 993.

Sulphomethyl polymyxins

By treatment with formalin and sodium bisulphite, some or all of the 5 amino-groups of the polymyxins can be replaced by sulpho-methyl groups. Sulphomethyl derivatives of both polymyxin B and of colistin (polymyxin E) are commercially available. The substituted compounds differ considerably in their properties from the parent antibiotics. They are relatively painless on injection, less toxic, less active antibacterially (Table 24), and more rapidly excreted by the kidney.

There has been some argument about the basis of these differences. The situation is complicated by the fact that the derivatives consist of undefined mixtures of the mono-, di-, tri-, tetra- and penta-substituted compounds—all of which might theoretically have different properties—and by the fact that the more substituted compounds readily dissociate in solution. The experimental toxicity of the sulphomethyl-colistin commercially available in America (ColyMycin) is so different from that available in this country (Colomycin) that the two compounds probably differ considerably in their degree of sulphomethylation.

Barnett, Bushby and Wilkinson (1964) showed that solutions of the compounds increase progressively in antibacterial activity on incubation until activity approaching that of the parent polymyxin is obtained. They argued from this and other evidence that the sulphomethyl derivatives are relatively non-toxic, inactive compounds which owe their effect to the liberation of the parent polymyxin. Beveridge and Martin (1967) confirmed that the sulphomethyl derivatives rapidly dissociate into more active compounds but found that the parent polymyxin was liberated only if the compounds were boiled. They conclude that the less substituted compounds must possess intrinsic antibacterial activity.

The liberation of more active compounds on incubation considerably complicates the determination of minimum inhibitory concentrations, since the results are compounded of the activities of substances liberated during incubation of the cultures. In a direct comparison of the antibacterial activity of colistin and polymyxin sulphates with their sulphomethyl derivatives, Eickhoff and Finland (1965) found the sulphates to be about eight times more active.

ANTI-BACTERIAL ACTIVITY

All the polymyxins have a similar anti-bacterial spectrum. Although there are slight quantitative differences in their activity *in vitro* (Eickhoff and Finland, 1965) there is effectively complete cross-resistance between them. Nearly all species of Gram-negative bacilli are highly sensitive to polymyxin and on a weight for weight basis are usually more sensitive to polymyxin than to any other antibiotic (Table 24). The main therapeutic importance of the polymyxins lies in their activity against *Pseudomonas*, the sensitivity of which has remained unchanged for 20 years (Adler and Finland, 1971). With the exception of some atypical strains (Goodwin *et al.*, 1971), all species of *Proteus* are resistant. Like the *El tor* vibrio, which is distinguished from classical *Vibrio cholerae* by being resistant to polymyxin B (Roy *et al.*, 1965), *Proteus* evidently owes its resistance to a peculiarity of cell-wall structure which renders it impermeable to the drug (Biswas and Mukergee, 1967; Sud and Feingold, 1970). It is possibly through modifica-

TABLE 24
Sensitivity of Bacteria to Polymyxins
M.I.C. μg. per ml.

	Colistin sulphate	Sulphomethyl-Colistin	Polymyxin B sulphate
Staph. aureus	(11) 75-300	(11) >100	(1·2) 50-200
Str. pyogenes	33	33	10->80
Str. faecalis	>100	>100	>100
Str. viridans	33->100	33->100	33->100
C. diphtheriae	—	—	10
Myco. tuberculosis	—	—	>80
N. meningitidis	4-33	>33	>100
H. influenzae	0·4-0·8	—	0·02
Br. abortus	>100	>100	>100
A. aerogenes	0·02-33 (>100)	0·4->100	0·02-11 (>100)
Kl. pneumoniae	0·01-1·2	0·01-3·7 (>100)	0·02-0·4
Esch. coli	0·01-25 (>100)	0·04->100	0·02-11 (>100)
Proteus spp.	>100	>100	>100
Ps. aeruginosa	0·14-10 (50)	1·2-33	0·02-3·7 (50)
Salmonella spp.	0·01-0·8 (4)	0·04-0·4 (4)	0·02-0·4 (1·2)
Shigella spp.	0·01-0·8 (3)	0·1-0·14 (16)	0·01-0·75

The minimum inhibitory concentrations reported for occasional exceptionally sensitive or resistant strains are shown in brackets.

Graber, C. O. *et al.* (1960). *Antibiot. Ann.* 1959-60, p. 77.
Ross, S. *et al.* (1960). *Ibid.*, p. 89.
Schwartz, B. S. *et al.* (1960). *Ibid.*, p. 41.
Wright, W. W. & Welch, H. (1960). *Ibid.*, p. 61.
Courtieu, A. L. *et al.* (1961). *Ann. Inst. Pasteur. Suppl.* 4, 14.
Postic, B. & Finland, M. (1961). *Amer. J. med. Sci.* 242, 551.
Fekety, F. R. *et al.* (1962). *Ann. intern. Med.* 57, 214.
Tavlor, G. & Allison, H. (1962). *Brit. med. J.* 2, 161.

tion of such a cell-wall component that *Proteus* growing in the presence of sulphonamide becomes susceptible to polymyxin (Holmgren and Muller, 1970) and that this is the mechanism of the well-known synergy between the two agents which can be extended to triple synergy against some strains by the addition of trimethoprim (Simmons, 1970).

Strong interaction between colistin and lipopolysaccharide components of Gram-negative cell wall is probably responsible for its depressant effect on phage attachment (Koike and Iida, 1971) and for its neutralizing effect on endotoxin shock (Corrigan and Bell, 1971).

The pathogenic Gram-negative cocci, *N. gonorrhoeae* and *N. meningitidis*, and nearly all species of Gram-positive bacteria and fungi are also resistant. *Candida tropicalis* is so exceptional in this regard that its sensitivity to 30-75 μg. colistin/ml. can be used as a screening test for its identification, and utilized therapeutically in eradicating it from the urine (Nichols, 1970). Because of its wide activity against Gram-negative organisms, polymyxin has been used in a number of selective media (see for example Orth and Anderson, 1970).

EFFECTS OF SERUM. Complex interactions occur with serum because polymyxins act synergically with the natural bactericidal systems against *Escherichia*, but are adversely affected by the calcium present in serum in their action against *Proteus* (Davis, Iannetta and Wedgwood, 1971).

PHARMACOKINETICS

Polymyxins are not absorbed from the alimentary tract and after parenteral administration of the sulphates blood levels are usually low. Somewhat higher levels are obtained in children, and by repeated administration, peak levels around 1·5 μg./ml. are obtained about an hour after a dose of 60 mg.

Substantially higher plasma levels are obtained from intramuscular injections of sulphomethyl polymyxins but (as in the determination of inhibitory concentrations, page 185) because the drug concentration has to be measured microbiologically there is an opportunity during incubation for the liberation of active agent which was not present in the serum at the time of collection of the samples. Levels reported by various authors are given in Table 25). A more recent study (Froman *et al.*, 1970) gives rather lower values for all the parameters: peak plasma levels of 5-6 μg./ml. at 1-2 hr. with a half-life of 2·75-3 hr. after an intramuscular dose of 150 mg. Ten minutes after a similar intravenous dose, the level was 18 μg./ml falling after 4 hr. to 2 μg./ml. Cox and Harrison (1971) treated some patients with urinary infection with an intravenous priming dose of 1·5-2·5 mg./kg. followed by continuous infusion of 4·8-6 mg./hr. for 20-36 hr. (after which they continued with intramuscular therapy). During the period of infusion they found steady-state levels around 5-10 μg./ml.

TABLE 25
Serum Levels of Sulpho-methyl Colistin in Man.

Dose i/m	Patients	Peak		Half life hrs.
		Hr.	μg. per ml.	
2 mg./kg. 4 mg./kg. 5 mg./kg.	Adult	2-3 3-5 4	6-15 17-25 25	6-12 6-10 5
2·5 mg./kg.	Children	1	5	2-3

Forni, P. V. & Guidetti, E. (1956). *Minerva Med.* **2**, *Suppl.* **77**, 823.
Ross, S. *et al.* (1960). *Antibiot. Ann.* 1959-60, p. 89.
Wright, W. W. & Welch, H. (1960). *Antibiot. Ann.* 1959-60, p. 61.
Colley, E. W. & Frankel, H. L. (1963). *Brit. med. J.* **2**, 790.

Polymyxins bind to both bacterial (p. 254) and mammalian cell membranes. Because of this binding, the agents persist in the liver, kidneys, brain, heart, muscle and lungs (at least of the rabbit) for as long as 72 hours (Kunin and Bugg, 1971). On repeated dosage the drugs accumulate in the tissues although they disappear from the serum. Such behaviour greatly complicates the general pharmacokinetics of the agents and may of course have special importance in relation to both toxicity and therapy of infection in the organs in which they accumulate. Binding is through the amino groups of the molecules and consequently only free colistin and not the sulpho-methyl derivatives, in which the amino groups are occluded, is bound.

Following a dose of 150 mg. sulphomethyl colistin intravenously, none could be detected in the amniotic fluid three hours later. Very low plasma levels (about 0·45 μg./ml.) were found in both mothers and infants born 6-20 hours later. A dose of 30-40 mg. injected into the amniotic fluid of patients not in labour was still present 18 hours later (MacAuley and Charles, 1967).

Excretion

Polymyxin sulphates are excreted mainly by the kidneys but after a considerable lag. With a daily dose of 3 mg./kg., only about 0·1 per cent of the dose is recovered in the first 12 hours, but concentrations varying from 40 to 400 μg./ml. can be found from 24 hours onwards.

The sulphomethyl derivatives are much more rapidly excreted and this accounts for their shorter half-lives. Froman *et al.* (1970) found that 67 per cent of an intramuscular dose and 75 excreted within 24 hours. Urinary levels around 100 to 200 μg./ml. were found at 2 hr. and 15-45 μg./ml. at 8 hr. A rather wider range of the same order (73-315 μg./ml.) was found by Cox and Harrison (1971) on their continuous intravenous regimen. Serum levels are not augmented by probenecid and extra-renal mechanisms probably take part in excretion (Baines and Rifkind, 1964), There is disagreement about the effect of peritoneal dialysis on the plasma half-life, but it is in any case insufficient for the management of overdosage for which Brown *et al.* (1970) successfully resorted to exchange transfusion. Described differences in the effect of haemodialysis may well depend on the membrane used (Curtis and Eastwood, 1968). There does not seem to be excessive retention of sulphomethyl colistin in the new-born (Lawson and Hewstone, 1964).

TOXICITY

Like other members of the family, but to a lesser degree, polymyxin B and colistin are nephrotoxic and neurotoxic. Possible hazards of their use must, therefore, be considered, but when appropriately given their therapeutic efficiency outweighs their nephrotoxicity since renal function improves as severe kidney infection is controlled (Atuk *et al.*, 1964).

Pain (and tissue injury) can occur at the site of injection of the sulphates but the sulphomethyl derivatives are less aggressive. Neurological symptoms such as paraesthesiae with typical numbness and tingling around the mouth, dizziness and weakness are relatively common and neuromuscular blockade, sometimes severe enough to impede respiration, occurs. In a review of 317 courses of treatment, Koch-Weser *et al.* (1970) found evidence of renal damage in 20·2 per cent, with acute tubular necrosis in 1·9 per cent. Neurotoxicity was encountered in 7·3 per cent with respiratory insufficiency in 2·1 per cent. Reactions appeared early in the course of treatment, often within the first four days. Most patients had received no more than conventional doses but toxic manifestations occurred more frequently in heavier patients. Apparently dosage on a direct weight basis results in such patients receiving toxic amounts of the drug. It is suggested that a dosage regimen based on the square root of the weight might ensure adequate treatment for the lighter patient and avoid overdosage in the heavier. The appearance of any evidence of deterioration of renal function or of neuromuscular blocade calls for immediate cessation of treatment. All the toxic manifestations appear to be reversible but complete recovery may be slow.

Nephrotoxicity

In the mouse, the sulphates and sulphomethyl derivatives differ considerably in their toxicity but the more toxic the compound, the more effective it is therapeutically. Nord and Hoeprich (1964) showed that polymyxin B was more toxic to white mice than colistin; that the sulphomethyl derivatives were considerably less toxic, and that the activity of the compounds against *Ps. aeruginosa* was in the same order as their toxicity. For a given antibacterial effect, an equally toxic dose of each of the compounds would have to be given. O'Grady and Pennington (1967) showed that the same was true of the sulphomethyl derivatives in the treatment of an experimental pseudomonas infection in the mouse. The LD_{50} for sulphomethyl colistin was almost three times that for sulphomethyl polymyxin B, but almost three times the dose of sulpho-methyl colistin had to be given to achieve the same therapeutic result.

In the dog, Vinnicombe and Stamey (1969) found a larger differential in the toxicity of the compounds as measured by depression of renal function. An intravenous dose of 5 mg./kg. polymyxin B sulphate, which produced average serum and urine levels of 30 and 60 μg./ml. depressed the G.F.R. and renal plasma flow by about 60 per cent. The same dose of sulphomethyl polymyxin B produced average serum and urine levels of 14·5 and 165 μg./ml. and depressed renal function by 20-25 per cent. In contrast, 40 mg./kg. of sulphomethyl colistin, which produced much higher serum and urine levels of 57 and 1020 μg./ml., had no depressant effect on renal function. When sulphomethyl polymyxin B was given in a dose (25 mg./kg.) which produced about the same urine levels (999 μg./ml.) but higher serum levels (143 μg./ml.), both the G.F.R. and renal plasma flow were reduced by more than 80 per cent.

In human volunteers studied by Caldwell *et al.* (1969) creatinine clearance was depressed less by sulphomethyl colistin than by sulphomethyl polymyxin B. In all subjects renal function returned to normal in 5 to 8 days. An effect on the renal tubules may have been responsible for the association described in leukaemic patients by Rodriguez *et al.* (1970) between polymyxin B therapy and low levels of sodium, potassium, chloride and calcium—sometimes with tetany.

Neurotoxicity. In addition to the common paraesthesiae, several cases of apnoea have been reported following polymyxin therapy, some with other pareses. This effect has not been described in patients with normal renal function (Lindesmith *et al.*, 1968) and presumably results from the high plasma levels which may develop (100 μg./ml. in one patient). It is possible that the cationic polymyxins, which owe their antibacterial effect to interaction with the lipid-rich anionic bacterial cell membrane, exert a similar effect on the lipid-rich synaptic membranes so interfering with conduction (Naiman and Martin, 1967). It is plainly unwise to give polymyxin to patients who are likely to receive muscle relaxants or anaesthetics, or to those suffering from hypoxia or impaired neuromuscular activity . A single dose of 150 mg. sulphomethyl colistin produced complete flaccid paralysis with respiratory arrest in an elderly man suffering from myasthenia gravis (Decker and Fincham, 1971) who subsequently recovered fully.

Histamine Liberation

Polymyxins liberate histamine and serotonin (Levy, 1967) and their intraperitoneal injection depletes the mast cells and in some way alters the peritoneal membrane so that absorption of the drug (and others) is facilitated (Reite and Hausken, 1970). Marschke and Sarauw (1971) observed two patients who developed acute respiratory distress on inhaling polymyxin B but concluded that this was due not to neuromuscular blockade but to airways obstruction possibly related to histamine liberation.

CLINICAL APPLICATIONS

Before the advent of gentamicin (p. 124) and carbenicillin (p. 81), polymyxins were unchallenged as the drug of choice for the treatment of infections due to *Ps. aeruginosa* and also in infections with some other resistant coliform bacilli.

Where systemic polymyxin therapy is indicated, relative painlessness on intramuscular injection and lower toxicity have caused sulphomethyl polymyxins to be generally used. Barnett, Bushby and Wilkinson (1964) have questioned the rationale of this on the ground that if the toxicity and antibacterial activity of the derivatives are due to the liberation of free polymyxin, therapy could be more accurately controlled by giving polymyxin sulphate intravenously. In addition, as the sulphomethyl derivatives are more rapidly excreted, tissue levels are likely to be lower than with polymyxin sulphate. As long as there is argument about the mode of action and pharmacokinetics of these compounds, many will still no doubt prefer to give the sulphomethyl derivatives by the more convenient intramuscular route.

For oral and local application, the more active polymyxin sulphate should be used.

Since the development of resistance to polymyxin is not a problem, and the antibiotic does not appear to damage healing wounds, it can be used as a spray, powder or cream, for the treatment of any superficial infection with *Ps. aeruginosa* such as superficial wounds, ulcers or otitis externa. A cream containing 1 mg. per g. polymyxin has had considerable success in preventing burns becoming colonized by *Ps. aeruginosa.*

PHARMACEUTICAL PREPARATIONS AND DOSAGE

COLISTIN SULPHATE (Polymyxin E Sulphate; Colomycin,* *Pharmax*; Coly-Mycin, *U.S.A.*)
    UNIT=0·00005128 mg. British Standard (1965)=19,500 units per mg. Tablets: 250,000 units; B.P. 1·5 mega units; Syrup: 250,000 units per 5 ml. Dose: oral: 9-18 mega units, daily in divided doses.

COLISTIN SULPHOMETHATE SODIUM (Sodium colistimethate, U.S.P., Colomycin* Injection, *Pharmax*, Colo-Mycin Injectable, *U.S.A.*)
    UNIT=0·00008 mg. British Standard (1965)=12,500 units per mg. Injection 0·5 and 1·0 mega units; U.S.P. equiv. 30 and 50 mg. colistin. Dose: i/m, i/v infusion: 3-9 mega units; Intra-thecal: 500-1,000 units per kg. per day in single dose.

POLYMYXIN B SULPHATE (Aerosporin *Burroughs Wellcome*) (Polymyxin M Sulphate, *U.S.S.R.* is similar)
    UNIT = 0·000127 mg. International Standard=7,874 units per mg. Tablets, U.S.N.F.: 250,000 and 500,000 units. Dose: 1-2 mega units per day. Injection, B.P.C., B.N.F.: 500,000 units. Dose: i/m: 500,000 units, 8 hourly.

SULPHOMYXIN SODIUM (Polymyxin B sodium methane sulphonate; Thiosporin, *Burroughs Wellcome*)
    Injection: equiv. 500,000 units polymyxin B sulphate. Dose: i/m: up to 500,000 units, 6 hourly.

* NOT Colimycin, *U.S.S.R.*—an aminoglycoside.

REFERENCES

ADLER, J. L. & FINLAND, M. (1971). *Appl. Microbiol.* **22**, 870.
AINSWORTH, G. C., BROWN, A. M. & BROWNLEE, G. (1947). *Nature (Lond.)* **160**, 263.
ATUK, N. O., MOSCA, A. & KUNIN, C. (1964). *Ann. intern. med.* **60**, 28.
BAINES, R. D. & RIFKIND, D. (1964). *J. Amer. med. Ass.* **190**, 278.
BARNETT, M., BUSHBY, S. R. M. & WILKINSON, S. (1964). *Brit. J. Pharmacol.* **23**, 552.
BENEDICT, R. G. & LANGLYKKE, A. F. (1947). *J. Bact.* **54**, 24.
BEVERIDGE, E. G. & MARTIN, A. J. (1967). *Brit. J. Pharmacol.* **29**, 125.
BISWAS, K. & MUKERJEE, S. (1967). *Proc. Soc. exp. Biol. N.Y.* **126**, 103.
BROWN, J. M., DORMAN, D. C. & ROY, L. P. (1970). *Med. J. Aust.* **2**, 923.
CALDWELL, A. D. S., MARTIN, A. J. & TRIGGER, D. J. (1969). *Brit. J. Pharmacol.* **37**, 283
CORRIGAN, J. J. & BELL, B. M. (1971). *J. lab. clin. Med.* **77**, 802.
COX, C. E. & HARRISON, L. H. (1971). *Antimicrob. Agents Chemother.* 1970, p. 269.
CURTIS, J. R. & EASTWOOD, J. B. (1968). *Brit. med. J.* **1**, 484.
DAVIS, S. D., IANNETTA, A. & WEDGWOOD, R. J. (1971). *J. infect. Dis.* **123**, 392.
DECKER, D. A. & FINCHAM, R. W. (1971). *Arch. Neurol.* **25**, 141.
DUBOS, R. J. (1939). *J. exp. Med.* **70**, 1.
DUBOS, R. J. & HOTCHKISS, R. D. (1941). *J. exp. Med.* **73**, 629.
EICKHOFF, T. C. & FINLAND, M. (1965). *Amer. J. med. Sci.* **249**, 172.
FROMAN, J., GROSS, L. & CURATOLA, S. (1970). *J. Urol.* **103**, 210.
GAUSE, G. F. & BRAZHNIKOVA, M. G. (1944). *Nature (Lond.)* **154**, 703.
GOODWIN, C. S. KLIGER, B. N. & DREWETT, S. E. (1971). *Brit. J. exp. Path.* **52**, 138.
HERR, E. B. JR. (1963). *Antimicrob. Agents Chemother.* 1962, p. 201.
HOLMGREN, J. & MÖLLER, O. (1970). *Scand. J. infect. Dis.* **2**, 121.
JOHNSON, B. A., ANKER, H. & MELENEY, F. L. (1945). *Science* **102**, 376.
KIMURA, Y., MURAI, E., FUJISAWA, M., TATSUKI, T. & NOBUE, F. (1969). *J. Antibiot.* **22**, 449.
KOCH-WESER, J., SIDEL, V. W., FEDERMAN, E. B., KANAREK, P., FINER, D. C. & EATON, A. E. (1970). *Ann. int. Med.* **72**, 857.
KOIKE, M. & IIDA, K. (1971). *J. Bact.* **108**, 1402.
KOYAMA, Y., KUROSASA, A., TSUCHIYA, A. & TAKAKUTA, K. (1950). *J. Antibiot. (Tokyo)* **3**, 457.
KUNIN, C. M. & BUGG, A. (1971). *J. infect. Dis.* **124**, 394.
LAWSON, J. S. & HEWSTONE, A. S. (1964). *Med. J. Aust.* **1**, 917.
LEVY, L. (1967). *Arch. int. Pharmacodyn.* **165**, 92.
LINDESMITH, L. A., BAINES, R. D., BIGELOW, D. B. & PETTY, T. L. (1968). *Ann. intern. Med.* **68**, 318.
MACAULAY, M. A. & CHARLES, D. (1967). *Clin. Pharmacol. Ther.* **8**, 578.
MARSCHKE, G. & SARAUW, A. (1971). *Ann. intern. Med.* **74**, 296.
NAIMAN, J. G. & MARTIN, J. D. Jr. (1967). *J. surg. Res.* **7**, 199.
NICHOLS, M. W. N. (1970). *J. med. Microbiol.* **3**, 529.
NORD, N. M. & HOEPRICH, P. D. (1964). *New Engl. J. Med.* **270**, 1030.
O'GRADY, F. & PENNINGTON, J. H. (1967). *Postgrad. med. J. Suppl.* (*March*) **43**, 72.
ORTH, D. S. & ANDERSON, A. W. (1970). *Appl. Microbiol.* **20**, 508.
PERLMAN, D. & BODANSZKY, M. (1966). *Antimicrob. Agents Chemothei.* 1965, p. 122.
REITE, O. B. & HAUSKEN, O. (1970). *Europ. J. Pharmacol.* **10**, 101.
REPORT (1969). *Joint Committee on the Use of Antibiotics in Animal Husbandry and Veterinary Medicine,* London: Her Majesty's Stationery Office.
RODRIGUEZ, V., GREEN, S. & BODEY, G. P. (1970). *Clin. Pharmacol. Ther.* **11**, 106.
ROUPE, G. & STRANNEGÅRD, Ö (1969). *Arch. Derm.* **100**, 450.

ROY, C., MRIDHA, K. & MUKERJEE, S. (1965). *Proc. Soc. exp. Biol. N.Y.* **119,** 893.
RUSSELL, D. W. (1960). *Biochim. biophys. Acta* **45,** 411.
SIMMONS, N. A. (1970). *J. clin. Path.* **23,** 757.
STANSLY, P. G., SHEPHERD, R. G. & WHITE, H. J. (1947). *Bull. Johns Hopk. Hosp.* **81,** 43.
SUD, I. J. & FEINGOLD, D. S. (1970). *J. Bact.* **104,** 289.
SUZUKI, T., HAYASHI, K., FUJKAWA, K. & TSUKAMOTO, K. (1964). *J. Biochem* **56,** 335.
SYMPOSIUM (1949). *Ann. N.Y. Acad. Sci.* **51,** 875, 879, 891, 897, 909, 952.
VAN DIJCK, P. J. (1969). *Chemotherapy* **14,** 322.
VAZQUEZ, D. (1967). *Antibiotics I: Mechanism in Action.* Ed. D. Gottlieb and P. D. Shaw, Springer-Verlag, Berlin, p. 387.
VINNICOMBE, J. & STAMEY, T. A. (1969). *Invest. Urol.* **6,** 505.
VOGLER, K. & STUDER, R. O. (1966). *Experientia* **22,** 345.

Chapter 12

VARIOUS ANTI-BACTERIAL ANTIBIOTICS

Here follow accounts of antibiotics not classifiable among the main groups described in other chapters. Those of some of the less important are necessarily brief, but some mention of them may be more helpful than none at all. Only those are included which have been used in human therapeutics (bacteriocines being an exception); we do not, for example, include tylosin, a macrolide, or nisin, a peptide, for which the only uses have been non-medical. Other exceptions are antibiotics used exclusively in tuberculosis, which are referred to in Chapter 26.

BACTERIOCINES

These interesting substances differ from antibiotics, and offer no known therapeutic possibilities, but some mention of them, however brief, seems called for.

Bacteriocines are substances formed by bacteria which inhibit the growth of other strains of the same or related species, an effect best demonstrated by cross-streaking on plates. A variable proportion of strains of a given species may be found to form such a substance: others form none. The bacteriocines formed by different strains are not identical: another strain may be inhibited by some and not by others. The best known and most extensively studied are the colicines, formed by *E. coli*, the existence of which was first detected by Gratia in 1925. Staphylococcines were described by Fredericq in 1946. Since then they have been observed in other enterobacteria, including *Salmonella* spp. (Agarwal, 1964; Hamon and Peron, 1966), enterococci (Brock *et al.*, 1963) group A streptococci, in which Kuttner (1966) found the property to be constant in strains of types 12, 4 and 49 derived from cases of nephritis, and a variety of other bacteria, including *Cl. welchii* and *Listeria monocytogenes*.

These substances are of practical interest in two directions. Their multiplicity within a species and different patterns of susceptibility to them afford an opportunity of identifying individual types among strains of the organism: examples are the colicine typing of *Sh. sonnei* and the pyocine typing of *Ps. aeruginosa*. Secondly, they may give rise to very puzzling appearances in diagnostic cultures, as when two staphylococci, one forming a staphylococcine to which the other is susceptible, are present together: the combined effect of the staphylococcine and of the antibiotic in a disc may be to produce a double zone of inhibition (Waterworth, 1956).

What part bacteriocines play in nature is almost unknown. Such evidence as there is of their activity within the body concerns only colicines. By repeated cultures of the faeces of five individuals during six months Branche *et al.* (1963) found that strains of *E. coli* forming colicines tended to persist, whereas non-colicine forming strains were frequently replaced by others. Friedman and Halbert (1960) showed that the growth of *Sh. flexneri* in the mouse peritoneum was antagonized by the addition of a colicine-producing *E. coli* to the inoculum. Braude and Siemienski (1965) injected colicine subcutaneously in mice and found their serum strongly bactericidal: these authors go so far as to suggest that colicines absorbed from the bowel or even the infected urinary tract may ' contribute to the heat-resistant bactericidal property of normal blood '.

REFERENCES

AGARWAL, S. C. (1964). *Bull. Wld Hlth Org.* **30**, 444.
BRANCHE, W. C. JR., YOUNG, V. M., ROBINET, H. G. & MASSEY, E. D. (1963). *Proc. Soc. exp. Biol. N.Y.* **114**, 198.
BRAUDE, A. I. & SIEMIENSKI, J. S. (1965). *J. clin. Invest.* **44**, 849.
BROCK, T. D., PEACHER, B. & PIERSON, D. (1963). *J. Bact.* **86**, 702.
FRIEDMAN, D. R. & HALBERT, S. P. (1960). *J. Immunol.* **84**, 11.
HAMON, Y. & PERON, Y. (1966). *Ann. Inst. Pasteur* **110**, 389.
KUTTNER, A. G. (1966). *J. exp. Med.* **124**, 279.
WATERWORTH, P. M. (1956). *J. med. Lab. Technol.* **13**, 385.

CYCLOSERINE

Cycloserine is a product of *Streptomyces orchidaceus* and other organisms, and has also been synthesized. Chemically it is D-4-amino-3-isoxazolidone, with a molecular weight of only 102, and thus perhaps the simplest known substance possessing antibiotic activity. A fairly wide range of bacteria, both Gram-negative and Gram-positive, including *Myco. tuberculosis,* are sensitive to it. Early studies of *in vitro* activity, such as those of Welch, Putnam and Randall (1955) produced discouraging results, but these were carried out before it was recognized that the action of cycloserine is specifically antagonized by D-alanine, a fact which provides the clue to its mode of action (Fig. 19). Tests in a medium free from this amino acid produce more realistic results. A majority of strains of *E. coli* were inhibited and some were killed, in such a medium by 25·5 μg. per ml. (Hoeprich, 1964): this paper contains similar observations on a variety of other bacteria.

Cycloserine is well absorbed after oral administration, attaining high and well sustained concentrations in the blood and being excreted unchanged in the urine (Anderson *et al.,* 1956). Its principal use is as a second-line drug for the treatment of tuberculosis, but it requires mention here because it also has advocates as a remedy for urinary tract infection including Hoeprich (1963) in the United States and Murdoch and his colleagues (Syme *et al.,* 1961; Gray *et al.,* 1967) in this country. *E. coli* infections are the most susceptible, *Proteus* less so and some others not at all. The dose commonly given is 250 mg. three times a day: Hoeprich advises up to 15-20 mg. per kg. daily in patients under 45, but at ages greater than this or if renal function is impaired it must be reduced. All authors advise blood assays to ensure that the concentration attained shall not exceed 20-25 μg. per ml. Of the two British papers cited, the first reports the results of 14-day courses for the treatment of existing infections, and the second those of long-term treatment with 250 mg. every other day for the prevention of recurrences, in which considerable success is claimed.

Cycloserine passes all toxicity tests in animals, and produces none of the side effects associated with other antibiotics in man, but a drawback to treatment with full doses is the possibility of effects on the central nervous system, ranging from headache and drowsiness to convulsions. The risk of these can be reduced by careful regulation of dosage, and no permanent damage appears to be caused. Sustained release preparations may be helpful in mitigating side effects; this and other aspects of the pharmacokinetics of this drug, as well as its therapeutic

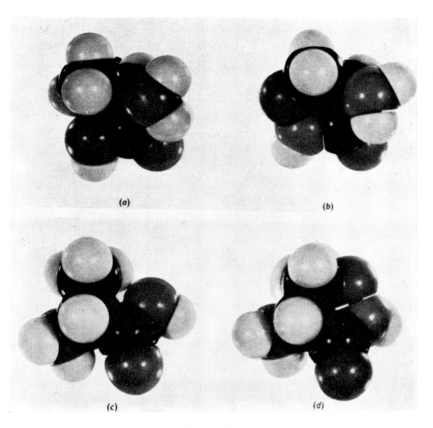

FIGURE 19

Two views of solid models of (a and c) d-alanine and (b and d) d-cyclo-serine (from Richmond, 1966).

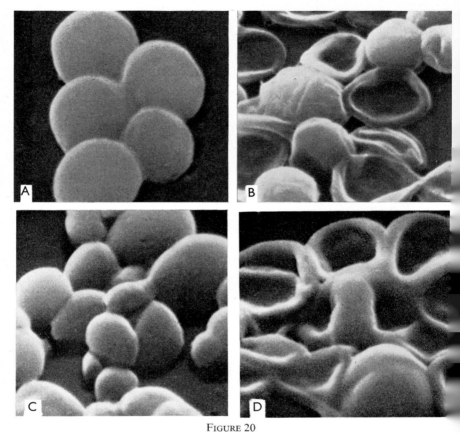

FIGURE 20

Staphylococcus aureus (A) before, and after $2\frac{1}{2}$ hours' exposure to (B) 3 µg. sodium fusidate per ml., (C) 3µg. novobiocin per ml. (D) 12 µg. lincomycin per ml.

(A and B stereoscan electron micrographs x 30,000 by David Greenwood, C and D from Greenwood, D. and O'Grady, F. (1972). *J. gen. Microbiol.* **70**, 263.)

use in tuberculosis, were discussed at an International Symposium (1970).

PHARMACEUTICAL PREPARATION AND DOSAGE

CYCLOSERINE (' Seromycin ' *Lilly*; ' Oxamycin ' *Merck*).
Capsules or Tablets of 250 mg. For dosage see text.

REFERENCES

ANDERSON, R. C., WORTH, H. M., WELLES, J. S., HARRIS, P. N. & CHEN, K. K. (1956). *Antibiot. Chemother.* **6**, 360.
INTERNATIONAL SYMPOSIUM (1970). *Scand. J. resp. Dis.* Suppl. 71, 13.
GRAY, J. A., GEDDES, A. M., WALLACE, E. T. & MURDOCH, J. McC. (1967). *Symposium on Pyelonephritis, Edinburgh,* 1966, p. 33. Edinburgh, E. & S. Livingstone.
HOEPRICH, P. D. (1963). *Arch. intern. Med.* **112**, 405.
HOEPRICH, P. D. (1964). *Amer. J. clin. Path.* **41**, 140.
RICHMOND, M. H. (1966). *Symp. Soc. gen. Microbiol.* **16**, 301.
STROMINGER, J. L. (1962). *Fed. Proc.* **21**, 134.
SYME, J., SLEIGH, J. D., RICHARDSON, J. E. & MURDOCH, J. McC. (1961). *Brit. J. Urol.* **33**, 261.
WELCH, H., PUTNAM, L. E. & RANDALL, W. A. (1955). *Antibiot. Med.* **1**, 72.

FUSIDIC ACID

Several antibiotics from different sources possess the basic cyclopentenophenanthrene skeleton of steroids but their stereochemistry is different. Three have received a fair amount of study: cephalosporin P_1, helvolic acid and fusidic acid (Figure 21). They have in common a narrow antibacterial range, synergic activity with penicillin and some other agents, and ready emergence of resistant mutants on passage *in vitro.* Their principal interest lies in their activity against penicillinase-

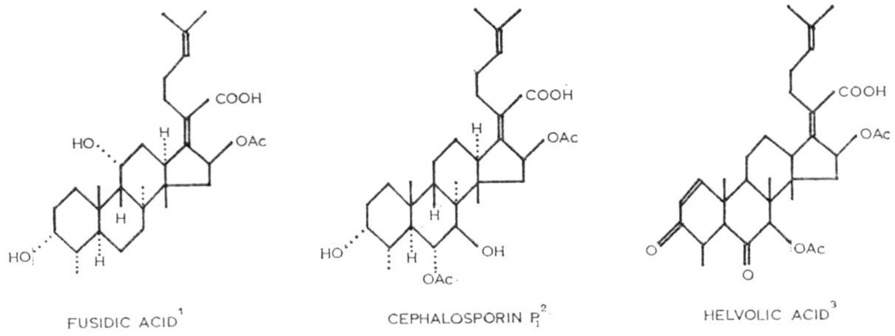

FUSIDIC ACID[1] CEPHALOSPORIN P[2] HELVOLIC ACID[3]

FIGURE 21
Structure of steroid antibiotics.

[1] Gotfredsen, W. O., *et al.* (1965). *Tetrahedron* **25**, 3505.
[2] Halsall, T. G., *et al.* (1966). *Chem. Comm.*—1966, p 685.
[3] Okuda, S., *et al.* (1964). *Chem. Pharm. Bull.* (Japan) **12**, 121.

producing staphylococci. Fusidic acid is about 10 times as active as the others and is the only one commercially available.

Fusidic acid is a colourless crystalline compound sparingly soluble in water, isolated from a strain of *Fusidium coccineum*. Fucidin is the sodium salt and is readily soluble in water (Godtfredsen *et al.*, 1962). The relationship between the structure of fusidic acid and its antibacterial activity has been studied by Godtfredsen *et al.* (1966).

Anti-bacterial Activity. Fucidin is active against species of Gram-positive bacteria and the Gram-negative cocci. Nearly all strains of *Staph. aureus*, regardless of their sensitivity to other antibiotics, are outstandingly sensitive to fucidin. It is bactericidal for many strains in concentrations close to the MIC (although a proportion of the cells, increasing with inoculum

TABLE 26

Minimum Inhibitory Concentrations of Fucidin in μg./ml.

*Staph. aureus**	0·03-0·16
Str. pyogenes	4·2-16·0
Str. viridans	1-6
Str. pneumoniae	2·0-16·0
Str. faecalis	1·0-5·0
N. meningitidis	0·06-0·25
N. gonorrhoeae	0·03-1·0
C. diphtheriae	0·004-0·005
Bacillus spp.	0·06-1·7
Clostridium spp.	0·016-0·59
Noc. asteroides	0·6-5·0
Myco. tuberculosis	0·5-1·6
Kl. pneumoniae	4·0-160·0
Enterobacteria	>100

* Including penicillin-resistant strains.
Godtfredsen, W. *et al.* (1962). *Lancet* **1**, 928; Barber, M. and Waterworth, P. M. (1962). *Lancet* **1**, 931. Black, W. A. and McNellis, D. A. (1971). *J. med. Microbiol.* **4**, 293.

size, always remains) and has been shown by stereoscan electron microscopy to exert a marked destructive effect on staphylococci (Fig. 20). *Nocardia asteroides* and some *C. diphtheriae* and many strains of *Clostridia* are also highly sensitive. Strains of *Myco. tuberculosis* have been shown to be partially inhibited by from 0·5 to 5·0 μg. per ml. Streptococci and pneumococci are relatively resistant and coliform bacilli and fungi are highly resistant (Table 26). The difference in sensitivity between streptococci and staphylococci has been utilized by Lowbury *et al.* (1964) in preparing a selective medium for the isolation of haemolytic streptococci.

Acquired Resistance. A large inoculum of most strains of *Staph aureus* contains a small number of resistant mutants and this appears to be responsible for the effect of inoculum size on the efficacy of fucidin. As would be expected from this, fucidin-resistant strains of *Staph. aureus* emerge rapidly *in vitro* and sometimes during clinical therapy. The growth rate, coagulase, haemolysin and penicillinase production of these mutants appears to be unimpaired. There is cross-resistance between fucidin and cephalosporin P_1.

Resistance appears often to be very unstable and in some poly-resistant strains reversion to the sensitive state on sub-culture may be accompanied by recovery of sensitivity to other agents (Evans and Waterworth, 1966) suggesting that the multiple resistance was plasmid-borne (p. 261). In 50 per cent serum the MIC may increase 50-100-fold. Fucidin is slightly more effective at pH 6-7 than at pH 8 (Stewart, 1964).

Interactions with Penicillins. Because fusidic acid-resistant mutants of staphylococci readily emerge *in vitro,* it has generally been recommended that this should be prevented as far as possible in patients by simultaneous administration of a penicillin or some other agent. As Waterworth (1963) showed, penicillin will kill any emergent resistant mutants while fusidic acid destroys the bulk of the bacterial population and thus prevents generation of sufficient penicillinase to destroy penicillin. The benefits of this peculiar form of ' synergy ' in controlling the minority population is clear, but the wisdom of giving fusidic acid and penicillins together has been questioned because the effect of the two agents on the bulk of the bacterial population can commonly be shown to be antagonistic·

Contradictory findings in the literature probably arise from the fact that different strains of staphylococci respond differently to the combination. Greenwood and O'Grady (1973) describe three distinct patterns of interaction. In the commonest, exhibited by more than half their penicillinase-producing

strains and almost all their penicillin-sensitive strains, there
was two-way antagonism: more staphylococci survived overnight incubation in the presence of fusidic acid and a penicillin
than in the presence of either agent alone. In the second kind
of interaction, least survivors were recovered after incubation
with a penicillin alone, more from the mixture and most from
fusidic acid. In this case there was one-way antagonism of
penicillin by fusidic acid. The remaining strains showed ' indifference ' in that the effect of the more bactericidal agent
(which against some strains was fusidic acid) prevailed. In the
in vitro situation, antagonism of one or other form is evidently
the commonest form of interaction between the two agents but
it is important to note that even where the effect of penicillin
against the bulk of the bacterial population was antagonised,
it always prevented the emergence of fusidic acid-resistant
mutants.

Absorption, Distribution and Excretion. Fucidin is well
absorbed after oral administration, a single dose of 500 mg. in
the adult producing peak plasma levels at about 4 hours of
15-20 μg./ml. In children the absorption is more rapid. Milk
appears to delay absorption, peak concentrations not being
reached for 4-8 hours. Because of slow elimination, considerable accumulation of the drug occurs on repeated administration of doses above 250 mg.: 500 mg. t.d.s. for four days
produced plasma concentrations of 11-41 μg. per ml. after 24
hours and 30-144 μg. per ml. after 96 hours. On doses of 3 g./
day (40 mg./kg.) Saggers *et al.* (1968) found plasma levels of
45-200 μg./ml. An intravenous form of the drug is available
for the treatment of patients in whom oral therapy is impossible.
Guttler and Tybring (1971) found that the relative concentrations in plasma and pus (20·8 and 17·2 μg./ml.) corresponded
with the ratio of their protein contents. The extravascular
albumen pool is as large as that of the plasma and together
with protein in oedema fluid and exudate constitutes an important depot of the drug. About 95 per cent is reversibly
bound to plasma protein.

Fucidin is well distributed in the tissues and most organs of
the body, but does not reach the cerebro-spinal fluid. Inhibitory
levels are obtained in muscle, kidney, lungs and pleural exu-

date Levels of 4-8 μg./ml. were found in bone (Stewart, 1964), and levels in excess of 7μg. per ml. have been demonstrated in aspirated synovial fluid from patients with osteo- or rheumatoid arthritis treated with 0·75 or 1·5 g. sodium fusidate daily after 3–7 days' treatment (Deodhar *et al.*, 1972). The drug has been detected in brain, milk and placenta which it crosses to reach the foetus. In patients treated with 1·5 g. per day, levels of 0·08-0·84 μg./ml. were found in the aqueous humour after one day and 1·2-1·28 μg./ml. after 3 days' treatment (Williamson *et al.*, 1970). Chadwick and Jackson (1969) found levels up to 2·0 μg./ml. and in contrast to other agents (p. 419), levels in the vitreous were 2-3 times as high.

It is excreted and concentrated in the bile where Godtfredsden and Vangedal (1966) detected seven metabolites. Much of the drug was in the form of glucuronides and very little unchanged. Although the stereochemical configuration of fusidic acid and the bile salts is different, the positioning of groups concerned with fat-solubilizing properties is similar. Carey and Small (1971) found fusidic acid to be similar to sodium taurocholate in its micellar properties and the only compound they have studied which was able to mimic the remarkable ability of bile salts to solubilize the biologically important lecithins. Fusidic acid (or conceivably less microbiologically potent congeners) may have a place in the treatment of bile-salt deficient states.

About two per cent of the administered dose can be recovered in active form in the faeces. Little or no active antibiotic is excreted in the urine: less than 1 per cent, producing concentrations of only 0·8 μg. per ml. after four days' treatment. Combined with the fact that very little of the drug is dialysed (no doubt because such a high proportion is bound to protein) this means that in anuric patients on haemodialysis dosage does not need to be modified (Hobby *et al.*, 1970).

Side Effects

When given by mouth fucidin appears to be well tolerated and apart from mild gastro-intestinal disturbance and occasional rashes no untoward symptoms have been reported.

The steroid skeleton of fusidic acid has excited speculation about possible metabolic effects. Wynn (1965) has clearly shown that no profound metabolic changes follow fucidin administration. It has a protein catabolic effect which is milder than that of tetracycline (p. 157) and unlikely to lead to clinical difficulty.

A number of workers have been sufficiently impressed by the rate at which staphylococcal infections heal to suggest that fucidin might exert a beneficial effect on healing, unrelated to its effect on the infection, but the experimental evidence is conflicting (Calnan and Fry, 1962; Cowan, 1965).

CLINICAL APPLICATION. Fucidin is a useful addition to the antistaphylococcal armoury. It has been successfully used for the treatment of a variety of severe staphylococcal infections often after other potent antistaphylococcal agents have failed. Particular benefit has been claimed for fucidin treatment of bone and joint infections in both the acute and intractable chronic forms of the disease (p. 340).

Several authors have reported outstanding success with combinations of fucidin and penicillins despite the fact that the mixture may show antagonism *in vitro* (p. 201). Jensen and Lassen (1969) found no evidence in treated patients that a combination of fucidin and methicillin was antagonistic and the presence of the penicillin is important in preventing the emergence of resistant mutants. Two findings in the study by Greenwood and O'Grady (1973) indicate that in the therapeutic situation this ' synergic ' aspect of interaction is likely to outweigh any antagonistic effect. Even where two-way antagonism was most marked, the combination still exerted a substantial bactericidal effect. Moreover the great difference between the half-lives of fusidic acid and penicillins means that (apart from the first dose) penicillin will be given when substantial concentrations of fusidic acid are already present. In these circumstances antagonism did not occur.

Nevertheless, the possibility of antagonism should be borne in mind when treating severe infections such as endocarditis. An imperfect response from this cause can only convincingly be demonstrated by improvement on withdrawal of one or other agent.

One other pharmacokinetic factor is likely to operate against significant interaction of the two agents *in vitro*. As discussed in the case of combined therapy with trimethoprim and sulphonamide, pairs of agents can only behave in the body as they do *in vitro* if they resemble one another closely in their absorption and distribution characteristics. Fusidic acid is apparently widely distributed in the body while, in the absence of active inflammation, penicillins commonly are not. It may therefore be argued that a second agent used with fusidic acid should follow its distribution more closely than do the penicillins. Erythromycin or lincomycin may be considered for this role, but their interaction with fusidic acid has not been sufficiently closely studied *in vitro* or *in vivo* to identify either as the correct choice.

Local therapy has been successfully used for a number of skin infections including erythrasma (p. 331).

PHARMACEUTICAL PREPARATIONS AND DOSAGE

SODIUM FUSIDATE (Fucidin, *Leo Laboratories*)
Capsules, B.P., B.N.F.: 250 mg. Mixture, B.N.F.: equiv. 175 mg. per 5 ml. Dose: 1·5 g., daily in divided doses.
Paedriatic suspension (Diethanolamine salt) equiv. 35 mg. fucidin/ml. Dose: 20-30 mg./kg./day in 3 equal doses. Intravenous (Diethanolamine salt) 500 mg. + 50 ml. sterile buffer. Freshly dilute in 500 ml. saline, administer over 2-4 hours. Dose: not more than 1·5 g./day.

REFERENCES

CALNAN, J. & FRY, H. J. R. (1962). *Brit. J. Pharmacol.* **19**, 321.
CAREY, M. C. & SMALL, D. M. (1971). *J. lipid. Res.* **12**, 604.
CHADWICK, A. J. & JACKSON, B. (1969). *Brit. J. Ophthal.* **53**, 26.
COWAN, A. (1965). *Irish J. med. Sci.* (6th Series), p. 125.
DEODHAR, S. D., RUSSELL, F., DICK, W. C., NUKI, G. & BUCHANAN, W. W. (1972). *Scand. J. Rheumatol.* **1**, 33.
EVANS, R. J. & WATERWORTH, P. M. (1966). *J. clin. Path.* **19**, 555.
GODTFREDSEN, W., ROHOLT, K. & TYBRING. L. (1962). *Lancet* **1**, 928.
GODTFREDSEN, W. O., ALBRETHSEN, C., V. DAEHNE, W., TYBRING, L. & VANGEDAL, S. (1966). *Antimicrob. Agents Chemother.*, 1965. p. 132.
GODTFREDSEN, W. D. & VANGEDAL, S. (1966). *Acta chem. Scand.* **20**, 1599.
GREENWOOD, D. & O'GRADY, F. (1973). *J. med. Microbiol.* In press.
GÜTTLER, F. & TYBRING, L. (1971). *Brit. J. Pharmacol.* **43**, 151.
HOBBY, J. A. E., BEELEY, L. & WHITBY, J. L. (1970). *J. clin. Path.* **23**, 484.
JENSEN, K. & LASSEN, H. C. A. (1969). *Quart. J. Med.* **38**, 91.
LOWBURY, E. J. L., KIDSON, A. & LILLY, H. A. (1964). *J. clin. Path.* **17**, 231.
SAGGERS, B. A., HARWOOD, H. F. & DAY, B. H. (1968). *Brit. J. clin. Pract.* **22**, 429.
STEWART, G. T. (1964). *Pharmacother.* **2**, 137.
WATERWORTH, P. M. (1963). *Clin. Med. Winnetka.* **70**, 941.
WILLIAMSON, J., RUSSELL, F., DOIG, W. M. & PATERSON, R. W. W. (1970). *Brit. J. Ophthal.* **54**, 126.
WYNN, V. (1965). *Brit. med. J.* **1**, 1400.

LINCOMYCIN

Lincomycin was isolated in the laboratories of the Upjohn Company from the fermentation products of a previously undescribed soil streptomycete, *Streptomyces lincolnensis* var. *lincolnensis* (Mason *et al.*, 1963).

Chemistry

Lincomycin is chemically unlike any other major antibiotic. Its structure is shown in Figure 22. The closely related celesticetin has only about 25-30 per cent of the antibacterial activity of lincomycin *in vitro*, and about 5 per cent *in vivo*. A number of derivatives of lincomycin have been prepared, the majority of which are less active than the parent compound, but clindamycin (7-chloro-7-deoxy-lincomycin) is substantially more active (p. 212).

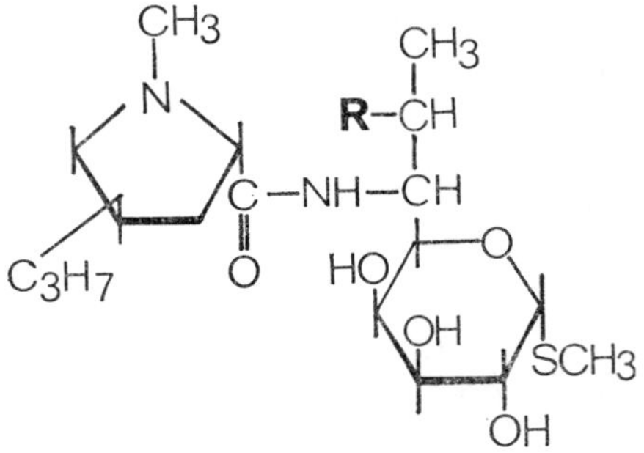

FIGURE 22

Structures of lincomycin (R = OH) and clindamycin (R = Cl).

Hoeksema, H. *et al.* (1964). *J. Amer. chem. Soc.* **86**, 4223.
Magerlein, B. J. *et al.* (1967).

Lincomycin is monobasic and is usually supplied as the hydrochloride (' Lincocin ') which is very soluble in water, soluble in methanol and ethanol, but relatively insoluble in less polar solvents. The free base is soluble in water and most organic solvents except hydrocarbons. The dry crystalline hydrochloride stored at 70°C. for six months showed no deterioration (Herr and Bergy, 1963).

Antibacterial Activity

Lincomycin closely resembles erythromycin in its activity against Gram-positive organisms, notably staphylococci, haemolytic streptococci and pneumococci. It also closely resembles the macrolides in showing a characteristic variety of cross-resistance (p. 170) and in its mode of action on the bacterial ribosome (p. 249). There are also some interesting differences.

TABLE 27

Minimum Inhibitory Concentrations of Lincomycins
(μg. per ml.)

	Lincomycin	Clindamycin*
Staph. aureus	0·36-2·8	0·1-1·5
Str. pyogenes	0·04-0·72	0·01-0·2
Str. pneumoniae	0·08-0·72	0·03
Str. viridans	0·17-0·92	0·03-0·06
Str. faecalis	1·4-46·0	0·06-50
B. anthracis	0·25-8·0	
Clostridium spp.	0·36-25·0	
A. israeli	0·12-0·6	
N. gonorrhoeae	10·0-40·0	0·4-3·0
N. meningitidis	>32	
H. influenzae	4·0-16	0·4-12·5
Enterobacteria	>100	64-100
B. fragilis	2-4	0·03-0·12
Veillonella spp.	<0·1-0·3	

Lewis, Clapp and Grady (1963); Barber and Waterworth (1964); Finegold *et al.* (1966). Magerlein *et al.* (1967); Garrison *et al.* (1968); Lerner (1968); Matsen (1971).
* 7-chloro-7-deoxy-lincomycin.

The enterobacteria are resistant to both lincomycin and the macrolides, but *Haemophilus* and *Neisseria*, which are sensitive to erythromycin, are resistant to lincomycin. The behaviour of *Neisseria* is particularly interesting since despite their Gram-negative staining they generally respond to antibacterial agents like Gram-positive organisms. *Mycoplasma hominis* is sensitive to lincomycin (0·4-1·6 μg./ml.) and resistant to erythromycin (100 μg./ml.); T-strain mycoplasma are sensitive to erythromycin (0·6-1·2 μg./ml.) and resistant to lincomycin (20-80 μg./ml.) according to Weström and Mardh (1971). *Streptococcus faecalis* is unusual amongst Gram-positive organisms in being resistant to lincomycin, but on the other hand, the faecal Gram-negative anaerobic bacilli (*Bacteroides*) and anaerobic cocci (*Veillonella*) are all sensitive. The minimum inhibitory concentrations of lincomycin for various species are shown in Table

27. The activity of lincomycin was not inhibited by the presence of up to 50 per cent serum (Lewis *et al.*, 1963).

Resistance

There have been wide geographical variations in the frequency with which lincomycin-resistant staphylococci have been found. In several series, 15-20 per cent of recently isolated,

TABLE 28

Serum Levels of Lincomycins in Man

Route	Dose	Peak		Half life hr.
		Hour	μg. per ml.	
LINCOMYCIN				
Oral	500 mg. 250 mg. 6 hourly 500 mg. 6 hourly	4	2-7 0·8-1·1 4·6-7·0	4-6
I.M.	200 mg. 600 mg.	1-2	3·5-4·2 8·0-18·0	4-6
I.V.	300 mg.	0	8·0-22·0	3-5·5
CLINDAMYCIN				
Oral	120 mg.	1-2	4·7-7·9	2-3

Ma *et al.* (1964).
Reinarz and McIntosh, (1966).
Vavra *et al.* (1964).

previously unexposed *Staph. aureus* have been resistant to lincomycin (Nunnery and Riley, 1965) yet Phillips *et al.* (1970) were impressed with the infrequency with which lincomycin-resistant staphylococci had been encountered in their hospital over a 4-year period. Lincomycin resistance is relatively easily induced by passage (Barber and Waterworth, 1964) especially in erythromycin-resistant strains, and has certainly been observed to emerge in the course of treatment, when such strains often show the dissociated resistance (p. 170) typical of macrolides (Duncan, 1968). There have also been reports from various parts of the world of lincomycin-resistant haemolytic streptococci and pneumococci and these strains are commonly also resistant to erythromycin (Weisblum, 1967; Lowbury and Kidson, 1968). Resistance of the oral viridans streptococci to both erythromycin and lincomycin was seen by Sprunt *et al.* (1970) to emerge in patients treated with either drug for as little as three days. They point out that patients receiving long-term penicillin for prophylaxis of rheumatic fever who require cover for dental extraction may be given erythromycin or lincomycin. Care should be taken to ensure that the patient has not received either agent in the preceding three weeks.

Pharmacokinetics

Lincomycin is readily absorbed when given by mouth. The drug is also promptly and completely absorbed from intramuscular sites. The serum levels obtained by various authors following administration by different routes are given in Table 28. Several authors have commented that constant, near maximum levels can be maintained on 4-6 hourly schedules. Much the same results have been obtained in children (Nunnery and Riley, 1965). Food significantly delays and decreases absorption of the oral dose, the mean peak serum level from a dose given immediately after a meal being only about half the fasting levels (McCall, Steigbigel and Finland, 1967).

The drug is widely distributed in the body. Ma *et al.* (1964) found its distribution space to approximate to the total body size. It does not appear to be concentrated in any particular organ (Meyer and Lewis, 1964). Medina *et al.* (1964) found low levels in C.S.F. (up to 1·2 μg. per ml.), and levels of 1·5-6·9 μg. per ml. in cord serum and amniotic fluid 2-4 hours after 600 mg. intramuscularly. Six hours after the last of 2×6 hourly doses of 0·5 g. they found levels in human milk of 0·5-2·4 μg. per ml. Holloway *et al.* (1964) found 1·1-6·6 μg. per g. of bone in patients successfully treated for osteomyelitis. The corresponding serum levels were 6-16·5 μg. per ml. Norden (1971) found very similar levels in experimental osteomyelitis of rabbits: 0·7-1·6 μg.ml. in normal and 1·4-2·5 μg./ml. in osteomyelitic bone when the plasma levels were 5·0-6·0 μg./ml.

He showed that the amount of drug in bone could not be accounted for by its blood content. There was no detectable drug in sequestra. Boyle *et al.* (1971) gave 75 mg. lincomycin (in 0·25 ml.) subconjunctivally to 27 patients without inflammatory ocular disease who were about to undergo elective surgery (usually for cataract extraction). Peak concentrations of 30-135 μg./ml. were found in the aqueous 1-2 hr. after injection in all but one case. Activity was still detectable 12 hr. later. Serum levels of the order of 2-3 μg./ml. appeared within 10 minutes of subconjunctival injection and persisted for 12 hr. Marked chemosis and subconjunctival haemorrhage frequently developed but there was little or no pain.

Excretion

Most workers have found the urinary levels of the drug to be low except after intravenous injection. (Vavra *et al.*, 1964; Ma *et al.*, 1964; Medina *et al.*, 1964). After oral administration only 3-5 per cent of the dose appeared in the urine over the next 24 hours but after intravenous injection up to 57 per cent was recovered. In patients with severe renal disease serum levels were 3-4 times normal and high levels persisted for over 24 hours but this has been said to result from the loss of normally important renal binding sites. Lincomycin appears to be virtually non-dialysable since its half-life in dialysed and undialysed azotaemic patients was approximately the same (Reinarz and McIntosh, 1966).

Finegold *et al.* (1966) found 0·9-6·8 μg. lincomycin per g. faeces after 1·5 g. orally and 1·6-9·6 μg. per g. after 4 g. orally. In the rat part of the unabsorbed drug is broken down in the caecum presumably as a result of bacterial action. In nonazotaemic patients with liver disease, Bellamy *et al.* (1967) found that the peak plasma level after a single intramuscular dose of 600 mg. was somewhat depressed (7·2-12·8 μg./ml.) and the plasma half-life increased from the 4·85 hr. found in their normal subjects to 8·96 hr.

Toxicity

Lincomycin appears to be an innocuous compound. Most authors have reported no side effects apart from diarrhoea which has commonly affected about 10 per cent of the patients and many more in some series (Price *et al.*, 1968). It has occasionally been so severe that therapy has had to be withdrawn. Much of the difference in incidence of diarrhoea may be explained by varying relation of drug administration to meals. If given with food much more of the drug remains unabsorbed to disturb the gut. The low toxicity of lincomycin has encouraged treatment with large and sometimes colossal doses. In some patients receiving large amounts of the drug by rapid intravenous injection, the blood pressure has fallen precipitately with nausea, vomiting and E.C.G. changes. This alarming effect can be avoided by giving the drug in a larger volume by slow intravenous infusion (Novak *et al.*, 1971). Vacek *et al.* (1970) suggest that the rate of infusion should not exceed 50 mg./kg. per hour. White (1966) concluded from experimental studies that lincomycin is of low antigenicity. In doses of 25-50 mg./kg. lincomycin depressed neuromuscular transmission in the rabbit but at low frequency stimulation the effect was much weaker than that of neomycin and it does not appear that any difficulty has been encountered clinically (Tang and Schroeder, 1968).

Clinical Use

Lincomycin has been used for the treatment of streptococcal pharyngitis, and for Gram-positive coccal otitis, pneumonia and pyoderma with very satisfactory results in both adults and children. It has also been satisfactorily used in more serious infections including diphtheria and staphylococcal septicaemia. Because of its penetration into bone, it has been particularly commended for the treatment of both acute and chronic osteomyelitis (p. 340).

Its antibacterial range, low toxicity, and clinical efficacy make lincomycin a suitable substitute for penicillin in Gram-positive coccal infections where penicillin is contraindicated—circumstances in which erythromycin might otherwise be used. It has been very successfully used for the treatment of bacteroides infections (p. 335) for which Tracy *et al.* (1972) describe it as the drug of choice.

The relatively ready emergence of resistance strongly suggests that lincomycin should not be widely used for conditions for which there are a number of satisfactory alternatives and that in the treatment of staphylococcal infection it should be combined with another anti-staphylococcal agent.

CLINDAMYCIN

This synthetic modification of lincomycin (Magerlein *et al.*, 1967) involving only the loss of an O and H and the addition of Cl (Fig. 22) is, to give its full chemical name, 7-chloro-7-deoxylincomycin hydrochloride hydrate. It is also known in the United States as Clinimycin and in this country as ' Dalacin C '. Both names are unfortunate since in Britain clinimycin is the name of a brand of oxytetracycline and there are no other Dalacins.

It appears from such studies as those of Wagner *et al.* (1968) and McGehee *et al.* (1968) to be many times more active than lincomycin against staphylococci, pneumococci and *Bacteroides* more active against *H. influenzae* (Matsen, 1971) and either more active or at least equally active against all other sensitive species (Table 27). Moreover it is better absorbed than lincomycin, producing substantially higher blood levels (Table 28), and this advantage is accentuated when doses are taken after a meal which impairs the absorption of lincomycin but merely slows that of the new derivative.

No countervailing disadvantages have been reported, and the available facts suggest that 7-chlorolincomycin should simply replace lincomycin in therapy, but both continue to be available. It should at least be recognized that 7-chlorolincomycin is not a new antibiotic, as its nomenclature and description suggest, but only a slight modification of an old one.

PHARMACEUTICAL PREPARATIONS AND DOSAGE

LINCOMYCIN HYDROCHLORIDE (Lincocin, *Upjohn*, Mycivin, *Boots*)
Capsules: Equiv. 500 mg.; Syrup equiv. 125 mg. per 5 ml. Dose: 500 mg., 6-8 hourly, between meals. Injection: 600 mg. in 2 ml. Dose: i/m 300-600 mg., 12 hourly; i/v infusion: 600 mg., 8-12 hourly in 250 ml. saline over 30 minutes.
CLINDAMYCIN (Dalacin C., *Upjohn*)
Capsules of 150 mg. and 75 mg. (paediatric).
Doses 150-300 mg. 4 times a day, but can be increased.
Also known as CLINIMYCIN in U.S.A. In the U.K. this name refers to a brand of oxytetracycline).
A parenteral preparation, clindamycin phosphate, is available in the United States of America, and may shortly be obtainable also in Great Britain.

REFERENCES

BARBER, M. & WATERWORTH, P. M. (1964). *Brit. med. J.* **2**, 603.
BELLAMY, H. M., BATES, B. B. & REINARZ, J. A. (1967). *Antimicrob. Agents Chemother.*—1966, p. 36.
BOYLE, G. L., LICHTIG, M. L. & LEOPOLD, I. H. (1971). *Amer. J. Ophthalmol.* **71**, 1303.
DUNCAN, I. B. R. (1968). *Antimicrob. Agents Chemother.*—1967, p. 723.
FINEGOLD, S. M., HARADA, N. E. & MILLER, L. G. (1966). *Antimicrob. Agents Chemother.*, 1965, p. 659.
GARRISON, D. W., DE HAAN, R. M. & LAWSON, J. B. (1968). *Antimicrob Agents Chemother.*—1967, p. 397.
HERR, R. R. & BERGY, M. E. (1963). *Antimicrob. Agents Chemother.*, 1962, p. 560.
HOLLOWAY, W. J., KAHLBAUGH, R. A. & SCOTT, E. G. (1964). *Antimicrob. Agents Chemother.*, 1963, p. 200.
LERNER, P. I. (1968). *Antimicrob. Agents Chemother.*—1967, p. 730.
LEWIS, C., CLAPP, H. W. & GRADY, J. E. (1963). *Antimicrob. Agents Chemother.*, 1962, p. 570.
LOWBURY, E. J. L. & KIDSON, A. (1968). *Brit. med. J.* **2**, 490.
MA, P., LIM, M. & NODINE, J. H. (1964). *Antimicrob. Agents Chemother.*, 1963, p. 183.
McCALL, C. E., STEIGBIGEL, N. H. & FINLAND, M. (1967). *Amer. J. Med. Sci.* **254**, 144.
MAGERLEIN, B. J., BIRKENMEYER, R. D. & KAGAN, F. (1967). *Antimicrob. Agents Chemother.*—1966, p. 727.
MATSEN, J. M. (1971). *J. lab. clin. Med.* **77**, 378.
McGEHEE, R. F. Jr., SMITH, C. B., WILCOX, C. & FINLAND, M. (1968). *Amer. J. med. Sci.* **256**, 279.
MASON, D. J., DIETZ, A. & DEBOER, C. (1963). *Antimicrob. Agents Chemother.*, 1962, p. 554.
MEDINA, H., FISKE, N., HJELT-HARVEY, I., BROWN, C. D. & PRIGOT, A. (1964). *Antimicrob. Agents Chemother.*, 1963, p. 189.
MEYER, C. E. & LEWIS, C. (1964). *Antimicrob. Agents Chemother.*, 1963, p. 169.
NORDEN, C. W. (1971). *J. infect. Dis.* **124**, 565.
NOVAK, E., VITTI, T. G., PANZER, J. D., SCHLAGEL, C. & HEARRON, M. S. (1971). *Clin. Pharmacol. Ther.* **12**, 793.
NUNNERY, A. W. & RILEY, H. D. (1965). *Antimicrob. Agents Chemother.*, 1964, p. 142.
O'CONNELL, C. J. & PLAUT, M. E. (1969). *Curr. ther. Res.* **11**, 478.
PHILLIPS, I., FERNANDES, R. & WARREN, C. (1970). *Brit. med. J.* **2**, 89.
PRICE, D. J. E., O'GRADY, F. W., SHOOTER, R. A. & WEAVER, P. C. (1968). *Brit. med. J.* **3**, 407.
REINARZ, J. A. & McINTOSH, D. A. (1966). *Antimicrob. Agents Chemother.*, 1965, p. 232.
SPRUNT, K., LEIDY, G. & REDMAN, W. (1970). *Pediatrics* **46**, 84.
TANG, A. H. & SCHROEDER, L. A. (1968). *Toxicol. appl. Pharmacol.* **12**, 44.
TRACY, O., GORDON, A. M., MORAN, F., LOVE, W. C. & McKENZIE, P. (1972). *Brit. med. J.* **1**, 280.
VACEK, V., TESAROVA-MAGROVA, J. & STAFOVA, J. (1970). *Arzneimitt. Forsch.* **20**, 99.
VAVRA, J. J., SOKOLSKI, W. T. & LAWSON, J. B. (1964). *Antimicrob. Agents Chemother.*, 1963, p. 176.
WAGNER, J. G., NOVAK, E., PATEL, N. C., CHIDESTER, C. G. & LUMMIS, W. L. (1968). *Amer. J. med. Sci.* **256**, 25.
WEISBLUM, B. (1967). *Lancet* **1**, 843.
WESTRÖM, L. & MÅRDH, P-A. (1971). *Acta obstet. gynaec. Scand.* **50**, 25.
WHITE, G. J. (1966). *Antimicrob. Agents Chemother.* 1965, p. 398.

NOVOBIOCIN

Cathomycin, isolated from a new species of actinomycete which was given the name *Streptomyces spheroides* (Wallick *et al.*, 1956) and streptonivicin isolated from *Streptomyces niveus* (Smith *et al.*, 1956) were shown to be identical and given the generic name novobiocin.

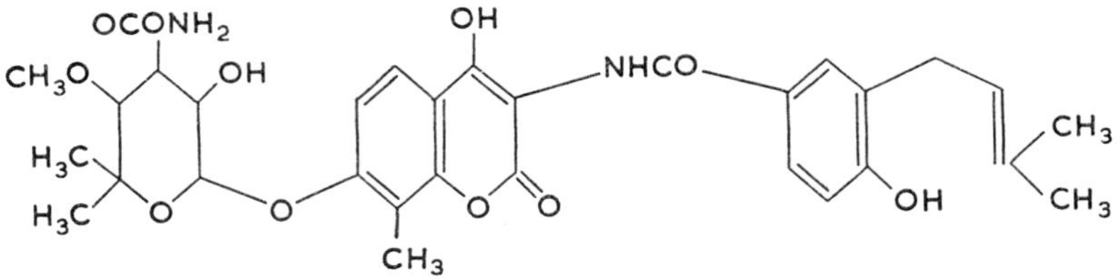

FIGURE 23

Structure of novobiocin (Hoeksema *et al.*, 1956, *J. Amer. Chem. Soc.* **78,** 2019; Shunk *et al.*, 1956, *ibid,* 1770).

Chemical Properties

Novobiocin is a dibasic acid usually supplied as the calcium or monosodium salt. The calcium salt is soluble at 3 mg./ml. water and 125 mg./ml. alcohol. The monosodium salt is much more readily soluble: 200 mg./ml. water, 140 mg./ml. ethyl alcohol and 350 mg./ml. methyl alcohol. With both salts a 2·5 per cent solution has a pH of 7·0 to 8·5. Both salts are moderately stable if kept dry, stored in the cold and protected from light.

Novobiocin combines with basic antibiotics (e.g. streptomycin, erythromycin) in stoichiometric proportion to form water-insoluble salts.

Anti-bacterial Activity

Novobiocin has a rather unusual anti-bacterial spectrum (Table 29). It is outstandingly active against *Staph. aureus*; other highly sensitive species are *Str. pneumoniae, C. diphtheriae, H. influenzae, N. gonorrhoeae* and *N. meningitidis.*

Novobiocin sensitivity (to a disk containing 5 μg.) serves to make very simply the taxonomic distinction between staphylococci, which are almost universally sensitive, and micrococci, which are almost universally resistant (Mitchell, 1968).

Some strains of *Pasteurella* and *Proteus*, particularly *Proteus vulgaris*, are sensitive to moderate concentrations but other enterobacteria are resistant.

Novobiocin is primarily a bacteristatic drug, but with highly sensitive species a concentration two to ten times that required for bacteristasis has a slow killing effect.

TABLE 29
Sensitivity of Bacteria to Novobiocin

Gram-positive Bacteria	MIC μg./ml.	Gram-negative Bacteria	MIC μg./ml.
Staph. aureus	0·1 - 2	H. influenzae	0·2 - 0·8
Str. pyogenes	0·5 - 4	N. meningitidis	0·5 - 4
Str. pneumoniae	0·2 - 2	N. gonorrhoeae	4
Str. faecalis	1 - 16	Pasteurella	2 - 16
C. diphtheriae	0·4	Proteus vulgaris	2 - 50
Cl. welchii	1·0	Proteus mirabilis	8 - 100
B. anthracis	1·0	Proteus morgani	16 - >100
Ery. insidiosa	>64	Proteus rettgeri	
L. monocytogenes	2·0	Escherichia, Klebsiella,	>100
Actino. israeli	2·0	Salmonella, Shigella	
Myco. tuberculosis	R	Pseudomonas	

Jones, W. F., Nichols, R. L. and Finland, M. (1956). *J. Lab. clin. Med.* **47**, 783.
Frost, B. M. *et al.* (1956). *Antibiot. Ann.* 1955-56, p. 918.
Schneierson, S. S. and Amsterdam, D. (1957). *Antibiot. Chemother.* **7**, 251.

A 1,000-fold increase in the size of inoculum causes a 4-8-fold increase in the M.I.C. of novobiocin for staphylococci and a much larger increase in the concentration necessary to sterilize the culture in 24 hours. The M.I.C. is 8 or more times greater at pH 8·0 than at pH 5·4, and markedly increased by the presence of 10 per cent or more serum or blood because about 90 per cent of the antibiotic is reversibly bound to serum albumin and the bound antibiotic is no longer active against bacteria.

Many species of bacteria initially sensitive to novobiocin readily develop resistance to it *in vitro* and a considerable increase in the resistance of the infecting staphylococcus during treatment has been recorded by several investigators. There is no cross resistance with other common antibiotics.

Absorption, Distribution and Excretion

Novobiocin is well absorbed from the alimentary tract, producing high blood levels (10·9 and 18·8 μg./ml. 1-4 hr. after doses of 250 and 500 mg.) which are long sustained. Wagner and Damiano (1968) found the plasma half-life to be 1·7-4 hours. After repeated doses partly due to biliary re-circulation there is also some accumulation and during treatment with full doses serum levels of 50 to over 100 μg./ml. may be reached.

Concentrations rather lower than that in the blood are found in serous effusions, but even when the blood level is high, cerebrospinal fluid contains very little or none. The amount found in the urine does not usually exceed three per cent of the dose and in single specimens of urine the concentration may be considerably lower than that in the blood.

Novobiocin is excreted mainly in the bile, in which the concentration is high. Biliary recirculation plays an important part in maintaining the high blood levels but much of the antibiotic eventually escapes by this route and high concentrations are found in the faeces.

Toxicity and side effects

Maculopapular, morbilliform or urticarial skin eruptions with or without fever are common, often developing about the ninth day. The rashes disappear on stopping the drug but may promptly re-appear if the drug is re-administered (Shelley, 1963) together with a prompt and profound fall in circulating basophils indicative of sensitization. Novobiocin may displace other substances from protein binding sites and one possible effect of this is to lower the plasma-bound iodine by displacing thyroxine (Takemura et al., 1966).

Eosinophilia and moderate transient leucopenia are occasionally seen. Thrombocytopenia which may be severe (Holswade et al., 1964) and haemolytic anaemia (Montgomery, 1963) have also been reported.

Novobiocin gives rise to a yellow pigment metabolite in the serum, which may give an indirect positive van den Bergh reaction, but there is no doubt that the drug exerts a profound effect on hepatic excretory function by interfering with uptake of various compounds by hepatic cells, inhibiting glucuronyl transferase—the enzyme concerned with glucuronide conjugation—and suppressing excretion of conjugates into the bile (Hargreaves and Lathe, 1963). Particularly severe effects may occur in the new-born where glucuronide formation is imperfectly developed (London, 1964).

Combination with Tetracyclines

It has several times been claimed that novobiocin and tetracycline act synergically (Masson and Kingsley, 1964) and this mixture is available commercially as, for example, 'Albamycin T'. However, Table 32 on page 284 shows that against the strain of *Staph. aureus* tested, so far from any synergy being demonstrable, the effect of this combination was not even additive, the inhibitory concentration of each remaining the same regardless of the presence of a sub-inhibitory concentration of the other.

In previous editions we mildly observed ' There seems no strong reason to suppose that this mixture is an exception to the rule that packaged antibiotic combinations are unlikely to provide the critical concentration relationships which are frequently required for synergic action between pairs of agents '. American experts have been much more severe: they have unanimously condemned the mixture according to Mintz (1969) who graphically tells the disturbing story of the battle to prevent the removal of the mixture from the U.S. market.

Clinical Application

Novobiocin is an interesting and active compound but its once useful place as an antistaphylococcal agent has been overtaken by numerous other agents. This, combined with its high-grade competition for albumin binding sites, its unequivocal depressant effect on hepatic function and its capacity to produce skin reactions with a frequency which many physicians regard as unacceptably high, makes it hard for the drug to look good in any risk/benefit analysis. Its activity against certain strains of *Proteus* has led to its continuing prescription for urinary tract infection—a use for which there is nowadays no possible justification.

PHARMACEUTICAL PREPARATIONS AND DOSAGE

NOVOBIOCIN (Streptonivicin, Albamycin*, *Upjohn;* Cathomycin, *Merck, Sharp and Dohme,* Cardelmycin, *U.S.A.;* and other proprietary names) Tablets: B.P., B.N.F.: equiv. 250 mg.; Suspension, U.S.N.F.: equiv. 2·5-3 per cent w/w. Syrup, B.N.F.: 125 mg. per ml. Dose: 1-2 g. daily in divided doses.

* NOT Albomycin (*U.S.S.R.*)—a basic peptide antibiotic from *Actinomyces subtropicus.*

REFERENCES

GREENWOOD, D. & O'GRADY, F. (1972). *J. gen. Microbiol.* **70**, 263.
HARGREAVES, T. & LATHE, G. H. (1963). *Nature (Lond.)* **200**, 1172.
HOLSWADE, G. R., DINEEN, P., REDO, S. F. & GOLDSMITH, E. I. (1964). *Arch. Surg.* **89**, 970.
JOHNSTON, K. H. & HOSHIKO, T. (1971). *Amer. J. Physiol.* **220**, 792.
LONDON, W. L. (1964). *N. Carolina Med. J.* **25**, 417.
MASSON, E. L. & KINGSLEY, V. V. (1964). *Antimicrob. Agents Chemother.* 1963, 624.
MINTZ, M. (1969). *Science* **165**, 875.
MITCHELL, R. G. (1968). *J. clin. Path.* **21**, 93.
MONTGOMERY, J. R. (1963). *New Engl. J. Med.* **269**, 966.
MORRIS, A. & RUSSELL, A. D. (1968). *Biochem. Pharmacol.* **17**, 1923.
SHELLEY, W. B. (1963). *Arch. Derm. (Chicago)* **88**, 759.
SMITH, C. G., DIETZ, A., SOKOLOSKI, W. T. & SAVAGE, G. M. (1956). *Antibiot. Chemother.* **6**, 135.
TAKEMURA, Y., YAMADA, T. & SHICHIJO, K. (1966). *Metabolism* **15**, 566.
WAGNER, J. G. & DAMIANO, R. E. (1968). *J. clin. Pharmacol.* **8**, 102.
WALLICK, H., HARRIS, D. A., REAGAN, M. A., RUGER, M. & WOODRUFF, H. B. (1956). *Antibiot. Ann.* (1955-6), p. 909.
WHITE, G. J. (1966). *Antimicrob. Agents Chemother.*, 1965, p. 398.

PRASINOMYCIN

This substance, derived from a strain of *Streptomyces prasinus* recovered from Colorado soil, was first described by Weisenborn *et al.* (1967). It acts exclusively on Gram-positive bacteria and appears of unique interest in that it contains phosphorus and that a single subcutaneous dose protects against inoculation with *Str. pyogenes* for as long as 28 days. Meyers *et al.* (1968) describe it as a diester of phosphoric acid, with a molecular weight of 1600 +, and mention that although streptococci and pneumococci are highly sensitive to it, *Sarcina lutea* is resistant. These authors assert that a single large dose renders mice refractory to inoculation with haemolytic streptococci for no less than 2 months, and report other interesting findings on the timing of medication in relation to curative effects in pneumococcal and staphylococcal infection.

It now appears that a similar if not identical phosphorus-containing antibiotic is formed by several other species of *Streptomyces*. Known originally as moenomycin and now as flavomycin, it is proposed for use as a growth-promoting food additive in livestock. The reasons for abandoning the study of this interesting antibiotic as a therapeutic agent have not been made clear.

REFERENCES

MEYERS, E., MIRAGLIA, G. J., SMITH, D. A., BASCH, H. I., PANSY, F. E., TREJO, W. H. & DONOVICK, R. (1968). *Appl. Microbiol.* **16**, 603.
WEISENBORN, F. L., BOUCHARD, J. L., SMITH, D., PANSY, F., MAESTRONE, G., MIRAGLIA, G. & MEYERS, E. (1967). *Nature* **213**, 1092.

RIFAMYCINS

The rifamycins are a family of antibiotics produced by *Streptomyces mediterranei* and studied in the laboratories of Lepetit, Milan. Rifamycin B is the most active, and its molecule has been modified with advantage in various ways, the derivatives recently studied and used in therapeutics being ' rifamycin SV ' and rifamycin B diethylamide (' Rifamide '). The principal account of these antibiotics is by Bergamini and Fowst (1965) who describe their structure, differing from that of other antibiotics, *in vitro* activity, pharmacology and clinical applications.

Rifamide

Extremely low concentrations (0·01 to 0·1 μg. per ml.) are said to inhibit the growth of staphylococci, streptococci (other than *S. faecalis*) and *Myco. tuberculosis*: Gram-negative species require 10-100 μg. per ml. or more. Welsch and Esther (1963) found the concentrations necessary to inhibit the growth of staphylococci and streptococci to be somewhat higher, and that results are affected by inoculum size and length of incubation: they also draw attention to the existence of small numbers of much more resistant cells in populations of staphylococci. The action is also bactericidal, and there is no cross-resistance with other antibiotics.

Rifamycin is little absorbed from the alimentary tract. Intramuscular injection of 500 mg. produces a therapeutic blood level for up to eight hours, but protein binding is extensive: with a blood level of 5 μg. per ml. only 14 per cent is said to be free. Elimination is mainly via the bile, in which a concentration as high as 2·8 mg. per ml. has been observed: some re-circulation occurs, but much is excreted in the faeces and little in the urine. On this account it has been described as ' the only specific antibiotic ' for cholecystitis (Stratford and Dixson, 1966). Bevan and Williams (1971) obtained good results with it in acute cholecystitis and from prophylactic use in patients undergoing biliary surgery.

Therapeutic applications have included the treatment of staphylococcal infections, both systemically and where applicable locally, of biliary tract infections, and of tuberculosis. Apparently the systemic treatment of tuberculosis in combination with other drugs has not been altogether successful, and greater emphasis is placed on local application, including the use of aerosols, intracavitary introduction in patients subjected to Monaldi drainage, and instillation into empyema cavities. A few encouraging results have also been obtained in leprosy.

Rifampicin

This derivative of rifamycin, 3-(4-methyl-piperazinyliminomethyl) rifamycin SV, represents perhaps the greatest advance over the original properties of an antibiotic which has yet been achieved by synthetic modification. It is one of 500 derivatives prepared by Ciba of Basel and Lepetit ot Milan in collaboration (Kradolfer, 1968). It has the same spectrum as other rifamycins but much higher activity, the M.I.C. for highly sensitive species being almost incredibly low (e.g. for *Staphylococcus aureus* 0·002 μg./ml.). Other bacteria are correspondingly more sensitive to rifampicin than to earlier rifamycin derivatives; 0·5 μg./ml. is actively bactericidal for *Myco. tuberculosis* and 20 μg./ml. for *E. coli*. According to Mandell and Vest (1972) rifampicin has a much superior bactericidal effect to that of any other antibiotic tested on intra-leucocytic staphylococci.

It is most important to recognize that large bacterial populations may contain a few resistant mutants. Hence the M.I.C. as determined in a fluid medium with a generous inoculum may be enormously higher than that in the plate dilution method with a light one (Atlas and Turck, 1968; McCabe and Lorian, 1968). A more important consequence is that, at least in treating most infections, rifampicin should never be given alone, but together with another drug to which the organism is sensitive.

PHARMACOKINETICS. The second advantage of rifampicin is that unlike other rifamycin derivatives it is well absorbed when administered orally. Not only is a high initial concentration reached in the blood, but, owing in part to entero-hepatic re-circulation, the subsequent fall is slow, a therapeutic level being maintained for 12 hours or more according to the dose.

Blood levels fall somewhat after the first week of treatment. The main excretory route is biliary, although concentrations in the bile are lower than those of rifamide, and biliary obstruction raises blood levels. The quantity normally excreted by the liver appears to be fixed, and any excess is dealt with by the kidney; thus the larger the dose the greater the proportion of it excreted in the urine. Renal insufficiency is said not to affect this. Haemodialysis does not reduce blood levels. An interesting fact with regard to distribution is that concentrations of 5-10 μg./ml. are demonstrable in sputum. An admirable account of these and other studies, including clinical, is given in a review with 847 references by Binda et al. (1971).

Much the most important use of rifampicin is for the treatment of tuberculosis, which is discussed from both experimental and clinical standpoints in Chapter 26. Some take the view that it should be reserved solely for this purpose. Among other uses for which it has been tried or examined are the following.

It may exceptionally be indicated in staphylococcal infection. One of us recently found rifampicin and erythromycin to be the most bactericidal of many antibiotic combinations for a strain of *Staph. aureus* from an infection of a patent interventricular septum in a child aged 3 (Peard et al., 1970). The fact that both drugs could be given orally was welcome at this age, and the infection was rapidly eliminated. The synergic effect of this combination on *Staph. aureus* has subsequently been demonstrated by Banić and Stropnik (1971). In this connection it should be recognized that rifamycins do not obey the Jawetz law on combined action; combination with another bactericidal antibiotic may be antagonistic, and with one which is only bacteristatic (such as tetracycline) may be synergic. Any combination proposed for clinical use should therefore be tested on the causative organism. Results from a single dose in gonorrhoea were good (Cobbold, Morrison and Willcox, 1968). Various other pulmonary, skin and soft tissue, bone and even intestinal infections have been treated, but there seems to be no clear reason for preferring rifampicin to other treatments for any of them. The treatment of leprosy is discussed on p. 451. Finally considerable activity against pox viruses and trachoma agent has been demonstrated (see Chapter 28.

There have been preliminary studies of the action of rifampicin on the causative organisms of gas gangrene (Schallehn, 1969) and melioidosis (Hobby *et al.*, 1969). A practical use to which the drug has been put is the treatment of meningococcus carriers. This is immediately very effective, but in each of four papers on this subject published within one year in the United States (e.g. Eickhoff, 1971; Weidmer *et al.*, 1971) it is acknowledged that the meningococcus may rapidly become highly resistant. Not only would this change soon deprive the treatment of efficacy, but the possible effect of mass administration on other bacterial species is a strong objection.

Side Effects. Various rashes and gastro-intestinal disturbances may occur. Hepatic dysfunction, manifested first by raised transaminase levels and then by a raised serum bilirubin, is not uncommon and not necessarily an indication for stopping treatment (Lal *et al.*, 1972); pre-existing liver disease predisposes to this effect. It is more common when the second drug given is isoniazid than when it is ethambutol (Lees *et al.*, 1971). An immune thrombocytopenia is liable to complicate intermittent treatment with large doses (Poole, Stradling and Worlledge, 1971).

PHARMACEUTICAL PREPARATIONS AND DOSAGE

Sodium Rifamycin B Diethylamide : Rifamide (Rifocin M, *Lepetit*)
Ampoules of 150 mg. in 3 ml.
Dose i.m. 1 every 6-12 hours.
Rifampicin (Rifadin, *Lepetit* : Rimactane, *Ciba* : Rifampin in U.S.A.)
Capsules of 150 and 300 mg.
Dose 600 mg. daily.

REFERENCES

Atlas, E. & Turck, M. (1968). *Amer. J. med. Sci.* **256,** 247.
Banič, S. & Stropnik, Z. (1971). *Zbl. Bakt. I. Orig.* **216,** 418.
Begg, R. J. (1967). *Tubercle* **48,** 149.
Bergamini, N. & Fowst, G. (1965). *Arzneimittel-Forsch.* **15,** 953.
Bevan, P. G. & Williams, J. D. (1971). *Brit. med. J.* **3,** 284.
Binda, G., Domenichini, E., Gottardi, A., Orlandi, B., Ortelli, E., Pacini, B. & Fowst, G. (1971). *Arzneimittel-Forsch.* **21,** 1907.
Cobbold, R. J. C., Morrison, G. D. & Willcox, R. R. (1968). *Brit. med. J.* **4,** 681.
Eickhoff, T. C. (1971). *J. infect Dis.* **123,** 414.
Hobby, G. L., Lenert, T. F., Maier-Engallena, J. & DeNoia-Cicenia, E. (1969). *Amer. Rev. resp. Dis.* **99,** 952.
Kradolfer, F. (1968). *Schweiz. med. Wschr.* **98,** 622.

LAL, S., SINGHAL, S. N., BURLEY, D. M. & CROSSLEY, G. (1972). *Brit. med. J.* **1**, 148.
LEES, A. W., ALLAN, G. W., SMITH, J., TYRRELL, W. F. & FALLON, R. J. (1971). *Tubercle* **52**, 182.
MANDELL, G. L. & VEST, T. K. (1972). *J. infect. Dis.* **125**, 486.
MCCABE, W. R. & LORIAN, V. (1968). *Amer. J. med. Sci.* **256**, 255.
MURDOCH, J. McC., SPEIRS, C. F., WRIGHT, N. & WALLACE, E. T. (1969). *Lancet* **1**, 1094.
PEARD, M. C., FLECK, D. G., GARROD, L. P. & WATERWORTH, P. M. (1970). *Brit. med. J.* **4**, 410.
POOLE, G., STRADLING, P. & WORLLEDGE, S. (1971). *Brit. med. J.* **3**, 343.
SCHALLEHN, G. (1969). *Schweiz. med. Wschr.* **99**, 1057.
STRATFORD, B. C. & DIXSON, S. (1966). *Med. J. Aust.* **1**, 1.
WEIDMER, C. E., DUNKEL, T. B., PETTYJOHN, F. S., SMITH, C. D. & LEIBOVITZ, A. (1971). *J. infect. Dis.* **124**, 172.
WELSCH, M. & ESTHER, H. (1963). *Chemotherapia (Basel)* **7**, 269.

SPECTINOMYCIN

This antibiotic, first known as actinospectacin, a product of *Streptomyces spectabilis*, was originally described by Mason and his colleagues (1961). It shows a moderate degree of *in vitro* activity (M.I.C. for most sensitive species of the order of 5-10 µg. per ml.) against a wide range of bacteria, both Gram-positive and Gram-negative (Lewis and Clapp, 1961). Staphylococci can become resistant to it fairly rapidly, but this capacity is not shared by other organisms. Administered by injection, it is more effective against various infections in mice than its *in vitro* activity would suggest. There are several reports on its clinical use, not only in urinary tract infections (Lindemeyer *et al.*, 1962), but in other infections including septicaemia and pneumonia (Romansky *et al.*, 1962). The conclusion appears to have been reached that although effective, it is no more so than other antibiotics, and its clinical use, except for gonorrhoea (p. 464) has been abandoned. It is now being used for growth promotion and the treatment of certain infections in farm stock.

REFERENCES

LEWIS, C. & CLAPP, H. W. (1961). *Antibiot. Chemother.* **11**, 127.
LINDEMEYER, R. I., TURCK, M. & PETERSDORF, R. G. (1962). *Amer. J. med. Sci.* **244**, 478.
MASON, D. J., DIETZ, A. & SMITH, R. M. (1961). *Antibiot. Chemother.* **11**, 118.
ROMANSKY, M. J., WALTERS, E. W., JOHNSON, A. C. & PECK, F. A. (1962). *Antimicrob. Agents Chemother.* 1961, p. 524.

VANCOMYCIN

Vancomycin, isolated in 1956 in the laboratories of Eli Lilly from strains of *Streptomyces orientalis*, is now a well recognized antibiotic with very limited if important uses, and calls for only a brief description.

Antibacterial Activity

The ' spectrum ' of vancomycin includes only Gram-positive organisms, and only its activity against staphylococci and streptococci is of clinical interest. The findings of various authors on the sensitivity of these and other organisms are shown in Table 30.

TABLE 30
Sensitivity of Bacteria to Vancomycin

	No. of Strains	Minimum Inhibitory Concentration ($\mu g./ml.$)
Staph. aureus[1]	10	0·8 - 1·6
Staph. aureus[1]	1	6·2
Staph. aureus[2]	41	0·156 - 1·87
Staph. aureus[2]	2	>10
Staph. aureus[3]	10	2·0 - 3·0
Str. pyogenes[2]	24	0·156 - 2·5
Str. pyogenes[3]	8	0·5 - 1·0
Str. pyogenes[2]	4	0·3 - 1·25
Str. pneumoniae[3]	6	0·5 - 1·0
Str. faecalis[2]	2	0·3 - 2·5
Str. faecalis[3, 4]	6	2·0 - 5·0
Bacillus spp.[1]	6	0·2 - 3·1
Corynebact. spp.[1]	4	0·4 - 0·8
Clostridium welchii[4]	3	0·39 - 0·625
Clostridium spp.[4]	9	0·625 - 5·0

All species of Gram-negative bacteria, Mycobacteria and fungi are resistant.

[1] McCormick *et al.* (1956).
[2] Griffith and Peck (1956).
[3] Kirby and Divelbiss (1957).
[4] Geraci *et al.* (1957).

The effect exerted is rapidly bactericidal in a concentration not much higher than that required for bacteristasis (Ziegler, Wolfe and McGuire, 1956; Geraci *et al.*, 1957).

Neither inoculum size nor pH within the range 6·5 to 8·0 affects activity, but the presence of 25 per cent horse serum has been shown to cause a two-fold increase in the bacteristatic concentration (Kirby and Divelbiss, 1957) and a two-fold increase in the bactericidal concentration (Geraci *et al.*, 1957).

Acquired resistance does not appear to be a problem. Early studies (McCormick, *et al.*, 1956; Griffith and Peck, 1956) recorded a few strains of *Staph. aureus* which were naturally resistant to five or more μg./ml. vancomycin but initially sensitive strains do not readily acquire resistance (Ziegler *et al.*, 1957; Garrod and Waterworth, 1956; Geraci *et al.*, 1957).

Pharmacokinetics

Vancomycin is not absorbed from the alimentary tract, and intramuscular injection causes pain and necrosis. Administration has therefore to be intravenous. Kirby and Divelbiss (1957) studied the blood levels after single and repeated intravenous injections of vancomycin. After a single dose the following levels were obtained :

Dose	*μg./ml. in Sera at Hours after Dose*						
	2	*4*	*6*	*8*	*12*	*24*	*48*
0·5 g.	10	3	3	1	0·5	0	—
1·0 g.	25	10	—	5	3	2	—
2·0 g.	50	33	—	10	10	3	0

When doses were repeated at 6- or 12-hour intervals there was slight accumulation. Therapeutic levels could be maintained by a regimen of 0·5 g. six-hourly, 1·0 g. 12-hourly, or 2·0 g. once a day. A regimen of 1·0 g. 12-hourly appeared to be the most satisfactory from the standpoint of ease of administration and effective blood levels.

In patients with impaired renal function much higher blood levels are obtained, and one such patient had a serum concentration of 5 μg./ml. nine days after vancomycin had been discontinued. Organ distribution shows no noteworthy features, except that little of the antibiotic is found in either cerebrospinal fluid or bile. A very high proportion (about 90 per cent) of a dose of vancomycin administered intravenously is excreted in the urine.

Toxic Effects

Thrombophlebitis and febrile reactions are common but the most serious risk is that of producing deafness. As usual with ototoxicity, the excessively high blood levels responsible are liable to be attained in patients with impaired renal function, and this unfortunately sometimes exists in patients requiring this treatment. Dosage should be controlled by blood assays: the aim should be to keep the level at between 5 and 25 μg./ml. Dutton and Elmes (1959) describe a rapid method for this purpose. The vancomycin level in the blood is little affected by renal dialysis (Lindholm and Murray, 1966); in spite of dialysis once or twice weekly 3 μg. per ml. was found in the blood three weeks after a 1 g. dose in a patient with ' end-stage kidney disease '.

Clinical Applications

The principal indication for vancomycin is the treatment of septicaemia, usually accompanied by endocarditis, caused by staphylococci or streptococci resistant to other antibiotics. This resistance may only be manifested *in vivo*. Vancomycin should be considered as an alternative when other treatment (despite its suitability as indicated by *in vitro* tests) is apparently failing.

The treatment of staphylococcal endocarditis has been most extensively studied at the Mayo Clinic (Geraci *et al.*, 1958; Geraci *et al.*, 1962), where divided intravenous doses totalling 2 g. daily have usually been given for up to three or four weeks, although a shorter course may sometimes be adequate. Eykyn, Phillips and Evans (1970) successfully treated staphylococcal shunt site infections in patients undergoing haemodialysis by giving 1 g. once a week. Enterococcal endocarditis has also been successfully treated (Romansky and Holmes, 1958) and occasionally *Str. viridans* infection clinically resistant to other treatment. Vancomycin is usually given alone; should anyone be tempted to combine it with another antibiotic he should know that its combined action against enterococci has been found antagonistic with penicillin (Stille and Rawer, 1970) and synergic with streptomycin (Mandell, Lindsay and Hook, 1970).

Another use recently reported on very favourably is oral administration for acute staphylococcal enterocolitis, usually resulting from treatment with other antibiotics. Wallace *et al.* (1965) successfully treated 7 such patients by giving 0·5 g. in 30 ml. water or fruit juice at 6-hour intervals. Khan and Hall

(1966) gave the same dose at 4- or 6-hour intervals to 45 patients with uniform success.

PHARMACEUTICAL PREPARATION

VANCOMYCIN (Vancocin, *Lilly*).
Vials of 500 mg. for solution for intravenous injection. Dose: see text.

REFERENCES

DUTTON, A. A. C. & ELMES, P. C. (1959). *Brit. med. J.* **1**, 1144.
EYKYN, S., PHILLIPS, I., EVANS, J .(1970). *Brit. med. J.* **3**, 80.
GARROD, L. P. & WATERWORTH, P. M. (1956). *Brit. med. J.* **2**, 61.
GERACI, J. E., HEILMAN, F. R., NICHOLS, D. R., WELLMAN, W. E. & ROSS, G. T. (1957). *Antibiot. Ann.* 1956-7, p. 90.
GERACI, J. E., HEILMAN, F. R., NICHOLS, D. R. & WELLMAN, W. E. (1958). *Proc. Mayo Clin.* **33**, 172.
GERACI, J. E., NICHOLS, D. R. & WELLMAN, W. E. (1962). *Arch. intern. Med.* **109**, 507.
GRIFFITH, R. S. & PECK, F. B. JR. (1956). *Antibiot. Ann.* 1955-6, p. 619.
KHAN, M. Y. & HALL, W. H. (1966). *Ann. intern. Med.* **65**, 1.
KIRBY, W. M. M. & DIVELBISS, C. L. (1957). *Antibiot. Ann.* 1956-7, p. 107.
LINDHOLM, D. D. & MURRAY, J. S. (1966). *New Engl. J. Med.* **274**, 1047.
MANDELL, G. L., LINDSEY, E. & HOOK, E. W. (1970). *Amer. J. med. Sci.* **259**, 346.
McCORMICK, M. H., STARK, W. M., PITTENGER, G. E., PITTENGER, R. C. & McGUIRE, J. M. (1956). *Antibiot. Ann.* 1955-6, p. 606.
ROMANSKY, M. J. & HOLMES, J. R. (1958). *Antibiot. Ann.* 1957-8, p. 187.
STILLE, W. & RAWER, F. (1970). *Deutsch. med. Wschr.* **95**, 2418.
WALLACE, J. F., SMITH, R. H. & PETERSDORF, R. G. (1965). *New Engl. J. Med.* **272**, 1014.
ZIEGLER, D. W., WOLFE, R. N. & McGUIRE, J. M. (1956). *Antibiot. Ann.* 1955-6, p. 612.

RISTOCETIN

This antibiotic was described at length in the same chapter as vancomycin in the first edition of this book. There are many similarities between them in range of activity, pharmacological behaviour, and indications for clinical use. Interesting differences between them are that ristocetin is active against *Mycobacteria*, whereas vancomycin is not, and toxic to the bone marrow, causing leucopenia, rather than to the eighth nerve.

We are informed by the discoverers, Abbott Laboratories, that the manufacture of ristocetin (' Spontin ') was discontinued several years ago.

CHAPTER 13

ANTI-FUNGAL ANTIBIOTICS

MOST of the major antibiotics are produced by fungi, and it is thus not surprising that others should be resistant to them. So resistant are they that quantities of penicillin and streptomycin enough to inhibit any bacterial growth can be added to culture media used for the isolation of pathogenic fungi: this is a useful proceeding in dealing with, for instance, material from secondarily infected lesions of histoplasmosis.

There is a single exception to this in the only systemic mycosis commonly occurring in Great Britain. *Actinomyces israeli* is usually highly sensitive to penicillin, and sufficiently so to several other antibiotics (Garrod, 1952; Blake, 1964). Actinomycosis in all its forms will usually respond to penicillin given in adequate doses for long enough: tetracyclines are the second choice, and their efficacy has been demonstrated, although not on the same scale.

All other mycoses, systemic or surface, are susceptible only to certain highly specialized antibiotics or other drugs, which in general have no anti-bacterial action. These have different specificities among the fungi themselves, very different pharmacological properties, and hence quite separate indications. Several are polyenes, but they now include two other antibiotics and two synthetic compounds.

Cycloheximide

This antibiotic, originally known as actidione, is β-[2-(3,5,-dimethyl-2-oxocyclahexyl)-2-hydroxyethyl] glutarimide, and is produced, usually together with other antibiotics, by several *Streptomyces* species. It is active against fungi but not bacteria, and has also some anti-protozoal and anti-tumour activity. It has been used with some success in a few cases of systemic mycotic infection, but toxic effects are a severe limitation: it has numerous applications in the control of plant diseases (Waksman and Lechevalier, 1962).

POLYENES

Nystatin

Originally named fungicidin, this antibiotic was the product of a soil survey by members of the staff of the New York State Department of Health (Hazen and Brown, 1951), and this is the derivation of its present name. It is formed by *Streptomyces noursei,* the original strain of which came from dairy farm soil in Virginia, and has a tetraene structure which is not very fully elucidated.

The very low solubility of nystatin has compelled investigators to work with suspensions prepared in various ways. Its discoverers used them not only to demonstrate *in vitro* activity, which is highest against yeast-like fungi, but therapeutically in animals by subcutaneous injection. In their experiments and those of Campbell *et al.* (1954, 1955) some effect was observed in infection by *Histoplasma capsulatum, Cryptococcus neoformans* and *Coccidioides immitis.* Drouhet (1955) not only had similar success from parenteral treatment of *Candida albicans* infection in rabbits, but good results from *oral* administration in 25 patients, some of whom had systemic infections. In human infections the primary and most extensive lesions are usually in the alimentary tract, where they are directly accessible, and it seems possible that when the organism is destroyed in these, the task of its elimination from inaccessible sites may become easier. How much of a systemic effect can be obtained with nystatin is now of less practical interest since the effect is certainly inferior to that obtainable with the more recently discovered amphotericin and perhaps with other drugs.

The local action of nystatin in controlling candidiasis involving any part of the alimentary tract from the mouth to the anus is now so generally familiar as to call for no further discussion. The only aspect of it on which there can be two opinions is whether or when it should be given together with tetracyclines as a preventive, since this class of broad spectrum antibiotic, with its suppressive action on the normal flora, is now probably the commonest cause of intestinal candidiasis. This question is discussed later (p. 233). Nystatin is available in suitable form for the local treatment of *Candida* infections elsewhere (skin, vagina, etc.).

Full purification of nystatin is impracticable, and it is usually prescribed in units, an average dose for candidiasis of the alimentary tract being 500,000 units administered three times a day: 3,500 units is the activity of 1 mg. of the pure substance.

Amphotericin B

This is the more useful of two antibiotics formed by a strain of *Streptomyces nodosus* found in soil from Templadora on the Orinoco river. It is a heptaene of not yet fully ascertained structure, insoluble in water but forming salts with a low solubility. It has a satisfactorily low acute toxicity in animals, and inhibits the growth of all yeast-like fungi causing systemic mycoses in a concentration not exceeding and sometimes considerably less than 0·5 μg./ml. Filamentous fungi are also susceptible: bacteria are not.

In early studies amphotericin B was shown to be effective in various mycotic infections in mice, including some caused by filamentous (e.g. *Aspergillus fumigatus, Rhizopus oryzae*) as well as yeast-like fungi. The intravenous route was chiefly used, but there is some evidence of an effect from much larger doses given orally. That there could be such an effect is shown by the human pharmacological studies of Louria (1958), who gave oral doses of 1·6 - 5·6 g. daily and found amounts up to 0·3 μg./ml. in the blood: on the other hand, an intravenous dose of about 1 mg./kg. gave blood levels of 0·5 to 3·5 μg./ml. and these were found still to be 0·5 to 1·5 μg./ml. 20 hours later, indicating very slow elimination. Very small amounts were found in the cerebro-spinal fluid, and urinary excretion accounted for only a small fraction of the dose given. An ingenious and highly sensitive method was used for these assays, depending on the difference between counts of *C. albicans* in known concentrations of the antibiotic with and without addition of the fluid to be tested.

Treatment by the intravenous route has now been shown to be effective in histoplasmosis, coccidioidomycosis, North American blastomycosis, and cryptococcal meningitis, for which additional small (0·5 mg.) intrathecal doses are advisable. Intravenous treatment is begun with doses of 1, 5 and 10 mg. increased to 1 mg./kg. on alternate days, continued if possible until 3 g. have been given (Andriole and Kravetz, 1962). More recently the antibiotic has been solubilized with sodium desoxycholate: in this form it is both more effective, giving higher blood levels, and more toxic. Various toxic effects are common, including fever and nausea and vomiting (which are usually mitigated by also giving aspirin and an antihistamine), local thrombophlebitis resulting from the injection, anaemia, hypokalaemia and a rise in blood urea. The latter is usually said to be ' reversible ', but Sanford *et al.* (1962) who performed renal biopsies on three successfully treated cases of coccidioidomycosis, found proliferative changes in glomeruli, degenerative tubular changes and interstitial deposits of calcium, indicative of some degree of permanent damage.

A conference at the National Institutes of Health, Bethesda (Utz *et al.*, 1964) on the toxic effects of amphotericin B includes two contributions in which effects on the kidney are fully described, in both patients and experimental animals. It is emphasized that some effect is invariable if a certain total dose is exceeded. A rise in blood urea and decreased clearance of creatinine may occur without albuminuria. In this paper and another from the same source (Tynes *et al.*, 1963) hydrocortisone is commended for reducing the frequency of immediate reactions such as fever and vomiting: its effect on actual tissue changes was not examined.

This is the only antibiotic used in the treatment of microbic infections of which so small a total dose can have such effects. It is therefore clear that this treatment should not be undertaken except in certainly diagnosed cases, and when, as in coccidioidomycosis, the severity of the infection is variable, only in the more severe and disseminated form.

Amphotericin B may also be indicated for systemic candidiasis. Its value for this has also been proved: indeed there are now several recorded instances of cure of *C. albicans* endocarditis, a condition which formerly was invariably fatal. Drouhet (1963) describes the treatment of 7 personal cases of *Candida* septicaemia, with successful results in 5.

The efficacy of this treatment is unquestioned but the course is difficult to administer, arduous for the patient, and not without risk. It will be interesting to see to what extent the use of several more recently discovered drugs, to be described later, can replace it.

Other Polyenes

Over 50 polyene antibiotics have now been discovered, a few of which have come into clinical use, although so far exclusively as local applications and principally for the treatment of candidiasis.

CANDICIDIN, a heptaene, formed by *Streptomyces griseus*, is more active than nystatin against *Candida* spp., but has been little used in therapeutics until recently, when good results have been obtained in vaginal candidiasis (Waksman *et al.*, 1965).

HAMYCIN, a heptaene from *Streptomyces pimprina* recovered from local soil in the Research Laboratories of Hindustan Antibiotics, is also said to be more active than nystatin against *Candida* (Thirumalachar *et al.*, 1961). *Aspergillus niger* is also sensitive, but *A. fumigatus* is resistant. Otomycosis due to *A. niger* was successfully treated by Atre *et al.* (1961). Maniar and Mavdikar (1963) have shown that repeated oral administration results in levels of 1-3 μg. per ml. in the blood and various organs of mice, and the same authors (1966) report that 100 or 200 mg. per kg. daily for 10 days eliminates *Cryptococcus neoformans* from the lungs of intravenously inoculated mice. Divekar, Vora and Khan (1966) contest some of the statements of the foregoing authors about the properties of hamycin, and claim themselves to have shown that it is indistinguishable from trichomycin. Several studies (e.g. that by Williams *et al.*, 1966) have shown that hamycin even when administered orally, is toxic, the main lesions being in the kidneys. Shadomy, Shadomy and Utz (1970) found it much more toxic as well as less effective than amphotericin B in the treatment of *C. neoformans* infection in mice.

PIMARCIN, a tetraene, so-called because *Streptomyces natalensis* forming it was derived from soil near Pietermaritzburg, (Struyk *et al.*, 1958) has been successfully used in vaginal candidiasis and has some effect also on trichomoniasis (Korteweg *et al.*, 1963). Bronchopulmonary aspergillosis and candidiasis were treated successfully in 7 out of 10 cases by inhalations (Edwards and La Touche, 1964). Fungal keratitis responded very well in 8 cases to the application of a 5 per cent suspension (Newmark *et al.*, 1971).

TRICHOMYCIN, a heptaene, so-called because of its activity against *Trichomonas vaginalis*, a product of *Streptomyces hachijoensis*, was discovered in Japan (Hosoya *et al.*, 1952). This property, together with the usual susceptibility of *Candida* to a polyene, enables this antibiotic to be used successfully for the treatment of both common forms of vaginitis (Magara *et al.*, 1954). Efficacy in vaginal candidiasis has been confirmed in the United States (Smith *et al.*, 1963) although only an 80 per cent cure rate is claimed, and some of the patients were also given trichomycin orally, whether in expectation of some systemic effect or merely to prevent re-infection from the bowel is not clear.

Prophylactic use of Polyenes

Several preparations are on the market in which a polyene, usually nystatin, is mixed with a tetracycline, with the object of preventing overgrowth of *Candida* in the alimentary tract. The merits of this combination require to be considered, and particularly the pros and cons of its regular use, as suggested by some manufacturers. This question was discussed at length in the previous edition, and the arguments now need only be summarized.

There are three objections to this practice. The first is that it usually fails to achieve any useful object. Almost all observers (e.g. Smits *et al.*, 1966) are agreed that giving the usual dose of 250,000 units of nystatin along with 250 mg. of tetracycline reduces the numbers of *Candida* in the bowel, but with a single exception (Larkin, 1959) no such study has revealed any difference in the frequency of side effects (Metzger *et al.*, 1957; Rein *et al.*, 1957). This lack of effect was confirmed in a more recent study (Report, 1968), an interesting feature of which is that in patients treated with tetracycline only, *Candida* was grown from rectal swabs in 37 and 38 per cent respectively of those with and without gastro-intestinal symptoms. In fact the common assumption that the ordinary side effects result from the proliferation of *Candida* is baseless. More extensive proliferation and actual tissue invasion can occur in debilitated patients, and in them only does the treatment appear to be indicated.

The second objection is one which applies to the indiscriminate and unnecessary use of any antibiotic: that it may lead eventually to increased microbic resistance. This has not yet been seen in clinical isolates of *Candida albicans,* but Hebeka and Solotorovsky (1965) trained this organism to a 60-fold increase in resistance to amphotericin B. There is evidence of cross-resistance among polyenes: Bodenhoff (1968) trained 5 strains of *Cryptococcus neoformans* to resistance to nystatin and amphotericin B, and with one exception the cultures resistant to one antibiotic were also resistant to the other. The margin between the present effective concentrations of amphotericin B and the maximum achievable blood levels is dangerously narrow, and even a small increase in the former might be disastrous.

A different objection applies to preparations, the first of which was intended only for administration to children, which contain tetracycline and amphotericin B. These have been shown to reduce the *C. albicans* population of the bowel, and are said to cause no ill effects (Stough *et al.,* 1959). On the other hand, amphotericin B is the most toxic antibiotic in therapeutic use: the studies of Louria (1958) already cited show that it is absorbed when administered orally, and therapeutic action from oral administration has been reported by Drouhet (1958) and O'Grady and Thompson (1961). The organ most likely to suffer damage is the kidney, and such damage would be undetected, since in discussing the nephrotoxicity of this antibiotic Butler (1964) states: ' Proteinuria . . . has been described in only a few patients, and is not considered characteristic.' In view of this possibility, however remote, and of the fact that severe forms of candidiasis are almost unheard-of in children, the advisability of using this preparation is questionable.

ANTI-MYCOTIC DRUGS OTHER THAN POLYENES

These include one antibiotic, griseofulvin, which is now a well established remedy solely for dermatomycoses, and three other recently discovered drugs, one being an antibiotic and two synthetic, the value of which cannot yet be fully assessed.

Saramycetin

This antibiotic, originally known as X-5079C, is a peptide with a high sulphur content, unique among peptides in having anti-fungal and no anti-bacterial activity (Grunberg, Berger and Titsworth, 1961). Emmons (1961) found it to be of low toxicity, highly effective in experimental histoplasmosis, rather less so in blastomycosis and coccidioidomycosis and ineffective in cryptococcosis. The first report on its clinical use by Utz, Andriole and Emmons (1961) concerns 27 patients, whose further progress together with results in 12 more, is reported on by Witorsch et al. (1966). The drug was injected subcutaneously at 6-hour intervals, 3-5 mg./kg. daily being usually given to a total dose of about 20 g. Of 16 patients with North American blastomycosis, 14 responded both clinically and with negative cultures, but 8 relapsed, and of 13 with histoplasmosis 6 failed to respond or relapsed. Both sporo-trichosis and aspergillosis responded in 2 out of 3 patients. Treatment failed in patients with coccidioidomycosis and in 3 severe *Candida* infections, 2 with endocarditis. To set against these unpromising or equivocal results is the fact that sara-mycetin is far better tolerated than amphotericin B, and could perhaps safely be given with better effect in larger doses.

5-Fluorocytosine

This substance, an anti-metabolite of the pyrimidine base cytosine, acts exclusively on certain yeast-like fungi and not at all on filamentous fungi or any bacteria. According to Shadomy (1969) it inhibits *Cryptococcus neoformans* in concentrations of 0.46-3.9 μg./ml. and kills it at 3.9-15.6 μg./ml. *Candida albicans* is about equally sensitive. Since the drug can be given orally in doses of 100 mg./kg. daily, and then attains concentrations in the blood and cerebro-spinal fluid of 10-30 and 8-20 μg./ml. respectively, an effect in these two infections is to be expected, and this has been confirmed clinically. *Histoplasma capsulatum* and *Blastomyces dermatitidis* are resistant.

Among reports of the successful use of this drug in cryptococcal meningitis, success has not always been complete (Fass and Perkins, 1971) and most patients had first been treated unsuccessfully with amphotericin B (McGill *et al.*, 1969), but one of the Gonzalez-Ochoa's (1970) patients was treated with 5-fluorocytosine only, and one of those described by Watkins *et al.* (1969) was so intolerant of amphotericin B that only 350 mg. had been given when it was abandoned. This patient was eventually given no less than 12 g. fluorocytosine daily without ill effects, a remarkable illustration of the non-toxicity of this drug. Duration of treatment has varied from a few weeks to as long as ten months, and recovery was complete in most of these patients. In some instances of therapeutic failure the organism has been found to have become highly resistant.

5-Fluorocytosine had also been used for *Candida* infections. Uncomplicated septicaemia has responded (Tassel and Madoff, 1968; Warner *et al.*, 1971), but endocarditis, although apparently controlled, has not been eradicated (Warner *et al.*, 1970; Record *et al.*, 1971). Since the drug is eliminated by the kidney, urinary candidiasis would be expected to respond, and this has been confirmed (Davies and Reeves, 1971). Good results are also claimed by Lopes *et al.* (1969) in chromoblastomycosis. This drug, with its great advantages of oral administration and almost total lack of toxicity, will be much preferred to amphotericin B for infections susceptible to it.

Clotrimazole (BAYb 5097)

This compound, bis-phenyl-(2-chlorphenyl)-1-imidazole methane, one of a long series of tritylimidazole derivatives prepared in the Bayer laboratories, is fully described by Plempel *et al.* (1969). It inhibits all the principal fungi causing systemic infections in concentrations of the order of 1 μg./ml. It is well absorbed from the alimentary tract. Blood levels are well sustained, and toxicity is very low. Some of the drug in the blood and that excreted in the urine is an inactive metabolite. Efficacy has been demonstrated in mice in *Candida, Histoplasma* and *Aspergillus* infections. Shadomy (1970) obtained less favourable results than these in experimental infections, and observed that pre-treatment worsened them; this paradoxical effect is confirmed by Waitz, Moss and Weinstein (1971), who found that after pre-treatment for 5 days the blood levels during subsequent post-inoculation treatment were much reduced. It seems therefore that habituation to the drug enables the body to dispose of it more rapidly. These authors also found it to be active against staphylococci, streptococci and even some enterobacteria, and that in the therapy of *C. albicans* infection in mice oral administration gave better results than parenteral. The wide range of anti-fungal activity of the drug, which includes dermatophytes, is shown in further *in vitro* studies by Shadomy (1971).

Few clinical results have yet been reported, but pulmonary aspergillosis has been successfully treated in two patients (Oberste-Lehn, Baggesen and Plempel, 1969; Evans, Watson and Matthews, 1971), and there are several accounts of successful use in candidiasis, including two severe systemic infections described by Malchow *et al.* (1972). Treatment has usually been prolonged, and at the rate of about 60 mg./kg. daily.

Griseofulvin

This antibiotic was discovered as a product of *Penicillium griseofulvum* by Oxford, Raistrick and Simonart (1939), who found it to be $C_{17}H_{17}O_6Cl$ and provisionally ascertained its structure, which has since been confirmed. It was re-discovered some years later as the product of a *Penicillium* in soil at Wareham Heath, Dorset, in which conifers grew poorly because of its action on mycorrhizal fungi: from its effect on these organisms it was called ' curling factor '. Its identity with a sample of griseofulvin supplied by Raistrick was verified by Grove and McGowan (1947). Its anti-fungal action was then further examined and exploited in the field of plant pathology. Clinical use was at first considered inadvisable because of the observation of an anti-mitotic effect, but this was produced by large doses given intravenously in animals, and there is not now believed to be any risk of such an effect from the doses employed clinically.

The highest activity of griseofulvin is against dermatophytes: yeast-like fungi are less susceptible, although O'Grady and his colleagues (1963), by giving large doses to mice, obtained a reduction in the size of *Candida* lesions in the mouse thigh, possibly by some indirect mechanism. Total inhibition of the growth of dermatophytes *in vitro* may require concentrations exceeding those obtainable at the site of infection, but much lower concentrations retard growth, and Jesenská and Danilla (1971) suggest determination of sensitivity by comparing colony diameters on solid media containing 0·1 to 3 μg./ml. with those on drug-free medium. A curative effect was first demonstrated in experimental *Microsporum canis* infection in guinea-pigs by Gentles (1958) who was also responsible (Gentles *et al.*, 1959) for showing that the antibiotic is actually in the hair of treated animals, some of it being only extractable with methanol. The fact that griseofulvin when administered orally is actually incorporated in keratin as it is formed explains its unique activity in fungus infections of the hair and nails.

The reader can now be referred to works on dermatology for details of clinical use. The results in *Microsporum audouini* and other infections of the scalp hair are uniformly good, and this treatment is now preferred to X-ray epilation. A good account of results in onychomycosis is given by Davies, Everall and Hamilton (1967). Treatment was continued for up to 2 years, 0·5 g. being given 3 times a day for one month and thereafter twice daily. Finger nail infections responded better than those of the toes, and *Trychophyton rubrum* infections better than *T. mentagrophytes,* the former being the more sensitive organism.

The antibiotic is better absorbed when in finely divided form, and its absorption is also said to be promoted by fat in the diet (Crounse, 1961). Blood levels are much reduced by administration of phenobarbitone, which apparently enables the liver to break down griseofulvin more rapidly (Busfield *et al.*, 1964). Other systems of dosage have been proposed for short courses. Atkinson *et al.* (1962) contest the suggestion made by others that scalp ringworm can be cured by a single massive dose, and showed that divided doses give higher blood levels than a single daily dose. Grin and Nadazdin (1965) observed effects by microscopy of hairs plucked at intervals, and confirmed that a single large dose is ineffective, but achieved economy by initial large doses (50 mg. per kg. daily) for five days followed by only 6·25 mg. per kg. daily for the remainder of a 28-day course.

Even long courses of treatment are usually well tolerated. Rashes, headache and gastric discomfort are uncommon and rarely severe. The disturbance of porphyrin metabolism and liver damage produced by large doses in mice (De Matteis and Rimington, 1963) appear to have little or no counterpart in patients given conventional doses.

PHARMACEUTICAL PREPARATIONS AND DOSAGES

NYSTATIN (' Fungicidin ', ' Mycostatin ', *Squibb*)
  Tablets 500,000 units: usual dose 1 t.d.s. Also in form of ointment, suspension, pessaries, etc.

AMPHOTERICIN B (' Fungizone ', *Squibb*)
  Vials containing 50 mg.+sodium desoxycholate and buffer for intravenous infusion: usual dose 0·1 mg. rising to 1 mg. per kg. body weight daily.

PIMARICIN (' Natamycin ', ' Myprozine ', ' Pimafucin ', *Brocades*)
  Sterile 2-5 per cent aqueous suspension for intrabronchial administration as aerosol: 2·5 mg. have been given t.d.s. Also as ointment, enteric-coated tablets and vaginal tablets.

GRISEOFULVIN (' Grisovin ', *Glaxo;* ' Fulcin Forte ' *I.C.I.*)
  Tablets of 125 or 250 mg.: usual dose 250 mg. 4 times a day.

REFERENCES

ANDRIOLE, V. T. & KRAVETZ, H. M. (1962). *J. Amer. med. Ass.* **180**, 269.
ATKINSON, R. M., BEDFORD, C., CHILD, K. J. & TOMICH, E. G. (1962). *Antibiot. Chemother.* **12**, 225.
ATRE, W. G., WAKANKAR, P. S. & PADHYE, A. A. (1961). *Hindustan Antibiot. Bull.* **3**, 172.
BLAKE, G. C. (1964). *Brit. med. J.* **1**, 145.
BODENHOFF, J. (1968). *Acta Path. Microbiol. scand.* **73**, 572.
BUSFIELD, D., CHILD, K. J. & TOMICH, E. G. (1964). *Brit. J. Pharmacol.* **22**, 137.
BUTLER, W. T. (1964). *Ann. intern. Med.* **61**, 344.
CAMPBELL, C. C., HODGES, E. P. & HILL, G. B. (1954). *Antibiot Ann.* 1953-54, p. 210.
CAMPBELL, C. C., O'DELL, E. T. & HILL, G. B. (1955). *Antibiot. Ann.* 1954-5, p. 858.
CROUNSE, R. G. (1961). *J. invest. Dermatol.* **37**, 529.
DAVIES, R. R., EVERALL, J. D. & HAMILTON, E. (1967). *Brit. med. J.* **3**, 464.
DAVIES, R. R. & REEVES, D. S. (1971). *Brit. med. J.* **1**, 577.
DE MATTEIS, F. & RIMINGTON, C. (1963). *Brit. J. Derm.* **75**, 91.
DIVEKAR, P. V., VORA, V. C. & KHAN, A. W. (1966). *J. Antibiot. (Tokyo) Ser.* A **19**, 63.
DROUHET, E. (1955). *Ann. Inst. Pasteur* **88**, 298.
DROUHET, E. (1958). *Bull. Soc. Path. exot.* **51**, 76.
DROUHET, E. (1963). *Antibiot. et Chemother. (Basel)* **11**, 21.
EDWARDS, G. & LA TOUCHE, C. J. P. (1964). *Lancet* **1**, 1349.
EMMONS, C. W. (1961). *Amer. Rev. resp. Dis.* **84**, 507.
EVANS, E. G. V., WATSON, D. A. & MATTHEWS, N. R. (1971). *Brit. med. J.,* **4**, 599.

240 ANTIBIOTIC AND CHEMOTHERAPY

FASS, R. J. & PERKINS, R. L. (1971). *Ann. intern. Med.* **74**, 535.
GARROD L. P. (1952). *Brit. med. J.* **1**, 1263.
GENTLES, J. C. (1958). *Nature (Lond.)* **182**, 476.
GENTLES, J. C., BARNES, M. J. & FANTES, K. H. (1959). *Nature (Lond.)* **183**, 256.
GONZALEZ-OCHOA, A. (1970). *Rev. Invest. Salud. Publica* **30**, 63.
GRIN, E. I. & NADAŽDIN, M. (1965). *Bull. Wld Hlth Org.* **33**, 183.
GROVE, J. F. & McGOWAN, J. C. (1947). *Nature (Lond.)* **160**, 574.
GRUNBERG, E., BERGER, J. & TITSWORTH, E. (1961). *Amer. Rev. resp. Dis.* **84**, 504.
HAZEN, ELIZABETH L. & BROWN, RACHEL (1951). *Proc. Soc. exp. Biol. (N.Y.)* **76**, 93.
HEBEKA, E. K. & SOLOTOROVSKY, M. (1965). *J. Bact.* **89**, 1533.
HOSOYA, S., KOMATSU, N., SOEDA, M. & SONODA, Y. (1952). *Jap. J. exp. Med.* **22**, 505.
JESENSKÁ, Z. & DANILLA, T. (1971). *Zbl. Bakt. I Orig.* **217**, 104.
KORTEWEG, G. C., SZABO, K. L. H., RUTTEN, A. M. G. & HOOGERHEIDE, J. C. (1963). *Antibiot. et Chemother. (Basel)* **11**, 261.
LARKIN, R. (1959). *Lancet* **1**, 1228.
LOPES, C. F., ALVARENGA, R. J., CISALPINO, E. O., MARTINELLI, B., SANTOS, P. U. & ARMOND, S. (1969). *O Hospital* **75**, 1335.
LOURIA, D. B. (1958). *Antibiot. Med.* **5**, 295.
MAGARA, M., YOKOUTI, E., SENDA, T. & AMINO, E. (1954). *Antibiot. Chemother.* **4**, 433.
MALCHOW, H., SEYBOLD, D., LANGE, H., FREUND, J. & RÜGER, K. (1972). *Dtsch. med. Wschr.* **97**, 935.
MANIAR, A. C. & MAVDIKAR, S. (1963). *Hindustan Antibiot. Bull.* **5**, 113.
MANIAR, A. C. & MAVDIKAR, S. (1966). *Canad. J. Microbiol.* **12**, 377.
McGILL, P. E., SEQUEIRA, R., JINDANI, A., NGULI, E. T., FORRESTER, A. T. T. & FULTON, W. F. M. (1969). *East African med. J.* **46**, 663.
METZGER, W. I., STEIGMANN, F., JENKINS, C. J., PAMUKCU, S. F. & KAMINSKI, L. (1957). *Antibiot. Ann.* 1956-57, p. 208.
NEWMARK, E., KAUFMAN, H. E., POLACK, F. M. & ELLISON, A. C. (1971). *Sth med. J.* **64**, 935.
OBERSTE-LEHN, H., BAGGESEN, I. & PLEMPEL, M. (1969). *Dtsch. med. Wschr.* **94**, 1365.
O'GRADY, F. & THOMPSON, R. E. M. (1961). *Antibiot. Chemother.* **11**, 26.
O'GRADY, F., THOMPSON, R. E. M. & COTTON, R. E. (1963). *Brit. J. exp. Path.* **44**, 334.
OXFORD, A. E., RAISTRICK, H. & SIMONART, P. (1939). *Biochem. J.* **33**, 240.
PLEMPEL, M., BARTMANN, K., BUCHEL, K. H. & REGEL, E. (1969). *Dtsch. med. Wschr.* **94**, 1356.
RECORD, C. O., SKINNER, J. M., SLEIGHT, P. & SPELLER, D. C. E. (1971). *Brit. med. J.* **1**, 262.
REIN, C. R., LEWIS, L. A. & DICK, L. A. (1957). *Antibiot. Med.* **4**, 771.
REPORT (1968). *Brit. med. J.* **4**, 411.
SANFORD, W. G., RASCH, J. R. & STONEHILL, R. B. (1962). *Ann. intern. Med.* **56**, 553.
SHADOMY, S. (1969). *Appl. Microbiol.* **17**, 871.
SHADOMY, S. (1970). *Antimicrob. Agents Chemother.* 169.
SHADOMY, S. (1971). *Infection Immunity*, **4**, 143.
SHADOMY, S., SHADOMY, H. J. & UTZ, J. P. (1970). *Infection Immunity* **1**, 128.
SMITH, A. G., TAUBERT, H. D. & MARTIN, C. W. (1963). *Amer. J. Obstet. Gynec.* **87**, 455.
SMITS, B. J., PRIOR, A. P. & ARBLASTER, P. G. (1966). *Brit. med. J.* **1**, 208.
STOUGH, A. R., GROEL, J. T. & KROEGER, W. H. (1959). *Antibiot. Med.* **6**, 653.
STRUYK, A. P., HOETTE, I., DROST, G., WAISVISZ, J. M., VAN EEK, T. & HOOGERHEIDE, J. C. (1958). *Antibiot. Ann.*, 1957-8, p. 878.
TASSEL, D. & MADOFF, M. A. (1968). *J. Amer. med. Ass.* **206**, 830.

THIRUMALACHAR, M. J., MENON, S. K. & BHATT, V. V. (1961). *Hindustan Antibiot. Bull.* **3**, 136.

TYNES, B. S., UTZ, J. P., BENNETT, J. E. & ALLING, D. W. (1963). *Amer. Rev. resp. Dis.* **87**, 264.

UTZ, J. P., ANDRIOLE, V. T. & EMMONS, C. W. (1961). *Amer. Rev. resp. Dis.* **84**, 514.

UTZ, J. P., BENNETT, J. E., BRANDRISS, M. W., BUTLER, W. T. & HILL, G. J. (1964). *Ann. intern. Med.* **61**, 334.

WAITZ, J. A., MOSS, E. L. & WEINSTEIN, M. J. (1971). *Appl. Microbiol.* **22**, 891.

WAKSMAN, S. A. & LECHEVALIER, H. A. (1962). *The Actinomycetes,* vol. III. London: Baillière.

WAKSMAN, S. A., LECHEVALIER, H. A. & SCHAFFNER, C. P. (1965). *Bull. Wld Hlth Org.* **33**, 219.

WARNER, J. F., MCGEHEE, R. F., DUMA, R. J., SHADOMY, S. & UTZ, J. P. (1971).*Antimicrob. Agents Chemother.*—1970, 473.

WATKINS, J. S., CAMPBELL, M. J., GARDNER-MEDWIN, D., INGHAM, H. R. & MURRAY, I. G. (1969). *Brit. med. J.* **3**, 29.

WILLIAMS, T. W., Jr., WITORSCH, P., HIGHMAN, B., EMMONS, C. W. & UTZ, J. P. (1966). *Antimicrob. Agents Chemother.* 1965, p. 700.

WITORSCH, P., ANDRIOLE, V. T., EMMONS, C. W. & UTZ, J. P. (1966). *Amer. Rev. resp. Dis.* **93**, 876.

CHAPTER 14

MODES OF ACTION

AN antibacterial agent suitable for human therapy must possess a remarkable array of attributes, but above all it must exhibit a high degree of selective toxicity—that is to say its detrimental effect on the infecting organism must greatly exceed any detrimental effect on the patient. Extreme degrees of selective toxicity depend on possession by bacteria of processes or structures (for example bacterial cell wall) which are not represented in man. Unacceptably low degrees of selective toxicity result from the fact that many essential processes (for example, protein synthesis) are common to widely separate species in which they differ only in detail. Antibacterial agents may be conveniently divided into four groups of which the effects centre about the synthesis of nucleic acid, of protein, of cell wall, or of cell membrane.

Nucleic Acid

Replication of the nucleic acids of the bacterial cell is prevented directly by nalidixic acid and rifamycins and remotely by sulphonamides and certain diaminopyrimidines.

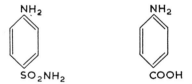

SULPHANILAMIDE   P-AMINOBENZOIC ACID

Para-aminobenzoate. Woods (1940) postulated that sulphonamides compete with the structurally similar para-aminobenzoic acid for the same enzyme. Para-aminobenzoic acid is incorporated into the co-enzyme folic acid (Hutner *et al.*, 1959) and considerable evidence has accumulated to show that sulphonamide-inhibited organisms exhibit the metabolic signs of folic acid deficiency. Synthesis of folic acid and its inhibition by sulphonamides has been demonstrated in living *E. coli*, and convincing confirmation of Woods' hypothesis has come from the demonstration that purified tetrahydropteroic acid synthetase—the enzyme which condenses para-aminobenzoic acid with 2-amino-4-hydroxy-tetrahydropteridine to form tetra-hydropteric acid, a step in the synthesis of folic acid—is competitively inhibited by sulphonamide.

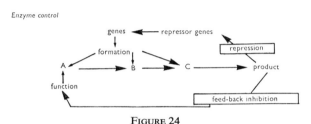

FIGURE 24

When sufficient product has accumulated, activity of the enzyme sequence, A, B, C is suppressed by (1) reduced activity of the first enzyme, A (with consequent substrate starvation of the rest) and (2) halt in production of the whole enzyme sequence.

Richmond (1966) has argued that for structural analogues to be successful antimicrobial agents, they must function as something more than simple competitive inhibitors. A compound may strongly inhibit an isolated, purified enzyme *in vitro*, but conditions *in vivo* are quite different. In the living cell, substrate is continuously supplied to the enzyme by the previous enzyme in the metabolic pathway, and its product removed by the next enzyme. In this balanced system a steady state is reached in which the quantities of substrate are insufficient to saturate the enzymes. If a competitive inhibitor is added to such a system, the competitor is taken up by the enzyme, and the natural precursor, of which the supply continues, accumulates. In time, the concentration of natural substrate becomes sufficiently high to reverse the effect of the inhibitor and the normal process is resumed—with the ' steady state ' concentration of substrate at a higher level. A successful competitive inhibitor has, therefore, either to have a much higher affinity for the enzyme than has the natural substrate (a very unusual state of affairs since the enzyme has evolved to handle the natural substrate—but evidently the case with sulphonamides), or it must act in some other way.

Control over microbial enzymes is exercised in two main ways: by feed-back inhibition and by repression (Fig. 24). The product inhibits the activity of the first enzyme of the pathway—a rapid effect—and also acts on the repressor genes to inhibit the formation of new enzymes, a slow effect since the existing enzymes continue to function. Structural analogues may mimic this effect, which cannot be overcome by increasing the concentration of the natural product, the supply of which is, in any case, cut off by this kind of inhibition. There is some evidence that sulphonamides may owe their action in part to such a mechanism (Richmond, 1966).

Tetrahydrofolate. From the precursors with which sulphonamides interfere, bacteria construct tetrahydrofolate which all cells use as a cofactor in the incorporation of 1-carbon fragments into the precursors of purines needed for nucleic acid synthesis. In the process tetrahydrofolate is oxidized to dihydrofolate and must be regenerated by reduction—a process which is brought about through the agency of the enzyme dihydrofolate reductase. Inhibition of this enzyme is a general property of 2:4 diaminopyrimidines which exhibit remarkable selectivity in that modification of the molecule can greatly increase the activity against the enzyme of one species while decreasing it against another (Hitchings, 1969).

Amongst therapeutically important examples of this class of agent, pyrimethamine inhibits mammalian and bacterial enzymes approximately equally but only in a concentration about 2000 times that needed to produce comparable inhibition of the plasmodial enzyme. In contrast, trimethoprim is extremely active against the bacterial enzyme, much less active against the plasmodial enzyme, and very feebly active against the mammalian enzyme which requires for comparable inhibition about 50,000 times the concentration which inhibits the bacterial enzyme, and 2000 times that which inhibits the plasmodial enzyme. Although its anti-plasmodial effect is plainly much less than its anti-bacterial effect, it is nevertheless sufficient to produce a useful degree of anti-malarial activity.

Differential affinity for the enzymes of different species is clearly of great importance in determining the selective toxicity of trimethoprim, but there is an additional important difference in the way in which animals and parasites obtain their folate requirements. Bacteria and protozoa synthesize folic acid from para-aminobenzoic acid, while man and animals utilize preformed folic or folinic acid (leucovorin) from the diet. These two processes appear to be mutually exclusive: parasites which synthesize folic acid cannot absorb it preformed, and man and animals which absorb it preformed cannot synthesize it.

This difference has two important consequences. Firstly, any depressant effect of diaminopyrimidines on human folate metabolism may be overcome by feeding tetrahydrofolate supplements which the parasite cannot utilize (Whitman, 1969). Secondly, since sulphonamides inhibit the incorporation by parasites of p-aminobenzoic acid into dihydrofolate, sulphonamides and trimethoprim act sequentially in the same metabolic pathway. As a result, their combined action is strongly synergic. There is about a 10-fold increase in activity when the agents are given together (Hitchings, 1961). Figure 25 shows the difference between parasite and human folic

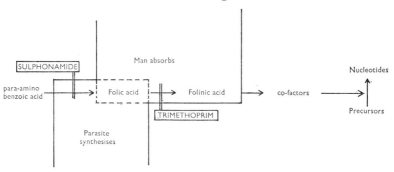

FIGURE 25

Sequential interruption of folate synthesis in parasites by sulphonamide and trimethoprim (based on Hitchings, 1961).

acid metabolism diagrammatically, and indicates the point at which sulphonamides and such folic acid antagonists as pyrimethamine and trimethoprim work.

DNA

The effect of sulphonamides and diaminopyrimidines is ultimately to deprive the cell of nucleic acid; the effect of nalidixic acid is to prevent its replication. Exposure to nalidixic acid causes specific degradation of the chromosome just behind its replication point which then extends rapidly backwards to involve previously formed DNA (Ramareddy and Rieter, 1969). Within minutes of removal of the drug, DNA replication is reinstated at the normal time (Ward *et al.*, 1970). By its effect on chromosomal replication nalidixic acid interrupts conjugation between enterobacteria if the male organism is sensitive but not if it is resistant (Hane, 1971).

RNA

Rifamycins specifically inhibit the bacterial enzyme concerned with replication of RNA. This effect is brought about by binding of one molecule of the antibiotic to one molecule of the enzyme (Lill *et al.*, 1970). The corresponding mammalian enzyme is unaffected by the antibiotic and this undoubtedly accounts for its selective toxicity (Umezawa *et al.*, 1968).

Protein

For bacterial growth to proceed all the biochemical events of the cell must be repeated cyclically: some over the long term from one division to the next, some over very short periods when a particular event has to recur many times in the course of construction of new material as, for example, in the linking together of the large number of amino-acids which make up a single molecule of protein. As each component makes its contribution to the cycle it is altered and must be regenerated before the cycle can begin again. Interruption of the cycle locks the process at that point and growth halts. Because of the continuation of unaffected processes the overall integration of cell metabolism is disrupted and the long-term effect of this may be so severe that the cell dies. On the DNA template the cell assembles three kinds of RNA: transfer-RNA (t-RNA), ribosomal-RNA (r-RNA) and messenger-RNA (m-RNA).

Ribosomal-RNA is utilized, with protein, in the construction of ribosomes—small bodies, lying free in the cytoplasm or attached to the cytoplasmic membrane, which are concerned with protein synthesis. Messenger-RNA takes from DNA to the ribosomes the code which fixes the order in which amino acids are assembled into protein.

In the metabolic pool, uncommitted ribosomes exist as separate 30S and 50S components (the figures indicate the speed at which the components sediment in the ultracentrifuge). On the end of a thread of m-RNA a 30S and a 50S component come together to form a functional ribosome on which there are two attachment sites for amino-acids. From the metabolic pool, amino-acids are transported to the ribosome, each kind of amino-acid being carried by its own specific t-RNA. The region of the messenger thread which is attached to the ribosome is ' recognized ' by the appropriate t-RNA which attaches to it and to the ribosome in such a way that the carried amino-acid is brought into contact with the first of the two ribosome sites. The energy required to effect this process of attachment is provided by ATP together with other factors, all of which have to be regenerated once the appropriate amino-acid has been attached to the ' receptor ' site of the ribosome and the carrier t-RNA released to collect another amino-acid. Once the amino-acid has been attached, the ribosome is moved to the next ' codon ' of the messenger which stipulates the amino-acid next to be added.

With this movement, called ' translocation ', the amino-acid is transferred to the second or ' donor ' site of the ribosome. The delivery and attachment process is now repeated so that the second specified amino-acid is brought onto the vacated receptor site. When both amino-acids are in position, the first is detached from the donor site and coupled to the free end of the newly attached amino-acid to form a dipeptide in a process called ' transfer '. The processes of translocation and transfer consume energy which is again supplied by cycling factors which must be regularly regenerated in each cycle.

In the meantime, a second ribosome is assembled from its two components at the first site on the messenger and the specified first amino-acid attached as before. In the second translocation move the dipeptide attached to the first ribosome

9

is transferred to the donor site and in due course transferred to the third amino-acid specified by the messenger.

This process continues until a ' polysome ' is assembled which consists of the messenger completely threaded with ribosomes the first of which, having traversed the whole length of the messenger, carries a completed protein. In its final move, the ribosome comes off the end of the messenger thread, re-releases the completed protein, dissociates into its two components and returns to the pool.

Sites of Antibiotic Action

The key step of initiation of polysome construction in which the first ribosome is attached to the messenger is halted by streptomycin and this is now thought to be the main mode in which it prevents protein synthesis. In high concentrations it also produces an extremely intriguing alteration in protein synthesis by causing the messenger code to be misread and the wrong amino acid to be incorporated into the growing peptide chain (Fig. 26 D).

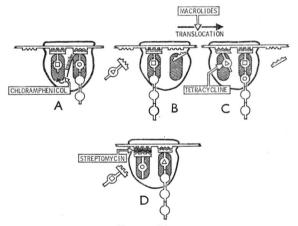

FIGURE 26

Protein synthesis: (A) The growing peptide chain is transferred to the amino acid which has recently attached to the ribosome. The t-RNA which attached the peptide is released and the m-RNA moves in relation to the ribosome (B→C) bringing the next codon in apposition to the amino acid site. The amino acid specified by the codon and carried by its specific t-RNA, attaches to the ribosome (C); the peptide chain is transferred to it and the whole cycle is repeated.

The degree of infidelity introduced into protein replication by this process is very small. Major deletions of amino-acid sequences do not occur and it appears that the lesion involves misplacement of a single amino-acid. Estimations of the numbers of streptomycin molecules required to inhibit protein synthesis strongly suggest that the specific biochemical lesion is brought about by attachment of a single streptomycin molecule to one of the nucleotides of the coding triplet. This very discrete lesion is sufficient for the continuation of the peptide sequence to fail, or for protein to be manufactured which is unable to fulfil its enzymic or structural function. The effect of streptomycin on cell growth is relatively slow and it is probable that considerable accumulation of faulty protein occurs before cell function ceases. Streptomycin produces a number of later effects on the cell, such as permeability changes and impairment of respiration, which might result from imperfections in the protein molecules concerned in those functions or might be independent effects of the drug. Either way it is probable that it is these effects, rather than the protein derangement itself, which are directly responsible for cell death.

As indicated in Fig. 26 C, tetracycline interrupts the cycle by which amino-acid is carried and attached to the ribosome. Transfer of the growing peptide chain to the newly attached amino-acid which is to be next added (Fig. 26 A) is interrupted by chloramphenicol (Teraoka, 1970). The process of translocation is prevented by macrolides, by lincomycin and by fusidic acid, which has been shown to fuse together the elements concerned in the translocation cycle so that the regenerative process which is essential to repetition of the cycle cannot occur (Brot *et al.*, 1971). Interestingly enough, the similarity of the translocation lesion produced by these three agents is reflected in the similarity of the characteristic morphological injury which they exert on staphylococci as seen in the stereoscan electron microscope (Fig. 20).

The translocation step may be peculiarly accessible to modification since all three agents which affect it are particularly liable to give rise to resistant mutants. It is not known why interruption of protein synthesis at the point of attack adopted by tetracycline and chloramphenicol halts bacterial growth while the effect of the agents which interfere with translocation is frequently lethal. Protein synthesis is absolutely essential to the cell's economy since the generation of both enzymes for metabolic processes and components for anatomical structures depend on it. Death of a cell involves a degree of irreversible structural organization which goes beyond a single biochemical event and it is no doubt secondary consequences of the biochemical lesion which are responsible for the cell's ultimate destruction. It is not at present possible even to speculate why the chain of events initiated by one kind of interference with protein synthesis is so much more serious than others.

The process of protein synthesis is essentially the same in all cells and the differential toxicity of antibacterial agents for different species (both in terms of selective toxicity and antimicrobial spectrum) depends either on differences in the ribosomes or on impermeability of the cell to the agent. The resistance of enterobacteria to lincomycin, erythromycin or fusidic acid (all of which will interfere with protein synthesis by the isolated ribosomes of E. coli—the biochemists' favourite tool) is due to failure of the agent to penetrate the cell. By using radioactively labelled antibiotics it is possible to show that the greater sensitivity of Gram-positive organisms to macrolides is due to the fact that they are not only permeable to the agents (which the resistant Gram-negative organisms are not) but actually concentrate the agent within the cell (Mao and Putterman, 1968). There is a good deal of evidence that this permeability barrier resides in the cell wall since wall-deficient forms are a great deal more sensitive than the parent enterobacteria (Greenwood and O'Grady, 1970).

The other reason why some cells are so sensitive and others not is that their ribosomes differ. Antibiotic action requires attachment to the ribosome and this occurs at a specific site which is carried on one of the 20 or more proteins which, together with ribosomal RNA, make up the ribosomes. Elegant biochemical analysis shows that antibiotic action occurs when one antibiotic molecule binds to one specific ribosomal protein binding site (Mao et al., 1970) and that absence of this particular protein renders the cell insusceptible (Otaka et al, 1970). It follows that the substitution of another protein for that carrying the specific binding site will render the cell resistant to the action of the antibiotic. This is precisely what happens in mutants highly resistant to streptomycin (Mazukawa, 1969).

Cell Wall

The outstanding difference between bacteria and mammalian cells is the tough thick cell wall external to the cell membrane which fixes the shape of bacterial cells and gives to them their extraordinary resistance to osmotic damage. This remarkable structure is absent from mammalian cells and any agent which interfered solely with its construction would be entirely without effect on a mammalian host. Several groups of antibacterial agents exert their effects through interference with cell wall synthesis, and setting aside the special problem of hypersensitivity the most important of them, the penicillins and cephalosporins, are amongst the most innocuous of therapeutic agents.

The walls of Gram-positive organisms consist largely of a characteristic wall component called mucopeptide, while those of Gram-negative bacteria, which are much thicker, consist of a sandwich of mucopeptide and lipoprotein. The steps by which mucopeptide is synthesized differ in detail between bacterial species but the sequence of events follows a similar general pattern (Strominger et al., 1971).

The process begins with the conversion of natural L-alanine into the D-form and the linking of two D-alanine molecules together. Both these events are inhibited by cycloserine which is a close structural analogue of alanine. Other amino-acids are linked to the di-alanine to create a short peptide which is united with a sugar characteristic of bacterial cell wall, acetylmuramic acid. This is coupled to a molecule of acetylglucosamine and a chain of 5-glycine residues attached to the peptide tail of the muramic acid. This complex constitutes the brick from which the wall is constructed. The hod which carries the brick across the cell membrane to the site of cell wall construction is a phospholipid which is released once the brick is in place and returns to carry more bricks (Fig. 27) until alternating acetylmuramic acid-acetylglucosamine molecules are united into long glycan strands with their trailing peptides. Layer upon layer of these strands are set down upon one another until the proper thickness of the wall is achieved.

In the final step—the one which gives the wall its shape-retaining rigidity—the glycine chains attached to the short peptides of one layer are fixed to the short peptides of the next (Fig. 27).

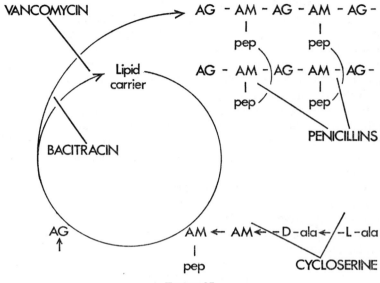

FIGURE 27

The cell-wall consists of layers of 'glycan' strands composed of units in which N-acetylglucosamine (AG)—made from alanine (ala)—is linked to N-acetylmuramic acid (AM) with a peptide tail (pep). The units are transported to the site of insertion into the wall by a lipid carrier which returns to carry more units. The wall is made rigid by joining the peptide tails together. The points of interruption by antibiotics are shown.

Apart from cycloserine, most antibiotics interfere with later stages of cell-wall synthesis. Vancomycin interferes with the release of the phospholipid carrier thus preventing further transport of new material, and bacitracin inhibits the next step in which the carrier, having delivered up its load, is regenerated in the active form. Penicillins and cephalosporins inhibit the final process of cross-linking between the layers.

The completed cell wall consists of a single giant bag-shaped molecule (Weidel and Peltzer, 1964) occupying the whole of the surface of the cell. For the cell to grow this tough envelope must be expanded in such a way that throughout the process its strength is preserved so that the cell does not succumb to osmotic damage, and when the time comes for division the shape of the original cell is reproduced in each of the progeny. Much elegant work has revealed a great deal about the structure and synthesis of the cell-wall polymer but the processes by which such remarkably controlled remodelling of the cell coat is achieved are at present unknown.

Two things are nevertheless plain. The first is that if the cell is to grow, the bonds which give the wall its strength must be opened in order to allow the insertion of fresh components as the cell expands. The second is that the process of expansion of the surface cell wall and the construction and ultimate cleavage of the septum when the cell divides are to an important extent separate. This is shown by the effect of low concentrations of penicillins or cephalosporins which interfere with septum formation but do not otherwise interfere with cell wall synthesis sufficiently to prevent cell growth. In such conditions Gram-negative bacilli continue to grow but instead of separating into new cells, expand into longer and longer filaments. In higher concentrations of these agents the cell membrane is progressively deprived of external support as the wall weakens and in conditions of low osmolality the cell ruptures. It is this osmotic or other external force which is directly responsible for the death of susceptible cells exposed to penicillins or cephalosporins. In conditions of suitably high osmolality—such as may occur in body fluids—the cell membrane remains intact and continues to grow. Through the weakened wall it may expand into a spherical cell covered only by membrane—a *protoplast*—or one which retains some cell-wall elements—a *spheroplast*. Being highly deficient in wall components these cells are unaffected by the continuing presence of penicillin and may remain dormant until therapy is stopped when synthesis of cell-wall can be resumed and infection re-emerges.

Such survival in the presence of penicillin has been held to account for the phenomenon of ' persisters ', the small number of cells first described by Bigger (1944) which survive when sensitive staphylococci are exposed to concentrations of penicillin to which the majority of the bacterial cells succumb. Such organisms are not resistant in the ordinary sense of the term since on subculture their progeny respond to exposure to penicillin in just the same way: the majority die and a few survive.

Similar persisting minorities can be demonstrated for a variety of other organism-antibiotic combinations and it does not appear that they can all be accounted for by conversion to spheroplasts. At least part of the persisting population evidently consists of cells which happen to be at a particular stage of their metabolic cycle at the moment of exposure, and in that stage are not accessible to the effect of the agent. Greenwood (1972) has suggested in the case of staphylococci exposed to penicillin that persisting cells are those which have just totally completed their walls and because there are no loose ends to their mucopeptides are frozen in their completed states until the penicillin is removed.

Cell Membrane

Beneath the cell wall is the lipoprotein layer of the cell membrane which corresponds with the limiting membrane of mammalian cells. It is this layer that is to a large extent concerned with the control of ingress and egress of material from the cells. The simplest model of the membrane sees it as bundles of lipoprotein molecules held together by magnesium ions in such a way that gaps are left through which molecules of suitable size can move. Chelating agents which compete with the membrane for its essential magnesium, increase the permeability of the cell bringing about direct lysis or permitting more ready access, and hence greater antibacterial effect, of other agents (Brown and Melling, 1969).

Some antibiotics unite with the membrane and function as ionophores—compounds which provide a way for abnormal movement of ions through the membrane. Many are composed of circular molecules and it has been fancifully suggested that they behave like false pores in the membrane. In fact, the distance that must be traversed from one side of the membrane to the other is so great compared with the size of ionophore molecules that it is much more likely that they function as transport for captured ions.

Therapeutically the most important agents which act on the membrane are the peptides. These consist of circular molecules (page 182) the attachment of which to the membrane modifies the ion flux and brings about lysis of the cell (Sebek, 1967). Subinhibitory doses of colistin make *Escherichia* susceptible to penicillin and erythromycin presumably by facilitating their entry to the cell (Kawamata and Nakajima, 1966).

Above the cell membrane is the cell wall and beneath it the point of attachment of the chromosome. Interference with the construction of the membrane may, therefore, affect these adjacent structures. Bacitracin, which interferes with cell wall synthesis (page 252), does so at the level of the membrane and because of this differs from penicillins and cephalosporins, which affect only mucopeptide synthesis, in being active against protoplasts.

Novobiocin also inhibits cell wall synthesis but the major effect of the drug is on the cell membrane (Morris and Russell, 1968) and it is from this site that it affects both the synthesis of the overlying cell wall and the replication of the underlying attached chromosome. The resulting incoordination of growth produces peculiar morphological changes in staphylococci not so far seen with any other agent (Greenwood and O'Grady, 1972). Incidentally this activity is not specific to *bacterial* cell membrane since Johnston and Hoshiko (1971) have shown that novobiocin profoundly increases the permeability of frog skin.

The study of the modes of action of antibiotics has contributed greatly to our understanding of cellular metabolism particularly to that of protein synthesis. Nevertheless much still remains to be done since agents which produce apparently similar effects on isolated enzyme or ribosomal systems commonly show marked differences in the degree or range of their activities against living bacteria. No doubt elucidation of the reasons for these differences will in due course be forthcoming and with that increased chance of synthesizing agents which possess precisely those properties which appear most desirable.

Details of the biochemical events outlined in this chapter and accounts of the mode of action of many individual agents can be found in Gottlieb and Shaw (1967) and Gale *et al.* (1972).

REFERENCES

BIGGER, J. H. (1944). *Lancet* **2,** 497.
BROT, N., SPEARS, C. & WEISSBACH, H. (1971). *Arch. Biochem. Biophys.* **143,** 286.
BROWN, M. R. W. & MELLING, J. (1969). *J. gen. Microbiol.* **59,** 263.

GALE, E. F., CUNDLIFFE, E., REYNOLDS, P. E., RICHMOND, M. H. & WARING, M. J. (1972). *The Molecular Basis of Antibiotic Action*, London, Wiley.

GOTTLIEB, D. & SHAW, P. D. (1967). *'Antibiotics*. Vol. 1: *Mechanism of Action'*, Berlin, Springer-Verlar.

GREENWOOD, D. (1972) *Lancet* 2, 465.

GREENWOOD, D. & O'GRADY, F. (1970). *Nature Lond.* 228, 457.

GREENWOOD, D. & O'GRADY, F. (1972). *J. gen. Microbiol.* 70, 263.

HANE, M. W. (1971). *J. Bact.* 105, 46.

HITCHINGS, G. H. (1960-1961). *Trans. N. J. Acad. Sci.* 23, 700.

HITCHINGS, G. H. (1969). *Postgrad. med. J.* 45 (Suppl. Nov.), 7.

HUTNER, S. H., NATHAN, H. A. & BAKER, H. (1959). *Vitamins and Hormones* 17, 1.

JOHNSTON, K. H. & HOSHIKO, T. (1971). *Amer. J. Physiol.* 220, 792.

KAWAMATA, J. & NAKAJIMA, K. (1966). *Antimicrob. Agents and Chemother.* 1965, p. 403.

LILL, H., LILL, W., SIPPEL, A. & HARTMANN, G. (1970). In *RNA Polymerase and Transcription*. Ed. L. Silvestri, Amsterdam, North-Holland, p. 55.

MAO, J. C. H. & PUTTERMAN, M. (1968). *J. Bact.* 95, 1111.

MAO, J. C. H., PUTTERMAN, M. & WIEGAND, R. G. (1970). *Biochem. Pharmacol.* 19, 391.

MASUKAWA, H. (1969). *J. Antibiot.* 22, 612.

MORRIS, A. & RUSSELL, A. D. (1968). *Biochem. Pharmacol.* 17, 1923.

OTAKA, E., TERAOKA, H., TAMAKI, M., TANAKA, K. & OSAWA, S. (1970). *J. molec. Biol.* 48, 499.

RAMAREDDY, G. & REITER, H. (1969). *J. Bact.* 100, 724.

RICHMOND, M. H. (1966). *Symp. Soc. gen. Microbiol.* 16, 301.

SEBEK, O. K. (1967). *Antibiotics I: Mechanism in Action.* Ed. D. Gottlieb and P. D. Shaw, N.Y., p. 142.

STROMINGER, J. L., BLUMBERG, P. M., SUGINAKA, H., UMBREIT, J. & WICKUS, G. G. (1971). *Proc. roy. Soc. Lond. B.* 179, 369.

TERAOKA, H. (1970. *Biochem. Biophys. Acta.* 213, 535.

UMEZAWA, H., MIZUNO, S., YAMAZAKI, H. & NITTA, K. (1968). *J. Antibiot.* (Jap.) 21, 234.

WARD, C. B., HANE, M. W. & GLASER, D. A. (1970). *Proc. nat. Acad. Sci. U.S.A.* 66, 365.

WEIDEL, W. & PELZER, H. (1964). *Adv. Enzymol.* 26, 193.

WHITMAN, E. N. (1969). *Postgrad. med. J.* 45, (Suppl. Nov.) 46.

WOODS, D. D. (1940). *Brit. J. exp. Path.* 21, 74.

CHAPTER 15

DRUG RESISTANCE

INTRODUCTION

THE adaptability of bacteria in the presence of poisonous agents has been well known since the early days of bacteriology and a paper on this subject appeared in the first volume of the *Annales de l'Institut Pasteur,* published in 1887, under the patronage of the master himself (Kossiakoff, 1887). Ehrlich, in his pioneer work on chemotherapy at the beginning of this century, appreciated the significance of this and attempted to cure syphilis with a single massive dose. As it affects antibiotics, this problem is of exceptional magnitude, since the degree of abnormal resistance which may appear is often enormously greater than that capable of being acquired to any other type of drug.

CHARACTERISTICS OF DRUG-RESISTANT STRAINS

Nature of Resistance

Drug-resistant bacteria can be divided into two fundamentally different types according to their response to the antibiotic. They are conveniently referred to as *drug-tolerant* and *drug-destroying.*

DRUG-TOLERANT bacteria are capable of growing in the presence of an increased concentration of an unchanged antibiotic. They may be indifferent to the drug, that is to say, capable of growing equally well in its presence or absence. Other strains, although capable of multiplication in the presence of the drug, grow more luxuriantly in its absence. Conversely in a few instances, particularly with streptomycin, the strain may be completely or partially addicted to the drug and is referred to as *drug-dependent.*

DRUG-DESTROYING BACTERIA. In clinical practice the most frequently encountered drug-destroying bacteria are penicillinase-producing staphylococci. These strains owe their resistance almost entirely to inactivation of penicillin by penicillinase, and are intrinsically almost as sensitive as a normal strain. The result of a tube dilution test of sensitivity is thus determined by the size of the inoculum: if this is heavy, it contains enough preformed penicillinase to destroy a concentration of penicillin 100 times or more greater than that which will inhibit the growth of a small inoculum.

Penicillin-inactivating enzymes are also produced by many coliform bacilli. *B. anthracis* and some strains of *Clostridia* also produce a penicillinase, but in both cases the individual bacteria, like staphylococci, are sensitive to benzyl penicillin, and in the case of *B. anthracis* so highly sensitive that treatment is fully effective.

Recently examples of resistance to other antibiotics have come to light which depend on drug inactivation. That in staphylococci to chloramphenicol is due to an enzyme which acetylates the antibiotic, and enzymes which acetylate or otherwise inactivate aminoglycosides are responsible for transmissible resistance to members of this group of drugs.

Stability of Resistance

DRUG-TOLERANT STRAINS. The stability of drug-resistance in drug-tolerant strains is very variable. Streptomycin-resistant organisms, whether isolated from *in vitro* experiments or from clinical infections, are usually highly stable and retain their resistance after prolonged passage in the absence of the antibiotic. Tetracycline- and chloramphenicol-resistant organisms are also fairly stable, especially when isolated from clinical infections. Erythromycin-resistant strains are often more labile and many, in the absence of the antibiotic, tend to revert to erythromycin sensitivity. Staphylococci trained to penicillin tolerance *in vitro* are highly unstable and rapidly revert to the sensitivity of the parent strain.

PENICILLINASE-PRODUCING STAPHYLOCOCCI. The capacity to produce penicillinase is usually a fairly stable characteristic, but there is a tendency for penicillin-destroying strains to yield a proportion of penicillin-sensitive cells, which completely fail to produce detectable amounts of the enzyme.

Changes in Sensitivity to Other Drugs

CROSS-RESISTANCE. With chemically related drugs there is usually almost complete cross-resistance. Thus bacteria which have developed resistance to one sulphonamide will show a corresponding increase in resistance to all sulphonamides. Similarly there is almost complete cross-resistance between the different tetracycline antibiotics. The erythromycin group are in a special category. Thus strains of staphylococci which have developed resistance by passage in one of the macrolides *in vitro* usually show a similar increase in resistance to all other members of the group. On the other hand, erythromycin-resistant staphylococci isolated from clinical infections are frequently sensitive to spiramycin and oleandomycin. (For a fuller discussion of this see Chapter 10.)

Moderate degrees of cross-resistance are sometimes seen with chemically unrelated antibiotics; these remain unexplained and are probably of little clinical importance. On the other hand a resistant variant obtained by *in vitro* training to one antibiotic may sometimes be found slightly more sensitive than before to another.

Associated Changes

Organisms trained to resistance *in vitro* often have a slower growth rate, with the result that during further transfers in drug-free broth of a mixture of resistant and sensitive cells the latter soon predominate. Accompanying changes may be diminished virulence and altered morphology. Most naturally occurring resistant variants usually show none of these changes: an exception are small-colony variants sometimes seen in cultures resistant to erythromycin and occasionally to other antibiotics.

MODE OF ORIGIN

Abnormal resistance to antibiotics and other drugs as seen in the clinical sphere may arise in at least four different ways.

Therapeutic selection

Here no change in bacteria themselves is involved. The extensive therapeutic use of a drug eliminates sensitive strains of an organism, but favours the spread of an originally very small minority of strains possessing natural resistance. It was thus that sulphonamide resistance in gonococci became prevalent within a few years of the introduction of this treatment. The outstanding example of this mechanism in the antibiotic field is penicillin resistance in staphylococci. An originally very small minority of strains forming penicillinase has multiplied to a majority in hospital environments.

Drug-tolerant Bacteria

In laboratory experiments drug-tolerant bacteria usually arise by a discontinuous process which suggests spontaneous mutation. In the first instance a few drug-resistant cells appear, which if not favoured by the environment are likely to be overgrown. But the presence of the antibiotic has a selective action so that the few resistant mutants are favoured at the expense of the sensitive cells until a pure culture of antibiotic-resistant cells is obtained.

It has been fashionable to attribute all drug resistance in a previously sensitive culture to mutation, and many ingenious methods have been devised to prove that this is so: among these perhaps the most convincing is the use of replica plating by Lederberg and Lederberg (1952) to prove the presence of resistant bacterial cells before exposure to an antibiotic. It should nevertheless be recognized that this proposition is not universally or wholly accepted. Hinshelwood and his colleagues have published a long series of studies, of which some of the more recent are by Dean and Hinshelwood (1964) and by Dean and Giordan (1965) providing evidence that increased bacterial resistance to various noxious agents, including some antibiotics, can arise by a process of adaptation.

Whatever the mechanism of the change, the fact remains that exposure to an antibiotic, whether *in vitro* or *in vivo*, may result in increased resistance to it in a bacterial population. The rapidity and extent of the change vary widely among different antibiotics. An organism may become highly resistant to streptomycin overnight ('single step' mutation), or within a few days to erythromycin or novobiocin, but to most other antibiotics the development of resistance is a more gradual process. In some cases the number of steps involved may be so great, and the increase in resistance with each step so slight, that the development of resistance may appear to be an almost continuous process. To some antibiotics, no substantial degree of resistance can develop at all: these include the peptides and vancomycin. It is also fortunate that in the clinical field no pathogenic species except the gonococcus and exceptionally the pneumococcus has yet shown itself capable of becoming resistant to penicillin.

The two remaining processes by which resistance may be acquired involve the transfer of genetic material from a resistant cell to a sensitive.

Transduction

The transmission of capacity to produce penicillinase by a phage to a penicillin-sensitive staphylococcus was first demonstrated by Ritz and Baldwin (1958). Since then the same mechanism has been shown capable of transmitting resistance to streptomycin, tetracycline, chloramphenicol and macrolides. In their study of the latter, Pattee and Baldwin (1962) were able to transduce resistance of both the ' double ' and ' dissociated ' types (Garrod, 1957) to sensitive staphylococci, and offer the first acceptable explanation of the difference between these types. This is that the enzyme system responsible for double resistance (i.e. resistance to oleandomycin and other macrolides as well as to erythromycin) is constitutive, whereas that conferring dissociated resistance (resistance to erythromycin only, but also to other macrolides in the presence of erythromycin) is inducible. Transducibility is governed by the phage type of the recipient: it occurs most readily between strains each of group I or group III, is less frequent from one of these groups to the other, and never succeeds from either to a strain of group II (McDonald, 1966). Co-transduction of resistances to two antibiotics can occur, as does that of the two properties of penicillinase formation and mercury resistance, which appear therefore to be genetically linked (Richmond and John, 1964).

There are strong reasons for believing that the elements transduced are plasmids: i.e. extra-chromosomal particles of genetic material (Novick and Richmond, 1965), although Asheshov (1966) describes an experiment with one strain in which it seems that the material must have been chromosomal. Transduction has also been achieved *in vivo*. Jarolmen *et al.* (1965)

inoculated mice intravenously with a sensitive staphylococcus, followed 6 days later by concentrated transducing phage from a strain resistant to both penicillin and tetracycline. Staphylococci resistant to tetracycline, but not to penicillin, were subsequently recovered from the kidneys, their numbers being increased by tetracycline treatment of the mice. The experiments of Novick and Morse (1967) are even more convincing: they inoculated mice intravenously with cultures of two strains of staphylococcus, a lysogenic strain possessing erythromycin resistance and another resistant to streptomycin, and recovered from the kidneys organisms resistant to both antibiotics, in numbers much greater when the mice were also treated with both. Linked penicillin-erythromycin resistance was also transduced *in vivo*.

Until recently a strain of staphylococcus described by Hashimoto *et al.* (1964) in which penicillinase formation is linked with erythromycin resistance, the two properties being regularly co-transduced (Novick and Richmond, 1965) was believed to be unique, but Evans and Waterworth (1966) have now observed two other such linkages. Among strains of staphylococci resistant to fusidic acid, one also resistant to penicillin lost both resistances together, and a second simultaneously lost resistance to tetracycline and kanamycin as well as to fusidic acid, but remained resistant to penicillin.

It is not certainly known whether and if so to what extent transduction is responsible for antibiotic resistance in clinical isolates of staphylococci, but the probability is very high that it plays a major part. Lacey (1971) achieved transference of resistance to neomycin in *Staph. aureus* to a sensitive strain not only in mixed culture but on the skin surface of volunteers, and adduces reasons for attributing this to transduction.

Drug resistance can also be transduced in various enterobacteria. Owing to the limited host range of phages, such transduction is for the most part intra-species, but the mechanism of transfer now to be described can operate between organisms of many different genera.

Episomal Transference by Conjugation (*Infectious Resistance*)

' Infectious ' resistance of this type was first observed in Japan in 1959 (for review of Japanese work see Watanabe,

1963), and reported in Europe first by Datta (1962) in England and by Lebek (1963) in Germany. Its recognition in the United States came late, the first descriptions (Smith and Armour, 1966; Kabins and Cohen, 1966) appearing in 1966. The earlier studies showed that in a mixed culture of a *Shigella* or *Salmonella* possessing multiple resistance (e.g. to sulphonamide, tetracycline, chloramphenicol and streptomycin) and a sensitive *E. coli*, this resistance may be transferred to a minority of cells of the latter organism, usually *en bloc* but sometimes in part. This organism can then re-transfer resistance to another pathogen. Clear clinical evidence of such transfer within the human bowel was obtained. It is now known that transfer can occur between organisms of all genera of the *Enterobacteriaceae*, and the transfer of resistance to *Serratia marcescens*, *Vibrio cholerae*, and *Pasteurella pestis* has also been observed. It is important to recognize that this mode of transference never occurs to or among any Gram-positive species.

The elements responsible, and transferred by conjugation, are again extra-chromosomal genetic particles (episomes or plasmids). These determine resistance in the cell possessing them, but can only be transferred to another when a second element is present, the ' resistance transfer factor ' (Anderson, 1965). Bacteria so capable of transmitting resistance are now described as possessing R factors. A full account of studies of the mechanism of transference by conjugation is given by Datta (1965).

MODE OF ACTION OF R FACTORS

The basis of resistance to some antibiotics transmitted in this way is now known to be the formation of an enzyme inactivating the antibiotic. Thus an organism so acquiring resistance to ampicillin can be shown to produce a β-lactamase. Other examples depend on enzymes acetylating or otherwise inactivating the antibiotic without breakdown of its main structure. Transmissible chloramphenicol resistance is due to the formation of chloramphenicol acetyltransferase. This enzyme is also responsible for resistance in staphylococci, and Shaw and Brodsky (1968) have found that the product of acetylation by the staphylococcal enzyme is indistinguishable from that obtained with a resistant *E. coli* carrying an R factor.

Transmissible resistance to aminoglycosides is also enzymic in nature, the process of inactivation being either acetylation, phosphorylation or adenylylation. Davies (1971) (see also Davies and Rownd, 1972) list the enzymes concerned as follows:

ENZYME	SUBSTRATE
Streptomycin phosphotransferase	Streptomycin
Streptomycin adenylyl synthetase	Streptomycin, spectinomycin
Kanamycin phosphotransferase	Kanamycin, neomycin, paromomycin, gentamicin A
Kanamycin acetyltransferase	Kanamycin, neomycin, gentamicin C_{1a}

Two of the products of these reactions, N-acetylated neomycin and gentamicin C_{1a}, retain substantial antibacterial activity.

It is now well recognized that the basis of transmissible resistance to tetracycline is inhibition of uptake of the antibiotic. For synthetic drugs and other agents the mechanism is unknown.

DRUGS TO WHICH RESISTANCE CAN BE TRANSMITTED. Among antibiotics these include penicillins, cephalosporins, aminoglycosides, tetracycline, chloramphenicol and fusidic acid (in specially sensitive *E. coli* mutants). Recognition sometimes came late; thus it was for some years believed that resistance to neomycin was non-transmissible, but this was emphatically disproved by Witchitz and Chabbert (1971). Among synthetic drugs, sulphonamides were the first of any to which transmissible resistance was studied. That to trimethoprim remained undetected for some time, and was first observed by Fleming, Datta and Grüneberg (1972) in 2 out of 6 resistant strains of *E. coli* and 1 of *Kl. aerogenes*, all from in-patients in one hospital. So also is that of nalidixic acid, a drug which in fact inhibits the transfer of resistance to other drugs between two organisms both of which are sensitive to it. Resistance to furazolidine is still believed to be non-transmissible. R factors can also confer resistance to phages, colicines, metal salts and UV light.

DURATION OF INFECTIOUS RESISTANCE. It is indeed fortunate that in the absence of further exposure to any of the drugs involved, this form of resistance is often spontaneously lost within weeks or months of its acquisition. It can well be imagined that but for this, resistance to commonly used drugs would by now be almost universal. Treatment with acridine dyes can also bring this about *in vitro* but no such process applicable *in vivo* is yet known.

INFECTIOUS RESISTANCE IN ANIMALS. The study of this form of resistance has passed through three phases: the original work in Japan mainly on human intestinal pathogens, an investigation in this country of such resistance in farm animals and its spread to man, and finally a much more widespread study of infectious resistance in human intestinal commensals and in organisms causing non-specific infections such as those of the urinary tract.

The study of farm animals owes much to the alarming revelations of Anderson and his colleagues (Anderson and Datta, 1965; Anderson and Lewis, 1965; Anderson, 1965, 1968). The later papers in this series deal with an epidemic of type 29 *S. typhimurium* infection in calves which lasted several years, during which the strain developed transferable resistance successively to six or more drugs. It also caused at least 500 human infections, its source being made certain not only by its phage type but by its resistance pattern, sometimes including furazolidone, a drug used only in animals. The main danger apprehended from such human infection by resistant animal pathogens was the transmission of resistance *via* human *E. coli* to organisms of the enteric group, notably *S. typhi*: the possible prospect of resistance in this species to both chloramphenicol and ampicillin was disastrous. Fortunately and strangely, transferable resistance to chloramphenicol in *S. typhi* has remained almost unknown until very recently, when an epidemic strain possessing it appeared in Mexico (Anderson and Smith, 1972). The outlook has also been improved by the advent of cotrimoxazole as an alternative treatment for typhoid fever (see p. 366).

At the same time the frequent existence of multiple infectious resistance in *E. coli* from calves and pigs, and less commonly lambs and fowls, was demonstrated by such studies as those of Walton (1966) and Williams Smith (1966). These findings were attributable to antibiotic feed supplementation, and a campaign to restrict this culminated in the report of the Swann Committee (Report, 1969) which proposed that the use of medical antibiotics for this purpose be prohibited (those hitherto permitted in this country were penicillin and oxy- and chlortetracycline only). These recommendations have been implemented, and it remains to be seen what the effects will be.

The extent of the contribution made by animal organisms to infectious resistance in the human intestinal flora has been the subject of much dispute. There is no question of the capacity of animal *Salmonella* to colonize the human bowel. Two other measures seem called for in this connection. The root cause of widespread animal salmonellosis is bad methods of animal husbandry, notably the wholesale trade in very young calves, conducted under conditions strongly favouring the spread of infection. Secondly, resistance in these organisms is attributable at least in part to therapeutic use; that to ampicillin which appeared in 1964 was clearly the result of attempts to control enteritis in calves with therapeutic doses. While feed supplementation has been prohibited, therapeutic use remains entirely uncontrolled, and is said often to be misdirected and ineffective. The single step of prohibiting the administration of chloramphenicol to animals would afford some reassurance, but the right of the medical profession to some say in the treatment of animals, which are an important source of human disease, although repeatedly asserted has never been acknowledged.

Any large scale transmission of resistance from animals to man must be *via* commensals such as *E. coli* which are found in meat and meat products (Shooter *et al.*, 1970; Cooke *et al.*, 1970), but unequivocal evidence of implantation from this source in the human bowel has not been obtained. The more frequent occurrence of resistant *E. coli* in country than in urban populations (Moorhouse, 1971; Linton *et al.*, 1972) has been adduced as an argument in this connection, but it must be remembered that the farming community handle antibiotics in preparing supplemented feeds, and the effect may be a direct one on their own flora; Schon *et al.* (1972), while confirming such findings, found an even higher frequency of resistance in workers in antibiotic production plants and in fodder plants where antibiotic supplements are mixed. It is interesting in this connection that Guinee, Ugueto and van Leeuwen (1970) found transmissible resistance in *E. coli* to be as frequent in vegetarians and in infants under 6 months as in either of two groups of meat eaters; indeed in one of these groups the frequency was decidedly lower.

Evidence has also been sought from deliberate implantation experiments such as those of Williams Smith (1969). Resistant strains of *E. coli* from pigs, oxen and fowls swallowed in large numbers by a human subject often failed to establish themselves at all, although two human strains were recoverable for periods up to 35 days later, and in the few instances in which transfer of resistance from an animal to the native human strain occurred, the resistant variant disappeared within a few days. Wiedeman, Knothe and Doll (1970), although using a resistant human strain, obtained similar results.

This question can only be decided by a large extension of such studies as these, but they need to be so laborious that reluctance to pursue them is not surprising. An implanted strain can only be recognized serologically, and if only 5 colonies are examined there can be no certainty either that it is not present among others or that it was not there originally. Nevertheless we need to know what variable characters, if any, in animal strains affect their capacity to multiply in the human bowel, and what numbers must be swallowed to achieve this. A character which might with advantage be taken into account is colicine production; the observations of Branche *et al.* (1963) suggest that this is a strong weapon in the competition for survival among different strains.

INFECTIOUS RESISTANCE IN HUMAN ENTEROBACTERIA. It seems strange that not until 1966 was any serious attempt made to discover how much drug resistance in human intestinal bacteria generally is infectious. From this time onwards a series of studies of strains from various sources has yielded remarkably consistent results. The proportion of drug-resistant strains has varied with both species and source (hospital strains being more often resistant than those from elsewhere), but a constant finding has been that transference has been achieved from over 50 per cent of cultures so tested. The organisms examined include *Salmonella* species (Schroeder, Terry and Bennett, 1967), *Shigella sonnei* (Davies, Farrant and Tomlinson, 1968), *E.*

coli, Klebsiella and *Proteus* exclusively (Smith and Armour, 1966) or mainly (Aandahl, 1968) from urinary tract infections, and *E. coli* both from infections and normal faeces (Gunter and Feary, 1968), from patients in a mental hospital and from a normal population (Lewis, 1968), and from adults (Datta, 1969) and infants (Moorhouse and McKay, 1968) on admission to hospital. The last-named paper also affords evidence suggesting that a free exchange of resistant bacteria takes place between infants in hospital.

Several of these studies have shown a higher frequency of infectious resistance, which is also more often multiple, in organisms from patients under treatment with antibiotics. This emerges from a comparison by Dailey, Sturtevant and Feary (1972) of the intestinal flora of infants in a well baby and a high risk nursery. The results of Datta *et al.* (1971) are interesting in showing the capacity of different drugs for selecting resistance. In the faeces of women treated for urinary tract infections, sulphonamide or ampicillin caused moderate increases in the frequency of resistance in *E. coli* only to the drug given, but during tetracycline treatment resistance to tetracycline itself was invariable, and usually accompanied by resistance to other drugs as well. Sensitive and resistant strains from the same patient were always of different serotypes.

Resistance transfer has been thought of as occurring only in the bowel, where purely physical factors impede it, although it unquestionably occurs. It is becoming recognized that it can occur, perhaps with more facility, elsewhere in the body. Roe, Jones and Lowbury (1971) have shown that it happens in burns, and Witchitz and Chabbert (1972) point out that peritoneal dialysis fluid is an ideal medium; in a patient undergoing this and being treated with gentamicin strains of 4 different species carrying an R factor determining resistance to this and several other drugs were recovered at different times from the dialysate. Other organisms carrying this factor were subsequently recovered from patients in this intensive care unit.

These studies have transformed our outlook on drug resistance in human enterobacteria and related organisms. Most of this is transmissible and much of it may have arisen by transference rather than by exposure to the drug itself. Although its existence severely limits the possibilities of anti-bacterial therapy, it is reassuring that of 95 strains of *Ps. aeruginosa* and 429 of enterobacteria from various infections in a general hospital, there were none which were not sensitive to at least one applicable antibiotic (Anderson, Datta and Shaw, 1972).

THE CLINICAL PROBLEM

Staphylococci

The staphylococcus is unlikely to show a change in sensitivity to a drug administered for a single short course unless the mutation rate to resistance to that drug is very high, as is the case with streptomycin and erythromycin. This, however, is not the whole story, since in hospitals where staphylococcal infections are nursed in large open wards, cross-infection is likely to occur. If in such a ward a given antibiotic is used extensively, the staphylococcus is in fact passaged from patient to patient in the presence of the antibiotic. Under these conditions staphylococci of enhanced virulence, resistant to all the extensively used antibiotics, have emerged *in vivo*.

PENICILLIN. It is known that rare strains of *Staph. aureus* isolated before the introduction of penicillin formed penicillinase. The increasing prevalence of such strains in the hospital environment after penicillin had come into general use was first described by our late co-author Mary Barber: the frequency of their occurrence was 14, 38 and 59 per cent in the successive years 1946-48 (Barber and Rozwadowska-Dowzenko, 1948). During the next few years similar reports followed from hospitals all over the world and by about 1950 the majority of staphylococcal infections in most general hospitals were penicillin-resistant. Resistance has since then become commoner than before in strains from the general population.

OTHER ANTIBIOTICS. Resistance has subsequently appeared in certain staphylococci to all the major antibiotics. Streptomycin and tetracyclines were first affected: triple resistance to these two and to penicillin has been common in epidemic strains, and resistance to tetracycline came to be regarded as the hall mark of a dangerous strain. Chloramphenicol resistance also appeared early, but diminished in frequency when consumption diminished following recognition of marrow toxicity (Kirby and Ahern, 1953). Resistance to erythromycin can develop rapidly, and according to Lepper *et al.* (1954) resistant strains can spread very rapidly in a hospital where the antibiotic is much used: more gradual spread is described by MacCabe *et al.* (1961) and by Forfar *et al.* (1966). Resistance is also readily produced to novobiocin, but it is not often seen because this antibiotic is little used.

It is not to be supposed that any staphylococcus can acquire these characters. Multiple resistance is largely confined to a few notorious types in phage groups I and III which are also those commonly responsible for epidemics of staphylococcal sepsis (for distribution of these types in epidemics, see Williams, 1959). Multiple resistance is also linked with mercury resistance (Moore, 1960) and with high penicillinase production (Richmond *et al.*, 1964). The selective effect of the therapeutic use of other antibiotics as well as penicillin has in fact been to bring into prominence what must have been an originally very small minority of staphylococci of a few phage types.

From time to time other resistances appear. That to methicillin and other penicillinase-resistant penicillins is discussed in Chapter 4. In 1963 an apparently new strain, described as of type 'A', appeared in Scotland and the north of England, possessing multiple antibiotic resistance, including resistance to neomycin and kanamycin, and said to be of exceptional virulence (Temple and Blackburn, 1963; Mitchell, 1964). Neomycin resistance has also been reported from elsewhere (see Chapter 7).

A progressive diminution in the frequency of antibiotic resistance in staphylococci during the past few years has been reported by Bulger and Sherris (1968) in Seattle and by Thabaut and Canayer (1969) of the French Army Medical Service in Germany. The frequency of multiple resistance has also diminished in strains isolated in St. Thomas' Hospital, London (Ridley *et al.*, 1970). All these authors attribute this change, at least in part, to suitably restricted and more rationally directed antibiotic therapy.

Streptococci

Strains of both *Str. pyogenes* and *Str. pneumoniae* resistant to sulphonamides were beginning to interfere with the efficacy of treatment and to cause grave apprehension for the future when penicillin came to the rescue. *Str. pyogenes* appears incapable of developing resistance to penicillin, and resistance in pneumococci has only been reported from the Antipodes, but resistance to tetracycline now occurs in both. *Str. viridans* is very variable in the degree of its natural resistance to penicillin: a moderate increase in this may occur during prolonged treatment for endocarditis.

STR. FAECALIS, although fairly constant in its moderate degree of sensitivity to penicillin, is liable to be abnormally resistant to streptomycin, tetracycline and other antibiotics.

Neisseria spp.

N. GONORRHOEAE. Sulphonamide resistance in this organism, a product of selection, has eventually been followed by the development of some degree of resistance to penicillin, evidently by a different mechanism, since resistant strains were unknown for many years: resistance to other antibiotics has also been observed. The therapeutic problem posed by these changes is discussed in Chapter 27.

N. MENINGITIDIS. For many years cerebrospinal fever remained the only acute bacterial infection for which treatment with sulphonamides remained equal or superior to that with antibiotics. Sulphonamide resistance of a degree precluding successful treatment was first reported in 1963 (Millar *et al.*) in a Naval Training Depot in California. A report from the same State (Leedom *et al.*, 1965) extends these observations to civilians. Of 106 strains isolated from patients with meningococcal infections in the Los Angeles County General Hospital, 35 (33 per cent) were inhibited only by 10 mg. sulphonamide per 100 ml. or more, whereas 59 were inhibited by 0·5 mg. per 100 ml. or less, only 12 giving intermediate results. A majority of strains from a large epidemic at Fort Lamy (Chad) in 1968 were sulphonamide-resistant (Lefevre *et al.*, 1969). Resistant strains have also been found in Norway (Holten *et al.*, 1969), Germany (Berger, 1971) and several other countries, but further information about their distribution is highly desirable (see p. 352).

All the Los Angeles strains were sensitive to penicillin and to ampicillin, with which the patients were treated. It is not to be expected that this alternative treatment will remain effective indefinitely. Miller and Bohnhoff (1947, 1948) showed long ago that meningococci could be trained to a high degree of penicillin resistance, not only *in vitro* but in experimentally infected mice. With the gonococcus as an example, resistance may be expected in the meningococcus at some time in the future.

Gram-negative Bacilli

Coliform bacilli form a group among which apparently increasing antibiotic resistance presents difficulties only exceeded by similar changes in staphylococci. No purpose would be served by reviewing the extensive and confused literature of this subject. Several processes have evidently been at work. Many authors have found that isolates in successive periods of the normally more drug-sensitive species, notably *E. coli,* show an increasing frequency of resistance. Secondly, the therapeutic use of antibiotics has favoured the survival and spread of organisms possessing a high degree of natural resistance, notably *Aerobacter, Pseudomonas,* and some species of *Proteus.* It seems impossible to determine whether organisms of this kind are more drug-resistant now than they were originally, but this seems highly probable. Thirdly, it now seems that a good deal of multiple resistance in intestinal bacteria may have been acquired by contact with other species (infectious resistance). However this situation may have arisen, Gram-negative infections, particularly those complicating other disease, and involving wounds, the bronchial tree or the blood-stream, are now among the most difficult to treat successfully. As they occur in the alimentary and urinary tracts, they are considered elsewhere (Chaps. 21 and 24).

Mycobacterium tuberculosis

This is another organism in which drug resistance menaces successful treatment, and has so far as possible to be prevented (see Chap. 26).

PREVENTION OF BACTERIAL RESISTANCE

Some measures by which an increase in the frequency of bacterial resistance may at least be discouraged are described on page 288.

REFERENCES

AANDAHL, E. H. (1968). *Acta Path. Microbiol. scand.* **74**, 26.
ANDERSON, E. S. (1965). *Brit. med. J.* **2**, 1289.
ANDERSON, E. S. (1968). *Brit. med. J.* **3**, 333.
ANDERSON, E. S. & DATTA, N. (1965). *Lancet* **1**, 407.
ANDERSON, E. S. & LEWIS, M. J. (1965). *Nature (Lond.)* **206**, 579.
ANDERSON, E. S. & SMITH, H. R. (1972). *Brit. med. J.* **3**, 329.
ANDERSON, F. M., DATTA, N. & SHAW, E. J. (1972). *Brit. med. J.* **3**, 82.
ASHESHOV, E. H. (1966). *Nature (Lond.)* **210**, 804.
BARBER, M. & ROZWADOWSKA-DOWZENKO, M. (1948). *Lancet* **2**, 641.
BERGER, U. (1971). *Dtsch. med. Wschr.* **96**, 578.
BRANCHE, W. C., YOUNG, V. M., ROBINET, H. G. & MASSEY, E. D. (1963). *Proc. Soc. exp. Biol. Med.* **114**, 198.
BULGER, R. J. & SHERRIS, J. C. (1968). *Ann. intern. Med.* **69**, 1099.
COOKE, E. M., SHOOTER, R. A., KUMAR, P. J., ROUSSEAU, S. A. & FOULKES, A. L. (1970). *Lancet* **1**, 436.
DAILEY, K. M., STURTEVANT, A. B., JR. & FEARY, T. W. (1972). *J. Pediat.* **80**, 198.
DATTA, N. (1962). *J. Hyg. (Lond.)* **60**, 301.
DATTA, N. (1965). *Brit. med. Bull.* **21**, 254.
DATTA, N. (1969). *Brit. med. J.* **2**, 407.
DATTA, N., FAIERS, M. C., REEVES, D. S., BRUMFITT, W., ØRSKOV, F. & ØRSKOV, I. (1971). *Lancet* **1**, 312.
DAVIES, J. (1971). *J. infect. Dis.* **124**, Suppl. Dec., 7.
DAVIES, J. E. & ROWND, R. (1972). *Science* **176**, 758.
DAVIES, J. R., FARRANT, W. N. & TOMLINSON, A. J. H. (1968). *J. Hyg. (Lond.)* **66**, 471, 479.
DEAN, A. C. R. & GIORDAN, B. L. (1965). *Proc. roy. Soc. B.* **161**, 571.
DEAN, A. C. R. & HINSHELWOOD, C. (1964). *Nature (Lond.)* **202**, 1046.
EVANS, R. J. & WATERWORTH, P. M. (1966). *J. clin. Path.* **19**, 555.
FLEMING, M. P., DATTA, N. & GRÜNEBERG, R. N. (1972). *Brit. med. J.* **1**, 726.
FORFAR, J. O., KEAY, A. J., MACCABE, A. F., GOULD, J. C. & BAIN, A. D (1966). *Lancet* **2**, 295.
GARROD, L. P. (1957). *Brit. med. J.* **2**, 57.
GUINÉE, P., UGUETO, N. & VAN LEEUWEN, N. (1970). *Appl. Microbiol.* **20**, 531.
GUNTER, A. C. & FEARY, T. W. (1968). *J. Bact.* **96**, 1556.
HASHIMOTO, H., KONO, K. & MITSUHASHI, S. (1964). *J. Bact.* **88**, 261.
HOLTEN, E., VAAGE, L., NEESS, C., MIDTVEDT, T. & JYSSUM, K. (1969). *Scand. J. infect. Dis.* **1**, 185.
JAROLMEN, H., BONDI, A. & CROWELL, R. L. (1965). *J. Bact.* **89**, 1286.
KABINS, S. A. & COHEN, S. (1966). *New Engl. J. Med.* **275**, 248.
KIRBY, W. M. M. & AHERN, J. J. (1953). *Antibiot. Chemother.* **3**, 831.
KOSSIAKOFF, M. G. (1887). *Ann. Inst. Pasteur* **i**, 465.
LACEY, R. W. (1971). *J. med. Microbiol.* **4**, 73.
LEBEK, K. (1963). *Zbl. Bakt. I. Abt. Orig.* **188**, 494.
LEDERBERG, J. & LEDERBERG, E. M. (1952). *J. Bact.* **63**, 399.
LEEDOM, J. M., IVLER, D., MATHIES, A. W., THRUPP, L. D., PORTNOY, B. & WEHRLE, P. F. (1965). *New Engl. J. Med.* **273**, 1395.
LEFEVRE, M., SIROL, J., VANDEKERKOVE, M. & FAUCON, R. (1969). *Bull. Wld Hlth Org.* **40**, 331.
LEPPER, M. H., MOULTON, B., DOWLING, H. F., JACKSON, G. C. & KOFMAN, S. (1954). *Antibiot. Ann.* 1953-54, p. 308.
LEWIS, M. J. (1968). *Lancet* **1**, 1389.
LINTON, K. B., LEE, P. A. RICHMOND, M. H., GILLESPIE, W. A., ROWLAND, A. J. & BAKER, V. N. (1972). *J. Hyg., Lond.* **70**, 99.
MACCABE, A. F., GOULD, J. C. & FORFAR, J. O. (1961). *Lancet* **2**. 7.
MCDONALD, S. (1966). *Lancet* **2**, 1107.

MILLAR, J. W., SIESS, E. E., FELDMAN, H. A., SILVERMAN, C. & FRANK, P. (1963). *J. Amer. med. Ass.* **186**, 139.
MILLER, C. P. & BOHNHOFF, M. (1947). *J. infect. Dis.* **81**, 147.
MILLER, C. P. & BOHNHOFF, M. (1948). *J. infect. Dis.* **83**, 256.
MITCHELL, A. A. B. (1964). *Lancet* **1**, 859.
MOORE, B. (1960). *Lancet* **2**, 453.
MOORHOUSE, E. (1971). *Ann. New York Acad. Sci.* **182**, 65.
MOORHOUSE, E. C. & MCKAY, L. (1968). *Brit. med. J.* **2**, 741.
NOVICK, R. S. & MORSE, S. I. (1967). *J. exp. Med.* **125**, 45.
NOVICK, R. S. & RICHMOND, M. H. (1965). *J. Bact.* **90**, 467.
PATTEE, P. A. & BALDWIN, J. N. (1962). *J. Bact.* **84**, 1049.
REPORT (1969). *Joint Committee on the Use of Antibiotics in Animal Husbandry & Veterinary Medicine.* London: Her Majesty's Stationery Office.
RICHMOND, M. H. & JOHN, M. (1964). *Nature (Lond.)* **202**, 1360.
RICHMOND, M. H., PARKER, M. T., JEVONS, M. P. & JOHN, M. (1964). *Lancet* **1**, 293.
RIDLEY, M., BARRIE, D., LYNN, R. & STEAD, K. C. (1970). *Lancet* **1**, 230.
RITZ, H. L. & BALDWIN, J. N. (1958). *Bact. Proc.* p. 40.
ROE, E., JONES, R. J. & LOWBURY, E. J. L. (1971). *Lancet* **1**, 149.
SCHÖN, E., WAGNER, V., WAGNEROVA, W., MANDLIKOVA, Z., ZIEGLEROVA, V. & DRNKOVA, V. (1972). *Rev. Czech. Med.* **18**, 1.
SCHROEDER, S. A., TERRY, P. M. & BENNETT, J. V. (1967). *J. Amer. med. Ass.* **205**, 903.
SHAW, W. V. & BRODSKY, R. F. (1968). *J. Bact.* **95**, 28.
SHOOTER, R. A., COOKE, E. M., ROUSSEAU, S. A. & BREADEN, A. L. (1970). *Lancet* **2**, 226.
SMITH, D. H. & ARMOUR, S. E. (1966). *Lancet* **2**, 15.
TEMPLE, N. E. I. & BLACKBURN, E. A. (1963). *Lancet* **1**, 581.
THABAUT, A. & CANAYER, H. (1969). *Rev. Hyg. Méd. Soc.* **17**, 563.
WALTON, J. R. (1966). *Lancet* **2**, 1300.
WATANABE, T. (1963). *Bact. Rev.* **27**, 87.
WIEDEMANN, B., KNOTHE, H. & DOLL, E. (1970). *Zbl. Bakt.* 1 Orig. **213**, 183.
WILLIAMS, R. E. O. (1959). *Lancet* **1**, 190.
WILLIAMS SMITH, H. (1966). *J. Hyg. (Lond.)* **64**, 465.
WILLIAMS SMITH, H. (1969). *Lancet* **1**, 1174.
WITCHITZ, J. L. & CHABBERT, Y. A. (1971). *J. Antibiot.* **24**, 137.
WITCHITZ, J .L. & CHABBERT, Y. A. (1972). *Ann. Inst. Pasteur* **122**, 367.

PART II

CHAPTER 16

GENERAL PRINCIPLES OF TREATMENT

NOT one of the drugs with which this book is concerned can be administered without some risk of ill effects. Many of them are costly, and many will preserve their value only if they are used with discrimination. For these and other reasons it is unjustifiable to prescribe a powerful anti-bacterial drug for most trivial infections. It is impossible to be fully dogmatic on this point, because admittedly some specially predisposing factor may convert a minor into a major infection unless steps are taken to prevent this. Such situations are exceptional, and it must regretfully be admitted that much prescribing for minor conditions goes on unnecessarily. If figures of consumption in relation to population were available, it would doubtless be found that some countries sin more gravely in this way than others.

Prescribing habits are revealed in a brilliant and tragic light in reports of fatalities from the administration of antibiotics. An astonishing proportion of deaths from penicillin shock have followed an injection given for what seems an inadequate indication, including even a common cold, toothache and a sprained toe. Likewise, some deaths from marrow aplasia have been caused by chloramphenicol administered for minor catarrhal conditions: in some instances this has even been self-administration from a left-over bottle kept in the bathroom. These are extreme examples, but they can be supported by thousands of others in which more harm than good has been done, and by untold millions in which the drug has merely been wasted because the condition treated is by nature insusceptible to it.

Clinical Diagnosis

Successful chemotherapy must be rational, and rational treatment demands a diagnosis. This may only be provisional, and it may later be proved wrong, but the treatment chosen should be based on some explicit assumption as to the nature of the disease process. This may or may not carry with it an implication that the cause is a particular micro-organism.

Bacteriological Diagnosis

This is in a sense more important, because treatment, to be successful, must be aimed at the micro-organism and not at the disease as such. There are fortunately many diseases which have only one microbic cause: if a clinical diagnosis of ery-sipelas, scarlet fever, typhoid fever, typhus or anthrax can be made, the microbic diagnosis is implicit in the clinical, and furthermore all the organisms concerned here are regularly susceptible to certain antibiotics. On the other hand pneumonia, meningitis, urinary tract infections and wound infections can be caused by any of a number of different bacteria, and the most astute clinician may sometimes be wrong if he has to guess with which of these he is dealing.

It is here that any writer on this subject is faced with his greatest difficulty. Given a patient in a hospital with a good laboratory service, a bacteriological diagnosis should soon be forthcoming. Where laboratory facilities are distant or even non-existent, how is treatment to be directed? It must be insisted that in the more serious of these infections of multiple causation, certainly in meningitis, suspected septicaemia or severe pneumonia, a bacteriological diagnosis must at all costs be made, but for the patient whose life is not in danger, it may often be necessary to dispense with laboratory aid. The choice of treatment may then be based on past experience in similar situations or on bacteriological guesswork. Some attempt will be made in this book to point to probabilities in the commoner of these situations.

Sensitivity Tests

A simple bacteriological diagnosis is not always enough. If the organism is a staphylococcus or one of the tougher coliform bacilli, there is no guarantee that it will be sensitive to the drug of obvious choice or indeed to any of those which would naturally be preferred for their usual efficacy, ease of administration and freedom from toxicity. Here again it may be a counsel of perfection to advise that an appropriate range of sensitivity tests be carried out, but there can be no certainty of effect unless this is done. Fortunately not all pathogenic bacteria are so unpredictable, and it is helpful to the clinician to know which should regularly be susceptible and which he should mistrust.

Choice of Drug

This depends in the first place on the causative organism being sensitive to the drug chosen. A comprehensive statement of normal sensitivities is given in Table 31.

There are few diagnoses which point unequivocally to a single drug for treatment. There is usually a choice, and it may be of either of two kinds.

Some infections, such as those caused by pneumococci and haemolytic streptococci, respond to a variety of drugs, including sulphonamides (usually), penicillin, and several other antibiotics. Because of the certainty and rapidity of its action, its harmlessness (except in sensitized patients), and incidentally its cheapness, penicillin is to be preferred for these infections. A suitable alternative in a sensitized patient would be erythromycin, a cephalosporin or cotrimoxazole (sulphamethoxazole + trimethoprim).

The second kind of choice is between a relatively harmless but less efficacious drug and one which is more potent but also more potentially toxic. This choice must take into account the severity of the condition, since naturally in a desperate situation risks not otherwise justifiable may rightly be taken, and secondly the likelihood that toxic effects will be produced. A vital factor in this is renal function: to the extent that this is already impaired, so do the chances increase of further renal damage by nephrotoxic drugs and of damage to the eighth nerve by those which are ototoxic. Adequate laboratory control of treatment, referred to in Chapter 29, can be a valuable safeguard against these effects.

Dosage and Route of Administration

The object of systemic treatment is to attain a drug concentration in the blood and tissues which is calculated to exert the effect desired, and to maintain this, either continuously or with only short intermissions, until the infection has been overcome. To devise effective treatment it is necessary to know (1) the minimum concentration of the drug necessary to inhibit or kill the infecting organism; (2) the concentration attained in the blood after a given single dose (which should exceed (1) by several-fold for most of the time between one dose and the next), and (3) the rate of elimination of the drug, on which the frequency of dosage must depend. This question therefore involves two other large subjects, the sensitivity of different microbic species, and the pharmacological behaviour of the drugs concerned, both of which are dealt with elsewhere in this book.

When there is a choice between the oral and parenteral routes of administration (as there is, for instance, for sulphonamides, penicillin and tetracyclines) the latter may be preferred in severely ill patients for the greater certainty of its effect, since the whole dose must be absorbed, whereas the whole of an oral dose never is; or to initiate treatment, since its effect is immediate. If the oral route only is used, a ' loading ' dose larger than those which follow may be advantageous, particularly with drugs which are more slowly and incompletely absorbed.

Necessary Accompanying Treatment

There are many kinds of condition in which chemotherapy cannot be expected to do the whole job of getting the patient well. It is most successful in acute uncomplicated infections, and least in those predisposed to by some structural abnormality. An obstructive lesion of the urinary tract or the bronchial dilatation and mucosal changes of bronchiectasis will cause the infection to recur unless they can be dealt with surgically. Chemotherapy does not obviate the necessity for draining an abscess or removing sequestra or calculi. General causes of diminished resistance to infection—nutritional, metabolic or due to disorders of blood formation—also require attention.

A minor example of accessory treatment which is often neglected is the control of urinary pH at the optimum for the drug administered in urinary tract infections. This is fully discussed in Chapter 24.

Laboratory Control of the Effects of Treatment

Whether treatment is succeeding is best judged by clinical criteria, but it is also useful to know whether the infecting organism has been eliminated: this is particularly helpful in deciding how long treatment should continue. Repeated cultures are therefore sometimes indicated if facilities for them are available. They are more decidedly called for when treatment is *not* succeeding, because one cause of failure is the replacement of the original sensitive organism by a resistant one requiring a different drug.

A more difficult service perhaps not within the competence of every laboratory is the assay of antibiotics in body fluids. This may be desirable to verify either that the concentration attained is adequate, or that it is not excessive. In the blood the level may prove inadequate if absorption from the alimentary tract is poor, or if long intervals between injections are adopted: in the cerebro-spinal fluid in meningitis treated without intrathecal injections it is reassuring to know that enough antibiotic is diffusing into the infected area. It is no less important to know that the blood level of a potentially toxic drug is not excessive: this possibility should be borne in mind when streptomycin, gentamicin, kanamycin or vancomycin have to be given to a patient with impaired renal function.

Treatment with Drug Combinations

There are five alleged indications for prescribing two antibacterial drugs together:

1. As a temporary expedient during the investigation of an obscure illness.
2. Mixed infections.
3. To permit reduction in dose of a potentially toxic drug.
4. To prevent the development of bacterial resistance.
5. To achieve a synergic effect.

10

TABLE 31

Sensitivity of Important Pathogenic Bacteria to the Principal Antibiotics
Usual Minimum Inhibitory Concentration (μg./ml.)

	Benzyl penicillin	Cloxacillin	Ampicillin	Carbenicillin	Cephaloridine	Cephalothin	Cephalexin	Erythromycin	Lincomycin	Clindamycin	Fucidin	Tetracycline	Chloramphenicol	Streptomycin	Kanamycin	Gentamicin	Polymyxin
Staph. aureus a.	0·03	0·12	0·06	0·5	0·12	0·25	2	0·12	0·5-2	0·1-1	0·06	0·12	4	2	0·5	0·06	32
Staph. aureus b.	R	0·25	R	R	5	0·5	8	0·12	0·5-2	0·1-1	0·06	0·12	4	2	0·5	0·06	32
Str. pyogenes	0·01	0·06	0·03	0·25	0·01	0·12	0·5	0·03	0·12	0·03	8	0·25	2	32	128	8	R
Str. faecalis	2	32	1	64	16	32-64	256	0·5	4-16	4-16	4	0·5	2	32	128	4	R
Str. pneumoniae	0·01	0·25	0·06	0·5	0·03	0·25	2	0·03	0·5	0·03	8	0·25	2	64	128	16	R
Cl. welchii	0·12	1	0·25	0·25	0·5	0·5-4		2	0·5-2	0·03-1	0·25	0·25	4	R	R	R	R
B. anthracis	0·01	0·25	0·06	0·25	0·12	0·5	2	0·25	0·25-8	0·01-0·1	0·5	0·12	4	1	1	0·06	R
Ery. insidiosa	0·03	0·25	0·12	0·5	0·25			0·06	4		0·12	0·12	8	16	R	R	R
L. monocytogenes	0·25	4	0·5	2	1			0·25	4		16	0·25	8	2	0·5	0·12	R
A. israeli	0·06	0·25	0·06		0·01			0·12	0·06		0·5	2	2	16	16		
Myco. tuberculosis	R	R	R	R	10			R	R		64	10	30	1	5	5	R
N. gonorrhoeae	0·01	0·5	0·04		0·2-8	0·2-4	0·2-4	0·06	32	4	0·5	1	1	4	8	2	R
N. meningitidis	0·03	0·5	0·06	0·06	0·1-1	0·5-2	0·5-4	0·5	>32		0·12	1	1	1	8	2	R

Organism																
Bord. pertussis	1	16	0.5	0.25	16	32	0.06	8		0.25	2	2	4	2	1	0.5
Esch. coli	32	16	8	4	8	8	R	R	R	R	1	2-8	2	2	1	0.25
Klebsiella-Aerobacter spp.	R	R	16-R	2-R	2-R	4-R	R	R	R	R	1-4	2-16	2	2	0.5	0.25
Pr. mirabilis a.	32	R	2	1	2	8	R	R	R	R	32	8	8	2	0.5	R
Pr. mirabilis b.	R	R	R	4	2	8	R	R	R	R	32	8	8	2	0.5	R
Pr. vulgaris	R	R	R	8	R	R	R	R	R	R	4-32	8	4	2	0.25	R
Pr. rettgeri	R	R	R	2	R	R	R	R	R	R	R	16-R	2	1	0.5	R
Pr. morgani	R	R	R	1-8	R	R	R	R	R	R	4-R	4-R	1	1	0.25	R
S. marsescens	R	R	8-R	4-R	R	R	R	R	R	R	16-R	8	4	2	0.5	R
Providencia	R	R	16-R	4-R	32-R	32-R	64-R	R	R	R	2-R	4-R	8	1-4	2-128	R
Salmonella spp.	4-16	R	1-8	2-8	2	4	8-R	R	R	R	1	2	2	1	0.25	0.25
Shigella spp.	16	R	8	2-8	2-8	8	8-R	R	R	R	1-2	8	4	2	0.25	0.25
Ps. aeruginosa	R	R	R	R	R	R	32	R	R	R	32-R	R	16-64	32	1	0.5
Br. abortus	2-8	R	1-4	8-16	4-8	16-64	1	4-16	R	4-16	1	2	2	1	0.25	8-16
Past. septica	0.5	1-8	0.5	2	0.5	2	1	0.5-4		1-8	0.5	0.5	2	1	1-4	0.5
Bact. fragilis	8-R	32	32	16	32	32	1-4		0.1-1	1-R	0.5-2	8	R	R	R	>16
Blood level †	0.5*	2.5	2.5*	5*	2.5	10	1.5	2.5	5	20	2.5	5	10	10	2.5	2

† These figures are necessarily arbitrary, but they are intended to represent a concentration which is exceeded in the blood after the usual ordinary full dose for at least half the inter-dose interval. It is assumed that administration is at short intervals as in the treatment of an acute infection.

* Much higher levels can be attained if necessary by giving larger doses.

Of these the blind treatment of (1) may obscure the diagnosis and so ultimately be detrimental, and is justifiable only in urgent situations and if specimens have been taken: (2) is a purpose which may sometimes be better served by a broad-spectrum antibiotic, and (3) is simply untrue if the dictum be accepted that in combined treatment each drug should be given in its normal independent dose.

The importance of combined treatment in delaying the emergence of bacterial resistance has been amply verified in tuberculosis. This is a special case, because treatment must be so prolonged: the argument from it applies little to acute self-limited infections, and of course not at all to those caused by bacteria, such as haemolytic streptococci and pneumococci, treated with an antibiotic such as penicillin, to which they do not become resistant. The main question here is how far this principle applies to the treatment of infection by staphylococci. There is some evidence that it does. Lowbury (1957), working in a burns unit where sepsis is almost inevitable and cross-infection very difficult to prevent, found that when erythromycin and novobiocin were used together, the appearance of strains resistant to either was delayed, although not indefinitely prevented. A clinical experiment involving an entire hospital is described by Barber *et al.* (1960): here the adoption of a general policy of combined treatment was followed by a substantial reduction in the frequency of multiple antibiotic resistance in staphylococci isolated from all sources. Other measures taken at the same time to combat cross-infection may have contributed to this.

Types of Combined Effect

The attainment of a synergic effect, when this is possible, may be the most important indication of all. This is only one of three possible types of combined action, according to the law formulated by Jawetz and Gunnison (1952) which distinguishes between combinations according to whether each component is bactericidal (e.g. penicillin, streptomycin, neomycin, kanamycin) or only bacteristatic (chloramphenicol, tetracycline, erythromycin, novobiocin). The law in simple terms is that:

Bacteristatic + bacteristatic is simply additive.

Bactericidal + bacteristatic may be antagonistic.

Bactericidal + bactericidal may be synergic.

BACTERISTATIC + BACTERISTATIC. Some degree of additive effect is usual when bacteristatic antibiotics are combined, but is not invariable. Synergy is very rare, although a clear example of it is the combined action of the two components of peptolide antibiotics (ostreogricin, pristinamycin, etc.). On the other hand, if synthetic drugs are included, some with perhaps not a purely bacteristatic effect, several types of combined action may be seen.

The best way of studying combined bacteristatic action is to add a series of concentrations of each drug to broth in every possible combination and to inoculate the tubes with a sensitive organism (' carré ' method). Four representative results from such tests are shown in Table 32. 'A' shows the result of a test with tetracycline and novobiocin acting on *Staph. aureus*, which is also referred to on p. 217. Each antibiotic behaves as if the other were not there, making no contribution to its effect whatever. ' B ' is a hypothetical result showing an additive effect: the same total amount in four different proportions has the same effect as each drug acting alone. ' C ' illustrates synergy: the total amount of sulphafurazole + trimethoprim required to inhibit growth is less than that of either drug acting alone. ' D ' is an example of antagonism: the action of nitrofurantoin on *Proteus* spp. over a wide range of concentrations is quantitatively neutralized by nalidixic acid.

BACTERICIDAL + BACTERISTATIC. The explanation of antagonism is that bactericidal antibiotics kill only multiplying bacteria, and if growth is prevented by a bacteristatic agent, the condition requisite for this action is removed. Such interference is readily demonstrable in experimental infections, and a clear clinical example of it is the much higher mortality in pneumococcal meningitis observed by Lepper and Dowling (1951) when chlortetracycline was given in addition to penicillin. That chloramphenicol also interferes with the bactericidal of penicillin in meningitis is shown by the experimental studies of Wallace *et al.* (1967). Giving chlortetracycline in addition to

TABLE 32
Results of Three Actual and One Hypothetical Tests of Combined Bacteristatic Action by the Carré Method
All concentrations in μg./ml. + = growth. − = no growth.

		TETRACYCLINE					
		0·5	0·25	0·12	0·06	0·03	nil
NOVOBIOCIN	0·5	−	−	−	−	−	−
	0·25	−	−	−	−	−	−
	0·12	−	−	+	+	+	+
	0·06	−	−	+	+	+	+
	0·03	−	−	+	+	+	+
	nil	−	−	+	+	+	+

A

		x	x/2	x/4	x/8	x/16	nil
	y	−	−	−	−	−	+
	y/2	−	−	−	−	+	+
	y/4	−	−	−	+	+	+
	y/8	−	−	+	+	+	+
	y/16	−	+	+	+	+	+
	nil	+	+	+	+	+	nil

B

		TRIMETHOPRIM					
		16	8	4	2	1	nil
SULPHAFURAZOLE	4	−	−	−	−	−	+
	2	−	−	−	−	−	+
	1	−	−	−	−	−	+
	0·5	−	−	−	−	+	+
	0·25	−	−	−	−	+	+
	nil	−	+	+	+	+	+

C

		NALIDIXIC ACID						
		32	16	8	4	2	1	nil
NITROFURANTOIN	128	−	−	−	−	−	−	−
	64	−	+	+	+	+	+	+
	32	−	−	+	+	+	+	+
	16	−	−	+	+	+	+	+
	8	−	−	−	+	+	+	+
	4	−	−	−	+	+	+	+
	2	−	−	−	−	+	+	+
	1	−	−	−	−	+	+	+
	nil	−	−	−	−	−	+	+

D

A—Indifferent. Tetracycline and novobiocin *v Staph. aureus*.
B—Additive. The two drugs have an equal effect in all proportions as the same concentration of each acting alone.
C—Synergic. Trimethoprim and sulphafurazole *v N. gonorrhoeae*.
D—Antagonistic. Nitrofurantoin and nalidixic acid *v Proteus mirabilis*.

penicillin for the treatment of streptococcal pharyngitis apparently interfered with the elimination of the organism from the throat, although therapeutic results were satisfactory (Strom, 1955). It is better in general to avoid administering any penicillin (and particularly methicillin) together with a tetracycline or chloramphenicol.

BACTERICIDAL + BACTERICIDAL. The synergy which may be exerted by such a combination is chiefly important for its total bactericidal effect on organisms, particularly *Str. faecalis* or other penicillin-resistant streptococci, causing bacterial endocarditis. Whatever definition of synergy may be preferred, an effect so different as total sterilization from the partial bactericidal action of the two components must surely deserve this description. These combinations are discussed in connection with the treatment of endocarditis in Chapter 18, where it is pointed out that staphylococcal as well as some streptococcal infections may call for this kind of treatment. Whenever it is proposed to use a combination for so serious a purpose as this its effect should be verified by appropriate *in vitro* test, and others should be examined if the effect is inadequate.

COMMERCIAL COMBINATIONS. The claims made for most commercial combinations are exaggerated, and the use of these preparations is in general to be discouraged. Many consist of penicillin and streptomycin, and although this has an important use just described, no one is likely to use such a commercial combination for treating endocarditis, since the proportions of the two constituents are wrong for this purpose: that of penicillin needs to be higher. These products are mainly used for purposes which often do not require such a combination at all, whether the ' blind ' treatment of infection of unknown nature, or as cover for surgical operations, including those for which no such precaution should be necessary. Many patients have quite unnecessarily suffered eighth nerve damage from streptomycin or dihydrostreptomycin in such combinations administered in this way: such damage is most likely to occur in those with unrecognized impairment of renal function, who fail to excrete the antibiotic at the normal rate. Naumann (1966) who roundly condemns these combinations for the reasons given here, adds information about the frequent

present-day resistance of Gram-negative species to streptomycin which deprives the combination of its expected broad
spectrum effect.

Most other commercial combinations contain bacteristatic
antibiotics, and there is no evidence in the extensive studies of
Finland and his colleagues (reviewed by Garrod, 1965) that
any of these exert an effect superior to that of the more active
of their constituents. In a separate category are mixtures of
tetracyclines with anti-fungal antibiotics, the merits of which
are discussed on p. 233.

Prophylactic Administration

This is subject on which much has now been written, and
no attempt will be made to review the literature, but only to
define some principles and to propose what we hope will be
considered a rational plan. Some accepted forms of prophylaxis are dealt with elsewhere in this book, including that of
rheumatic fever (p. 380) and of bacterial endocarditis (p. 319)
and pre-operative bowel preparation (p. 372).

Antibiotics have often been given in clinical situations which
involve a special risk of autogenous infection, especially of the
lungs. These include inhalation anaesthesia in elderly and
' chesty ' patients, and particularly for operations on the upper
abdomen which limit the depth of subsequent respiration. In
the medical field, supposed indications have been virus infections such as measles, and various comatose and paralytic
states. We are aware of no evidence that any of these proceedings is beneficial; indeed, studies have usually shown a higher
infection rate in treated than in control patients. The principle
involved here is that treatment does nothing to remove the
predisposing cause; if this is strongly operative infection will
always follow, and all that the antibiotic does is to select a
resistant pathogen. In place of, say, a pneumococcus, infection
due to which, if it does occur, is amenable to treatment, the
more likely cause is a *Klebsiella* or some other Gram-negative
organism relatively resistant to any treatment.

In the surgical field prophylaxis aimed at the wound itself
is a different matter. An imperative indication for it is a serious
risk of gas gangrene, as in extensive trauma with gross soiling
of the wound, or thigh amputation for obliterative arterial

disease, when *Cl. welchii* may be derived from the peri-anal skin and the disease itself for which the operation is undertaken ensures the reduced tissue oxygen tension to enable its spores to germinate. There is also general agreement that antibiotic cover is advisable for open heart surgery. At the other extreme are commonplace clean operations involving no risk of sepsis, for which most surgeons, in this country at least, consider antibiotic cover quite superfluous, yet serious harm has commonly been caused by such treatment (see preceding section).

Between these two extremes lies debatable ground. Various particular operations have been thought to require cover, usually because highly susceptible tissues are exposed, or because bacterial contamination cannot be prevented, or because the consequences of any infection can be particularly disastrous. We would only suggest that, the decision having been made, it should further be decided exactly what the antibiotic is intended to do. If the aim is to destroy bacteria accidentally implanted in the wound during operation, what purpose is served by starting treatment 24 hours beforehand? Yet this is very common practice. A logical aim would be to maintain an adequate concentration of a bactericidal antibiotic throughout the operation and for a few hours after it. That such simple treatment can be effective is supported by the findings of Campbell (1965), who gave 10 mega units of penicillin intravenously 15 minutes before the operation began, repeated 2-hourly, with a final dose at the time of suture. A similar short period of administration is advocated by Bernard and Cole (1964), who gave a mixture of penicillin, methicillin and chloramphenicol 1-2 hours before, during and within 4 hours after the operation, and claim a reduction in wound infections following abdominal surgery from 25 to 5 per cent. Polk and Lopez-Mayer (1969) greatly reduced the frequency of infection following abdominal operations by giving 1 g. cephaloridine immediately before and 5 and 12 hours after operation. (Pollock and Tindal (1972) failed in this object by giving a single intravenous dose of 500 mg. ampicillin at operation, but do not say how many infections were caused by penicillin-resistant staphylococci, against which little protection would have been afforded.)

So short a course as this may not provide for all situations, but it may well be adequate for many, and those in the habit of continuing antibiotic prophylaxis for days—or even, in connection with heart surgery, for weeks—might perhaps with advantage ask themselves what exactly the later stages of such a course are supposed to be achieving. If some fresh autogenous infection is feared it is likely, owing to the selective effect of such treatment on the normal flora of the body, to be due to a highly resistant organism.

A general policy in prophylaxis should be to restrict it to the few patients clearly requiring it. There is abundant evidence that the lavish use of antibiotics favours the spread of resistant species. A remarkable illustration of this is reported by Price and Sleigh (1970) from a neuro-surgical intensive care unit in which *Klebsiella aerogenes* infection was endemic and had caused numerous chest and urinary infections and 8 deaths from meningitis. The occurrence of these infections was abruptly halted by stopping all antibiotic treatment, both therapeutic and prophylactic; the antibiotic largely used for the prophylaxis of both chest and wound infections had been ampicillin. Restricted use was resumed four months later.

We are not so much concerned here with local application, but there is apparently sound evidence that several forms of this are beneficial. Three differing examples are intraperitoneal instillation of a solution of kanamycin and bacitracin at operation for perforating lesions of the alimentary tract (Noon *et al.*, 1967), post-operative infiltration of the area with penicillin solution after operation for external hernia (Ryan, 1967) and the application of ampicillin powder to the possibly soiled wound in operations on the colon after peritoneal closure (Nash and Hugh, 1967).

Concerted Policies in Antibiotic Prescribing

This chapter has hitherto been concerned with the welfare of the individual patient. The community has also to be considered, since it has been abundantly proved that the more some antibiotics are used, the less useful do they become, because the frequency of bacterial resistance to them increases correspondingly. To counter this tendency, policies in prescribing have been adopted in hospitals or hospital groups, in areas, and in one instance at least, throughout an entire country. They are of four kinds: (1) *restriction,* the use of an antibiotic being reserved for cases in which nothing else will serve; (2) *rotation,* an antibiotic being used until resistance appears and then replaced by another with similar action: while the second is being used, resistance to the first will diminish again; (3) *diversification,* or the prescribing of a wide variety, no single antibiotic being used enough to provoke frequent resistance; (4) *combinations,* an apparently successful application of which has already been cited.

These measures were mainly designed to ensure that there shall always be an effective antibiotic for treating severe staphylococcal infections. There are now so many antibiotics available for this purpose, including the new penicillins unaffected by penicillinase, that the danger of having to stand with folded hands before the bed of such a patient has receded into at least a fairly distant future. The deliberate adoption of any of these policies may now therefore seem less urgent, although the danger of selecting staphylococci of high virulence by the process which selects drug-resistant strains (see p. 269) must be borne in mind. However, none of them can rival in the importance of its effects a general restriction of the antibiotics, particularly in prophylaxis, to really necessary purposes.

An altogether new situation has been created by the discovery that drug resistance, often multiple, can readily be transferred by contact between various Gram-negative bacteria, notably from *E. coli* to intestinal pathogens. It so happens that in this country this mode of acquiring resistance has been most actively studied in *S. typhimurium* in farm animals, whence infection by resistant strains has spread on a considerable scale to man (see Chapter 15). It has been suggested that this menacing situation demands a review of the use of antibiotics in animals and perhaps the imposition of restrictions on this. These have already been applied to the use of medical antibiotics for growth promotion. In view of the fact that animal pathogens are much more able than commensals to colonise the human bowel, steps to limit the indiscriminate and often ineffective use of antibiotics for treating enteritis in farm animals might be helpful.

REFERENCES

BARBER, M., DUTTON, A. A. C., BEARD, M. A., ELMES, P. C. & WILLIAMS, R. (1960). *Brit. med. J.* i, 11.
BERNARD, H. R. & COLE, W. R. (1964). *Surgery* **56**, 151.
CAMPBELL, P. C. (1965). *Lancet* **2**, 805.
GARROD, L. P. (1965). *S. Afr. med. J.* **39**, 607.
JAWETZ, E. & GUNNISON, J. B. (1952). *Antibiot. and Chemother.* **2**, 243.
LEPPER, M. H. & DOWLING, H. F. (1951). *Arch. intern. Med.* **88**, 489.
LOWBURY, E. J. L. (1957). *Lancet* ii, 305.
NASH, A. G. & HUGH, T. B. (1967). *Brit. med. J.* **1**, 471.
NAUMANN, P. (1966). *Dtsch. med. Wschr.* **91**, 1152.
NOON, G. P., BEALL, A. C., JORDAN, G. L., RIGGS, S. & DE BAKEY, M. E. (1967). *Surgery* **62**, 73.
POLK, H. C. & LOPEZ-MAYER, J. F. (1969). *Surgery* **66**, 97.
POLLOCK, A. V. & TINDALL, D. S. (1972). *Brit. J. Surg.* **59**, 98.
PRICE, D. J. E. & SLEIGH, J. D. (1970). *Lancet* **2**, 1213.
RYAN, E. A. (1967). *Brit. J. Surg.* **54**, 324.
STROM, J. (1955). *Antibiot. Med.* **1**, 6.
WALLACE, J. F., SMITH, R. H., GARCIA, M. & PETERSDORF, R. G. (1967). *J. Lab. clin. Med.* **70**, 408.

CHAPTER 17

DOSAGE

NORMAL doses are specified in appendices to earlier chapters, and some indications for increasing these are mentioned in the text. We are here concerned with situations in which normal dosage needs to be modified, and with other problems of administration.

DOSAGE IN CHILDREN

In general, dosage is related to that for the adult on a basis of body weight or of surface area, using one of a number of standard formulas. Although methods based on estimation of surface area are of disputed validity and are little used in Britain in their direct form, the ' Percentage Method ' of Catzel (1966) which is a simplified form of a surface area method, is widely used for its convenience. The dose is given as a percentage of adult dose appropriate to the child's age; for example, at birth a child receives 10 per cent of the adult dose, at one year 25 per cent, at 7 years 50 per cent. Different considerations apply in premature infants and in the full time neonate during the first week of life, when excessive or even moderate doses of many drugs, including antimicrobial agents, such as chloramphenicol and sulphonamides, can have disastrous effects (Nyhan, 1961). In these infants the dose should be limited to one half to two thirds of that calculated in the usual way, even if no special information is available about limitation of dosage. The reasons for these effects lie mainly in the undeveloped state of hepatic and renal function in the premature infant and neonate. Detoxification mechanisms in the liver are inadequate, and deficiency of glucuronyl transferase in particular renders the infant incapable of rapidly detoxifying drugs such as chloramphenicol and novobiocin (p. 216). A number of drugs, such as sulphonamides, may compete for binding sites to albumin in plasma, thus causing a rise in serum bilirubin and a consequent increased risk of kernicterus. Renal function, too, is not fully developed in the first weeks of life and deficient renal excretion accounts for higher blood levels and a slower rate of decline than in older patients. Other enzyme systems may be genetically deficient and a low concentration of glucose 6-phosphate dehydrogenase leads to increased likelihood of haemolysis when drugs such as nitrofurantoin and sulphonamides are administered.

The difficult task of studying this behaviour of antibiotics in the neonatal period has been tackled recently in Germany and the United States. Von Harnack et al. (1964, 1965) administered single doses of oxacillin to infants of different ages, older children and adults, and found that in the first week of life a standard dose based on body surface area produced blood levels 4 times higher than those attained in older children: at 2-4 weeks the level attained was already lower. Boe et al. (1967) found the blood levels attained after a dose of methicillin based on body weight to be very high in the first 24 hours of life, falling progressively at 4-5, 8-9, 13-15 and 26-30 days. An even more rapid increase in the capacity to excrete benzyl penicillin was demonstrated by Abramowicz et al. (1966), with differences between the findings in 12 hours, 13-14 hours, 26-62 hours and thence to 7 days. Axline, Yaffe and Simon (1967) determined the half-life of ampicillin in infants aged 2-7, 8-14, 15-30 and 31-68 days to be 4·0, 2·8, 1·7 and 1·6 hours respectively. Similar results were obtained with methicillin, oxacillin and neomycin, but not with colistin, the half-life of which remained unchanged throughout the neonatal period. McCracken et al. (1971) found the half-life of gentamicin in infants under one week old was directly related to birth-weight, being $11\frac{1}{2}$ hours in infants with birthweights less than 1500 g., 8 hours for those weighing 1500-2000 g. at birth, and $4\frac{1}{2}$-5 hours in those with birthweights over 2000 g. From one week to six months of age the half-life was 3-3·5 hours. These authors suggest suitable schemes of dosage for gentamicin in various neonatal infections, and suitable doses for the use of kanamycin in premature and full-term infants have been proposed by Eichenwald (1966).

Since penicillins are non-toxic, even at this age, this slow elimination is an advantage: shortly after birth a 12-hour interval between doses will give a sustained effect, shortened through 8- and 6-hours to the usual 4-hourly schedule at 4 weeks of age (Boe *et al.*, 1967). Reduced daily doses are naturally imperative for antibiotics causing toxic effects. Most of the authors responsible for these studies have included premature infants in their tests, and found, as would be expected, that elimination in them is even slower.

ANTIBIOTICS IN RENAL FAILURE

It is often necessary to administer antibacterial drugs in patients with impaired renal function, either for the treatment of infection of the renal tract itself, or for infection at other sites. The likelihood of accumulation and the consequent chance of toxic effects is influenced by a number of factors, which differ in their relative importance with different drugs. Most important is the mode of elimination of the antibiotic. The risks of toxicity associated with renal failure are in general higher for those drugs, such as the aminoglycosides, of which a high proportion is excreted in the urine than for those, for example, the macrolides, in which renal excretion plays a small part in their elimination. An important exception to this rule must be made for some drugs whose metabolites, although antibacterially inactive (and therefore undetectable by assay systems relying on their biological effects) are excreted by the kidney and therefore accumulate in renal failure. In this situation the possible toxicity of the inactive metabolites must be considered, as well as that of the undegraded antibiotic. There is much variation in the stability of different antimicrobial drugs in the body, and this factor, together with the ratio between toxic and therapeutic levels, again affects the likelihood of toxic effects. Among the antibiotics, those which are known to be nephrotoxic must be regarded with particular caution in renal failure. An additional factor has to be evaluated when antibacterial drugs are used for the treatment of urinary infection, since the urinary concentration of a drug may be greatly affected by declining renal function. Finally, antibiotics must often be given to patients with conditions such as septicaemic shock, in which renal function is threatened and may decline rapidly during the course of treatment; it is therefore essential to monitor renal function constantly, and to modify dosage of antibiotics where necessary, in patients who are seriously ill. This diversity of factors affecting the relationship between antimicrobial drugs and renal function often leads to practical difficulties of administration in renal failure. At one extreme no limitation is imposed by the presence of renal failure on the dosage of a drug, such as fusidic acid, which is handled entirely by non-renal mechanisms. For other drugs, renal excretion accounts for a small proportion of the administered dose, and only moderate restriction of dosage is required in renal failure. This is also true for the penicillins, despite the importance of renal excretion in their elimination, because the ratio of therapeutic to toxic concentration is so great. The dose of many antimicrobial drugs, however, must be severely modified in patients with renal failure, and unfortunately this group includes several which are often needed for infections associated with renal disease.

The serum concentration of most antibiotics, after reaching a peak, usually declines exponentially at a rate characteristic of the particular drug. Thus, although the pharmacokinetics of the different agents vary widely, the serum half-life of the drug is a useful general measure of its duration of action, and is prolonged in renal failure when an appreciable proportion of the drug is eliminated by the kidney. The degree to which the half-life is prolonged offers, for many antibiotics, a useful guide to dosage in renal failure. General factors bearing on the use of antibiotics in renal failure have been reviewed by O'Grady (1971). Administration of antibiotics in renal failure must often be monitored by frequent assay of plasma concentration of the drug, and suitable methods are described in Chapter 29, including recently introduced techniques of rapid assay.

Individual Antimicrobial Drugs and Renal Failure

General factors bearing upon the use of individual antibiotics in renal failure are considered in the following paragraphs. Table 33 gives a summary of antibiotic use in renal failure, detailed dose schemes in various circumstances are given in Table 34, and dose schedules for patients on haemodialysis are provided in Table 35.

Antibiotics are sometimes added to peritoneal dialysis fluid for the prevention or treatment of peritonitis. Not only a local but a systemic effect can be secured by this proceeding (Bulger, Bennett and Boen, 1965; Buck and Cohen, 1968).

Penicillins

Penicillins are eliminated by both glomerular filtration and tubular secretion, and the serum half life is much prolonged in renal failure. Even in anuria, however, serum levels do slowly decline by virtue of non-renal elimination. Since the margin of safety in dosage is very great, and penicillin encephalopathy is associated with very high serum levels, only modest adjustments of dosage are required in renal failure.

TABLE 33

Limitations on Antibiotic Prescribing in Renal Failure

Normal doses in renal failure
    Erythromycin and other macrolides
    Novobiocin
    Sodium fusidate

Slight adjustment of dose
    Penicillins
    Cephalothin
    Cephalexin
    Lincomycin
    Clindamycin
    Isoniazid
    Cotrimoxazole*

Major adjustment of dose
    Streptomycin, kanamycin, gentamicin
    Colistin
    Vancomycin
    Para–amino salicylic acid
    Amphotericin

Avoid in renal failure
    Tetracyclines (except doxycycline)
    Nitrofurantoin
    Cephaloridine (if frusemide given also)
    Chloramphenicol

* but see p. 298.

Cephalosporins

Serum half-lives of cephaloridine and of cephalexin are greatly increased in renal failure, but that of cephalothin is only slightly prolonged. Cephaloridine is potentially nephrotoxic in doses of 6 g. or more daily, and there is danger of renal damage when cephaloridine is given together with frusemide. Evidence

TABLE 34

Antimicrobial Drugs in Renal Failure

Drug	Serum Half-life in Hours		Dose		
	in Normal	*in Severe Renal Failure*	*Normal*	*Moderate Renal Failure*	*Severe Renal Failure*
Penicillin	0·5	7-10	Variable	No reduction	Reduce interval to 12 hourly
Ampicillin	1·8	8	Variable	No reduction	0.25 g. 6-12 hourly
Cloxacillin	1·5		Variable	No reduction	1 g. 8-12 hourly
Carbenicillin	1·0	16	Variable	No reduction	2 g. 8-12 hourly
Cephalothin	0·85	3	1 g. 6 hourly	No reduction	1 g. 8 hourly
Cephalexin	1·0	21	0·5-1·0 g. 6 hourly	8-12 hourly	0.25 g. every 24-48 hours
Lincomycin	4·8	8-12	600 mg. 8-12 hourly	No reduction	200 mg. 8-12 hourly
Streptomycin	2·5	Up to several days	1 g. daily	Reduction of dose and/or increase in interval between doses essential. Frequent estimation of serum concentration essential (see Text).	
Kanamycin	5		0·5 g. 12 hourly		
Gentamicin	2·5		60-80 mg. 8 hourly		
Colistin	2		150 mg 12 hourly		
Vancomycin	6	many days	0·5 g. 6 hourly		

Based on the findings of Eastwood and Curtis (1968), Hoffman *et al.* (1970), Kunin and Finkelberg (1970), Kabins *et al.* (1970), Kunin and Atuk (1966), McKay and Kaye (1964), Eykyn *et al.* (1970), Reinarz and McIntosh (1966), Kunin and Finland (1959), Curtis and Eastwood (1968), Goodwin and Friedman (1968), Gingell and Waterworth (1968), McHenry *et al.* (1971), Cutler and Orme (1969).

of deteriorating renal function has been obtained occasionally in patients receiving cephalothin, particularly in very large doses, but cephalexin has not so far been definitely associated with renal damage. If a cephalosporin is indicated in a patient with threatened or established renal failure, cephalothin or cephalexin should be given rather than cephaloridine (Kabins *et al.*, 1970; Curtis and Marshall, 1970; Kunin and Atuk, 1966).

Tetracyclines

The dangers of tetracyclines in renal failure are well documented (p. 157). Clinical and biochemical deterioration may follow their use in patients with previously well compensated renal failure, and they are generally contraindicated in renal impairment. The effects are caused by the anti-anabolic action of this group of drugs, and it is important to note that the

TABLE 35

Provisional Dosage Schedules* in Patients on Haemodialysis

Drug	Dose to be Given after each Dialysis
Carbenicillin	2 g.
Cephalexin	0·5 g.
Streptomycin	Removal variable. Monitor serum concentrations frequently
Kanamycin	0·5 g.
Gentamicin	80 mg.
Colistin	150 mg.
Vancomycin	0·5-1 g. every 7 to 10 days.
Penicillin	
Ampicillin	
Cloxacillin	Not removed or slowly removed
Cephalothin	Dosage as in severe renal failure in patients not on dialysis.
Lincomycin	
Fucidin	

* See also Schreiner and Teehan (1971).

maximal effect is often delayed for some days, so that deterioration of renal function may not be linked with the episode of tetracycline treatment.

The effects are not related in any direct way to prolongation of action of the drug; although the serum half-life of tetracycline and oxytetracycline is prolonged in renal failure, that of chlortetracycline is little affected, but all are potentially dangerous in renal failure. Doxycycline appears to provide an exception, although it must be remembered that the dose of this drug is much smaller than that of other tetracyclines. The long half-life of this drug, about 17 hours, is usually, but not always, unaffected in renal failure. More importantly, a number of patients with renal failure have received this tetracycline without showing ill effects. We conclude that tetracyclines are, in general, contraindicated in renal failure. If it is essential to use this group of drugs, doxycycline should be given, but it would be prudent to monitor serum levels of the drug at appropriate intervals.

Sulphonamides

Williams *et al.* (1968) found that the renal clearance of sodium sulphadimidine was greater in patients with renal failure than in normal subjects. This was attributable to the lower plasma concentration found in the patients with renal failure, itself presumably related to the increased volume of distribution for the drug. Sharpstone (1969) also found little relationship between the clearance of sulphamethoxazole and creatinine clearance. By contrast Fischer (1972) found the mean clearance of sulphadimidine much reduced in renal failure, with significant prolongation of plasma levels in the uraemic patients. The urinary concentration of sulphonamide in renal failure usually exceeds the M.I.C. for most sulphonamide-sensitive pathogens.

Short-term administration of sulphonamides is probably safe in renal failure, but plasma levels should be monitored if the drug is given for more than a few days.

Trimethoprim

Clearance of this agent is closely correlated with creatinine clearance, but declines at a lesser rate than does creatinine clearance with falling renal function, and concentrations in the urine are greater than those required for urinary pathogens even in advanced renal failure. The renal clearance of trimethoprim rises with increasing urinary acidity (Sharpstone, 1969).

Cotrimoxazole

Kalowski *et al.* (1973) observed 16 patients in whom renal function deteriorated in association with treatment by this drug combination. Deterioration continued in some in spite of modification of dose and they suggest that cotrimoxazole should not be used if the serum creatinine is greater than 2 mg. per 100 ml.

Nitrofurantoin

The serum half-life of this drug in normal subjects is short, about 20 minutes, no doubt reflecting an important extra-renal component in its metabolism. Sachs *et al.* (1968) found that very little nitrofurantoin appeared in the urine of patients with renal failure, the concentrations not reaching the M.I.C. for most urinary pathogens. In addition, peripheral neuropathy as a complication of nitrofurantoin treatment has developed chiefly in patients with renal failure.

For these reasons nitrofurantoin is contraindicated in renal failure.

Nalidixic Acid

Only a small proportion of the administered dose, 4-7 per cent, is found as biologically active drug in the urine, and serum concentrations rise little in renal failure. Nevertheless, adequate concentrations for the inhibition of most urinary pathogens are achieved even in advanced renal failure (Adam and Dawborn, 1971; Stamey *et al.*, 1969). Unfortunately clearance of the inactive conjugates, mainly the glucuronide, is closely related to renal function, and the serum concentration of these compounds rises in renal failure. Their toxic effects are uncertain, but unwanted effects of nalidixic acid are encountered more commonly in renal failure. Nalidixic acid should be avoided if possible in renal failure, but, if there are strong reasons for it, it should be given for the shortest possible time.

Chloramphenicol

The situation is very similar to that described for nalidixic acid. The duration of action of the active compound is not much changed in renal failure, but the metabolic products accumulate significantly (Kunin *et al.*, 1959). At very low glomerular filtration rates, maximal excretion is 10-20 μg. per ml. of urine (Lindberg *et al.*, 1966), a concentration which is too low for the treatment of most urinary infections.

Streptomycin, Kanamycin, Gentamicin

The serum concentrations of these drugs are greatly influenced by renal function, they have relatively low margins of safety, and they may be needed for infections which patients with renal failure may suffer. A number of studies have provided data on the relationship of serum half-life to creatinine clearance for each of these drugs, but it is nevertheless essential to monitor any treatment lasting for more than a day or two with frequent assays of serum concentration, partly because of individual variations in drug handling, and partly because the antibiotics have often to be prescribed in conditions of rapidly changing renal function.

Many schemes recommend increasing the interval between doses, each individual dose remaining the same as in patients with normal function. For example, kanamycin, normally given as a dose of 0·5 g. 12-hourly, would be given in the same dose at intervals of one to two days in a patient with moderate impairment of renal function, or of three to four days in a patient with severe renal failure. This type of regimen may leave long periods in which the serum drug concentration is negligible and the alternative method, of giving smaller doses at more conventional intervals, may be preferable (O'Grady, 1971). The relationship of different levels of impaired renal function to dosage of streptomycin has been examined by Kunin and Finland (1959), and data relating kanamycin half-life to serum creatinine concentration has been provided by Cutler and Orme (1969). Gentamicin dose in renal impairment has been studied by Gingell and Waterworth (1968), and by McHenry *et al.* (1971).

Polymyxins

These drugs accumulate in renal failure, and are potentially nephrotoxic. A high incidence of renal failure has been reported in patients receiving large doses of colistin sulphomethate sodium (Price and Graham, 1970). Serious restriction of dose is imposed by renal failure, and a number of dose schedules have been described (MacKay and Kaye, 1964; Curtis and Eastwood, 1968; Goodwin and Friedman, 1968). As with other potentially toxic drugs, initial dose schemes are provisional and should, if necessary, be modified following estimation of serum levels. Contradictory results have been obtained by different workers in estimating the effect of peritoneal and haemodialysis on blood levels of colistin and here too serum concentration must be monitored.

Antituberculous Drugs

Streptomycin has already been discussed. Isoniazid levels are somewhat prolonged in renal failure. Ogg *et al.* (1968)

found a half life of 17 hours in a patient on intermittent dialysis, and found a significant fall in plasma concentration across the dialyser. This suggests the usual dose should be reduced somewhat, to 150 mg. daily.

P.A.S. is eliminated entirely by the kidney and accumulates in renal failure. It will in general be avoided in patients with renal failure, but can be given provided assays of plasma concentration are performed. The patient on haemodialysis reported by Ogg *et al.* (1968) required 2-3 g. after each dialysis.

Rifampicin (and rifamide) do not accumulate in renal failure and can be given in normal dose (McGeachie *et al.*, 1970). Ethambutol, however, is excreted largely by the kidney and dose restriction in renal failure is necessary.

Fucidin

Very little of the administered dose can be found in the urine and normal doses can be given in the presence of impaired renal function.

Lincomycin

The half-life in renal failure is about three times that in normal subjects, and the drug is not significantly removed by dialysis (Reinarz and McIntosh, 1965).

INCOMPATIBILITIES AND INTERACTIONS

When a patient receives an antimicrobial drug by intravenous injection it is necessary to ensure its compatibility with the infusion fluid, and with other drugs, including other antimicrobials, which may be administered at the same time.

A recent series of publications (Meisler and Skolaut, 1966; Patel and Phillips, 1966; Fowler, 1967; Webb, 1969; Lynn, 1970) provides much information about the compatibilities of anti-bacterial and many other drugs: some of these findings together with data from Martindale (1972) and with information kindly supplied to us by manufacturers* are condensed in Table 36. Published data are based largely on the physical effects of mixing solutions, and a more subtle change than the

* We are indebted for this to Aspro-Nicholas Ltd., Beecham Pharmaceutical Division, Eli Lilly & Co., Glaxo Research Ltd. and Upjohn Ltd.

TABLE 36

	Ampicillin sodium	Carbenicillin sodium	Cephalothin sodium	Cephaloridine	Chloramphenicol sodium succinate	Cloxacillin sodium	Colistimethate	Erythromycin lactobionate	Fucidin (as diethanolamine fusidate)	Gentamicin sulphate	Kanamycin sulphate	Lincomycin sodium	Methicillin sodium	Novobiocin sodium	Penicillin G	Polymyxin B sulphate	Streptomycin sulphate	Tetracycline hydrochloride	Vancomycin hydrochloride	Heparin sodium	Hydrocortisone sodium
Ampicillin sodium																					
Carbenicillin sodium	C																				
Cephalothin sodium	—	C																			
Cephaloridine	C	C	C																		
Chloramphenicol succinate	—	—	—	—																	
Cloxacillin sodium	—	—	—	C	—																
Colistimethate	—	—	—	C	—	C															
Erythromycin lactobionate	C	C	C	C	C	—	C														
Fucidin (as diethanolamine (fusidate))				—																	
Gentamicin sulphate	C	C	C	—	—	—	C	—													
Kanamycin sulphate	C	C	C	—	—	C	C	C	—												
Lincomycin hydrochloride	—	—	—	—		—	C	—	—												
Methicillin sodium			—	C	—	—	—	—	C	C	—										
Novobiocin sodium	—	—	—	—	C	—	C	—	—	C	—	C									
Penicillin G	C	—	C	—	—	C	—	—	C	—	—	—	C	—							
Polymyxin B sulphate	—	C											—	—	C						
Streptomycin sulphate	—	—											—	—	C						
Tetracycline hydrochloride	—	—												—	—		—				
Vancomycin hydrochloride	C	C												—	C		—				
Heparin sodium		—																C			
Hydrocortisone sodium succinate	Ct	Ct	C	C	C	C	C	C	C	C	C	C	C	—	C	C	C	C	C	C	C
Isotonic saline solution	Ct	Ct	C	C	C	C	C	C	C	C	C	C	C	—	C	C	C	C	C	C	—
5% Dextrose in water	I*	Ct	C	—	—	C	—	C	—	—	—	C	—	—	C	—	C	Ct	C	—	—
Amino acid solution	C	C	C	C	C	C	C	C	—	C	C	—	C	C	C	C	C	C	C	—	—

formation of a visible precipitate cannot always be excluded. Thus Lynn (personal communication, 1970) determined the effect of mixing solutions of methicillin and kanamycin by actual assays of antibiotic activity, and found that although kanamycin was unaffected, there was rapid loss of methicillin activity (20-30 per cent in 15 minutes). The data in Table 36, although extensive, are incomplete, but they may serve as some guide to what is possible and what should be avoided. The antagonistic effect of carbenicillin on gentamicin in solutions containing both drugs has attracted some interest recently, especially since there is much evidence, both in man and in experimental animals, that this combination may be synergic (p. 82). Whether the action of carbenicillin (and of ampicillin) in lowering the concentration of gentamicin *in vitro* is also significant *in vivo* is doubtful but it is certain that the two drugs should not be mixed in intravenous fluids (McLaughlin and Reeves, 1971; Noone and Pattison, 1971).

Another factor bearing on the use of antibiotics by the intravenous route is the choice of intravenous infusion or bolus injection. As regards efficacy there is little evidence on which to decide which method is superior, but pharmaceutical factors may also be important, and Simberkoff *et al.* (1970) have shown that penicillins lose activity rapidly in solutions containing glucose sucrose or dextran together with bicarbonate. In general we prefer, when antibiotics are given intravenously, to inject them at intervals into the infusion, but the following antibiotics should be given by continuous slow infusion; amphotericin B, diethanolamine fusidate, and the tetracyclines.

The term ' incompatibility ' refers to an adverse relationship between two drugs *in vitro,* but increasing attention is now being directed to interactions between different drugs *in vivo*. The forms of interaction between various antimicrobial drugs are referred to in a number of chapters, but interactions between antimicrobial and other drugs must also be considered. These may operate before absorption, for example, the chelating effect of a number of metallic ions tends to diminish tetracycline absorption. After absorption, competition for serum binding sites may be important, and has been especially referred to in discussing antibiotic dosage in the neonate (p. 291), while interactions related to inhibition or stimulation of hepatic enzymes responsible for drug inactivation have also assumed growing importance. Again, this form of interaction is especially important in the newborn. Interaction related to competition in the renal tubule may be used to therapeutic advantage.

The forms of interactions between antibiotics themselves and between antibiotics and other drugs have recently been reviewed by Kabins (1972).

LOCAL ADMINISTRATION

It may be good practice to introduce a solution, usually of an antibiotic, into an infected cavity, such as a thoracic empyema. A special instance of such treatment is intrathecal injection, the pros and cons of which are discussed in describing the treatment of meningitis (q.v.). Different considerations apply to the local treatment of a superficial infected surface. The application of sulphonamide powders to wounds, and of antibiotic creams to burns and areas of dermatitis, has been abandoned by some because such application is believed to carry a special risk of causing sensitization. It is therefore advised that only antibiotics which are unlikely to be employed systemically should be applied in this way, and those often chosen are bacitracin, neomycin and polymyxin. (It should not too lightly be assumed that any of these, and polymyxin in particular, will never be needed for systemic use.)

Assuming that this idea of a special reactivity in the skin is correct, does it also exist in other epithelial surfaces? Penicillin and other antibiotics can be used locally for the treatment of conjunctivitis (or the prevention of ophthalmia neonatorum), and they have been sprayed into the nose and the bronchi. Penicillin pastilles were first recommended for the treatment of Vincent's and other infections in the mouth by MacGregor and Long (1944), and penicillin chewing gum has been used for the same purpose by Emslie et al. (1962). Should applications like these also be frowned on because of a risk of sensitization? The idea that they should derives largely from an emphatic statement by Guthe, Idsøe and Willcox (1958) in a paper concerned with reactions to penicillin in patients treated for venereal disease. They say: ' Its topical use should be abandoned. The inclusion of penicillin in toothpaste, chewing gum and similar substances is indefensible.' In so far as this refers to preparations like toothpaste freely available to the public, everyone will agree with this statement, but as a general condemnation of all legitimate topical use it may be disputed. In the overwhelming majority of patients sensitized to penicillin there is a history of previous parenteral treatment, and the few examples cited by these authors in which there was a history of local application have little evidential value. Unless evidence can be produced that topical use sensitizes more often than parenteral it seems unjustifiable to prohibit some unquestionably useful forms of topical therapy. Some inquiry also seems advisable into the relative degrees of sensitizing effect of application to different kinds of body surface. If mucous membranes are to be equated with the skin, then presumably all oral administration should come under the same ban.

REFERENCES

ABRAMOWICZ, M., KLEIN, J. O., IGNALL, D. & FINLAND, M. (1966). *Amer. J. Dis. Child.* **111**, 267.

ADAM, W. R. & DAWBORN, J. K. (1971). *Aust. N.Z. J. Med.* **1**, 126.

AXLINE, S. G., YAFFE, S. J. & SIMON, H. J. (1967). *Pediatrics* **39**, 9.

BOE, R. W., WILLIAMS, C. P. S., BENNETT, J. V. & OLIVER, T. K. (1967). *Pediatrics* **39**, 194.

BUCK, A. C. & COHEN, S. L. (1968). *J. clin. Path.* **21**, 88.

BULGER, R. J., BENNETT, J. V. & BOEN, S. T. (1965). *J. Amer. med. Ass.* **194**, 1198.

CATZEL, P. (1966). *The Paediatric Prescriber, Third Edition.* Oxford, Blackwell.

CURTIS, J. R. & EASTWOOD, J. B. (1968). *Brit. med. J.* **1**, 484.

CURTIS, J. R. & MARSHALL, M. J. (1970). *Brit. med. J.* **2**, 149.

CUTLER, R. E. & ORME, B. M. (1969). *J. Amer. med. Ass.* **209**, 539.

EASTWOOD, J. B. & CURTIS, J. R. (1968). *Brit. med. J.* **1**, 486.

EICHENWALD, H. F. (1966). *Ann. N.Y. Acad. Sci.* **132**, 984.

EMSLIE, R. D., CROSS, W. G. & BLAKE, G. C. (1962). *Brit. dent. J.* **112**, 320.

EYKYN, S., PHILLIPS, I. & EVANS, J. (1970). *Brit. med. J.* **3**, 80.

FISCHER, E. (1972). *Lancet* **2**, 210.

FOWLER, T. J. (1967). *Amer. J. Hosp. Pharm.* **24**, 450.

GINGELL, J. C. & WATERWORTH, P. M. (1968). *Brit. med. J.* **2**, 19.

GOODWIN, N. J. & FRIEDMAN, E. A. (1968). *Ann. intern. Med.* **68**, 984.

GREENBERG, P. A. & SANFORD, J. P. (1967). *Ann. intern. Med.* **66**, 465.

GUTHE, T., IDSØE, O. & WILLCOX, R. R. (1958). *Bull. Wld Hlth Org.* **19**, 427.

HOFFMAN, T. A., CESTERO, R. & BULLOCK, W. E. (1970). *Ann. intern. Med.* **73**, 173.

KABINS, S. A. (1972). *J. Amer. med. Ass.* **219**, 206.

KABINS, S. A., BELNER, B., WALTON, E. & GOLDSTEIN, E. (1970). *Amer. J. med. Sci.* **259**, 133.

KALOWSKI, S., NANRA, R. S., MATHEW, T. H. & KINCAID-SMITH, P. (1973). *Lancet* **1**, 394.

KUNIN, C. M. (1967). *Ann. intern. Med.* **67**, 151.

KUNIN, C. M. & ATUK, N. (1966). *New Engl. J. Med.* **274**, 654.

KUNIN, C. M. & FINKELBERG, Z. (1970). *Ann. intern. Med.* **72**, 349.
KUNIN, C. M. & FINLAND, M. (1959). *J. clin Invest.* **38**, 1509.
KUNIN, C. M., GLAZKO, A. J. & FINLAND, M. (1959). *J. clin. Invest.* **38**, 1498.
LINDBERG, A. A., SON NILSSON, L. H., BUCHT, H. & KALLINGS, L. O. (1966). *Brit. med. J.* **2**, 724.
LYNN, B. (1970). *J. Hosp. Pharm.* **28**, 71.
MACGREGOR, A. B. & LONG, D. A. (1944). *Brit. med. J.* **2**, 686.
MACKAY, D. N. & KAYE, D. (1964). *New Engl. J. Med.* **270**, 394.
MCCRACKEN, G. H., CHRANE, D. F. & THOMAS, M. L. (1971). *J. infect. Dis.* **124**, Supp. p. 214.
MCGEACHIE, J., GIRDWOOD, R. W. A., BURTON, J. A. & KENNEDY, A. C. (1970). *Scottish med. J.* **15**, 257.
MCHENRY, M. C., GAVAN, T. L., GIFFORD, R. W. J. R., GEURKINK, N. A., VAN OMMEN, R. A., TOWN, M. A. & WAGNER, J. G. (1971). *Ann. intern. Med.* **74**, 192.
MCLAUGHLIN, J. E. & REEVES, D. S. (1971). *Lancet* **1**, 261.
MARTINDALE, [W]. (1972). *The Extra Pharmacopoeia,* Ed. R. G. Todd, 26th Ed. London Pharmaceutical Press.
MEISLER, J. M. & SKOLAUT, M. W. (1966). *Amer. J. Hosp. Pharm.* **23**, 557.
NOONE, P. & PATTISON, J. R. (1971). *Lancet* **2**, 575.
NYHAN, W. L. (1961). *J. pediat.* **59**, 1.
OGG, C. S., TOSELAND, P. A. & CAMERON, J. S. (1968). *Brit. med. J.* **2**, 283.
O'GRADY, F. (1971). *Brit. med. Bull.* **27**, 142.
PATEL, J. A. & PHILLIPS, G. L. (1966). *Amer. J. Hosp. Pharm.* **23**, 409.
PRICE, D. J. E. & GRAHAM, D. I. (1970). *Brit. med. J.* **4**, 525.
REINARZ, J. A. & MCINTOSH, D. A. (1966). *Antimicrob. Agents Chemother.* 1965, p. 232.
RUEDY, J. (1966). *Canad. med. Ass. J.* **94**, 257.
SACHS, J., GEER, T., NOELL, P. & KUNIN, C. M. (1968). *New Engl. J. Med.* **278**, 1032.
SCHREINER, G. E. & TEEHAN, B. P. (1971). *Trans. Amer. Soc. for Artificial Internal Organs.* **17**, 513.
SHARPSTONE, P. (1969). *Postgrad. med. J.* **45**, Suppl. p. 38.
SIMBERKOFF, M. S., THOMAS, L., MCGREGOR, D., SHENKEIN, I. & LEVINE, B. B. (1970). *New Engl. J. Med.* **283**, 116.
SØRENEN, A. W. S., SZABO, L., PEDERSEN, A. & SCHARFF, A. (1967). *Postgrad. med. J.* Suppl. May, 37.
STAMEY, T. A., NEMOY, N. J. & HIGGINS, M. (1969). *Invest. Urol.* **6**, 582.
VON HARNACK, G. A., NAUMANN, P., BLUNCK, W., MAI, K. & WINTZER, G. (1964). *Dtsch. med. Wschr.* **89**, 2321.
VON HARNACK, G. A., NAUMANN, P., MAI, K. & BLUNCK, W. (1965). *Dtsch. med. Wschr.* **90**, 1433.
WEBB, J. W. (1969). *Amer. J. Hosp. Pharm.* **26**, 31.
WILLIAMS, D. M., WIMPENNY, J. & ASSCHER, A. W. (1968). *Lancet* **2**, 1058.

CHAPTER 18

SEPTICAEMIA AND ENDOCARDITIS

THERE has been a profound change in the bacterial aetiology of septicaemia in recent years. Blood-stream infection by haemolytic streptococci, formerly common, is now very rarely seen, because of the complete control which penicillin exerts over the earliest stages of infection by this organism. Staphylococcal infections have not been so well controlled, and in the experience of Finland *et al.* (1959) at the Boston City Hospital, there has been a large increase in septicaemia due to various coliform bacilli. The nett result of these changes, and of the substitution of infections more refractory to treatment for those prevalent before, has in Finland's experience been an actually higher mortality from septicaemia than that recorded in 1935.

In proposing treatment for septicaemia, everything depends on an exact bacteriological diagnosis, and much on the sensitivities of the organism, which should be accurately determined to individual appropriate antibiotics and if necessary to combinations. The following are provisional suggestions for each causative organism, some of which can only be tentative, since optimum treatment must be based on laboratory studies of the individual strain.

STREPTOCOCCUS PYOGENES (group A). This now most uncommon infection should always respond to benzyl penicillin.

STAPHYLOCOCCUS AUREUS. Treatment should be begun with cloxacillin as soon as the diagnosis is verified or even strongly suspected, since the strain is likely to be penicillin-resistant. Should it subsequently prove sensitive, it is better to change to benzyl penicillin. Should the patient not respond, treatment directed as for *Staph. aureus* endocarditis (q.v.) is advisable.

COLIFORM INFECTIONS. These, unless transitory and incidental to an infection of the urinary tract from which recovery is possible, tend to occur in patients gravely ill from other

308 ANTIBIOTIC AND CHEMOTHERAPY

causes, and the prognosis is consequently poor. For each type of organism which may be responsible there are alternative treatments, and experience with some of these is so far too limited for assessment of their relative merits. Degrees of bacterial sensitivity to some of these drugs are not constant e.g. sensitivity to ampicillin in *E. coli* varies considerably), and all the resources of the laboratory should be mobilized to provide accurate information as soon as possible. Among antibiotics, those likely to be indicated are for : —

E. coli—ampicillin, cephaloridine, gentamicin, kanamycin, polymyxin.

Proteus—ampicillin, cephaloridine (in each case for some species or strains only), gentamicin, kanamycin.

Klebsiella—polymyxin, cephaloridine (some strains only), gentamicin, kanamycin (also variable).

Pseudomonas—polymyxin, gentamicin, carbenicillin.

Serratia—gentamicin (Wilfert, Barrett and Kass, 1968; Martin *et al.*, 1969).

According to Cox and Harrison (1971) and Holloway and Taylor (1971) gentamicin gave results at least as good as kanamycin, alone or combined with polymyxin, in miscellaneous series or Gram-negative septicaemias (75 and 70 cases respectively). A combination may be considered safer, and Bryant *et al.* (1971), in a study of 218 patients affording useful conclusions about factors affecting prognosis, commend initial treatment with penicillin (or ampicillin or cephalothin, either of which seems more appropriate), kanamycin and sodium colistimethate.

Cotrimoxazole has also been successfully used in the first two of these infections.

A special variety of this type of infection is ' *bacteriaemic shock* ', severe hypotension of sudden onset assumed to be produced by endotoxin from large numbers of bacteria in the circulation. It occurs most commonly after surgical interference with an already infected urinary tract, often transurethral prostatic resection, but sometimes no more than cystoscopy or the blockage or removal of a catheter (Talbot, 1962). Among other procedures, pelvic operations are a cause.

In the extensive series reported by Weil, Shubin and Biddle (1964) shock accompanied 169 out of 692 cases of Gram-negative bacteriaemia, with a mortality of 82 per cent. The commonest infecting organism is *E. coli*; *Klebsiella Aerobacter* spp. come next, then *Proteus* spp.; *Ps. aeruginosa* is a rare cause. This condition calls for immediate anti-bacterial treatment even before verification by blood culture, and the most appropriate antibiotic is gentamicin, which should be administered 8-hourly for the first two days, pending laboratory results. Its bactericidal effect on most of the commonly causative bacteria commends it in preference to chloramphenicol and oxytetracycline, which are suggested by Weil *et al.* on the basis of static sensitivity tests on their strains. Polymyxin may be given in addition to afford even broader cover. Kanamycin is a possible alternative to gentamicin and has been used. It should be recognized that shock may also occur in a Gram-positive septicaemia.

CANDIDA ALBICANS. Septicaemia is sometimes caused by this organism, usually in patients in whom its overgrowth in the respiratory or alimentary tract has followed treatment with tetracyclines. Some good can be done by the application of nystatin to the primarily infected surface, but a systemic effect can best be exerted with amphotericin B. 5-Fluorocystosine (p. 235) is a better tolerated but rather less effective alternative.

Acute Endocarditis

This condition is liable to complicate almost any uncontrolled septicaemia, and much that has already been said therefore applies to it. Since it will be necessary to kill all the bacteria embedded in vegetations, the choice of a bactericidal drug is even more imperative, and treatment will need to be longer continued. Gonococcal and pneumococcal endocarditis, not hitherto mentioned, were sometimes classified as acute: they are now very rarely seen. Each of these infections and the endocarditis sometimes complicating ' chronic ' meningococcal septicaemia, should respond to benzyl penicillin, again with the proviso that in the treatment of endocarditis the course of treatment must be greatly extended.

Subacute Endocarditis

Antibiotics have transformed the outlook in this disease more than in any other. Formerly invariably fatal, the infection can now be cured in most patients by well-directed treatment, although severe residual damage to valves may limit the period of survival.

The diagnosis must be verified, if possible, by blood culture, and the organism found should be exactly identified. Further, this is a disease in which something more than ordinary antibiotic sensitivity tests is called for. If penicillin appears to be the antibiotic of choice, its minimum inhibitory concentration should be determined by a tube dilution test with no more than two-fold differences. If this concentration proves to be unduly high, it cannot be assumed that penicillin will be fully bactericidal, and tests should be undertaken to determine how such an effect can be achieved: a combination will often be necessary (Chap. 29).

Consideration in further detail must be in relation to the causative organisms.

STREPTOCOCCUS VIRIDANS. This is not really a species, but a highly heterogeneous group of streptococci having little else necessarily in common except the property of alpha-haemolysis. In addition an endocarditis may be caused by streptococci, presumably derived from the mouth, which are non-haemolytic or have some other peculiar character: some, for instance, are micro-aerophilic. What follows refers to any streptococcus which is neither *Str. pyogenes* nor *Str. faecalis*.

Such organisms are usually highly sensitive to penicillin. Of 339 strains quantitatively tested in the extensive collaborative study reported on by Cates and Christie (1951), 291 were not more than twice as resistant as the Oxford staphylococcus: *i.e.*, they were inhibited by about 0·05 unit (0·03 μg.) per ml. or less. Various systems of treatment have been used, now too familiar to call for detailed description. The choice lies between benzyl penicillin given 6-hourly or by infusion, procaine penicillin given twice daily, or even an acid-resistant penicillin given in adequate doses (if these are tolerated) orally. Phenoxymethyl penicillin has so been used; Gray *et al.* (1964) were successful in 9 out of 10 cases with propicillin. If one of these is used the exact degree of sensitivity to it of the causative streptococcus should be determined, and not merely that to benzyl penicillin. Such treatment can be reinforced with probenecid, and/or by also giving streptomycin.

The necessary duration of these treatments has always been in some doubt; courses have sometimes been continued for 6 weeks. Valuable guidance on this is afforded by the studies of the late Morton Hamburger of Cincinnati and his colleagues (Tan *et al.*, 1971). Over a period of years they treated three groups of patients, each for 2 weeks only. Of 13 given benzyl penicillin only in doses of 15-20 mega units daily 2 relapsed but responded to a second course. Each of the other groups received 0·5-1 g. streptomycin twice daily, one composed of 9 patients also receiving parenteral benzyl penicillin, the second of 27 patients all given 600-750 mg. phenoxymethyl penicillin orally at 4-hour intervals. No patient in either of these groups relapsed, and numerous specimens of serum from the last group were highly inhibitory for the causative streptococcus. This system of treatment, requiring few injections and a relatively short hospital stay, has evidently much to commend it. It removes any need for maintaining a continuous intravenous drip, which has been known to lead to disastrous secondary infection (Darrell and Garrod, 1969).

These instructions apply only to normally penicillin-sensitive strains. Higher degrees of resistance bring the organism into the same therapeutic category as the following species.

STREPTOCOCCUS FAECALIS. Endocarditis due to this organism has been said to occur in women of 25 and men of 60, the respective sources of infection being the uterus after abortion and the urinary tract, and our experience tallies closely with this statement. It occurs occasionally in other kinds of patient, including even children. The antibiotics to which the streptococcus is most sensitive *in vitro* are almost always the tetracyclines, but treatment with these, or with erythromycin or chloramphenicol, almost invariably fails. These are bacteristatic drugs, and it should be an axiom that for the treatment of endocarditis generally a bactericidal antibiotic or combination is essential. Unless the vegetation is sterilized—even if a singe coccus remains, damaged but viable —relapse is likely to follow.

11

Penicillin in optimal concentration (6 μg./ml.) is bacteri-cidal, but not completely so : some survivors remain (Jawetz, 1952). Jawetz and Sonne (1966) report that penicillin was was totally bactericidal for two out of ten strains, but support this with no clinical evidence : all their nine patients were treated with combinations of penicillin and other antibiotics.

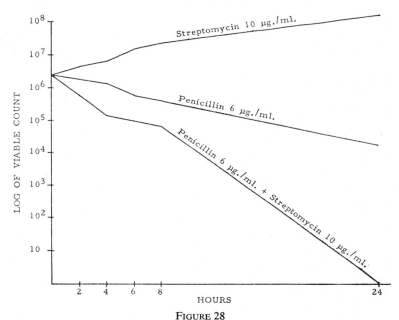

FIGURE 28

Viable counts in broth containing an optimal concentration of penicillin (6 μg./ml.), streptomycin (10 μg./ml.) or both, and inoculated with a strain of *Str. faecalis* (G.F.) from the blood of a patient with bacterial endocarditis. Penicillin causes only a slow fall in the viable count. Streptomycin fails to prevent growth (M.I.C. was 16 μg./ml.): the combination sterilizes the preparation. This combination was used successfully in treating not only the original attack of endocarditis but a recurrence eight months later.

Two out of nine cases described by Toh and Ball (1960) were successfully treated with penicillin alone, but the sensitivity of these strains to penicillin was so exceptional (M.I.C. 0·1 and 0·05 μg./ml.) that they must have been highly atypical. The experience of others has been that penicillin alone will not eradicate this infection. It appears that the same is true of ampicillin, to which the organism is rather

more sensitive (a difference of about two-fold). Gray *et al.*
(1964) refer to it as ' the penicillin of choice ' for this infection,
but of their two patients treated with it, one was also given
erythromycin throughout, and the other relapsed and had to
be re-treated with ampicillin + streptomycin. Kayser (1971),
on the basis of extensive *in vitro* studies, concludes that ampicillin should not be used alone, but suggests that it may be
preferable to penicillin as a combination with streptomycin.

The fact that penicillin and streptomycin together will
exterminate a population of *Str. faecalis*, whereas neither alone
is capable of doing so, has long been recognized; it will do so
even when the concentration of streptomycin used is incapable
when acting alone even of inhibiting growth, as is shown in
Fig. 28. This outstanding example of synergy has frequently
been demonstrated by *in vitro* methods, and the fact that a
similar action is exerted *in vivo* is shown by the study of
Sapico, Keys and Hewitt (1972) of the effect of these antibiotics,
singly and together, on the bacteriaemia accompanying experimental enterococcal endocarditis in the dog. This combination
has been the regular treatment for this infection for over twenty
years (Robbins and Tompsett, 1951; Cates, Christie and Garrod,
1951), but it may be modified in two ways; ampicillin may be
preferable to penicillin and another aminoglycoside to streptomycin.

Str. faecalis is sometimes highly resistant to streptomycin;
the M.I.C for the strain from a case reported by Havard,
Garrod and Waterworth (1959) was 50,000 μg./ml., and no
synergy with penicillin was demonstrable, but penicillin +
neomycin was totally bactericidal. This combination was therefore used, and recovery achieved at the cost of almost total
loss of hearing. Tompsett and Pizette (1962) were successful
with the usual combination in treating two patients infected
with highly streptomycin-resistant strains, but now that alternative aminoglycosides are available, the dependability of such
treatment need not be further tested. Kanamycin is the second
choice, and in contrast to the fate of the earlier patient given
neomycin, Case 8 of Garrod and Waterworth (1962a), given an
almost identical course of penicillin + kanamycin, recovered
with no loss of hearing. Gentamicin should also now be considered; Watanakunakorn (1871), studying one hundred strains,

found none resistant to it, and a synergic bactericidal effect with penicillin was invariable, whereas penicillin + streptomycin had no such effect on more than a third of the strains so tested, most of which were highly streptomycin-resistant.

Although combinations including other antibiotics may occasionally seem indicated (Jawetz and Sonne, 1966), treatment with a penicillin and an aminoglycoside will almost always be the best available. The combination to be used must be chosen on the basis of tests of combined bactericidal action *in vitro*, preferably carried out by an expert in these methods, which are described in Chapter 29. The penicillin should be given in a dose calculated to maintain the optimum bactericidal concentration in the blood, which for benzyl penicillin is 6 μg./ml. and for ampicillin rather less; about 10 mega units of benzyl penicillin daily by continuous infusion, perhaps reinforced with probenecid, will achieve this. Streptomycin or kanamycin are given intramuscularly, ideally at 8-hour intervals, suitable total daily doses being respectively 1·5 and 1·0 g; the dose of gentamicin should be lower. Whether the duration of such treatment, hitherto rarely given for less than 4 weeks, can safely be reduced is not known, but might justifiably be subjected to trial.

STAPHYLOCOCCUS AUREUS. Endocarditis caused by this organism is of two kinds. An acute form is a complication of uncontrolled septicaemia and can probably attack normal valves. The subacute form occurs only in patients with predisposing rheumatic or congenital lesions, and may be of more insidious onset, the source of the infection being sometimes a trivial lesion such as a boil, although it usually runs a more rapid course with higher fever than a true ' endocarditis lenta '.

Penicillin, if the strain is sensitive to it, methicillin, an isoxazolyl penicillin or cephalothin (see p. 91) if not, should be the mainstay of treatment, but since a total bactericidal effect is often not achieved even by an antibiotic to which the strain is fully sensitive, full tests of bactericidal action by single antibiotics and combinations should be carried out. It may well be found that the addition of, for instance, streptomycin or kanamycin to the penicillin will convert incomplete bactericidal effect to complete, and if so this combination should unhesitatingly be used. For a methicillin-resistant strain such a combination is essential, and Bulger (1967) has shown that kanamycin together with methicillin or cephalothin exerts a synergic effect against such organisms. Even to such a combination the response may be poor; among 31 cases of staphylococcal septicaemia caused by methicillin-resistant strains, only 6 of whom had endocarditis, reported by Acar, Courvalin and Chabbert (1971) 11 out of 18 treated with cephaloridine or cephalothin + kanamycin or gentamicin still had positive blood cultures after three days. These are exceptionally discouraging results, the reasons for which are not clear. Successful treatment of one case of this infection, involving a prosthetic valve, with cotrimoxazole, accompanied for the first 2 weeks of the course by penicillin, is reported by Shafqat, Shah and Syed (1971).

STAPHYLOCOCCUS ALBUS. This is an infection the existence of which may be overlooked because the organism in a blood culture is taken for a contaminant. A helpful sign that the finding is significant is flocculent growth, due to the action of agglutinin which has always been formed by the time a culture is made: we have rarely seen uniform turbidity in a genuinely positive blood culture, even one containing *E. coli*.

This infection occurs in two types of patient. It has always been recognized as an uncommon variety of endocarditis of usually unknown origin in predisposed subjects. Recently it has also been seen as a direct sequel of open heart operations, most often mitral valvotomy, when it may be supposed that implantation occurs during the operation itself. Infections so produced are also sometimes due to *Staph. aureus*. Quinn and Cox (1964) describe 16 *Staph. albus* infections, nine of the first type and seven of the second. In all the idiopathic cases the staphylococcus was sensitive to penicillin, and penicillin, usually with streptomycin, cured the eight treated. From the ' post-cardiotomy ' cases six of the seven strains were penicillin-resistant, and despite a variety of antibiotic treatments, three of these patients died. No series has hitherto been published which enables optimum treatment for a penicillin-resistant *Staph. albus* infection to be defined. Each case demands full laboratory investigation on the lines already indicated.

A peculiar form of infection commonly caused by *Staph. albus* is the colonization of Spitz-Holter valves. Bruce *et al.* (1963) saw 19 patients with persistent bacteriaemia among 300 subjected to ventriculo-caval shunt operations employing this device. *Staph. albus* was cultivated from the blood in eight, *Staph. aureus* in six patients in whom the valve had become exposed by pressure necrosis, and *Serratia marcescens* in four. Despite treatment which sterilizes the blood-stream and is calculated to deal with infection involving any living tissue, bacteria persist in the valve, and the only effective treatment is its removal.

HAEMOPHILUS spp. *H. influenzae,* or, it is said, more usually *H. parainfluenzae,* is an uncommon cause of endocarditis, and not enough cases have been reported in recent years for it to be possible to define optimum treatment. Ampicillin, as a bactericidal antibiotic to which these organisms are usually highly sensitive, if necessary combined with streptomycin, would be a logical first choice.

MISCELLANEOUS INFECTIONS. Those due to *Neisseria* spp and *Erysipelothrix rhusiopathiae* should respond to penicillin. The treatment of *Brucella* endocarditis is as for undulant fever, but with a longer course and perhaps higher dosage. Coliform infections are usually fatal: antibiotics likely to be indicated are mentioned in the section on Septicaemia at the beginning of this chapter. Fowle and Zorab (1970) cured an *Esch. coli* endocarditis with trimethoprim-sulphamethoxazole after appropriate antibiotics had failed. *Candida albicans* endocarditis should be treated with amphotericin B: several successes have been recorded.

COXIELLA BURNETI is now being increasingly recognized as a cause of endocarditis. This occurs mainly in rheumatic subjects and at varying intervals after an attack of Q fever. Males preponderate and the aortic valve is that usually affected. A high titre of complement-fixing antibody for phase 2 antigen of *C. burneti* enables the diagnosis to be made (Marmion, 1962). Treatment with tetracycline delays the progress of the infection, but does not eradicate it. Surgical treatment becomes essential, and replacement with a prosthesis is preferable to a homograft (Kristinsson and Bentall, 1967): four patients undergoing this operation were successfully treated thereafter with tetracycline to prevent recurrence, this having continued in one of them for two years at the time of reporting.

CAUSE UNKNOWN. Repeatedly negative blood cultures in the face of strongly suspicious clinical features present a difficult problem. According to Griffith and Levinson (1949) it can be of little use to go on repeating blood cultures: in their series of 140, 129 were positive at the first and all but two of the remainder at the second attempt. Nevertheless one should perhaps not be content with less than 8-10 cultures made over a period of several days before admitting defeat. It is assumed that all appropriate laboratory tricks have been tried, including the use of liquoid, pour plates, anaerobiosis and extra CO_2. The possibility of *Chlamidia psittaci* infection should also be considered when the patient has a pneumonitis or gives a history of contact with birds (Levison *et al.*, 1971).

The response to penicillin in 34 patients with negative blood cultures in Cates and Christie's (1951) series was poor. Probably the best ' blind ' treatment for a supposed bacterial infection would be with penicillin and streptomycin, but this would be without effect on a rickettsial infection, for which serological tests should be carried out in any suspicious case

It is often extremely difficult to obtain a positive culture in a patient who has had inadequate preliminary treatment with penicillin, as by a practitioner before hospital admission: the two gravest sins committed in connection with this disease are to ignore the possibility of it despite strongly suggestive signs until it is far advanced, and to start treatment before attempting to verify the diagnosis by blood culture. After a full course of treatment cultures may also be negative at first although relapse is taking place.

Treatment of Penicillin-sensitive Patients

Penicillins play at least an important part in the optimum treatment of almost all forms of endocarditis, and nothing can fully replace them. If a patient with endocarditis is said to be penicillin-sensitive, this should first be verified by a cautious test dose, and may be proved untrue. If the condition is verified, there are two alternatives. One is to find a substitute.

Most other bactericidal antibiotics, such as streptomycin and the neomycin group, have an inadequate effect on streptococci when acting alone, but may serve in combination with erythromycin or cephaloridine in *Str. viridans* infections. The second, and in our view preferable, course is to administer penicillin and protect the patient against reaction to it, either with antihistamines, as originally advocated by Maslansky and Sanger (1952) or with steroids. Prednisone in doses not exceeding 60 mg. daily served to protect three patients described by Raper and Kemp (1965) during courses of treatment with penicillin or ampicillin. Green, Peters and Geraci (1967) describe extensive experience with these methods.

An alternative is treatment with vancomycin, which may also be resorted to because other treatment has failed. Friedberg, Rosen and Bienstock (1968) report six successfully treated cases, four infected with *Str. faecalis,* two treated from the outset with vancomycin because of penicillin sensitivity and the remainder because reactions occurred to initial treatment with penicillin and streptomycin: in some of them this treatment must at least have contributed to recovery. Mandell, Lindsey and Hook (1970) demonstrated strong synergy between vancomycin and streptomycin in their action on *Str. faecalis,* but do not discuss the advisability or otherwise of combining two ototoxic drugs.

Laboratory Control of Treatment

Blood cultures should be repeated if the response to treatment is inadequate, although they are likely to remain positive only if the antibiotic is singularly ineffective, as in the staphylococcal infection treated with cephaloridine described by Burgess and Evans (1966).

If any system of treatment is being used which justifies doubt about the attainment of adequate blood levels, the antibiotic should be assayed in the blood, preferably at times when maximum and minimum levels are to be expected. This doubt is most likely to arise during oral treatment, when appropriate times would be at one and four hours after a dose, i.e. at the peak following absorption and immediately before a further dose is due. Assays are also required to determine that excessive levels, particularly of streptomycin, kanamycin or vancomycin, are not being maintained in patients with possibly impaired renal function. If administration is at six-hour intervals and blood is taken at the end of this period, the level of either of these antibiotics should have fallen to not >10 μg./ml.

A third control procedure, largely employed in the United States but less commonly in this country and deserving more frequent use, is to determine the maximum dilution in which the patient's serum retains a bactericidal effect on his own organism. A method for doing this is described in Chapter 29.

Prophylaxis

Dental extraction, tonsillectomy and other operations causing bacteriaemia should not be undertaken in predisposed patients i.e., past sufferers from rheumatic fever or those with a known predisposing congenital abnormality) without antibiotic ' cover '. The object of this is to destroy bacteria which enter the circulation before they can colonize a valve, and penicillin, which kills the great majority of a susceptible bacterial population within four hours, is very suitable for the purpose. Penicillin should therefore be given at such a time that the maximum concentration in the blood after the first dose is being reached at the time of the operation : appropriate intervals are a few minutes before if ' soluble ' penicillin is given, or one to two hours for procaine penicillin. A single dose containing both these forms of penicillin, such as Fortified Procaine Penicillin Injection B.P. (300 mg. procaine penicillin and 60 mg. benzyl penicillin) given immediately before extraction provides both an immediate high level and a persistent effect, and should not require repetition.

Some have taken the view that the object should be so far as possible to sterilize the area of operation (mouth, throat, etc.) to which end penicillin administration is begun several days beforehand. This is an extremely dangerous policy, because the effect of such treatment is to eliminate the sensitive streptococci from the mouth and to permit a small minority of much more resistant strains to multiply in their place. These highly resistant streptococci are constantly present in the saliva of patients having penicillin treatment, and appear within two days of its being started. Garrod and Waterworth (1962b) who report these findings, which have since been verified by Naiman and Barrow (1963) and by Tozer, Boutflower and Gillespie (1966), also describe two cases of endocarditis due to such organisms, one immediately following dental extraction which was preceded by several days of penicillin ' cover ', the other an evident re-infection following dental extraction during a full course of treatment for an endocarditis caused originally by a sensitive streptococcus. It is often said that suspicious teeth are best extracted during a course of treatment for endocarditis because this treatment affords protection: if these findings and their interpretation are accepted this belief must be abandoned. It is better that a full dental examination and any necessary treatment should be carried out as soon as the diagnosis is suspected and while positive blood cultures are awaited.

If dental extraction is necessary in patients receiving small doses of penicillin for the prophylaxis of rheumatic fever, cover may be afforded by an injection of 1 mega unit of penicillin + 0·5 g. streptomycin, a combination which is usually bactericidal for the moderately resistant streptococci found in the mouths of such patients. If large doses of penicillin are being given, and particularly if streptomycin is being given in addition, as in the actual treatment of endocarditis, it seems from the findings of Tozer *et al.* (1966) that cover is best afforded by an injection of 0·5 g. cephaloridine. This can be repeated, or followed by a short course of erythromycin. This proceeding may also be preferred for patients on low prophylactic doses. It should also be employed in patients who have had a therapeutic course of penicillin at any time during the preceding six weeks, since the reversion of the mouth flora from penicillin resistance to sensitivity is a slow process.

Vancomycin, originally suggested by Garrod and Waterworth (1962b) should also be effective according to the findings of Tozer *et al.*, but is much more inconvenient to administer.

Antibiotic cover is also required for procedures in other parts of the body. Outstanding among these are operations on the heart itself, including mitral valvotomy and the insertion of artificial valves. A five-day course of penicillin + streptomycin is commonly given, and should be capable of eliminating any staphylococci, but has apparently not always succeeded. Holswade *et al.* (1964) tried five different antibiotic combinations in 300 open-heart operations, and conclude by recommending methicillin alone (1 g. six-hourly). Some strains of *Staph. albus* are resistant to methicillin, and might not be disposed of by this treatment. Nelson *et al.* (1965) obtained their best results with the combination of penicillin, streptomycin and oxacillin. The best method of protecting these patients has perhaps yet to be defined. If the object is simply to destroy any staphylococci accidentally implanted at operatoin a 3- or 4-day course started at the time of operation should suffice, and a logical choice would be a penicillinase-resistant penicillin (or cephalosporin) + an aminoglycoside.

In predisposed subjects various forms of surgical interference with the urinary tract, including even dilatation of a urethral stricture, may be followed by *S. faecalis* endocarditis. Penicillin + streptomycin should afford appropriate cover.

Undulant Fever (Brucellosis)

The subject of this and the succeeding section are included here for the possibly inadequate reason that both diseases are accompanied by bacteriaemia.

Early specific treatment of *Brucella* infections with, first, sulphonamides and then with streptomycin, was only partially successful: combined treatment with both was more so. The advent of the broad spectrum antibiotics altered the outlook profoundly, because thenceforth an easily administered treatment regularly brought about defervescence within a few days, usually with relief of all symptoms and apparent cure. Unfortunately relapse was common, but usually responded to a further course.

Although there are isolated reports of the successful use of other antibiotics, tetracyclines have been the mainstay of treatment of this disease for many years. Which of this group to use, in what doses and for how long, and whether to reinforce its action with streptomycin (although this forms a theoretically antagonistic combination) are subjects discussed in previous editions of this book, and repetition here seems unnecessary. Of more immediate interest is the question whether this treatment should be replaced with cotrimoxazole.

According to Lal *et al.* (1970) although *Br. abortus* is only moderately sensitive to trimethoprim, it is highly so to its combination with sulphamethoxazole (M.I.C. 0·05 and 1·0 μg./ml. respectively of the two drugs together). They treated four cases of acute *Br. abortus* infection with this combination with successful results, although the outcome was doubtful in one who for a time was given trimethoprim alone because of a sulphonamide rash. Hassan *et al.* (1971) treated 8 cases of *Br. melitensis* infection in Cairo with a good immediate response in all of them to a 3-week course of 10 and 50 mg./kg. daily of trimethoprim and sulphamethoxazole respectively. Of 3 relapses 2 responded to a further 6-week course; one was given tetracycline and streptomycin because of suspected spondylitis. W. K. Daikos, in a hitherto unpublished report on a series of 50 cases in Greece, also strongly commends this treatment. There is general agreement on the simplicity, safety and freedom from side effects of this treatment, and on its rapid relief of symptoms. Although optimum dosage remains to be defined, and even allowing for some initial over-enthusiasm, it seems likely that cotrimoxazole may replace antibiotics for this purpose.

Tularaemia

This disease responds well to streptomycin, a course lasting about seven days eradicating the infection. Chloramphenicol or tetracyclines have a similar immediate effect, but with some tendency to relapse. The fact that streptomycin, by virtue of its bactericidal action, eliminates the organism, whereas chloramphenicol only suppresses it, has been shown by preventive administration to volunteers inoculated subcutaneously. A report by Overholt *et al.* (1961) concerns 42 cases occurring in laboratory staff at Fort Detrick despite previous vaccination: the infection was acquired by inhalation, and was therefore of the 'typhoidal' type with pulmonary lesions, although of very varying severity. A streptomycin-resistant strain was responsible for 75 per cent. Treatment with 2 g. tetracycline daily for 10 days or more was followed by relapse in five out of 15 cases treated during the first week, but in none of 16 in whom it was begun after this time, suggesting that an adequate immune response combines to render tetracycline alone effective. On the other hand, Knothe and Helpap (1965) in patients treated with tetracycline during an epidemic in Schleswig-Holstein, obtained good results when the antibiotic was given early and less satisfactory when it was delayed. These authors' poor results with streptomycin may have been due in some patients to inadequate dosage, but it also seems possible that American and European strains of *Br. tularensis* differ in their drug susceptibility.

REFERENCES

ACAR, J. F., COURVALIN, P. & CHABBERT, Y. A. (1971). *Antimicrob. Agents and Chemother.* 1970, p. 280.

BRUCE, A. M., LORBER, J., SHEDDEN, W. I. H. & ZACHARY, R. B. (1963). *Develop. Med. Child Neurol.* 5, 461.

BRYANT, R. E., HOOD, A. F., HOOD, C. E. & KOENIG, M. G. (1971). *Arch. intern. Med.* 127, 120.

BULGER, R. J. (1967) *Lancet* 1, 17.

BURGESS, H. A. & EVANS, R. J. (1966). *Brit. med. J.* 2, 1244.

CATES, J. E. & CHRISTIE, R. V. (1951). *Quart. J. Med.* 20, 93.

CATES, J. E., CHRISTIE, R. V. & GARROD, L. P. (1951). *Brit. med. J.* 1, 653.

COX, C. E. & HARRISON, L. H. (1971). *J. infect. Dis.* 124, Dec. Suppl., 156.

DARRELL, J. H. & GARROD, L. P. (1969). *Brit. med. J.* 2, 481.

EVANS, A. D., POWELL, D. E. B. & BURRELL, C. D. (1959). *Lancet* i, 864.

FINLAND, M., JONES, W. F, JR. & BARNES, M. W. (1959). *J. Amer. med. Ass.* 170, 2188.

FOWLE, A. S. E. & ZORAB, P. A. (1970). *Brit. Heart J.* 32, 127.

FRIEDBERG, C. K., ROSEN, K. M. & BIENSTOCK, P. A. (1968). *Arch. intern. Med.* 122, 134.

GARROD, L. P. & WATERWORTH, P. M. (1962a). *J. clin. Path.* 15, 328.

GARROD, L. P. & WATERWORTH, P. M. (1962b). *Brit. Heart J.* 24, 39.

GRAY, I. R., TAI, A. R., WALLACE, J. G. & CALDER, J. H. (1964). *Lancet* ii, 110.

GREEN, G. R., PETERS, G. A. & GERACI, J. E. (1967). *Ann. intern. Med.* 67, 235.

GRIFFITH, G. C. & LEVINSON, D. C. (1949). *Calif. med.* 71, 403.

HASSAN, A., ERIAN, M. M., FARID, Z., HATHOUT, S. D. & SORENSEN, K. (1971). *Brit. med. J.* 3, 159.

HAVARD, C. W. H., GARROD, L. P. & WATERWORTH, P. M. (1959). *Brit. med. J.* 1, 688.

HOLLOWAY, W. J. & TAYLOR, W. A. (1971). *J. infect. Dis.* 124, Dec. Suppl., 180.

HOLSWADE, G. R., DINEEN, P., REDO, S. F. & GOLDSMITH, E. I. (1964). *Arch. Surg.* 89, 970.

JAWETZ, E. (1952). *Arch. intern. Med.* 90, 301.

JAWETZ, E., GUNNISON, J. B. & SPECK, R. S. (1951). *New Engl. J. Med.* 245, 966.

JAWETZ, E. & SONNE, M. (1966). *New Engl. J. Med.* 274, 710.

KAYSER, F. H. (1971). *Ztschr. med. Mikrobiol. Immunol.* 156, 125.

KNOTHE, H. & HELPAP, B. (1965). *Dtsch. med. Wschr.* 90, 2361.

KRISTINSSON, A. & BENTALL, H. H. (1967). *Lancet* 2, 693.

LAL, S., MODAWAL, K. K., FOWLE, A. S. E., PEACH, B. & POPHAM, R. D. (1970). *Brit. med. J.* 3, 256.

LEVISON, D. A., GUTHRIE, W., WARD, C., GREEN, D. M. & ROBERTSON, P. G. C. (1971). *Lancet* 2, 844.

MANDELL, G. L., LINDSEY, E. & HOOK, E. W. (1970). *Amer. J. med. Sci.* **259,** 346.
MARMION, B. P. (1962). *J. Hyg. Epidem. (Praha)* **6,** 79.
MARTIN, C. M., CUOMO, A. J., GERAGHTY, M. J., ZAGER, J. R. & MANDES, T. C. (1969). *J. infect. Dis.* **119,** 506.
MASLANSKY, L. & SANGER, M. D. (1952). *Antibiot. and Chemother.* **2,** 385.
NAIMAN, R. A. & BARROW, J. G. (1963). *Ann. intern. Med.* **58,** 768.
NELSON, R. M., JENSON, C. B., PETERSON, C. A. & SANDERS, B. C. (1965). *Arch. Surg.* **90,** 731.
OVERHOLT, E. L., TIGERTT, W. D., KADULL, P. J. & WARD, M. K. (1961). *Amer. J. Med.* **30,** 785.
QUINN, E. L. & COX, F. (1964). *Antimicrob. Agents and Chemother.,* 1963, p. 635.
RAPER, A. J. & KEMP, V. E. (1965). *New Engl. J. Med.* **273,** 297.
ROBBINS, W. C. & TOMPSETT, R. (1951). *Amer. J. Med.* **10,** 278.
SAPICO, F. L., KEYS, T. F. & HEWITT, W. L. (1972). *Amer. J. med. Sci.* **263,** 128.
SHAFQAT. S. H., SHAH, S. A. A. & SYED, S. A. (1971). *Brit. Heart J.* **33,** 974.
TALBOT, C. H. (1962). *Lancet* **i,** 668.
TAN, J S., TERHUNE, C. A. JR., KAPLAN, S. & HAMBURGER, M. (1971). *Lancet* **2,** 1340.
TOH, C. C. S. & BALL, K. P. (1960). *Brit. med. J.* **2,** 640.
TOMPSETT, R. & PIZETTE, M. (1962). *Arch. intern. Med.* **109,** 146.
TOZER, R. A., BOUTFLOWER, S. & GILLESPIE, W. A. (1966). *Lancet* **i,** 686.
WATANAKUNAKORN, C. (1971). *J. infect. Dis.* **124,** 581.
WEIL, M. H., SHUBIN, H. & BIDDLE. M. (1964). *Ann. intern. Med.* **60,** 384.
WILFERT, J. N., BARRETT, F. R. & KASS, E. H. (1968). *New Engl. J. Med.* **279,** 286.

CHAPTER 19

INFECTIONS OF SKIN, SOFT TISSUES AND BONES

ANTIBACTERIAL preparations for topical application to the skin should have a wide spectrum since many superficial infections have a mixed bacterial flora. Local applications are very liable to lead to the development of drug-resistance, so that agents to which bacteria rapidly become resistant should be avoided.

The agent must be non-irritating and non-toxic to leucocytes and other phagocytic cells and granulation tissue, and antibacterial drugs liable to give rise to hypersensitivity should not be used. Antibiotics suitable for systemic administration should be avoided, so that if drug-resistance or skin hypersensitivity should occur the patient is not thereby deprived of the benefits of a valuable drug for systemic treatment should this become necessary. The skin is neither entirely impervious to topically applied antibiotics nor unaffected by systemically administered agents. In an experimental system, fucidin penetrated the skin at a rate comparable with that of glucocorticoids (Vickers, 1969). Penicillin, tetracycline and erythromycin penetrated at lower rates and ampicillin very slowly (Knight, Vickers and Percival, 1969). Marples and Kligman (1971) review the ways in which antibacterial agents reach the skin and discuss the resulting effects on the microflora.

Preparations

Many antibacterial agents are available in proprietary preparations as creams, ointments, powders, lotions and sprays. The attributes of wide antibacterial spectrum, little chance of emergent resistance and very limited parenteral usage are provided in various combinations of bacitracin (or its relatives), neomycin (or its relatives) and polymyxin.

Amongst those commercially available are:

BACITRACIN AND NEOMYCIN. Neomycin and bacitracin ointment B.N.F. contains neomycin sulphate 5 mg. and bacitracin zinc 500 units per g. Numerous similar proprietary preparations are available some of which *e.g.* Cicatrin (Calmic: powder and aerosol) contain added amino acids which are said to promote wound healing. Graneodin (Squibb) is a similar preparation in which bacitracin is replaced by gramicidin; in Ecomytrin (Warner) bacitracin is replaced by amphomycin (a peptide antibiotic produced by *Streptomyces canus* principally active against Gram positive cocci). Soframycin (cream and ointment) contains framycetin 1·5 per cent and gramicidin 0·005 per cent.

BACITRACIN, NEOMYCIN AND POLYMYXIN. Available as creams, *e.g.* Polybactrin (Calmic): bacitracin zinc 400 units, neomycin sulphate 3,300 units and polymyxin B 5,000 units per g.; as powders or as sprays: Polybactrin (Calmic); Rikospray Antibiotic (Riker); Trispray (Pigot and Smith) and others. Framspray (Fisons) is a similar mixture with framycetin substituted for neomycin.

Several other combinations of neomycin with polymyxin, or bacitracin with polymyxin and many similar mixtures with added corticosteroids are also available.

It may not be widely known that antibiotics are incorporated in some cosmetics and deodorants (Carney, 1963). The presence of neomycin in such preparations may contribute to the development of sensitization and the emergence of resistant strains.

Antiseptics

There is, in addition, a very wide choice of antiseptics, singly or in combination, for local application. They include:

CETRIMIDE (Cetavlon, *I.C.I.,* and numerous other proprietary preparations) B.P., B.N.F.: 0·5 per cent cream.

CHLORHEXIDINE (Hibitane, *I.C.I.*) cream B.P.C., B.N.F.: 1 per cent. Naseptin (*I.C.I.*) contains chlorhexidine hydrochloride 0·1 per cent and neomycin sulphate 0·5 per cent. It is most commonly used for application to the nose in treatment of nasal carriers of staphylococci.

DIBROMO-PROPAMIDINE ISETHIONATE B.P. (Brulidine *M. and B.*); Propamidine isethionate, B.P.C.: 0·15 per cent creams.

POLYNOXYLIN (Anaflex, *Geistlich*) 10 per cent cream and paste.

QUINOLINES: Clioquinol (Vioform, *Ciba*) 3 per cent cream. Halquinol (Quinolor, *Squibb*) 0·5 per cent ointment; Potassium hydroxyquinoline sulphate, B.P.C. (Quinoderm, *Quinoderm Ltd.*) 0·5 per cent cream.

Many preparations for local dermatological use also contain steroids, and numerous warnings have been given about the possible facilitation of superinfection, especially with fungi. While the danger is undoubtedly real and must be watched for, it appears that in the majority of cases the benefits of inflammation control outweigh any deleterious effect on infection (Davis *et al.,* 1968).

SUPERFICIAL INFECTIONS

Impetigo Contagiosa

This is an infection of the superficial layers of the epidermis which occurs in two forms (Dillon, 1968). The commoner is the vesicular, golden-crusted variety which is primarily of streptococcal origin but is commonly superinfected with staphylococci (Markowitz *et al.*, 1965). Less common is the bullous variety, a pure staphylococcal infection, which may occur in hospital nurseries in the severe epidemic form called impetigo (or pemphigus) neonatorum. The streptococci and staphylococci are often of unusual types peculiar to skin infections. Most mild cases respond fairly readily to local treatment. After removal of heavy crusting with warm water the lesions should be treated two or three times a day with ointments or sprays containing neomycin and bacitracin.

In more severe cases, the results of systemic erythromycin therapy (250 mg. 6-hourly for 5 days) are generally superior to those of topical treatment (Hughes and Wan, 1967). Topical erythromycin is ineffective.

Dodge *et al.* (1968) say that mild cases respond to antibacterial soaps and that systemic erythromycin should be reserved for severe cases and those in whom topical treatment fails. Systemic treatment should be supplemented by an antibacterial soap to limit the possibility of relapse.

In some patients with mild crusted impetigo it may be felt that systemic treatment is necessary in order to prevent the sequelae of streptococcal infection. It is currently unsettled whether the unusual streptococcal types peculiar to skin infections are important in this respect but some patients are infected with classical nephritogenic strains. Hughes and Wan (1967) had one case of overt glomerulonephritis and three of asymptomatic haematuria amongst those topically treated in their group of 62 children. Derrick and Dillon (1970) confirm that while oral penicillin and erythromycin are clinically effective, systemic benzathine penicillin is superior in eradicating streptococci. Of their 708 cases of streptococcal skin infection, 91 yielded nephritogenic strains and amongst patients infected with those strains, five developed acute nephritis.

Where erythromycin-resistant staphylococci are involved cloxacillin is required.

Impetigo Neonatorum (*Pemphigus neonatorum*). Milder
cases of this staphylococcal infection in the new-born may
respond to local treatment as for *Impetigo contagiosa,* but the
condition occurs in a severe epidemic form, in which case early
systemic treatment is essential and measures to control the
outbreak are required (Albert *et al.,* 1970). Since in this
hospital-acquired disease the infecting staphylococcus is likely
to be resistant to penicillin, while waiting for laboratory reports treatment should be started at once with cloxacillin,
clindamycin or fucidin.

Sycosis Barbae. Mild and early cases usually respond to
local treatment as for *Impetigo contagiosa,* but relapses are
frequent. The source of infection is sometimes nasal carriage, in
which case the nose should be treated as described on page 332.
Quinoline derivatives, e.g. iodochlorhydroxyquinoline (Vioform) may be helpful in intractable cases. Adult pyoderma (also
due to streptococci and staphylococci acting alone or in concert) was successfully managed by McMillan and Hurwitz
(1969) with phenoxymethyl penicillin (oxacillin in those
infected with penicillin-resistant staphylococci) 500 mg. 6-
hourly.

Erysipeloid of Rosenbach (*Erythema serpens*). This is an
acute infection of the skin by *Erysipelothrix rhusiopathiae.*
The organism is very widely distributed in nature and infection in man usually occurs in those who handle meat, particularly pork, or fish. The disease tends to be limited and in the
absence of treatment usually clears up in three or four weeks,
but may persist for longer. The condition responds rapidly to
benzyl penicillin or the tetracyclines. Sulphonamides and
streptomycin are said not to be effective.

Acne Vulgaris

Increasing evidence suggests that normal follicular bacteria,
including coagulase-negative staphylococci and *Corynebacterium acnes* (Izumi *et al.,* 1970) split the triglycerides of sebum
liberating free fatty acids causing the inflammation of acne
(Ray and Kellum, 1971). Suppression of the lipolytic activity

of these organisms may be responsible for the improvement which occurs on tetracycline 250 mg. 6-12 hourly for one or two weeks reduced progressively to the smallest effective maintenance dose. Tetracycline has been shown to lower the fatty acid content of sebum (Beveridge and Powell, 1969) but a placebo effect also occurs and the efficacy and mode of action of tetracycline in this condition are disputed (Juhlin and Liden, 1969). Penicillin, to which the implicated organisms are also sensitive, has no effect on acne and it may be that tetracyclines owe their effect to concentration in the sebaceous glands and follicular epithelium (Marks and Davies, 1969). Cotterill *et al.* (1971) found co-trimoxazole (1 tablet daily for three months) just as effective as tetracycline and showed that treatment reduced the titratable acidity of sebum. They concluded, however, that the site of action must differ from that of tetracycline since co-trimoxazole was effective in some patients who had previously failed long-term tetracycline treatment.

Cutaneous Anthrax

B. anthracis is highly sensitive to benzyl penicillin which, like streptomycin, is superior to tetracycline or chloramphenicol in the treatment of experimental infection (Jones *et al.*, 1967). Cutaneous anthrax responds well to penicillin (4-6 mega units per day for 10-12 days). Of 197 cases reviewed by Brachman (1966) 8 died. Penicillin therapy reduced the total inflammation and the systemic symptoms but it did not affect the evolution of the typical local lesion and eschar, even though in the majority of cases the exudate was sterile after 24 hr. Excision of the lesion increased and prolonged both the local and the systemic manifestations and evidently has no place in treatment. Knight, Wynne-Williams and Willis (1969) were dissatisfied with the response in the first 24 hours of one of their two patients to penicillin and added streptomycin for 5 days.

Fungal Infections

Before starting treatment accurate identity of the fungus should be established. Griseofulvin, the most important agent for dermatophyte infections, has no effect on *Candida, Malassezia furfur* (the causative organism of pityriasis versicolor), or other non-dermatophytes which occasionally infect the skin.

CANDIDA INFECTIONS. Numerous local agents are available but all are less effective than nystatin (p. 230). This is not absorbed by mouth and is applied locally usually as a cream containing 100,000 units per g. Preparations with added steroids or antibacterial agents are available for use in patients with underlying eczematous conditions or concurrent bacterial infections. Amphotericin B, as a 3 per cent lotion or cream, or other polyene-containing creams sometimes succeed where nystatin has failed. On the basis of *in vitro* studies, Caplan and Clabaugh (1969) suggest that the corticosteroids contained in many local dermatological preparations may modify the response to antifungal agents in a complex way. Lehner and Ward (1970) discuss the distinction between iatrogenic candida infection which follows steroid therapy from that which follows tetracycline.

TINEA CAPITIS. Fungal infections of the scalp hair due to *Microsporum canis, Microsporum audouini* or *Microsporum gypseum* respond well to oral treatment with griseofulvin. This should be given, as the fine particle preparation, in a daily dose of 0·5-1 g. for adults and older children or 0·25 g. for children under four years. Treatment should be continued for 2-3 months. For infections of the glabrous skin three to four weeks are usually enough.

Griseofulvin is similarly effective in scalp ringworm due to the trichophyton fungi but recognition of carriers and elimination of the source of infection may be more difficult. In Britain at least epidemics occur more frequently with *Trichophyton tonsurans var. sulphureum* than with the microsporum group.

TINEA PEDIS AND FUNGAL INFECTION OF NAILS. Although early reports suggested that griseofulvin would cure athlete's foot, this has not been borne out by further experience and the same is true of fungal infection involving nails. Clinical improvement may occur but relapses are frequent and the fungus is rarely eradicated, although the finger nails may respond to 6-9 month's treatment. Success may follow treatment for one to two years but some dermatologists doubt whether such prolonged treatment is justified. Local fungicides must be used for these infections whether or not griseofulvin is given.

Two recent preparations, tolnaftate (naph-2-yl-*N*-methyl-*N*-*m*-tolyl thiocarbamate), and pecilocin (an antibiotic obtained from a species of paecilomyces and marketed in an ointment containing 3000 units per g. under the name Variotin) have both had successful trials (Robinson and Raskin, 1965; Holti *et al.*, 1966) but Wethered *et al.* (1967) were unable to demonstrate any benefit from either substance in the treatment of *Trichophyton rubrum* infection. Neither is active against candida.

Erythrasma

This is caused by *Corynebacterium minutissimum* which possesses keratolytic properties (Montes, Black and McBride, 1967). Corynebacteria capable of attacking hair also appear to be the principal occupants of the pigmented incrustations on the axillary hairs in trichomycosis axillaris (McBride *et al.*, 1968). The infected skin in erythrasma shows a striking pink fluorescence when viewed in ultra-violet light. In recent years standard treatment has been with oral erythromycin (250 mg. 6-hourly for two weeks) but in a controlled trial Seville and Somerville (1970) put benzoic acid ointment and framycetin ointment above erythromycin in order of efficacy. In a later study (Somerville *et al.*, 1971) they found 2 per cent sodium fusidate ointment to be as effective as benzoic acid ointment in clearing the fluorescent lesions and more effective in eliminating the organism, but less effective in de-scaling the lesions. This supports the successful use of sodium fusidate ointment by MacMillan and Sarkany (1970) who were unable to confirm previous claims that *C. minutissimum* is sensitive to tolnaftate or that erythrasma is benefited by treatment with it.

Boils

Boils do not require systemic antibiotic therapy, which exerts no significant effect on their rate of resolution (Price *et al.*, 1968; Rutherford *et al.*, 1970). Nevertheless there is a suspicion that antibiotic therapy has contributed to the reduced severity of superficial staphylococcal lesions seen in recent years and it should be instituted if there is evidence of local or lymphatic spread. Local applications of one of the preparations listed on page 326 or of gentian violet paint may be useful in limiting spread to adjacent skin. Infections severe enough to require surgery deserve systemic therapy beginning immediately before operation. Boils on the face should be treated because of the possibility of the grave complication of cavernous sinus thrombosis.

The choice of possible agents is wide. Unless the lesion is sufficiently serious to warrant admission to hospital, oral therapy is obviously desirable. For out-patients, an oral penicillin may well be the drug of choice, although the penicillin sensitivity of the infecting staphylococcus can no longer be relied upon. Erythromycin (250 mg. 6-hourly), flucloxacillin (250 mg. 6-hourly), clindamycin (300 mg. 6-hourly), and various other antistaphylococcal agents have all been successfully used. The drugs should be continued until the lesion heals. Failure to respond is an indication for bacteriological and surgical reassessment.

Recurrent Boils

The cropping of recurrent boils can usually only be stopped if vigorous and persistent efforts are made to control the carrier state. Swabs from the usual carrier sites should be taken from the patient and all his family. Positive carrier sites should be treated with naseptin or other suitable cream or spray. Where neomycin-resistant strains are prevalent, or sensitization to neomycin proves troublesome, chlorhexidine, gentamicin, or chloramphenicol may be used. The patient and carriers in the family should substitute for their normal toilet-soap a soap containing hexachlorophene which they should use for all washing and bathing. The patient's underclothes and sheets should be changed at frequent intervals (initially daily), and boiled. A dusting powder containing hexachlorophene (' Ster-Zac ') may also be used with advantage. This process should be continued for two months after the last boil has cleared.

In cases troublesome enough to justify this regimen, systemic antibiotic therapy is usually required initially. The choice of available agents is wide; we have been successful with erythromycin or, more recently, clindamycin. In particularly troublesome cases it may be worth giving the patient a small supply of the drug to take as soon as signs of a fresh lesion appear. The interesting state of affairs where some physicians continue to be convinced of the value of staphylococcal vaccines in the absence of any convincing scientific evidence of their value is discussed by Greenberg (1968).

Aerobic Wound Infections

ACCIDENTAL WOUNDS may be infected by one or more of a variety of bacteria of which the most frequent are *Staph. aureus, Str. pyogenes, E. coli, Proteus* species and *Ps. aeruginosa.* In healthy individuals the infection is usually only superficial and local treatment with a spray containing one of the combinations of antibiotics recommended at the beginning of the chapter is usually adequate. If deep-seated infection develops, systemic treatment may be necessary, in which case the choice of drug will depend on the sensitivity of the infecting organism or organisms.

OPERATION WOUNDS. The most likely organisms to infect clean operation wounds in hospital are *Staph. aureus, Ps. aeruginosa* and *E. coli.* As with accidental wounds local treatment is often sufficient. If infection is deep-seated or becomes generalized appropriate systemic treatment must be given. One superficial infection which has produced septicaemia often enough to cause concern is the entry wound for plastic indwelling intravenous catheters (Moran *et al.*, 1965). Movement of the catheter in the wound facilitates ingress of skin organisms and fixation is one important preventive measure. In addition, the entry site should be cleansed daily and treated with one of the preparations listed on page 326. Corso *et al.* (1969) discuss the general aseptic management of intravenous catheters.

INFECTION WITH PASTEURELLA SEPTICA. This may follow the bite of cats, dogs or other animals. Constitutional upset is frequent and systemic treatment should be given. Benzyl penicillin, or possibly ampicillin, is the drug of choice. Most strains are also sensitive to the sulphonamides, erythromycin and the tetracyclines.

ANAEROBIC INFECTIONS

Anaerobic infections fall generally into three groups in which the principal organisms are clostridia, bacteroides, and anaerobic streptococci. Bornstein *et al.* (1964) describe the clinical manifestations and general management of these conditions. Altemeier and Fullen (1971) describe 54 cases with a mortality rate of 14·8 per cent and discuss the clinical differentiation of clostridial and non-clostridial crepitant lesions.

Gas Gangrene. This term denotes an acute rapidly spreading myositis with gas formation (detectable by crepitus) caused most often by *Cl. welchii*, and terminating, if unchecked, in a rapidly fatal septicaemia. It is most likely to result from gross trauma, when the wound is contaminated with soil or dirt, as in battle wounds or farm accidents. It very rarely arises in operation wounds, with one exception: amputation through the thigh for obliterative arterial disease; here the source of infection is the skin in the neighbourhood of the anus, and the low oxygen tension in the tissues resulting from the poor blood supply permits spore germination. Nearly all the serious infections reported by Parker (1969) arose in this way. Attention has again been drawn to the dangers of gas gangrene following injection into the buttock of compounds (notably depot adrenaline preparations) which impair the local blood supply (Editorial, 1968).

The most important step in preventing clostridial infection of traumatic wounds is surgical debridement with the removal of foreign material and the excision of grossly traumatized tissue, in which alone the initial multiplication of clostridia can occur in the otherwise healthy subject. Any patient seriously at risk (and this includes patients about to undergo amputations through the thigh or orthopaedic operations between the waist and the knees) should also have the benefit of prophylactic penicillin, the value of which was amply demonstrated in Allied casualties from D-day 1944 onwards. Although all the toxigenic clostridia are sensitive to penicillin, the degree of sensitivity is only about one-tenth of that of a Group A streptococcus; hence at least two million units a day in divided doses should be given for several days, by intramuscular injection. In less severely injured and possibly ambulant patients, phenoxymethyl penicillin in very large oral doses may be substituted. Because of the emergence of resistant strains, tetracycline can no longer be relied upon for this purpose (Johnstone and Cockcroft, 1968) and it appears from one case reported by Parker (1969) that ampicillin should not be used. Erythromycin (250 mg. 6-hourly, if necessary intramuscularly) is generally held to be the best alternative for patients sensitive to penicillin.

It has been repeatedly emphasized that the treatment of clostridial myonecrosis is primarily surgical and that wide excision of the affected tissues or amputation is urgently required. If accumulating experience of hyperbaric oxygen continues to be as favourable, these mutilating procedures may no longer be necessary. The treatment is not without dangers, but with its use a number of authors have achieved high survival rates with limited surgery (Colwill and Maudsley, 1968). Treatment with penicillin, 10-20 mega units a day, is still required and local irrigation with antibiotics and hydrogen peroxide is recommended by some.

Many authors side-step the issue of the place of antitoxin in the treatment of gas gangrene by concluding that it is of questionable value, recounting its dangers and then reciting the dose. We have not recommended the use of antitoxin in the few patients we have seen in recent years and have no reason to believe that the prognosis suffered. We await convincing evidence that it contributes materially to the benefit of the multipronged therapeutic attack which is necessary in this disease.

Bacteroides Infections

These small Gram-negative anaerobic bacilli (the most numerous organisms in faeces and present also in the mouth) are responsible, either alone or in concert with other anaerobic organisms, for infections at many sites (Gelb and Seligman, 1970) most often in the air passages or abdomen, but including even bones and joints (Pearson and Harvey, 1971). Some species are sensitive to penicillin; others, including *B. fragilis,* are resistant to this and often to other antibiotics. If Gram-stained films of putrid material reveal organisms morphologically resembling bacteroides, an antibiotic directed against them is indicated. Uudoubtedly the antibiotic with the highest activity against this group is clindamycin; lincomycin has the same range of activity but is less potent. Successful treatment with these antibiotics has been reported by Tracy *et al.* (1972), Bartlett, Sutter and Finegold (1972) and Haldane and van Rooyen (1972).

Anaerobic Streptococcal Infections

These organisms, which are normal inhabitants of the mouth, gut and vagina, are most frequently responsible for infections around the perineum, but they are important causes of putrid lung abscess, sinusitis and brain abscess, and may cause a myositis clinically resembling gas gangrene. They are also implicated in post-operative synergic gangrene (Meleney's gangrene). This rare condition usually follows abdominal operations (de Jongh *et al.*, 1967). A gangrenous area develops in the vicinity of the wound and rapidly spreads to destroy much of the skin and subcutaneous tissue of the abdominal wall. It is a mixed infection with anaerobic streptococci, *Staph. aureus* and enterobacteria, or sometimes other organisms. Chemotherapy should be instituted as for clostridial myonecrosis but prompt wide excision of the affected tissues has also been essential. Morgan *et al.* (1971) discuss the management of patients in whom very extensive forfeiture of abdominal skin, muscle and fascia is necessary. Whether this condition will respond to hyperbaric oxygen remains to be seen.

Actinomycosis

Although *Actinomyces israeli* is highly sensitive to many chemotherapeutic drugs (p. 280; Blak, 1964) the chemotherapy of actinomycosis can be difficult, because the granulomatous and fibrotic tissue involved is not readily penetrated. Cervicofacial actinomycosis is relatively amenable to treatment and we, and others (Caron and Sarkany, 1964) have successfully managed this form of the disease with oral phenoxymethyl penicillin (2 g. per day). At least six weeks' treatment is usually necessary. Successful therapy has also been reported with tetracycline (3 g. per day for 28 days; or 3 g. per day for 10 days and 2 g. per day for a further 18 days) and with erythromycin (300 mg. 6-hourly for six weeks).

Thoracic, abdominal, and disseminated actinomycosis (and similar infections with ' anaerobic diphtheroids ') can be very difficult to eradicate. Penicillin is generally regarded as the antibiotic of choice, given in doses of 0·5 to 1·0 mega unit procaine penicillin b.d. for periods of two to three months. There is no advantage in adding sulphonamides (Seabery and Dascomb, 1964). Because of their powers of penetration, fucidin and lincomycin, both of which are highly active against *Actinomyces* (p. 280, Blake, 1970, personal communication) should be considered. Our own experience accords with that of Mohr *et al.* (1970) who obtained rapid improvement in four patients treated with lincomycin. It may be that prolonged therapy is more important than high dosage since there have been several reports of relapse after a few weeks' therapy followed by satisfactory response to further treatment with the same dosage. Surgical treatment is necessary to open and drain abscesses or an empyema and to remove infected bone.

Co-bacteria of Actinomyces. In actinomycotic lesions, the *Actinomyces* is commonly, perhaps regularly, accompanied by small anaerobic Gram-negative bacilli, *Actinobacillus actinomycetem comitans,* and a haemophilus-like organism *Haemophilus aphrophilus.* These may also be found alone as rare causes of endocarditis or of infections arising from the upper respiratory tract (Page and King, 1966). Their therapeutic interest is that they are relatively insensitive to penicillin, but sensitive to tetracycline. It has occasionally been shown that the actinobacillus persists in actinomycotic lesions after treatment with penicillin. The common presence of penicillin-resistant potential pathogens has been used as an argument for treating actinomycosis with tetracycline.

INFECTION IN BURNS

Prophylaxis

It cannot be too strongly emphasised that chemoprophylaxis is not a substitute for physical methods to prevent infection of burns in hospital. Overwhelming infection remains the greatest threat to the survival of badly burned patients. The organisms most likely to infect burns are *Str. pyogenes, Staph. aureus* or *Ps. aeruginosa.* Of the septicaemias arising from infected burns seen by MacMillan (1967) *Staph. aureus* was responsible for 6, *Proteus* and other Gram-negative bacilli for 11, and *Pseudomonas* for 29.

From 1960-65 Gram-negative bacilli became increasingly important. Mortality from Gram-positive infections was 50 per cent, and from Gram-negative infection 75 per cent. The importance of preventing burn sepsis is obvious. Most authors agree that systemic antibiotics should not be given prophylactically although several believe penicillin should be given over the first few hours to prevent the establishment of haemolytic streptococci. Larson *et al.* (1966) have shown that penicillin distribution through burned areas is satisfactory.

Two previously abandoned antibacterial agents, silver nitrate and sulfamylon (marfanil), have been resuscitated and proved to be of great benefit in the management of burns. Moyer *et al.* (1965) found that application of 0·5 per cent silver nitrate solution to large burns delayed sepsis and reduced mortality from 81 to 33 per cent. Monafo (1967) found that in patients treated early, *Staph. aureus, Proteus* and *Pseudomonas* were infrequently recovered from the burned areas and nearly 40 per cent were sterile. As treatment progressed, *Klebsiella, Aerobacter,* and *Providencia* appeared and persisted until the wounds healed. *Pseudomonas* appeared only after several weeks' treatment and seldom predominated. In contrast, in patients in whom treatment was delayed, *Pseudomonas* was isolated from every case and was not eliminated; *Staph. aureus* was isolated from all but one, but promptly disappeared on silver nitrate treatment.

The success of this therapy has been confirmed by a number of workers but it has several times been commented that it requires diligent and exact management (Price and Wood, 1966). Sulphamylon, as a 10 per cent cream, has been held to be equally effective and easier to manage. Switzer (1967) reduced the mortality in patients with 30-40 per cent burns from 41·1 to 3 per cent and in those with 40-50 per cent burns from 63·6 to 19 per cent. There was no improvement in patients with more than 60 per cent burns. Sulphamylon and its major metabolite are both potent inhibitors of carbonic anhydrase. In patients with extensive burns, and especially in those with renal failure, local application results in substantial blood levels of the drug with resulting inhibition of red-cell and renal carbonic anhydrase (White and Asch, 1971). The urine becomes persistently alkaline and urinary potassium levels can increase

4-5 fold. With maintenance of good pulmonary ventilation, however, little overall disturbance of acid-base balance occurs and the drug should not be withdrawn unless absolutely essential as cessation may be followed by overwhelming infection. Sulphamylon has been held to be at a disadvantage compared with silver nitrate because of skin sensitization and development of bacterial resistance. Yaffee and Dressler (1969) obtained cutaneous reactions in 9·5 per cent of 400 patients treated with sulphamylon but it did not interfere with completion of therapy in any case. Two patients developed erythema multiforme.

It has been claimed that the benefits of silver nitrate solution together with the advantages of ease of application can be obtained from silver nitrate cream (Bouterie and McLean, 1971) and that the combined benefits of silver nitrate and sulphonamide can be obtained from silver sulphadiazine cream (Fox, 1968). Topical gentamicin has been shown to be equally or more effective (MacMillan, 1969; Jefferson and McKnight, 1969). In a review of the present situation, Moncrieff (1969) concludes that each of the treatments has advantages and disadvantages and that the most important conclusion is that the value of topical antibacterial therapy is now well established. As always with topical therapy, superinfection is a possible hazard and Nash *et al.* (1971) report a ten-fold increase since 1964 in the frequency of colonization of burns with fungi. This colonization was not ordinarily of any clinical significance but they point out that the organisms involved —phycomycetes and aspergillus—are those responsible for the rare clinical infections which occur.

Treatment

Treatment of a burn already infected must depend on the infecting microbe or microbes and its sensitivity to antibiotics. Since *Str. pyogenes* is not infrequently present in a burn in association with a penicillin-resistant strain of *Staph. aureus,* it is worth pointing out that in such cases benzyl penicillin is liable to be inactivated before it can affect the streptococcus. Thus if penicillin-resistant *Staph. aureus* is isolated in association with *Str. pyogenes* the patient should be given systemic treatment with cloxacillin. This is probably better than methicillin, since it is more active against *Str. pyogenes.*

If a penicillin-resistant *Staph. aureus* is present alone no treatment is necessary unless there are signs of infection. In this case systemic treatment with cloxacillin or fucidin plus penicillin is indicated.

In the treatment of *Pseudomonas* septicaemia in burned patients, Stone (1967) found gentamicin more effective than colistin, but it was essential to combine systemic therapy with local applications of the drug to the burned area.

PYOGENIC INFECTIONS OF BONES AND JOINTS

Acute Osteomyelitis

The infecting organism is nearly always *Staph. aureus.* Haemolytic streptococci and *Salmonella* are each responsible for a few per cent, and *Proteus* and other enterobacteria, *Haemophilus* and other organisms for occasional cases. In the infant, haemolytic streptococci have been the commonest cause, but in the series studied by Lindblad *et al.* (1965) *Staph. aureus* was the only organism isolated. Children with sickle cell anaemia (and perhaps other haemolytic anaemias) appear to be peculiarly susceptible to salmonella infections (Engh *et al.,* 1971).

Since infection is likely but not certain to be due to staphylococci, attempts should be made to obtain material for bacteriological examination before instituting treatment. In cases not needing surgery this can be obtained by aspiration from the affected metaphysis, from any evident primary focus of infection, often the skin, or blood culture which is positive in a high proportion of early cases.

Before antibiotic therapy, up to 50 per cent of the patients died and a high proportion of the survivors were left with chronic discharging sinuses. Of 73 patients treated with penicillin in 3 series between 1945 and 1947, none died and only two developed complications (Gilmour, 1962). Since the advent of penicillin-resistant staphylococci, the situation has to some extent reverted to that of the pre-penicillin era. The incidence of acute osteomyelitis has increased, and while the mortality in patients treated with broad-spectrum antibiotics has remained low, the complication rate has risen and in several series there has been the impression that low grade persistent ' smouldering ' osteomyelitis has become more frequent. Of 15 penicillin-sensitive infections treated with penicillin by Meyer *et al.* (1965) none drained spontaneously, required drainage, or relapsed. In contrast, of 14 penicillin-resistant infections treated with appropriate agents, 8 developed chronic osteomyelitis. It has several times been suggested that this imperfect response is the result of using bacteristatic agents such as chloramphenicol or tetracycline.

As soon as adequate specimens have been obtained, treatment should begin with a mixture of benzyl penicillin (which is the most active agent against penicillinase-negative staphylococci) and an agent active against penicillin-resistant staphylococci. The choice lies between cloxacillin, a cephalosporin, fucidin and lincomycin. There has been no extensive direct comparison and their therapeutic efficacy appears to be so similar that there is at present no reason for preferring one to the others. Each has certain theoretical advantages and disadvantages. Cloxacillin and the cephalosporins are the most actively bactericidal *in vitro* and lincomycin the least. Clindamycin is more actively bactericidal than the parent lincomycin but is not yet available in a form suitable for parenteral administration. Both fucidin and lincomycin have the advantage of unusual penetration into bone (Evascus *et al.*, 1969) but the disadvantage that resistant mutants emerge relatively easily, especially to fucidin.

If the staphylococcus proves to be penicillin-sensitive the other agent should be discontinued. If the staphylococcus proves to be penicillin-resistant, in a patient treated with cloxacillin and penicillin, the penicillin should be discontinued. With lincomycin and fucidin combined treatment with penicillin should continue since this will be effective against any mutants resistant to the second agent which might appear. Clawson and Dunn (1967) comment on the need to correct anaemia if optimum benefit is to be obtained from antibiotic therapy.

Craven *et al.* (1970) treated six severely ill patients infected with penicillin-resistant staphylococci, four of whom had multiple bone lesions, with co-trimoxazole and obtained prompt and satisfactory responses.

The work of Dawkins and Hornick (1967) and Engh *et al.* (1971) indicates that salmonella osteomyelitis should be treated with chloramphenicol. In patients in whom salmonella appears likely—for example those suffering from salmonella infections elsewhere or sickle-cell anaemia—chloramphenicol should be given until the bacteriological diagnosis is established. In patients suffering from osteomyelitis of other aetiology the treatment must be guided by the bacteriological findings.

Antibiotics must be given in large doses in order to ensure adequate levels at the site of infection. After the first few days the frequency of injections can be reduced to six- or eight-hourly and after the first week or so oral therapy can be substituted for injections if the response is satisfactory. Benzyl penicillin should be given in a daily dose of 6 mega units, initially as 4-hourly injections or continuous infusion. Cloxacillin should be given in doses of 0·5 to 1·0 g. every four to six hours (children: 25 mg. per kg., 4-hourly). Fucidin and lincomycin should be given in a dose of 500 mg. 6-hourly (children: 50 mg./kg./day). The absorption of lincomycin, which is affected by food, may be uncertain and the drug can be given parenterally over the crucial first 48 hours. Oral therapy may then profitably be continued with the more regularly absorbed and more active clindamycin in a dose of 300 mg. 6-hourly (children: 15 mg./kg./day).

If treatment is started at the onset of disease the response to penicillin is usually obvious within 24 hours and Blockey and Watson (1970) suggest that if X-ray on the tenth day shows only osteoporosis without erosion of the cortex or new bone formation, therapy can be stopped. If on the other hand there is evidence of continuing activity they continue therapy for a total of three weeks when in the absence of local tenderness or pain on moving the limb treatment may be discontinued. If daily examination reveals acute local tenderness or a sense of deep fluctuation surgery is required.

Chronic Osteomyelitis

Chronic osteomyelitis may follow incomplete resolution of acute osteomyelitis or be the sequel to penetrating wounds (West *et al.*, 1970). The treatment is the same in both instances. Most cases are again due to staphylococci but other organisms, including Gram-negative bacilli, are more frequent and mixed infections are not uncommon (Clawson and Dunn, 1967; Agranat, 1969). Quite apart from complex bacteriology, chemotherapy is difficult because sequestra have no blood supply and the masses of dense fibrous tissue surrounding the affected bone have a very poor blood supply. There is, however, not the same urgency to begin treatment and as surgery is always necessary, antibiotic treatment can be guided by bacteriological examination. Kelly *et al.* (1970b) obtained the best results when saucerization of the lesion was combined with closed irrigation (usually with the same antibiotic as that given systematically) and suction. Amongst the Gram-negative rods which may superinfect chronic bony lesions is *Pseudomonas*. Shroeder *et al.*, (1970) describe three cases which followed internal fixation of femoral fractures. In two, good results were obtained from treatment with gentamicin once the pin had been removed In the third, prolonged gentamicin treatment while the pin remained *in situ* was of no avail.

Where staphylococci are responsible, combined fucidin plus penicillin may be particularly valuable: Rowling (1970) describes 29 patients in 86 per cent of whom he obtained primary healing.

Septic Arthritis

This condition, which may arise spontaneously, as for example in rheumatoid arthritis (Karten, 1969), or complicate trauma, resembles chronic rather than acute osteomyelitis in its bacteriology. *Staph. aureus* is responsible for not much more than half of the cases; streptococci of various kinds, enterobacteria, and mixed infections (sometimes including anaerobes) are all found (Kelly *et al.*, 1965). In children *H. influenzae* is a more common cause than is generally realized (Wall and Hunt, 1968) and accounted for most of the cases under the age of two reported by Nelson (1972).

Aspiration of the joint may be necessary to establish the diagnosis, but blood culture is positive in a high proportion of cases. Open surgical drainage may be preferable to repeated aspiration in the management and is held to be essential in infection of the hip joint (Kelly *et al.*, 1970a; Clawson and Dunn, 1967). Systemic treatment with cloxacillin and ampicillin in full dosage should be instituted until the bacteriological diagnosis is established after which the optimum therapy can be planned on the basis of *in vitro* sensitivity tests. There is a division of opinion on the value and wisdom of re-aspirating the joint and instilling anti-bacterial agents. There are potential dangers in aspiration (not the least being superinfection with a resistant organism) and it has been claimed that many of the antibiotics likely to be useful in this condition reach adequate levels in infected joints on systemic administration (Nelson, 1972).

REFERENCES

AGRANAT, B. J. (1969). *J. oral surg.* **27**, 293.
ALBERT, S., BALDWIN, R., CZEKAJEWISKI, S. VAN SOESTBERGEN, A., NACHMAN, R. & ROBERTSON, A. (1970). *Amer. J. Dis. Child.* **120**, 10.
ALTEMEIER, W. A. & FULLEN, W. D. (1971). *J. Amer. med. Ass.* **217**, 806.
BARTLETT, J. G., SUTTER, V. L. & FINEGOLD, S. M. (1972). *New Engl. J. Med.* **287**, 1006.
BEVERIDGE, G. W. & POWELL, E. W. (1969). *Brit. J. Derm.* **81**, 525.
BLAKE, G. C. (1964.) *Brit. med. J.* **1**, 145.
BLOCKEY, N. J. & WATSON, J. T. (1970). *J. Bone Jt Surg.* **52-B**, 77.
BORNSTEIN, D. L., WEINBERG, A. N., SWARTZ, M. N. & KUNZ, L. J. (1964). *Medicine (Balt.)* **43**, 207.
BOUTERIE, R. L. & McLEAN, D. H. (1971). *Amer. J. Surg.* **121**, 576.
BRACHMAN, P. S. (1966). *Antimicrob. Agents Chemother.*—1965, p. 111.
CAPLAN, R. M. & CLABAUGH, W. (1969). *J. invest. Derm.* **52**, 247.
CARNEY, R. G. (1963). *J. Amer. med. Ass.* **186**, 646.
CARON, G. A. & SARKANY, J. (1964). *Brit. J. Derm.* **76**, 421.
CLAWSON, D. K. & DUNN, A. W. (1967). *J. Bone Jt Surg.* **49(A)**, 164.
COLWILL, M. R. & MAUDSLEY, R. H. (1968). *J. Bone Jt Surg.* **50(B)**, 732.
CORSO, J. A., AGOSTINELLI, R. & BRANDRISS, M. W. (1969). *J. Amer. med. Ass.* **210**, 2075.
COTTERILL, J. A., CUNLIFFE, W. J., FORSTER, R. A., WILLIAMSON, D. M. & BULUSU, L. (1971). *Brit. J. Derm.* **84**, 366.
CRAVEN, J. L., PUGSLEY, D. J. & BLOWERS, R. (1970). *Brit. med. J.* **3**, 201.
DAVIS, C. M., FULGHUM, D. D. & TAPLIN, D. (1968). *J. Amer. med. Ass.* **203**, 298.
DAWKINS, A. T. & HORNICK, R. B. (1967). *Antimicrob. Agents Chemother.* —1966, p. 6.
DE JONGH, D. S., SMITH, J. P. & THOMA, G. W. (1967). *J. Amer. med. Ass.* **200**, 557.
DERRICK, C. W. & DILLON, J. C. JR. (1970). *J. Pediat.* **77**, 696.
DILLON, H. C. (1968). *Amer. J. Dis. Child.* **115**, 530.
DODGE, B. G., KNOWLES, W. R., McBRIDE, M. E., DUNCAN, W. C. & KNOX, J. M. (1968). *Arch. Derm.* **97**, 548.
EDITORIAL (1968). *Brit. med. J.* **1**, 721.
ENGH, C. A., HUGHES, J. L., ABRAMS, R. C. & BOWERMAN, J. W. (1971). *J. Bone Jt Surg.* **53-A**, 1.
EVASKUS, D. S., LASKIN, D. M. & KROEGER, A. V. (1969). *Proc. Soc. exp. Biol. Med.* **130**, 89.
FOX, C. L. (1968). *Arch. Surg. (Chicago)* **96**, 184.
GELB, A. F. & SELIGMAN, S. J. (1970). *J. Amer. med. Ass.* **212**, 1038.
GILMOUR, W. N. (1962). *J. Bone Jt Surg.* **44(B)**, 841.
GREENBERG, L. (1968). *Bull. N.Y. Acad. Med.* **44**, 1222.

HALDANE, E. V. & VAN ROOYEN, C. E. (1972). *Canad. med. Ass. J.* **107,** 1177.
HOLTI, G., LYELL, A., McCALLUM, D. I. & MORGAN, J. K. (1966). *Brit. J. Derm.* **78,** 661.
HUGHES, W. T. & WAN, R. T. (1967). *Amer. J. Dis. Child.* **113,** 449.
IZUMI, A. K., MARPLES, R. R. & KLIGMAN, A. M. (1970). *Arch. Derm.* **102,** 397.
JEFFERSON, J. & McKNIGHT, A. G. (1969). *Brit. J. clin. Pract.* **23,** 133.
JOHNSTONE, F. R. C. & COCKCROFT, W. H. (1968). *Lancet* **1,** 660.
JONES, W. I. JR., KLEIN, F., LINCOLN, R. E., WALKER, J. S., MAHLANDT, B. G. & DOBBS, J. P. (1967). *J. Bact.* **94,** 609.
JUHLIN, L. & LIDEN, S. (1969). *Brit. J. Derm.* **81,** 154.
KARTEN, I. (1969). *Ann. intern. Med.* **70,** 1147.
KELLY, P. J., MARTIN, W. J. & COVENTRY, M. B. (1965). *J. Bone Jt Surg.* **47(A),** 1005.
KELLY, P. J., MARTIN, W. J. & COVENTRY, M. B. (1970a). *J. Amer. med. Ass.* **213,** 1843.
KELLY, P. J., MARTIN, W. J. & COVENTRY, M. B. (1970b). *J. Bone Jt Surg.* **52(A),** 1595.
KNIGHT, A. G., VICKERS, C. F. H. & PERCIVAL, A. (1969). *Brit. J. Derm.* **81** (Suppl. 4), 88.
KNIGHT, A. H., WYNNE-WILLIAMS, C. J. E. & WILLIS, A. T. (1969). *Brit. med. J.* **1,** 416.
LARSON, D. L., MEYER, J. V., LYNCH, J. B. & LEWIS, S. R. (1966). *Amer. Surg.* **32,** 453.
LEHNER, T. & WARD, R. G. (1970). *Brit. J. Derm.* **83,** 161.
LINDBLAD, B., EKENGREN, K. & AURELIUS, G. (1965). *Acta paediat. (Uppsala)* **54,** 24.
MACMILLAN, B. G. (1967). *J. Trauma* **7,** 88.
MACMILLAN, B. G. (1969) *J. infect. Dis.* **119,** 492.
MACMILLAN, A. L. & SARKANY, I. (1970). *Brit. J. Derm.* **82,** 507.
MARKOWITZ, M., BRUTON, H. D., KUTTNER, A. G. & CLUFF, L. E. (1965). *Pediatrics* **35,** 393.
MARKS, R. & DAVIES, M. J. (1969). *Brit. J. Derm.* **81,** 448.
MARPLES, R. R. & KLIGMAN, A. M. (1971). *Arch. Derm.* **103,** 148.
MEYER, T. L., KIEGER. A. B. & SMITH, W. S. (1965). *J. Bone Jt Surg.* **47(A),** 285.
McBRIDE, M. E., FREEMAN, R. G. & KNOX, J. M. (1968). *Brit. J. Derm.* **80,** 509.
McMILLAN, M. R. & HURWITZ, R. M. (1969). *J. Amer. med. Ass.* **210,** 1734.
MOHR, J. A., RHOADES, E. R. & MUCHMORE, H. G. (1970). *J. Amer. med. Ass.* **212,** 2260.
MONAFO, W. W. (1967). *J. Trauma* **7,** 99.
MONCRIEF, J. A. (1969). *Clin. Pharmacol. Ther.* **10,** 439.
MONTES, L. F., BLACK, S. H. & McBRIDE, M. E. (1967). *J. invest. Derm.* **49,** 474.
MORAN, J. M., ATWOOD, R. P. & ROWE, M. I. (1965). *New Engl. J. Med.* **272,** 554.
MORGAN, A., MORAIN, W. & ERAKLIS, A. (1971). *Ann. Surg.* **173,** 617.
MOYER, C. A., BRENTANO, L., GRAVENS, D. L., MARGRAF, H. W. & MONAFO, W. W. (1965). *Arch. Surg. (Chicago)* **90,** 812.
NASH, G., FOLEY, F. D., GOODWIN, M. N. JR., BRUCK, H. M., GREENWALD, K. A. & PRUITT, B. A. JR. (1971). *J. Amer. med. Ass.* **215,** 1664.
NELSON, J. D. (1972). *Pediatrics* **50,** 437.
PAGE, M. I. & KING, E. O. (1966). *New Engl. J. Med.* **275,** 181.
PARKER, M. T. (1969). *Brit. med. J.* **3,** 671.
PEARSON, H. E. & HARVEY, J. P. (1971). *Surgery Gynec. Obstet.* **132,** 876.
PRICE, D. J. E., O'GRADY, F. W., SHOOTER, R. A. & WEAVER, P. C. (1968). *Brit. med. J.* **3,** 407.

PRICE, W. R. & WOOD, M. (1966). *Amer. J. Surg.* **112,** 674.
RAY, T. & KELLUM, R. E. (1971). *J. invest. Derm.* **57,** 6.
ROBINSON, H. M. & RASKIN, J. (1965). *Arch. Derm.* **91,** 372.
ROWLING, D. E. (1970). *J. Bone Jt Surg.* **52-B,** 302.
RUTHERFORD, W. H.. CALDERWOOD, J. W., HART, D. & MERRETT, J. D.
    (1970). *Lancet* **1,** 1077.
SCHROEDER, S. A., CATINO, D.. TOALA, P. & FINLAND, M. (1970). *J. Bone Jt
    Surg.* **52-A,** 1611.
SEABURY, J. H. & DASCOMB, H. E. (1964). *J. Amer. med. Ass.* **188,** 509
SEVILLE, R. H. & SOMERVILLE, D. A. (1970). *Brit. J. Derm.* **82,** 502.
SOLOMON, S. & BLUEFARB, S. M. (1969). *Indust. Med.* **38,** 54.
SOMERVILLE, D. A., NOBLE, W. C., WHITE, P. M., SEVILLE, R. H. & SAVIN,
    J. A. (1971). *Brit. J. Derm.* **85,** 450.
STONE, H. H. (1967). *J. Trauma* **7,** 109.
SWITZER, W. E. (1967). *J. Trauma* **7,** 110.
TRACY, O., GORDON, A. W., MORAN, F., LOVE, W. C. & MCKENZIE, P. (1972).
    Brit. med. J. **1,** 280.
VICKERS, C. F. H. (1969). *Brit. J. Derm.* **81,** 902.
WALL, J. J. & HUNT, D. D. (1968). *J. Bone Jt Surg.* (A) **50,** 1657.
WEST, W. F., KELLY, P. J. & MARTIN, W. J. (1970). *J. Amer. med. Ass.* **213,**
    1837.
WETHERED, R. R., HEELER, W. R. & WARIN, R. P. (1967). *Brit. J. Derm.* **79**.
    352.
WHITE, M. G. & ASCH, M. J. (1971). *New Engl. J. Med.* **284,** 1281.
YAFFEE, H. S. & DRESSLER, D. P. (1969). *Arch. Derm.* **100,** 277.

Chapter 20

MENINGITIS

Primary Bacterial Meningitis

The common causes of bacterial meningitis, except in the neonate, are *N. meningitidis, H. influenzae,* and *Str. pneumoniae.* Their frequency differs in different age groups; in early childhood all three organisms are found, with a predominance of *H. influenzae* and *N. meningitidis. H. influenzae* meningitis may be increasing in frequency (Editorial, 1971). This form becomes rare by school age, although it is occasionally found even in adults (Nordern *et al.,* 1970). *N. meningitidis* is the predominant causal organism in school age children and young adults, while in older age groups the pneumococcus becomes predominant.

Neonatal Meningitis

In the neonate the situation is completely different. Most cases are caused by enterobacteria, notably *E. Coli, Klebsiella-Aerobacter, Pseudomonas,* and *Proteus,* and most of the remaining cases are caused by streptococci and staphylococci. An enormous variety of organisms are capable of causing meningitis in the neonate, of which *Listeria monocytogenes* and *Salmonella* species are especially notable, while the three species commonly found at older ages also occasionally are responsible.

Secondary Bacterial Meningitis

When meningitis supervenes in chronic ear infection, is associated with congenital defects of the central nervous system, or follows trauma, operation or lumbar puncture, the infecting organisms resemble those of neonatal meningitis, with a large proportion caused by staphylococci, streptococci, enterobacteria and pseudomonas, while the pneumococcus is also represented in this group especially in association with meningitis following fracture of the skull. Mixed infections, sometimes including anaerobic organisms, are also found.

347

Diagnosis

Early diagnosis of bacterial meningitis is essential for successful treatment. The age of the patient is of some value in indicating which of the common bacteria is responsible, but the only sign commonly helpful on physical examination is the characteristic rash found in some patients with severe meningococcal infections. Because of this paucity of clinical evidence, early bacteriological diagnosis is of the utmost importance, and an expert opinion on a Gram-stained film of a specimen of cerebro-spinal fluid should be regarded as one of the few bacteriological emergencies. Meningococci can usually be recognized with certainty although a considerable search may be needed to find them in the film. Recognition of scanty organisms, especially in patients who have already received some treatment, may be facilitated by immuno-fluorescent staining (Fox *et al.*, 1969). Similarly, pneumococci, streptococci and haemophilus organisms can in most cases be recognized. If coliform bacilli are seen, although it is impossible to identify the species or even the genus, the observation is nevertheless a guide in the choice of early chemotherapy. As well as cultures of C.S.F. blood cultures should also be done.

No organisms can be recovered from the C.S.F. in some cases of purulent meningitis; the proportion varies between 12 and 25 per cent in different series. One reason for this shortfall in causal diagnosis, although not the only one, is previous antibiotic treatment. In one extensive study (Dalton and Allison, 1968) pre-treatment had the effect of reducing the number of positive C.S.F. Gram-stained films by 20 per cent, the number of positive C.S.F. cultures by 30 per cent, and the number of positive blood cultures by nearly two-thirds. There is, however, no good evidence that such pre-treatment makes the prognosis worse, and some that it may improve prognosis, presumably since the patients have received treatment at an earlier stage of the disease (Harter, 1963; Heycock and Noble, 1964). Infants with partially treated meningitis may, however, present with puzzling illnesses presenting some difficulty in diagnosis (Heycock, 1959).

Treatment

Despite the susceptibility of the common causes of bacterial meningitis to many potent agents, the results of treatment are often disappointing. Mortality in the neonate, in the elderly, and in patients with underlying disease, is very high, and neurological sequelae are common in neonates (de Lemor and Haggerty, 1969). The overall mortality in a series of 356 cases treated between 1960 and 1965 was 11 per cent (Jensen et al., 1969). The death rate from meningococcal meningitis was 2·9 per cent, from *Haemophilus* meningitis 18 per cent and from pneumococcal meningitis 21 per cent. Poor response to treatment is associated not only with the factors already specified, but with delay in diagnosis and initiation of treatment. Antibiotic factors implicated in poor results are failure to achieve the necessary drug concentration in the C.S.F., antagonism between antibacterial agents, and occasionally, sequestration of infection at sites inaccessible to host defence mechanisms.

Antagonism

The evidence that pairs of drugs may operate antagonistically in the treatment of meningitis is derived from the classic observations of Lepper and Dowling (1951) who found that of 43 patients treated with massive doses of penicillin 13 (30 per cent) died; of 14 patients treated with the same dose of penicillin plus chlortetracycline (previously successfully used alone) 11 (79 per cent) died. Similarly, Mathies *et al* (1968) found the fatality in patients with bacterial meningitis treated with ampicillin alone to be 4·3 per cent and in those treated with ampicillin plus chloramphenicol and streptomycin 10·5 per cent.

Wallace *et al* (1966) studied the interaction of penicillin and chloramphenicol against pneumococci and found that, both *in vitro* and in the treatment of experimental pneumococcal meningitis in the dog, penicillin alone or penicillin given before chloramphenicol rapidly killed the pneumococci while chloramphenicol inhibited growth of the organisms and consequently the action of simultaneously or later administered penicillin, the lethal effect of which is only exerted on growing organisms.

Antibiotic Concentration in C.S.F.

The intrathecal concentrations of antibacterial agents are determined by: 1. Plasma concentration of the agent, 2. diffusion, 3. active cellular transport (in or out of the C.S.F.), 4. entry with other plasma constituents in the course of inflammation, 5. bulk transport (that is to say removal of fluid without change of composition) of the agent in the C.S.F. through the arachnoid villi. Protein binding may be important in both limiting normal diffusion and facilitating access with protein entry in the course of inflammation.

The Table gives a guide to the percentages of the plasma levels of various agents to be found in the C.S.F.

TABLE 37

Penetration of Antimicrobial Agents into C.S.F.

	% plasma level found in C.S.F.
Sulphadiazine	40-80
Sulphadimidine	30-80
Sulphamethoxazole	25-33
Trimethoprim	50
Chloramphenicol	30-50
Tetracycline	10
Penicillin Ampicillin Cephaloridine	Therapeutic concentrations achievable by high doses I.V. or I.M. See text.
Streptomycin Gentamicin Kanamycin Polymyxin	C.S.F. concentrations low or very low. Intrathecal administration may be necessary. See text.

Duration of Treatment

The response to treatment in cases of acute meningitis is usually extremely rapid. Except with coliform infections and tuberculous meningitis (p. 447), if uncomplicated cases are treated early, the cerebro-spinal fluid is often sterile within 24 hours of the onset of treatment and almost invariably within a week. It is rarely necessary for treatment to exceed 10 days.

INTRATHECAL INJECTIONS. It seems reasonable to attempt to supplement inadequate C.S.F. levels resulting from systemically administered drug by direct intrathecal injection. Unfortunately it appears that the distribution of agents administered in this way is often erratic (Schanker, 1966) and there is no good evidence that the results are significantly improved by these injections. With increasing experience of treating meningitis, several authors have abandoned intrathecal therapy on the grounds that the risks of medullary coning, local toxicity, and the frequency of subdural effusions outweigh the doubtful therapeutic advantage.

There are, nevertheless, a few situations in which intrathecal treatment may be indicated. Those patients with neonatal meningitis who require antibiotics diffusing poorly into the C.S.F., notably polymyxin, gentamicin, and sometimes kanamycin, often need intrathecal treatment. An intrathecal injection of penicillin or ampicillin at initial lumbar puncture may reasonably be given to very ill patients with purulent C.S.F. Similarly very ill patients with pneumococcal meningitis may likewise be given an initial intrathecal injection of penicillin. The role of intrathecal treatment in tuberculous meningitis is discussed on p. 447. If intrathecal injections are necessary, the irritant effect of introducing a foreign substance into the theca must be remembered. The purest available material must be used : the dose must not be higher than necessary to obtain the appropriate bactericidal effect; and the number of injections must be kept to a minimum. The following doses are those usually recommended :

Penicillin	10,000-20,000 units (6-12 mg.) reduced proportionately for children.
Streptomycin	50-100 mg., reduced proportionately for children.
Polymyxin	10,000-50,000 units; under 2 years up to 16,000 units
Ampicillin	10-40 mg. for adults : 3-5 mg. for children.
Gentamicin	5 mg., 1 mg. for infants.
Cephaloridine	50 mg., children 25 mg., infants 12·5 mg.

Injections should not be given more than once daily.

TREATMENT OF SPECIFIC INFECTIONS

Meningococcal Meningitis

Until recently, meningococcal meningitis was successfully treated with sulphadiazine. Since 1963, when they first appeared, sulphonamide-resistant meningococci have made rapid strides. By 1969, 70 per cent. of meningococcal infections in the United States were due to sulphonamide-resistant strains (Artenstein, 1969). Although still uncommon, sulphonamide-resistant strains have been detected in Great Britain and in many other countries, and it must be anticipated that their prevalence will increase. Abbott and Graves (1972) found that 6 per cent of strains isolated from a number of parts of Britain from 1966-71 were resistant. As a result, sulphonamides can no longer be relied upon for the initial treatment of meningococcal meningitis. Treatment should be initiated with benzyl penicillin, two mega units given four hourly by intramuscular or intravenous injection. In areas where sulphonamide resistance is still rare, a long period of parenteral treatment can be avoided by changing to sulphadiazine, sulphadimidine or sulphafurazole as soon as the isolated strain is reported sensitive to sulphonamide, and when the patient is emerging from the phase of serious illness and can properly be treated by the oral route. The initial dose of sulphonamide should be 50 mg./kg., followed by a dose of 100 mg./kg./day in adults, or 200 mg./kg./day in infants.

The results of penicillin treatment do not appear to be improved by the addition of sulphonamide (Carpenter and Petersdorf, 1962). In the series treated with penicillin plus sulphonamide by Anglin et al. (1965) 10·5 per cent died. Of those treated by Mathies et al. (1966) with penicillin alone 9·1 per cent died. It is evident both from the in vitro sensitivity of the organism and the poor results of treatment that cephalothin should not be used for the treatment of meningococcal meningitis (Southern and Sanford, 1969).

Prophylaxis of Meningococcal Meningitis

Outbreaks of meningococcal meningitis in closed communities, especially of military recruits, are well recognized, but spread within family groups may also occur. Greenfield and Feldman (1967) described three cases in first cousins, and found that 11 of 25 contacts of the extended family were meningococcal carriers, as also were 12 of their 60 primary contacts. The carrier rate in unrelated populations was 3 per cent.

Sulphadiazine has been very effective for chemoprophylaxis in contrast to other agents successfully used for the treatment of meningitis which have been largely ineffective in prophylaxis. As a result, the emergence of sulphonamide-resistant strains has posed a considerable problem. It appears that rifampicin is a suitable substitute for sulphadiazine, being markedly more effective than penicillin, ampicillin, tetracycline or erythromycin in controlling the carriage of sulphonamide-resistant strains. Treatment with rifampicin 600 mg. daily for four days produced a reduction in the carrier rate of 84 per cent (Beam *et al.*, 1971), but 73 per cent of the strains isolated just after treatment were resistant, the proportion of resistant strains falling to 30 per cent by the time trainees left camp. In another study 17 of 62 carriers who received rifampicin possessed resistant strains (Guttler *et al.*, 1971). It is clear that widespread use of rifampicin is likely to be followed by an increase in strains resistant to this drug. Rifampicin may, however, be properly used to treat family contacts of sporadic cases of meningococcal meningitis or septicaemia caused by sulphonamide-resistant strains. If the organism is sulphonamide–susceptible, family contacts should be given 1·0 g. sulphadimidine or sulphadiazine three times daily for three days. Moderate success in controlling meningococcal carriage has also been achieved with a tetracycline, minocycline (Guttler *et al.*, 1971; Devine *et al.*, 1971).

Pneumococcal Meningitis

Despite the extreme sensitivity of *Str. pneumoniae* to the agents commonly used in the treatment of meningitis, the mortality from pneumococcal meningitis remains disappointingly high. In most series treated with massive doses of penicillin, with or without sulphonamide, the mortality rate has been 20-30 per cent (Mathies, *et al.*, 1966; Anglin *et al.*, 1965). Part of the excess mortality is undoubtedly due to the extreme age, poor general condition and associated diseases of the patients. In Carpenter and Petersdorf's (1962) patients, 60 per cent had concurrent pneumonia and 25 per cent were alcoholic.

Penicillin should be given in doses of 2 mega units 2-hourly. This is best achieved by injecting the doses into an intravenous infusion. After the first few days of treatment. when the interval between doses can be increased to four-hourly, it becomes practical to change to the intramuscular route. Treatment should be continued for at least ten days. Success has also been reported with cephaloridine. Love *et al.* (1970) gave 100 mg./kg./day up to 6 g. daily in eight–hourly intramuscular injections, together with daily or alternate daily intrathecal injection (50 mg. for adults 25 mg. for children, 12·5 mg. for infants): 49 patients were treated with 7 deaths (14 per cent), and neurological sequelae in 5 of the survivors.

Haemophilus Meningitis

This infection is almost invariably due to *H. influenzae,* Pittman type b. Until recently chloramphenicol was unquestionably the drug of choice. It inhibits the growth of the infecting organism in a concentration of less than 1 μg./ml. and, unlike its action on other species, it is bactericidal in concentrations which can readily be achieved in the C.S.F.

It then appeared that ampicillin was equally effective (Barrett *et al.,* 1966) and being free from the possible haematological toxicity of chloramphenicol, became the drug most commonly used, especially in the U.S.A. Since then increasing numbers of examples of poor response or relapse have been described after ampicillin treatment, not all of which can be attributed to inadequate dosage. Many of the patients then recovered after subsequent treatment with chloramphenicol (Young *et al.,* 1968; Sanders and Garbee, 1969). It is clear that if ampicillin is to have the best results in *Haemophilus* meningitis, it must be given parenterally, and in high dosage, for the whole course of treatment. The tendency to reduce the dose as treatment progresses must be resisted, since ampicillin passage into the C.S.F. is likely to be impaired as meningeal inflammation subsides. The minimum dose is 150 mg./kg./day, given by intravenous injection at four-hour intervals for the first 48 hours, and then continuing by intravenous or intramuscular injection to a total of at least 10 days. This need for prolonged intravenous therapy or the frequent i.m. injection of large volumes of antibiotics is itself a serious disadvantage of ampicillin treatment in the group of infants and small children who experience this variety of meningitis. Chloramphenicol treatment is much easier to administer. It is given by intravenous or intramuscular injection for the first 48 hours, after which oral therapy can be started if the patient's condition allows it. The dose is 75 mg./kg./day (but see p. 291 for dose in younger children).

As regards efficacy there is little to choose between the two methods. A direct comparison (Schulkind *et al.*, 1971) gave very similar results except for a longer average duration of fever with ampicillin therapy. Shackelford *et al.* (1972) found ampicillin inferior to chloramphenicol both as to duration of fever and liability to relapse, which was noted in six of 136 ampicillin-treated patients, but in none of 116 treated with chloramphenicol. The only serious disadvantage of chloramphenicol, the rare possibility of marrow aplasia, must be set against those of ampicillin, namely the psychological and technical difficulties of prolonged injection treatment, and failure of response in a small proportion of cases. Prolonged intravenous therapy is itself not without risk, and i.v. catheters are a common cause of prolonged fever in meningitis (Balagtas *et al.*, 1970).

We conclude that both forms of treatment are generally affective and acceptable. The choice between them will be based on individual preference and technical factors such as the availability of veins.

Cephaloridine should not be given for the treatment of *H. influenzae* meningitis. The organism is relatively resistant to the agent *in vitro* and Walker and Collins (1968) treated three cases with intravenous cephaloridine in doses up to 600 mg./ kg. daily without sterilizing the C.S.F.

Initial Treatment When Bacteriological Diagnosis is Unknown

Treatment begins as soon as the gram-stained smear of the C.S.F. deposit has been examined. In seriously ill patients in whom purulent fluid is obtained at lumbar puncture, it is reasonable to begin treatment at once by instilling 20,000 units of pure benzyl penicillin or 10 mg. ampicillin (adult doses) into the theca (see p. 357). If no bacteria are seen or the findings are uncertain, initial treatment must cover as far as possible the likely infecting species. The best method of treating patients with pyogenic meningitis of uncertain cause is in dispute. Until recently a common policy was to initiate treatment with penicillin, chloramphenicol and a sulphonamide (' triple therapy ') and good results have been obtained with such a scheme (McKendrick, 1968). On the other hand, the patient is thus exposed to the unwanted effects of three drugs, and the antagonism between penicillin and chloramphenicol (p. 283) is also a potential disadvantage. All the three common bacterial causes are susceptible to chloramphenicol, and it is possible to use this drug alone for meningitis of unknown cause. The other method, which has gained favour in recent years, is to give large doses of ampicillin intravenously. The advantages and disadvantages of ampicillin and chloramphenicol have been discussed in the section on *Haemophilus* meningitis and the same considerations apply to patients with undiagnosed pyogenic meningitis. There is little evidence that the addition of a sulphonamide will enhance the response to either chloramphenicol or ampicillin.

Patients who are allergic to penicillin suffering from any of the three common causes of bacterial meningitis should be treated with chloramphenicol, or, in the case of sulphonamide-sensitive meningococcal infection, by sulphonamide.

Neonatal Meningitis

Meningitis is a frequent accompaniment of neonatal septicaemia, and carries a high mortality and a high incidence of residual neurological damage (Gotoff and Behrman, 1970). The variety of organisms which may be responsible has been described on p. 347. Factors predisposing to neonatal meningitis (Overall, 1970) are low birth weight, complications during labour, and maternal puerperal infection, while other cases are associated with meningomyelocoele or other neurological defects. The gram-negative organisms commonly responsible have a wide variety of antibiotic sensitivity patterns, and it is particularly important in this group to obtain guidance from the laboratory as soon as possible. Blood cultures as well as C.S.F. cultures should always be done, and the organism tested against gentamicin, kanamycin, streptomycin, ampicillin, polymyxin, carbenicillin, cephaloridine, chloramphenicol and cotrimoxazole. The choice of initial treatment will be influenced by knowledge of the prevalent gram-negative flora, or by concurrent cases of neonatal sepsis in the hospital concerned. In the past a wide variety of drugs, especially ampicillin and kanamycin, have been used as initial treatment when gram-negative rods are seen in the film, but recent experience with gentamicin has been especially promising (Klein et al., 1971). Gentamicin has the advantage of including most strains of Pseudomonas in its antibacterial activity, but the disadvantage, shared with the polymyxins, that treatment must usually be supplemented by intrathecal injections to ensure adequate C.S.F. levels (Newman and Holt, 1971). Gentamicin should be given to the neonate in a dose of 3-6 mg./kg./day, with daily intrathecal injections of 1 mg. If no organisms are seen on the smear it is wise to initiate treatment with a cephalosporin or a penicillin as well as gentamicin, since the latter drug is relatively inactive against streptococci, a significant cause of meningitis in infancy, and a wider range of antibacterial cover is achieved.

The great difficulties in treating neonatal enterobacterial meningitis warrants further study of the value of cotrimoxazole, especially under conditions in which parenteral treatment and intrathecal injections are impracticable. Favourable results have been reported both in E. coli neonatal meningitis (Morzaria et al., 1969), and in other forms of purulent meningitis at various ages (Bolletti and Bertaggia, 1971; Felix, 1971).

Streptococcal and Staphylococcal Meningitis

Like enterobacterial infections, these may be secondary to trauma, surgery, or ear or sinus infections, or arise de novo usually in very young infants (Maher and Irwin, 1966). If the stained film of C.S.F. deposit shows Gram-positive cocci which can be positively identified as streptococci, penicillin treatment, as described under pneumococcal meningitis, should be immediately instituted. If the cocci cannot be identified, or are identified as staphylococci, similar penicillin treatment should be given together with cloxacillin 1 g. 3-hourly (children 100 mg./kg./day) intravenously. When the identity and sensitivities of the infecting organism are known, the inappropriate agent can be stopped or the treatment changed as necessary.

Listeria Meningitis

Listeria meningitis is probably less uncommon than was previously thought (Moore and Whitmore, 1960). It occurs in the newborn when it appears to result from latent genital tract infection in the mother (Rappaport *et al.,* 1960). It is also encountered in adults; some patients have no underlying disease, but listeria meningitis is especially associated with lymphoreticular diseases, and with pregnancy, diabetes and alcoholism. Strains of listeria are in general susceptible to most of the main groups of antimicrobial drugs except the poly-myxins, but variation among individual strains has been recorded, especially in relation to penicillins and sulphonamides (Buchner and Schneierson, 1968), and it is important to establish the sensitivity pattern of the isolated strain. A number of schemes of treatment have been used successfully. Seeliger *et al.* (1967) and Buchner and Schneierson (1968) regard tetracyc-line as the drug of choice, but its lack of bactericidal effect and, in children, its effects on the teeth and bones, are disadvantages. Ampicillin is effective against a greater number of strains than is benzylpenicillin and good results have been reported from its use. Lavetter *et al.* (1971) treated 19 patients with penicillin alone or in combination, of whom 17 survived, and Weingartner and Ortel (1967) treated 57 infants with ampicillin with 9 deaths (16 per cent). English and McCafferty (1965) successfully treated listeria meningitis in adults with penicillin and erythromycin.

The treatment of choice appears at present to be ampicillin alone, given in large doses intravenously in the manner de-scribed for *Haemophilus* meningitis. In adults the clinical syndrome may be that of meningo-encephalitis, encephalitis or brain abscess rather than one of acute meningitis; in these patients it may be necessary to add intrathecal ampicillin to the regimen, and to continue treatment for a prolonged period. Other antibiotic schemes may be chosen on the basis of the resistance pattern of the isolated strain.

Amoebic Meningo-encephalitis

Acute and rapidly fatal purulent meningitis associated with amoebic infection of the C.N.S. has been reported from a number of countries, mainly in children and young adults after swimming in inland water in hot weather. (Fowler and Carter, 1965). The causative agent appears to be *Naegleria* although *Hartmanella* (*Acanthamoeba*) species were at first thought to be responsible. If such a diagnosis is established or suspected amphotericin B should be given, and the report from Apley *et al.* (1970) provides suggestive evidence that such treatment may have been effective in a patient developing the disease. Recovery from the fully established infection seems to be extremely rare.

ASSESSMENT OF RESPONSE TO TREATMENT IN MENINGITIS

Difficulties are often encountered in judging the progress of treatment in meningitis. In particular, fever may be prolonged, and neurological signs or disturbance of consciousness may persist for a variable time during treatment. If progress is unsatisfactory, it is essential to review the evidence for the initial diagnosis, the basis on which the antibiotic regimen was chosen, and the dose and route of administration of the drugs. But prolonged fever seldom results from antibiotic failure, and it is rare to recover organisms from the C.S.F. within 48 hours of starting treatment. Repeat lumbar punctures are therefore unnecessary if progress is satisfactory. The most common cause of prolonged fever in patients receiving intravenous treatment is phlebitis at injection sites (Balagtas *et al.*, 1970). and similarly patients receiving intramuscular injections may have fever associated with inflamed areas of muscle. Occasionally fever may be associated with metastatic foci of infection, such as arthritis in meningococcal septicaemia, while focal neurological complications such as subdural effusion, sinus thrombosis or brain abscess must be considered. The fever of infection may be supplanted by that of drug hypersensitivity, and very rarely a second organism may be introduced at lumbar puncture. Once antibiotic failure has been excluded, it is often best to stop treatment after 10-14 days, and to observe the patient's progress and temperature thereafter. Once therapy is established on a rational basis it is unnecessary and confusing to make frequent changes of treatment because fever persists. It is often found that the temperature returns to normal as soon as chemotherapy is discontinued.

REFERENCES

ABBOTT, J. D. & GRAVES, J. F. R. (1972). *J. clin. Path.* **25**, 528.

ANGLIN, C. S., FUJIWARA, M. W., HILL, D., JAMES, W., McARTHUR, R. & SELIGMAN, G. (1965). *Appl. Ther.* **7**, 1091.

APLEY, J., CLARKE, S. K. R., ROOME, A. P. C. H., SANDRY, S. A., SAYGI, G., SILK, B. & WARHURST, D. C. (1970). *Brit. med. J.* **1**, 596.

ARTENSTEIN, M. S. (1969). *New Engl. J. Med.* **281**, 678 (Ed).

BALAGTAS, R. C., LEVIN, S., NELSON, K. E. & GOTOFF, S. P. (1970). *J. Pediat.* **77**, 957.

BARRETT, F. F., EARDLEY, W. A., YOW, M. D. & LEVERETT, H. A. (1966). *J. Pediat.* **69**, 343.

BARRETT, F. F., TABER, L. H., MORRIS, C. R., STEPHENSON, W. B., CLARK, D. J. & YOW, M. D. (1972). *J. Pediat.* **81**, 370.

BEAM, W. E., NEWBERG, N. R., DEVINE, L. F., PIERCE, W. E. & DAVIES, J. A. (1971). *J. infect. Dis.* **124**, 39.

BOLLETTI, M. & BERTAGGIA, A. (1971). *Gazz. med. Ital.* **130**, 171.

BUCHNER, L. H. & SCHNEIERSON, S. S. (1968). *Amer. J. Med.* **45**, 904.

CARPENTER, R. R. & PETERSDORF, R. G. (1962). *Amer. J. Med.* **33**, 262.

DALTON, H. P. & ALLISON, M. J. (1968). *Amer. J. clin. Path.* **49**, 410.

DE LEMOS, R. A. & HAGGERTY, R. J. (1969). *Pediatrics* **44**, 30.

DEVINE, L. F., JOHNSON, D. P., HAGERMAN, C. R., PIERCE, W. E., RHODE, S. L. & PECKINPAUGH, R. O. (1971). *Amer. J. Epidem.* **93**, 337.

EDITORIAL (1971). *New Engl. J. Med.* **285**, 666.

ENGLISH, J. C. & McCAFFERTY, J. F. (1965). *Med. J. Aust.* **2**, 332.

FELIX, H. (1971). *Rev. Med.* **23**, 1503.

FOWLER. M. & CARTER, R. F. (1965). *Brit. med. J.* **2**, 740.

FOX, H. A., HAGEN, P. A., TURNER, D. J., GLASGOW, L. A. & CONNOR, J. D. (1969). *Pediatrics* **43**, 44.

GOTOFF, S. P. & BEHRMAN, R. E. (1970). *J. Pediat.* **76**, 142.

GREENFIELD, S. & FELDMAN, H. A. (1967). *New Engl. J. Med.* **277**, 497.

GUTTLER, R. B., COUNTS, G. W., AVENT, C. K. & BEATTY, H. N. (1971). *J. infect. Dis.* **124**, 199.

HARTER, D. H. (1963). *Trans. Amer. neurol. Ass.* **88**, 179.

HEYCOCK, J. B. (1959). *Brit. med. J.* **1**, 629.

HEYCOCK, J. B. & NOBLE, T. C. (1964). *Brit. med. J.* **1**, 658.

JENSEN, K., RANEK, L. & ROSDAHL, N. (1969). *Scand. J. infect. Dis.* **1**, 21.

KLEIN, J. O., HERSCHEL, M., THERAKAN, R. M. & INGALL, D. (1971). *J. infect. Dis.* **124**, Suppl. 224.

LAVETTER, A., LEEDOM, J. M., MATHIES, A. W., IVLER, D. & WEHRLE, P. F. (1971). *New Engl. J. Med.* **285**, 598.

LEPPER, M. H. & DOWLING, H. F. (1951). *Arch. intern. Med.* **88**, 489.

LOVE, W. C., McKENZIE, P., LAWSON, J. H., PINKERTON, I. W., JAMIESON, W. M., STEVENSON, J., ROBERTS, W. & CHRISTIE, A. B. (1970). *Postgrad. med. J.* **46**, (Suppl. Oct.), 155.

MAHER, E. & IRWIN, R. C. (1966). *Pediatrics* **38**, 659.

MATHIES, A. W. JR., LEEDOM, J. M., THRUPP, L. D., IVLER, D., PORTNOY, B. & WEHRLE, P. F. (1966). *Antimicrob. Agents Chemother.*—1965, p. 610.

MATHIES, A. W. JR., LEEDOM, J. M., IVLER, D., WEHRLE, P. F. & PORTNOY, B. (1968). *Antimicrob. Agents Chemother.*—1967, p. 218.

McKENDRICK, G. D. W. (1968). *J. Neurol. Neurosurg. Psychiat.* **31**, 528.

Moore, S. & Whitmore, D. N. (1960). *Brit. med. J.* **2**, 1572.
Morzaria, R. N., Walton. I. G. & Pickering, D. (1969). *Brit. med. J.* **2**, 511 (C).
Newman, R. L. & Holt, R. J. (1971). *J. infect. Dis.* **124**, Suppl. 254.
Norden, C. W., Callerame, M. L., Baum, J. (1970). *New Engl. J. Med.* **282**, 190.
Overall, J. C. (1970). *J. Pediat.* **76**, 499.
Rappaport, F., Rabinovitz, M., Toaff, R. & Krochik, N. (1960). *Lancet* **1**, 1273.
Sanders, D. Y. & Garbee, H. W. (1969). *Amer. J. Dis. Child.* **117**, 331.
Schanker, L. S. (1966). *Antimicrob. Agents Chemother.*—1965, p. 1044.
Seeliger, H. P. R., Laymann, U. & Finger, H. (1967). *Dtsch. med. Wschr.* **92**, 1095.
Schulkind, M. L., Altemeier, W. A. & Ayoub, E. M. (1971). *Pediatrics* **48**, 411.
Shackelford, P. G., Bobinski, J. E., Feigin, R. D. & Cherry, J. D. (1972). *New Engl. J. Med.* **287**, 634.
Southern, P. M. & Sandford, J. P. (1969). *New Engl. J. Med.* **280**, 1163.
Wallace, J. F., Smith, R. H., Garcia, M. & Petersdorf, R. G. (1966). *Antimicrob. Agents Chemother.*—1965, p. 439.
Weingartner, L. & Ortel, S. (1967). *Dtsch. med. Wschr.* **92**, 1098.
Young, L. M., Haddow, J. E. & Klein, J. O. (1968). *Pediatrics* **41**, 516.

CHAPTER 21

INFECTIONS OF THE ALIMENTARY TRACT

The Mouth

STOMATITIS is much more often an indication for stopping antibiotic treatment than for starting it. The condition is produced by the excretion of antibiotics in the saliva with consequent suppression of the normal flora and its replacement by resistant species. This is the only area in which penicillin can cause such a change: the substituted flora is mainly coliform, although it may include *Candida,* and symptoms are uncommon unless very large doses are given or penicillin is employed locally. Tetracyclines, if given in full doses for more than a few days, are more liable to lead to an overgrowth of *Candida albicans.* There are three stages in the resulting process: soreness without visible lesions, redness, and frank thrush. In severe cases this may extend to the fauces and even to the bronchi.

Thrush is in fact the only specific form of stomatitis for which antibiotic treatment is indicated. Nystatin, administered in the form of a suspension which comes in contact with the lesions, is highly effective.

VINCENT'S GINGIVITIS. This otherwise intractable condition merits treatment with penicillin, to which the causative organisms are highly sensitive. Two doses of a mixed potassium and procaine preparation on successive days will usually eradicate the infection. Success has also been claimed for local treatment. This was introduced by MacGregor and Long (1944) who used penicillin in pastilles with a gelatin base. It has been revived by Emslie, Cross and Blake (1962), who strongly advocate the use of a chewing gum containing penicillin, and contest the idea that short-term topical application in the mouth involves any special risk of sensitization (see p. 304). Metronidazole in doses of 200 mg. three times a day for seven days also gave good results in the hands of

362

Davies, McFadzean and Squires (1964). It attains concentrations in the saliva as well as in the blood calculated to exert a direct anti-bacterial effect.

Acute Parotitis in its most severe form is usually a staphylococcal infection, and many require surgical treatment. An antibiotic should also be helpful, and methicillin or cloxacillin is indicated in the first instance, pending the results of sensitivity tests, particularly in cases arising in hospital. There appears to be no evidence as to the utility of chemotherapy in chronic catarrhal infections of the salivary glands, the secretion in which (only obtainable in suitable form for culture by catheterising the duct) usually contains a pneumococcus.

The Stomach

The main question involved here is whether antibiotic ' cover ' is advisable for gastric operations. Several studies of its effects (reviewed by Taylor, 1960) have led to the conclusion that it is actually detrimental, untreated controls having a lower incidence of infection, both at the operation site and in the lungs. The combination of penicillin and streptomycin which has commonly been used also predisposes to staphylococcal enterocolitis (see p. 369). These unfavourable results have followed treatment continued for several days, and a better case can perhaps be made for treatment at the time of operation only. Bernard and Cole (1964) gave three doses only of a mixture of penicillin, methicillin and chloramphenicol, before, during and after gastric and other abdominal operations, and thus reduced the rate of operation site infections from 25 per cent in controls to 5 per cent (see also p. 287).

The Biliary Tract

The literature contains numerous reports of the successful use of various anti-bacterial drugs in infections of the bile passages. These are presumably based on symptomatic improvement, since evidence of the nature of the infection and of any effect of treatment on it is only obtainable by duodenal intubation. Moreover, the usual cause of either cholecystitis or cholangitis is obstruction by a gall-stone, and treatment directed merely at the consequences of this can clearly be only palliative. The uncertainty of this subject in its clinical aspects is such that attention is better directed to two aspects which are factual, namely, the nature of the infections concerned, and the concentrations attained by different drugs in the bile, which vary widely.

Bile is a medium congenial to some bacteria, notably the typhoid bacillus, and highly inimical to others, notably the more virulent of the pyogenic cocci, *Str. pyogenes* and *Str. pneumoniae*. Hence most infections in this area are due to coliform bacilli, which are in general bile-resistant: the only Gram-positive organism likely to be found is *Str. faecalis*. Thus, in the absence of direct bacteriological evidence a logical choice would be a drug active against the coliform group.

From the point of view of concentration in the bile, the available drugs are sharply divisible into two classes. Sulphonamides, chloramphenicol, streptomycin and neomycin are excreted only in low concentrations, usually less than those occurring at the same time in the blood. Others are concentrated in the bile, some of them owing the maintenance of the blood level after an individual dose to reabsorption after excretion by this route. Antibiotics excreted in larger amounts in the bile but nevertheless mainly via the kidney are tetracyclines and penicillins (Harrison and Stewart, 1961), particularly ampicillin (Acred *et al.*, 1962): it should be noted that the very high ampicillin bile levels found in experimental animals are not equalled by those in man, and when any obstruction is present they are further reduced even to *nil* (Ayliffe and Davies, 1965; Mortimer, Mackie and Haynes, 1969). Cephalexin, according to Sales, Sutcliffe and O'Grady (1972) attains substantial levels in the bile, which can be increased by also giving probenecid. They point out that although some bacteria implicated in biliary tract infections are resistant to this antibiotic, *S. typhi* is highly sensitive, and suggest a trial in the treatment of typhoid carriers. Erythromycin and novobiocin are also excreted mainly in the bile.

Much the highest biliary concentrations, according to Acocella *et al.* (1968) are attained by derivatives of rifamycin, and although this antibiotic has only moderate activity against enterobacteria, the high levels attained compensate for this. There are enthusiastic reports of its efficacy in biliary tract infections by Bergamini and Fowst (1965) and Stratford (1966).

The treatment of biliary typhoid carriers is discussed in the following section.

INTESTINAL INFECTIONS

Enteric Fever

The recognized treatment for typhoid fever for over twenty years has been with chloramphenicol. Marmion (1955) recommends a total daily dose (administration being at four- or six-hour intervals) of 50 mg. per kg. until defervescence, and half this dose for a further 14 days. Woodward and Smadel (1964) recommend a dose of 3 g. daily reduced to 2 g. when the temperature falls and continued for 14 days, with the alternative of two five-day courses of this dosage separated by an interval of eight days. In severe cases cortisone or prednisolone may also be given (Rowland, 1961): defervescence is then more rapid and accompanied by a greater sense of well-being.

This treatment has several disadvantages. These are the risk of marrow damage, the frequency of relapse and total lack of bactericidal effect, with the result that a carrier state may persist: it has even been suggested that subsequent carriage is favoured. Moreover it seems that the response of the disease has become slower: Chakraborty (1961) in India and Omar and Wahab (1967) in Cairo both report that the mean period to defervescence, formerly about three days, has more recently extended to about six. It would be interesting to know whether this is attributable to diminished bacterial sensitivity, but in neither of these studies was this possibility examined. Both also report results of treatment with furazolidone, which appears to have been moderately effective.

As an alternative, great hopes were centred on ampicillin, since it is not only more active than chloramphenicol *in vitro* against the typhoid bacillus, but has two additional advantages in being bactericidal and safe to administer in larger doses, but results have been disappointing.

In Sanders' (1965) series given 4 g. ampicillin daily, six out of 10 patients with attacks rated as severe had to be given chloramphenicol ' because their condition was worsening after periods of treatment with ampicillin varying from four to eight days '. Patel (1964) found this necessary in fewer patients, and relates the degree of success with ampicillin to the stage of the disease at which it started : whereas chloramphenicol is effective at any stage, ampicillin brings down fever within a few days only when given early. This difference, and a better effect from ampicillin in mild infections, are evident from the experience of others. Scioli, Giusti and Balestrieri (1964) compared the effect on typhoid fever of 15 days' treatment with either 2 g. of chloramphenicol or 8 g. of ampicillin: the average times to defervescence were 3·6 and 6·1 days. They were also three and six days in patients with paratyphoid B fever given 2 g. chloramphenicol and 6 g. ampicillin by Sleet, Sangster and Murdoch (1964). In a non-comparative trial by Manriquez et al. (1965) the results were again judged inferior to those obtained with chloramphenicol. There seems to be no clear evidence that treatment with ampicillin reduces the frequency of relapse, and there is little information about its effect on the subsequent carrier state.

Typhoid fever seems to be the disease *par excellence* in which *in vitro* antibiotic activity is no guarantee of therapeutic success. Dawkins and Hornick (1967) treated experimental disease in prisoners with various antibiotics bactericidal for *S. typhi in vitro* in concentrations lower than that in which chloramphenicol is merely bacteristatic. Cephaloridine, gentamicin and polymyxin E failed even to achieve negative blood cultures. Ampicillin (6 g. daily) produced defervescence in two patients in five and 13 days: in two others chloramphenicol had to be substituted. It must be concluded that, except in infection by a chloramphenicol-resistant strain, ampicillin has no place in the treatment of any but perhaps mild cases of typhoid. An exception may be its use in combined treatment. De Ritis, Giammanco and Manzillo (1972) obtained a 29 per cent reduction in duration of fever by giving 4 g. daily in addition to 2 g. chloramphenicol in a total series of 100 patients.

Much more promising results have been obtained from treatment with cotrimoxazole, originally reported on by Akinkugbe et al. (1968), in whose small series defervescence was more rapid than in cases on chloramphenicol. More recently Kamat (1970) in Bombay studied 220 cases, all with positive blood cultures, treated either with chloramphenicol or with cotrimoxazole: mean periods to defervescence were 4·3 and

4·0 days respectively, but there was a much greater difference in the duration of ' toxaemia ' and weakness, which persisted longer in chloramphenicol-treated patients, 10 of whom also had a ' toxic crisis '. Sardesai, Melinkere and Diwate (1971), who treated 40 cases in Poona, also obtained uniformly good results, and there are several enthusiastic reports on smaller series from Italy. On the other hand, Scragg and Rubidge (1971), who treated 103 children in Durban, confirm the ' rapid improvement in well being ', but on all other counts found cotrimoxazole inferior to chloramphenicol. These included the persistence of fever, and in 19 out of 80 cases of a positive blood culture, a higher relapse rate, more frequent subsequent carriage, and in some cases evidence of bone marrow depression. Geddes *et al.* (1971) obtained satisfactory results in 21 out of 23 cases of typhoid fever, but express only guarded approval of the treatment. Further experience of it may help to explain the discordance between results obtained in different parts of the world.

TREATMENT OF CARRIERS. Here ampicillin has had much more success. Whereas tetracyclines or large doses of penicillin have in the past cleared only about 25 per cent of cases, ampicillin has been successful in 80 per cent or more. Christie (1964) cleared seven out of eight by three months' treatment with initially large doses reduced to 3 g. orally daily, together with probenecid and continued for 12 weeks. Münnich, Békési and Uri (1965/66) succeeded in 11 out of 12 cases by giving ampicillin parenterally (500 mg. four times a day) together with oral probenecid for up to six weeks. Simon and Miller (1966) gave 75-100 mg./kg. daily for four weeks or more to 15 cases, clearing 13. Scioli, Fiorentino and Sasso (1972) cleared every one of 19 longstanding cases (all followed up for 16-24 months), 5 of whom had gall stones and 8 non-functioning gall bladders, by giving 1 g. intravenously 8-hourly for 15 days. These findings confirm that success may be achieved regardless of gall bladder abnormalities, and suggest that parenteral administration may enable the course to be shortened.

Other Salmonella Infections

The treatment of paratyphoid fever is the same as that for typhoid. Chloramphenicol is also effective in acute *Salmonella* enteritis of the food-poisoning type, but in the previously healthy subject this is a self-limited disease of very short duration, and it is extremely doubtful whether treatment of this nature is necessary or even justified. On the other hand, in infancy or old age or in the presence of other disease, and if a systemic infection has been demonstrated by blood culture or is suspected from the clinical condition, it should be given.

There is strong evidence that unnecessary antibiotic treatment of mild *Salmonella* enteritis actually prolongs the subsequent carrier state. This was originally observed by Dixon (1965) and was confirmed in an extensive epidemic reported by Aserkoff and Bennett (1969) in which treatment with various antibiotics not only delayed elimination of the organism but in some cases led to its becoming resistant to one or more drugs, this resistance usually being transferable. In a controlled study of the action of oral neomycin, its only effect was to increase the frequency of the subsequent carrier state (Report, 1970). A strange episode is reported by Rosenthal (1969): a youth who had recovered from a mild attack of diarrhoea was found to have *S. typhimurium* in his faeces and was given ampicillin, which caused a recurrence much more severe than the original attack. The strain proved to be ampicillin-resistant, and it is suggested that suppression of the normal flora by the antibiotic enabled it to multiply ' unrestrainedly '. Loss of restraint by the normal flora—including that depending on bacteriocine production—may contribute to continued excretion of a pathogen when antibiotics are given.

Acute Infantile Gastro-enteritis

Correction of fluid loss and of electrolyte imbalance are the essential features of treatment and this is all that may be necessary in many cases. The infection is confined to the gut, without systemic invasion, which is the clearest indication for chemotherapy in other forms of acute enteritis. Locally acting antibiotics have chiefly been used in recent years. Oral neomycin or kanamycin had their advocates until bacterial resistance appeared; this is evidently not universal, since Nelson (1971) found all his strains sensitive to neomycin. He gave 100 mg. per kg. daily for either 2-4$\frac{1}{2}$ or 10 days to 113 cases, and obtained better results from the shorter course. Kahn, Stein and Wayburne (1963) commend paromomycin, and Coetzee and Leary (1971) gentamicin, given both orally and intramuscularly. In an epidemic the sensitivities of the strain to all applicable drugs, perhaps including polymyxin and cotrimoxazole, should be accurately determined, and any such treatment thought advisable should be directed accordingly.

Acute Staphylococcal Enterocolitis

This dangerous condition seems to be much less common than formerly. It occurred mainly in surgical patients treated with a broad spectrum antibiotic (tetracycline, and occasionally oral neomycin) or combination (penicillin + streptomycin) acting in an empty bowel (hence its frequent occurrence after gastrectomy), coupled with the unfortunate presence in the environment of a virulent staphylococcus with multiple antibiotic resistance.

Treatment consists of stopping the responsible antibiotic(s), generous fluid replacement, and the administration of an antibiotic to which the staphylococcus is sensitive. Penicillinase-resistant penicillins have been used successfully. Khan and Hall (1966) make a strong case for vancomycin, given orally in 0·5 g. doses every 4-6 hours: in 45 patients so treated there were no deaths from the enterocolitis, whereas in 54 treated with other antibiotics and 10 given none there were eight and three such deaths respectively.

Intestinal Candidiasis

' Superinfection ' of the bowel consequent on suppression of the normal flora by broad spectrum antibiotics is of three kinds, staphylococcal, coliform (resistant strains of *Pseudomonas, Proteus,* etc.), which is rarely accompanied by anything more than mild diarrhoea, and that due to *Candida albicans.* This also is accompanied by diarrhoea which is liable to be more intractable, and by pruritus ani. Oral nystatin may be indicated as a preventive and also affords the best treatment.

Bacillary Dysentery

The average mild infection due to *Sh. sonnei* does not require specific treatment, and it seems inadvisable that routine reports of the isolation of this organism should include information about drug sensitivities, since this may seem to encourage such treatment. Moreover, *Sh. sonnei* is now frequently drug-resistant. This is a species in which multiple transferable resistance has been studied for years, and Farrant and Tomlinson (1966) describe an epidemiological study suggesting that such transference is occurring on a large scale in this country. The great majority of strains isolated in London are now resistant not only to sulphonamides but to ampicillin (Davies, Farrant and Uttley, 1970).

Specific treatment may be required for more severe infections by other *Shigella* species, and the choice of an antibiotic should depend on laboratory tests either of the patient's own strain or of previous isolates in an epidemic. The results of these vary considerably in different parts of the world. Nelson and Haltalin (1967) in the United States and Tong *et al.* (1970) in Vietnam found most strains sensitive to ampicillin and obtained beneficial clinical effects from its use. Two recent papers commend cotrimoxazole: Freiberg (1971) in Germany, dealing with a *Sh. flexneri* epidemic among mental defectives, emphasizes its capacity to eliminate the organism from the bowel, for which chloramphenicol sometimes failed, and Lexomboon *et al.* (1972) in Thailand not only confirm this, but observed more rapid recovery than in patients treated with furazolidone. All their strains, mostly of *Sh. flexneri*, were sulphonamide-resistant, but synergy with trimethoprim was nevertheless demonstrated.

Amoebic Dysentery

This infection is outside the scope of this book, and we are not in a position to judge the merits of various antibiotics and synthetic drugs which now appear to be replacing emetine and its derivatives. Among the former paromomycin appears to be the most useful, and the latter now include metronidazole, which in doses of 750 mg. 3 times a day for 10 days is effective in all stages of the disease and particularly so for liver abscess (Medical Letter, 1972).

Cholera

Recognition that chemotherapy can be effective in cholera came late. Carpenter *et al.* (1964) in India and Greenough *et al.* (1964) in Pakistan have shown that tetracycline in moderate doses, the first few intravenous and thereafter oral, rapidly eliminates *V. cholerae* from the bowel, greatly reduces both stool volume and the requirement for intravenous fluid, and enables patients to be discharged in three days instead of seven. The economy in intravenous fluids and in bed occupancy is important in enabling more patients to be treated in an epidemic. Furazolidone (Chaudhuri *et al.,* 1968; Pierce *et al.,* 1968) is a cheaper and apparently effective alternative.

Travellers' Diarrhoea

More questions are asked about this common and troublesome condition than about many more serious diseases. Prophylaxis rather than treatment is the objective, and the choice of suitable drugs is impeded by ignorance of the aetiology in different parts of the world, in some of which it seems possible that causative organisms may exist which have yet to be identified.

Assuming an enterobacterial cause, prophylaxis should be feasible, since it is much easier to prevent the growth of a small number of bacteria than of the vast numbers present in established infection, particularly with sulphonamides. Several controlled studies, in which the attack rate was substantially reduced, appear to confirm this. Kean and Waters (1959) and Kean *et al.* (1962) conducted double-blind trials in North American students spending the summer session at the University of Mexico, and obtained good results with either neomycin or sulphathalidine, the placebo used being lactose; iodochlorhydroxyquinoline (Entero-Vioform), perhaps the most commonly used drug and apparently a good prophylactic for amoebiasis, had no effect. Moreover, this drug is now under suspicion because of its possible relationship to subacute myelo-optic neuropathy (Editorial, 1971). Turner (1967) in a similar study in B.O.A.C. personnel going abroad, found both the attack rate and the severity of such attacks as occurred to be reduced by a combination of streptomycin and triple sulphonamides (Streptotriad), although the same sulphonamides together with a larger dose of neomycin only had the second of these effects. Nelson, Jones and Ross (1962) greatly reduced the attack rate in R.A.F. personnel east of Suez with furazolidone. It seems possible that some of these results might be improved by more frequent administration than twice a day, in order to ensure more uniform distribution in the intestinal contents. For intelligent visitors at risk for only a few days this should not be unduly burdensome.

Therapeutic Suppression of the Normal Bowel Flora

The commonest indication for this is an operation on the colon, which it facilitates by diminishing both gaseous distension and liability to subsequent peritonitis. The less soluble sulphonamides were first used for this purpose, and later tetracyclines: these have a more profound effect, but were abandoned because they predispose to dangerous superinfections. The most popular antibiotic is now neomycin. It is not necessary, and indeed highly undesirable, to give this in large doses or for long periods, as described by Jacobson *et al.* (1960), who found that such treatment caused mucosal changes and malabsorption. Provided that the bulk of the intestinal contents has been reduced by suitable diet and aperients, two days' treatment should suffice. Various combinations of neomycin with other drugs have been used. In the only recent trial in which any of us has been concerned, Sellwood *et al.* (1969) found a combination of neomycin, bacitracin and nystatin more effective than sulphathalidine in preventing post-operative infections, and a correspondingly much greater reduction in numbers of the principal bowel flora was demonstrated.

A body of surgical opinion, particularly in the United States, seems to be moving against such proceedings. Altemeier, Hummel and Hill (1966) compared five regimens involving pre-operative oral medication with sulphathalidine, sulphathalidine + neomycin or paromomycin, with or without post-operative parenteral treatment with penicillin and tetracycline, and obtained the best results with post-operative treatment only, but the group so treated numbered only 17, and the total cases in the five groups only 93. Polacek and Sanfellipo (1968) gave 'a sulfonamide preparation' or 'a neomycinsulfonamide preparation' post-operatively in unstated doses to 78 and 112 patients, in whom the subsequent infection rate was 23 per cent, whereas in 73 controls it was only 4 per cent, but this comparison is vitiated by several days' post-operative treatment of the controls only with penicillin and chloramphenicol. The authors of both of these papers complain that pre-operative bowel preparation leads to an overgrowth of staphylococci, which caused some of the subsequent wound infections, and in the hands of Azar and Drapanas (1968), when pre-operative neomycin + sulphathalidine was followed by post-operative treatment with chloramphenicol, tetracycline, or penicillin with either of the foregoing or streptomycin, there was a 14 per cent incidence of staphylococcal enterocolitis. In none of these papers is any reference made to the fact that staphylococcal growth can almost certainly be prevented by including bacitracin in the pre-operative oral mixture. Vancomycin would probably serve the same purpose well. Such an addition is advisable wherever neomycin-resistant staphylococci exist; there can be no possible objection to ' shot-gun ' treatment for so short a period, by an innocuous route, and when each ingredient in the mixture has a defined purpose.

Possibly the only indication for much more prolonged treatment of this kind is hepatic failure, the effects of which can be mitigated by administering an antibiotic, usually neomycin or kanamycin, for considerable periods. In patients also suffering from renal failure, the small amounts of antibiotic absorbed may accumulate in the blood and cause damage to the eighth nerve, and possibly further damage to the kidneys (Last and Sherlock, 1960; Kunin et al., 1960). As the less ototoxic, kanamycin may be preferable to neomycin for such patients. According to Berk and Chalmers (1970) this risk is not confined to patients with damaged kidneys; 2 out of 5 becoming deaf after treatment with 3 g. neomycin daily for 8-28 months had normal renal function. It is usually believed that ulceration enhances absorption, but Breen et al. (1972), who measured absorption of neomycin by assaying urinary output, could not confirm this in patients with active peptic ulceration, regional ileitis or ulcerative colitis.

Peritonitis

The treatment of peritonitis due to a perforated viscus depends in the first place on the level at which this occurs. If the site is in the stomach or duodenum the comparatively few bacteria liberated originate mainly in the mouth, where the flora is generally penicillin-sensitive. If the lower bowel is involved, the flora is entirely different and immensely varied, and in the individual case has in the past been imperfectly identified, particularly in laboratories which make only aerobic cultures. The exudate will usually contain *E. coli* and *Str. faecalis*, probably *Cl. welchii* (although the importance once attached to this species in the effects produced is no longer admitted), but it is now widely recognized that the most numerous organisms are often *Bacteroides* spp., and any anti-bacterial treatment must take these into account. These include *B. fragilis*, which is highly resistant to penicillin, and more so than other species to several other antibiotics.

Popular treatments in the past have been with penicillin + streptomycin or with a tetracycline; both involve a risk of causing staphylococcal enterocolitis, and the original very broad spectrum of tetracyclines has been badly eroded by acquired bacterial resistance. Present-day opinion, recognizing the exceptional sensitivity of *Bacteroides* to lincomycin and clindamycin, particularly the latter, favours the use of one of these antibiotics; the parenteral form of clindamycin, when it becomes available, will be preferable. This may with advantage be combined with gentamicin for its action on coliforms. These recommendations refer to parenteral treatment; local application may also be of value, and a solution of kanamycin has been commended for instillation at operation for a perforated appendix (see p. 122).

REFERENCES

ACOCELLA, G., MATTIUSSI, R., NICOLIS, F. B., PALLANZA, R. & TENCONI, L. T. (1968). *Gut* 9, 536.

ACRED, P., BROWN, D. M., TURNER, D. H. & WILSON, M. J. (1962). *Brit. J. Pharmacol.* 18, 356.

AKINKUGBE, O. O., LEWIS, E. A., MONTEFIORE, D. & OKUBADEJO, O. A. (1968). *Brit. med. J.* 3, 721.

ALTEMEIER, W. A., HUMMEL, R. P. & HILL, E. O. (1966). *Arch. Surg.*, 93, 226.

ASERKOFF, B. & BENNETT, J. V. (1969). *New Engl. J. Med.* 281, 636.

AYLIFFE, G. A. J. & DAVIES, A. (1965). *Brit. J. Pharmacol.* 24, 189.

AZAR, H. & DRAPANAS, T. (1968). *Amer. J. Surg.* 115, 209.

BERGAMINI, N. & FOWST, G. (1965). *Arzneimittel forsch.* 15 (Suppl.), 951.

BERK, D. P. & CHALMERS, T. (1970). *Ann. intern. Med.* 73, 393.

BERNARD, H. R. & COLE, W. R. (1964). *Surgery* 56, 151.

BREEN, K. J., BRYANT, R. E., LEVINSON, J. D. & SCHENKER, S. (1972). *Ann. intern. Med.* 76, 211.

CARPENTER, C. C. J., SACK, R. B., MONDAL, A. & MITRA, P. P. (1964). *J. Indian med. Ass.* 43, 309.

CHAKRABORTY, G. (1961). *Indian J. Pediat.* **28,** 357.
CHAUDHURI, R. N., NEOGY, K. N., SANYAL, S. N., GUPTA, R. K. & MANJI, P. (1968). *Lancet* **1,** 332.
CHRISTIE, A. B. (1964). *Brit. med. J.* **1,** 1609.
COETZEE, M. & LEARY, P. M. (1971). *Arch. Dis. Child.* **46,** 646.
DAVIES, J. R., FARRANT, W. N. & UTTLEY, A. H. C. (1970). *Lancet* **2,** 1157.
DAVIES, A. H., MCFADZEAN, J. A. & SQUIRES, S. (1964). *Brit. med. J.* **1,** 1149.
DAWKINS, A. T. & HORNICK, R. B. (1967). *Antimicrob. Agents and Chemother.*—1966, p. 6.
DE RITIS, F., GIAMMANCO, G. & MANZILLO, G. (1972). *Brit. med. J.* **4,** 17.
DIXON, J. M. S. (1965). *Brit. med. J.* **2,** 1343.
EDITORIAL (1971). *Brit. med. J.* **2,** 291.
EMSLIE, R. D., CROSS, W. G. & BLAKE, G. C. (1962). *Brit. dent. J.* **112,** 320.
FARRANT, W. N. & TOMLINSON, A. J. H. (1966). *J. Hyg. (Lond.)* **64,** 287.
FREIBERG, T. (1971). *Arzneimittel-Forsch.* **21,** 599.
GEDDES, A. M., FOTHERGILL, R., GOODALL, J. A. D. & DORKEN, P. R. (1971). *Brit. med. J.* **3,** 451.
GREENOUGH, W. B. III., GORDON, R. S., ROSENBERG, I. S., DAVIES, B. I. & BENENSON, A. S. (1964). *Lancet* **1,** 355.
HARRISON, P. M. & STEWART, G. T. (1961). *Brit. J. Pharmacol.* **17,** 420.
JACOBSON, E. D., PRIOR, J. T. & FALOON, W. W. (1960). *J. Lab. clin. Med.* **56,** 245.
KAHN, E., STEIN, H. & WAYBURNE, S. (1963). *Lancet* **2,** 703.
KAHN, M. Y. & HALL, W. H. (1966). *Ann. intern. Med.* **65,** 1.
KAMAT, S. A. (1970). *Brit. med. J.* **3,** 320.
KEAN, B. H., SCHAFFNER, W., BRENNAN, R. W. & WATERS, S. R. (1962). *J. Amer. med. Ass.* **180,** 367.
KEAN, B. H. & WATERS, S. R. (1959). *New Engl. J. Med.* **261,** 71.
KUNIN, C. M., CHALMERS. T. C., LEEVY, C. M., SEBASTYEN, S. C., LIEBER, C. S. & FINLAND. M. (1960). *New Engl. J. Med.* **262,** 380.
LAST, P. M. & SHERLOCK, S. (1960). *New Engl. J. Med.* **262,** 385.
LEXOMBOON, U., MANSUWAN, P., DUANGMANI, C., BENJADOL, P. & MCMINN, M. T. (1972). *Brit. med. J.* **3,** 23.
MACGREGOR, A. B. & LONG, D. A. (1944). *Brit. med. J.* **2,** 686.
MANRIQUEZ, L., SALCEDO, M., BORGONO, J. M., MARZULLO, E., KRALJEVIC, R., PAREDES, L. & VALDIVIESO, R. (1965). *Brit. med. J.* **2,** 152.
MARMION, D. E. (1955). *Med. ill. (Lond.)* **9,** 214.
MEDICAL LETTER (1972). The Medical Letter on Drugs and Therapeutics, **14,** 39.
MORTIMER, P. R., MACKIE, D. B. & HAYNES, S. (1969). *Brit. med. J.* **3,** 88.
MÜNNICH, D., BÉKÉSI, I. & URI, J. (1965/6). *Chemotherapia* **10,** 253.
NELSON, J. D. (1971). *Pediatrics* **48,** 248.
NELSON, J. D. & HALTALIN, K. C. (1967). *Ann. New York Acad. Sci.* **145,** 414.
NELSON, S. R. C., JONES, H. L. & ROSS, J. B. (1962). *Practitioner* **188,** 654.
OMAR, M. E. S. & WAHAB, M. F. A. (1967). *J. trop. Med. Hyg.* **70,** 43.
PATEL, K. M. (1964). *Proc. IIIrd Int. Congr. Chemother.,* Vol. 1, p. 416. Stuttgart: Thieme.
PIERCE, N. F., BANWELL, J. G., MITRA, R. C., CARANASOS, G. J., KEIMOWITZ, R. I., THOMAS, J. & MONDAL, A. (1968). *Brit. med. J.* **3,** 277.
POLACEK, M. A. & SANFELLIPO, P. (1968). *Arch. Surg.* **97,** 412.
REPORT (1970). Joint Project by Members of the Association for the Study of Infectious Diseases, *Lancet* **2,** 1159.
ROSENTHAL, S. L. (1969). *New Engl. J. Med.* **280,** 147.
ROWLAND. H. A. K. (1961). *J. trop. Med. Hyg.* **64,** 101.
SALES, J. E. L., SUTCLIFFE, M. & O'GRADY, F. (1972). *Brit. med. J.* **3,** 441.
SANDERS, W. L. (1965). *Brit. med. J.* **2,** 1226.
SARDESAI, H. V., MELINKERE, R. D. & DIWATE, A. B. (1971). *Trans. roy. Soc. trop. Med. Hyg.* **65,** 189.
SCIOLI, C., FIORENTINO, F. & SASSO, G. (1972). *J. infect. Dis.* **125,** 170.

SCIOLI, C., GIUSTI, G. & BALESTRIERI, G. (1964). *Postgrad. med. J.* **40,** (Suppl.) 87.
SCRAGG, J. N. & RUBIDGE, C. J. (1971). *Brit. med. J.* **3,** 738.
SELLWOOD, R. A., BURN, J. I., WATERWORTH, P. M. & WELBOURN, R. B. (1969). *Brit. J. Surg.* **56,** 610.
SIMON, H. J. & MILLER, R. C. (1966). *New Engl. J. Med.* **274,** 807.
SLEET, R. A., SANGSTER, G. & MURDOCH, J. McC. (1964). *Brit. med. J.* **1,** 148.
STRATFORD, B. C. (1966). *Med. J. Aust.* **1,** 7.
TAYLOR, G. W. (1960). *Brit. med. Bull.* **16,** 51.
TONG, M. J., MARTIN, D. G., CUNNINGHAM, J. J. & GUNNING, J-J. (1970). *J. Amer. med. Ass.* **214,** 1841.
TURNER, A. C. (1967). *Brit. med. J.* **4,** 653.
WOODWARD, T. E. & SMADEL, J. E. (1964). *Ann. intern. Med.* **60,** 144.

Chapter 22

INFECTIONS OF THE AIR PASSAGES

ANTIMICROBIAL drugs are prescribed with enormous frequency in acute respiratory infections, but in no part of medicine is rational chemotherapy more difficult. The syndromes of respiratory infection are of widely varied aetiology, and clinical and laboratory evidence often offer limited guidance about the causal organism in a particular patient. For example, acute sore throat may have viral, mycoplasmal or a number of bacterial causes, but only occasionally can the cause be accurately deduced from the clinical findings. Moreover, the frequency and significance of secondary bacterial infection in syndromes of primary viral origin are often quite uncertain.

Colds

The great majority of colds are viral in origin, and are not at present susceptible to any direct form of chemotherapeutic attack. The possible rôle of secondary bacterial infection in prolonging and worsening the effects of the illness has been in dispute for many years; so too has the value of antimicrobial drugs in mitigating these effects. Ten double-blind trials, mostly involving the use of a tetracycline, were reviewed by Davis and Wedgewood (1965). Many trials gave negative results, but in those of Ritchie (1958) and McKerrow *et al.* (1961) the average duration of illness was shortened with small doses of tetracycline taken in lozenge form.

The evidence of benefit derived from a few of the trials is on the whole outweighed by the likelihood of promoting, by widespread use, an increased incidence of pathogens resistant to the agents. This policy applies to patients with normal chests; by contrast the use of an antimicrobial agent, usually tetracycline or co-trimoxazole, is indicated at the onset of a cold in patients with chronic bronchitis. Exacerbations of bronchitis are often induced by viral infection (Lambert and Stern, 1972), especially by rhinoviruses (Stenhouse, 1967) but in this susceptible group it is best to assume the likelihood of secondary bacterial infection, difficult as it is to provide clear evidence of this.

Influenza

Antiviral chemotherapy is discussed on p. 477. As with the common cold, antibacterial chemotherapy is not indicated in previously healthy subjects. In those at special risk treatment should be given and should take account of secondary bacterial invaders known to be prevalent in the particular epidemic. If no special information is available, a penicillinase-resistant penicillin should be included, since staphylococci are especially dangerous in association with influenza virus. Other organisms such as *H. influenzae* may also be important in patients with chronic respiratory disease who develop influenza, so a suitable scheme of treatment for such patients is provided by ampicillin and cloxacillin. Those at special risk, for whom antibiotics should be given during an attack of influenza, include patients with chronic bronchitis, those with chronic heart disease, the elderly, and pregnant women.

Acute Sore Throat

Many acute sore throats are caused by virus infection, but an important group is caused by *Str. pyogenes*. This organism accounted for 30 per cent of acute sore throats in a recent study in Scotland (Ross *et al.*, 1971). In some countries diphtheria remains important, while Vincent's angina is found especially, but not exclusively, in association with gingival sepsis. Clinical signs are often unreliable as a guide to aetiology. Haemolytic streptococci are more likely to be found in association with high fever, follicular tonsillitis, tender anterior cervical glands and neutrophilia in the peripheral blood, but may be grown profusely from patients with mild sore throat or, indeed, from symptomless carriers. Conversely, bad sore throat even with pharyngeal exudate, may be viral in origin. For these reasons antibiotic treatment of acute sore throat is most satisfactory if based on examination of a throat swab. The use of suitable transport medium makes this practicable in the community as well as in hospital.

The most appropriate treatment for streptococcal sore throat is penicillin. This can be given orally as phenoxymethylpenicillin 250 mg. four times daily. Because of erratic taking of medicine, especially by children, more satisfactory results may be achieved by initiating treatment with one injection of procaine penicillin or fortified procaine penicillin (containing 300 mg. of procaine penicillin and 60 mg. benzylpenicillin per unit volume), continuing treatment thereafter with phenoxymethyl penicillin by mouth. Treatment makes little difference to the rate at which symptoms subside and the aim of therapy is eradication of streptococci from the nasopharynx. In order to ensure this in a high proportion of patients, it is necessary to continue penicillin for 10 days. This is rarely achieved in practice, since patients feel well again in a few days and do not complete the course. Patients hypersensitive to penicillin can be treated by erythromycin. Cephalosporins have also been used for this purpose but since there are some examples of cross allergy with the penicillins, cephalosporins should not be given when the history of penicillin allergy is well-documented or one of severe reaction. Stillerman *et al.* (1972) found that treatment by oral cephalexin was followed by a lower relapse rate than treatment with phenoxymethyl penicillin. For those working in circumstances which do not allow examination of swabs in cases of sore throat, it is useful to have a policy for the use of penicillin which, while including most patients likely to have streptococcal infection, avoids its widespread use in predominantly viral syndromes. In these circumstances penicillin can be given on the following indications:

1. Scarlet fever. Its exact aetiology is implicit in the diagnosis, so that penicillin is indicated.
2. Follicular tonsillitis with fever and tender anterior cervical glands.
3. Bacterial complications of acute pharyngitis such as peritonsillar abscess (quinsy), otitis media, and suppurative cervical lymphadenitis.
4. Acute sore throat in a patient with rheumatic heart disease.
5. Acute sore throat in a family or community setting in which there is known to be a high prevalence of streptococcal infection.

Chronic Carrier States in the Nasopharynx

The prevention of streptococcal throat infections in patients subject to rheumatic fever is best achieved with penicillin. The most successful method is a monthly injection of benzathine penicillin. Two disadvantages of this method are the need for repeated injections, albeit infrequently, and the likelihood that any allergic reactions will be of long duration. In this country the most widely used method is oral phenoxymethyl penicillin 250 mg. twice daily. The treatment of meningococcal carriers is discussed on p. 352.

Diphtheria

Antibiotics are an essential part of treatment but do not obviate the need for antitoxin. *C. diphtheriae* is moderately sensitive to penicillin, and is also sensitive to ampicillin, erythromycin, rifampicin and clindamycin. Seven-day courses of penicillin and of erythromycin were found equally effective both clinically and bacteriologically (McCloskey *et al.*, 1971). Erythromycin has been mainly used in the treatment of carriers, but in the same study a single injection of benzathine penicillin was equally effective, both methods showing a failure rate of 11 per cent.

Acute Epiglottitis

This rapidly progressive and life-threatening cause of croup is encountered mainly in children, but has also been increasingly recognized in adults. It is caused by infection with *H. influenzae* type B which may often be cultivated from the blood as well as from the local lesion. Treatment is as much concerned with maintaining the airway as with control of the infection. Chloramphenicol and ampicillin have both been used successfully on different occasions, and the relative rarity of the condition does not allow an objective judgment between them. Since, however, ampicillin acts more slowly and less certainly than chloramphenicol in a number of acute infections in which they have been compared, we agree with Addy *et al.* (1972) that parenteral chloramphenicol is the drug of choice. The general practitioner may more probably have intramuscular ampicillin to hand, and he should administer this on suspicion of acute epiglottitis without attempting to take throat cultures or to delay until the patient reaches hospital.

Acute Otitis Media

The milder catarrhal forms often resolve without chemotherapy, and Fry (1958) used penicillin only in a minority of his cases. The predominant organisms found in otitis media severe enough to need myringotomy are *Str. pneumoniae*, *Haemophilus influenzae* and *Str. pyogenes*. The proportion of cases caused by the latter organism varies greatly in different series, while *H. influenzae* is found mostly in children less than five years old, although Howie *et al.* (1970) found it equally commonly in older children. *Staph. aureus* is found more commonly, as are coliforms and less common organisms, in discharge from the ear contaminated by organisms in the external meatus. An interesting observation in many series is the cultivation of *N. catarrhalis* in pure culture in a small (1·3-5 per cent) but significant number of exudates, taken directly from the middle ear with careful technique to avoid contamination: in such cases intracellular gram-negative diplococci may sometimes be seen in the exudate (Kamme, 1970).

The results of recent antibiotic trials, together with studies of antibiotic concentrations in middle ear exudates, correlate well with the bacteriological findings. Bass *et al.* (1967), in a double blind trial involving 400 children, found no significant difference between ampicillin and two regimens of penicillin + sulphafurazole. Oxytetracycline treatment was associated with a higher relapse rate. Nilson *et al.* (1969) were able to relate the results of treatment to bacterial aetiology; overall, ampicillin gave similar results to a penicillin + sulphonamide scheme, but ampicillin was superior for the group caused by *H. influenzae*. In a smaller trial in milder forms of disease encountered in private practice (Laxdal *et al*, 1970), the order of merit observed was ampicillin, followed by penicillin, followed by placebo, but only the ampicillin versus placebo difference attained conventional levels of significance. Coffey (1968) showed that good levels of ampicillin were obtained in middle ear exudate following injections of ampicillin, and

Kamme *et al.* (1969) clearly demonstrated the relation of dose of phenoxymethylpenicillin to the concentration found in serum and middle ear exudate in acute otitis media of childhood. Doses of 13 mg./kg. gave inadequate levels to inhibit most strains of *H. influenzae*, but 26 mg./kg. produced concentrations in the exudate of up to 4 μg./ml. which approximates to the M.I.C. for this relatively resistant organism. A three times daily scheme of $13 + 13 + 26$ mg./kg. was successful in 86 per cent of patients.

It appears that phenoxymethyl penicillin, with injections of penicillin at the beginning of treatment in severe cases, provides satisfactory treatment for otitis media in the school age child and adult. For the younger children, in whom *H. influenzae* otitis is common, treatment with ampicillin in a dose of 50 mg./kg./day may be preferable, although phenoxymethyl penicillin may also be effective, provided an adequate dose, 50-75 mg./kg./day, is given. For patients hypersensitive to penicillin, erythromycin may be given. Adequate concentrations for inhibiting pneumococci and *Str. pyogenes* can be achieved in purulent exudate by doses of 12·5 mg./kg. six hourly, but some strains of *H. influenzae* would not be inhibited (Bass *et al.*, 1971). Lincomycin was shown to achieve similar results to penicillin in acute otitis media by Taylor *et al* (1969) but with a higher incidence of unwanted reactions, mainly diarrhoea. Trakas and Lind (1966) achieved good results with lincomycin in eight of 14 patients with chronic otitis media and mastoiditis.

Acute Sinusitis

Most investigations of sinusitis have found pneumococci and *Str. pyogenes* as the dominant organisms, for which penicillin is the most suitable treatment. Some investigators have also found a high incidence of *H. influenzae* and Nylen *et al.* (1972) observed that after 10 days' treatment with phenoxymethylpenicillin *H. influenzae* was often still present in the middle meatus, and that re-isolation was more common in the patients whose course was unsatisfactory. Full doses of penicillin, by injection at first and later orally, should be administered to patients with acute sinusitis. If *H. influenzae* is grown from the pus, ampicillin should be used instead.

PNEUMONIA

A wide variety of organisms may cause pneumonia, but the causal diagnosis is only occasionally evident at the time when the clinical and radiological diagnosis is made. Florid illness, lobar distribution, and a neutrophilia favour a bacterial cause but antibiotic treatment before admission to hospital often mutes the features of a bacterial pneumonia, while viruses and *Mycoplasma pneumoniae* may cause severe illnesses and lobar consolidation. Examination of sputum may be disappointing but a sputum smear should be gram-stained and examined soon after admission. Blood as well as sputum cultures should be taken, since an appreciable number of patients with pneumococcal pneumonia have positive blood cultures. Although a large number of bacteria can cause pneumonia, many of them do so only rarely, and in special circumstances. For example, in 1,032 patients with pneumonia drawn from the indigent population of Detroit, Tillotson and Lerner (1968) found only 38 with pneumonia caused by gram-negative organisms, of whom 36 had serious chronic illnesses. Since accurate information about the causal organism is so often hard to come by early in the illness or even throughout its course, it is useful to consider the likely bacterial pathogens in relation to the patient's age and to the setting in which the pneumonia occurs.

Pneumonia in Previously Healthy Adults and Children

The predominant bacterial pathogen is *Str. pneumoniae*. Although less commonly isolated than formerly, it is still by far the most common isolate (Table 38), and benzyl penicillin is therefore the drug of choice. Treatment should be by injection initially, but oral penicillin can be given after the first day or two. Tetracycline is no longer suitable as a universal treatment for all pneumonias, since strains of pneumococci resistant to this drug as well as to erythromycin and to lincomycin have emerged. These drugs should now be reserved for patients hypersensitive to penicillin. Resistance to cotrimoxazole has also been reported (Howe & Wilson, 1972). Anderson *et al.* (1968) showed that lincomycin was as effective as penicillin in mild or moderately severe pneumonia.

The other common agent in this group is *Mycoplasma pneumoniae*. It may be suspected in patients with atypical pneumonia associated with other similar cases within a family or residential institution, and about half the patients show cold agglutinins in their serum. The definitive diagnosis rests on serological tests or cultivation of the organism from the sputum or naso-pharynx. Appropriate antimicrobial treatment shortens the duration of illness and the period during which the chest radiograph is abnormal, but results in civilian communities

TABLE 38

Causes of Adult Pneumonia

Source	Year	No. of Cases	Pneumo-coccal %	Other Bacteria %	Unknown %
Humphrey et al.	1948	267	73	5	21
M.R.C.	1951	351	79	6	15
Bath et al.	1964	193	55	11	34
Fiala	1969	156	57		38

TABLE 39

Efficacy of Different Antibiotics against Organisms concerned in Bronchopneumonia

Species of Organism	Antibiotic						
	Penicillins			Ceph-alori-dine	Tetra-cyclines	Ery-thro-mycin	Chlor-amphe-nicol
	Benzyl	Ampi-cillin	Methi-cillin				
Str. pneumoniae	+	+	(+)	+	±	+	(+)
Str. pyogenes	+	+	(+)	+	±	+	(+)
Staph. aureus	±	±	+	+	±	±	(±)
H. influenzae	(+)	+	—	(+)	+	+	+
Kl. pneumoniae	—	±	—	±	+	—	+
Psittacosis virus	—	—	—	—	+	—	+
R. burneti	—	—	—	—	+	—	+
Mycoplasma pneumoniae	—	—	—	—	+	+	(+)
+ = full therapeutic effect.							
± = variable therapeutic effect.							
(+)= lesser therapeutic effect.							
— = no therapeutic effect.							

have been less impressive than in Army Camps, possibly be-cause treatment is begun earlier in the latter group. Kingston *et al.* (1961) showed the efficacy of demethylchlortetracycline in a double blind trial, while Shames *et al* (1970) showed that erythromycin, tetracycline, methacycline, demethylchlortetra-cycline and triacetyloleandomycin all showed a beneficial effect compared with a control group who received penicillin or no antimicrobial drug. If the initial evidence leaves the clinician in doubt between a bacterial and mycoplasmal cause for pneu-monia, it is best to ensure that the likely bacterial causes are treated, since bacterial pneumonia is a much greater hazard than mycoplasmal. While pneumococcal strains resistant to it remain rare, erythromycin is suitable to treat both pneumo-coccal and mycoplasmal pneumonia. The sensitivities to seven antibiotics of a variety of causal organisms in pneumonia are given in Table 39. The rare cases caused by *Kl. pneu-moniae* (Friedlander's bacillus) present a particular problem, and antibiotic sensitivity tests are especially important. Indi-vidual strains may be susceptible to streptomycin, sulphon-amides, tetracycline, chloramphenicol, aminoglycosides, cephalosporins and co-trimoxazole. If the clinical situation and gram-stained film of the sputum suggest this diagnosis, treatment may be started with gentamicin, or with kanamycin and a cephalosporin, pending further information.

Q fever and psittacosis are both treated by tetracycline. A dose of 2 g. daily continued for 10 days or for three days after the fever subsides is usually recommended but it might be wiser to continue treatment for a longer period in the hope of pre-venting chronic infections.

Pneumonia in Infancy

Most pneumonias in infancy are viral in origin, but a possible bacterial cause must be assumed in the absence of specific evidence to the contrary, since the bacterial pneu-monias may be life-threatening. In addition to the pneumo-coccus, *Staph. aureus* must be considered as a now uncommon but potentially serious cause. Pertussis is considered elsewhere (p. 387). Precise evidence of aetiology is especially hard to establish in this group, since children rarely produce sputum except in pertussis, and organisms cultivated from throat swabs poorly represent the bronchial flora. For these reasons it is customary to treat infants with pneumonia by broad spectrum as well as anti-staphylococcal drugs; a combination of ampicillin and cloxacillin, or cephaloridine alone, is widely used.

Acute bronchitis in infancy is commonly caused by respiratory syncytial virus without evidence of additional bacterial infection. Antimicrobial drugs are not indicated if this diagnosis is established by the typical clinical picture, or by identification of the agent by immunofluorescent microscopy of pharyngeal aspirate or material from the throat swab. Controlled trials have shown no benefit from antibiotics in this condition.

Acute laryngotracheobronchitis in infancy is also commonly viral in origin and antimicrobial drugs are not necessary, but other causes of croup especially acute epiglottitis and diphtheria (q.v.) must always be considered since they demand urgent treatment including antibiotics.

Pneumonia in Patients with Chronic Bronchitis

The factors which influence choice of treatment are the same as in severe exacerbations of chronic bronchitis, and are not greatly influenced by whether or not the patient has areas of pulmonary consolidation warranting a diagnosis of pneumonia. This problem is discussed on p. 388.

Pneumonia Developing in Hospital or in Patients with Lowered Resistance

Patients developing pneumonia while in hospital are at special risk of infection with unusual organisms. They are often also in a state of lowered resistance by reason of their underlying disease and of the treatment with drugs such as corticosteroids and antimetabolites which they may be receiving. Antibiotic choice in this group must take account of pneumonia caused by hospital staphylococci, and by a variety of gram-negative organisms including *Klebsiella* and *Pseudomonas*. Initial treatment must be guided by these possibilities and by knowledge of the prevalent hospital flora. When no useful information is at first available treatment can be initiated in seriously ill patients by a combination of gentamicin with a cephalosporin.

Pertussis

Antibiotic treatment of pertussis is generally disappointing, although *Bordetella pertussis* is susceptible *in vitro* to the penicillins, chloramphenicol, tetracyclines, and polymyxin. An early M.R.C. trial (1953) showed some benefit from chloramphenicol and chlortetracycline in patients treated early in the disease, but the advantages were not dramatic even in this group, and it is difficult to make a firm diagnosis of pertussis during its early stages. Ampicillin has been used in pertussis more recently; Nelson *et al.* (1966) claimed that it eliminated the organism in four patients but contradictory results have been recorded by other workers. Bass *et al.* (1969) treated and carefully observed ten cases each with ampicillin, chloramphenicol, erythromycin, oxytetracycline and no antibiotics. No effect was observed on the course of the disease by any of the antibiotics and ampicillin failed to eliminate the organism, whereas erythromycin achieved this rapidly. Strangert (1969) compared ampicillin and chloramphenicol in 148 children with pertussis, finding that cultures were more often negative, and that the number of coughing bouts was somewhat fewer, following treatment with chloramphenicol.

There is probably little to be gained by the use of antibiotics in children with mild pertussis. Children with more severe attacks should be given ampicillin as a relatively non-toxic agent for which benefit has sometimes been claimed. Children whose lives are threatened by severe pertussis bronchopneumonia would best be treated by chloramphenicol.

Acute Bronchitis

In a previously normal subject acute bronchitis is most commonly viral in origin. If the illness is severe, secondary bacterial infection must be assumed and tetracycline or ampicillin given. The former drug, or erythromycin, will be preferred if there is any reason to believe the bronchitis is caused by *Mycoplasma pneumoniae*. This organism more often causes bronchitis or upper respiratory tract infection than pneumonia (p. 385).

Chronic Bronchitis

The rôle of antimicrobial drugs in chronic bronchitis has been especially difficult to assess since the disease varies so greatly in its rate of progress, and especially in its propensity to acute exacerbations. *H. influenzae* and the pneumococcus are the most common bacterial isolates from sputum, staphylococci may be found and *Klebsiella, Pseudomonas* and other gram-negative species may become predominant after antibiotic treatment.

Antibacterial drugs have been given in chronic bronchitis with three main objects; the treatment of exacerbations when they occur, long-term prophylaxis aimed at preventing exacerbations and suppressive treatment in advanced cases with constantly purulent sputum.

The benefits attained by long-term treatment throughout the winter have been explored in a number of trials, the results of which were reviewed in previous editions of this book and by Stuart-Harris (1968). Tetracyclines have been used most commonly for this purpose, but ampicillin and penicillin V have also been employed. In most studies a reduction in time off work was achieved, usually by a diminution in the duration rather than the number of exacerbations, but little or no change in the rate at which respiratory function deteriorated was demonstrated in three 5-year trials of tetracycline treatment (M.R.C., 1966; Calder *et al.*, 1968; Johnston *et al.*, 1969). Two of these studies gave convincing evidence to support the common view that long-term treatment was beneficial in that group of patients, representing only a small proportion of those with chronic bronchitis, who suffer frequent acute exacerbations during the winter. Treatment throughout the winter is now prescribed for few patients, but the early treatment of acute exacerbations is widely practised. Malone *et al.* (1968), giving antibiotics at the first sign of a ' chest cold ' to outpatients at three chest clinics, found ampicillin, tetracycline and methacycline equally effective. Pines *et al.* (1968), after extensive trials in purulent exacerbations of bronchitis, suggest that tetracycline or oxytetracycline should be used if the daily dose is 2 g. or less, but that lymecycline is better tolerated if larger doses are needed, as they may be in severe exacerbation. A recent addition to the drugs useful in exacerbation of bronchitis is cotrimoxazole, found superior to ampicillin by Hughes (1969) and to tetracycline by Lal and Bhalla (1969) and by Pines *et al.* (1972a). The drugs of most value in the home treatment of exacerbations are therefore cotrimoxazole, the tetracyclines and ampicillin. The choice between them will depend on the patient's previous treatment, his experience of unwanted effects of the different drugs, and occasionally on the results of laboratory tests.

Treatment by injection is often used in severe exacerbations requiring treatment in hospital and in advanced cases. Pines *et al.* (1971) found cephaloridine, 6 g. daily, marginally better than ampicillin 4 g. daily, while a smaller dose of cephaloridine, 4·5 g. daily, gave no advantage over ampicillin. The large dose of cephaloridine was associated with a high incidence of urinary casts. Cephaloridine is not very effective against *H. influenzae*, the M.I.C. for most strains being about 8 μg./ml., and often fails to eliminate this organism from the sputum. These reasons, together with the large number of injections required, limit the value of this drug in severe purulent bronchitis. The rôle of chloramphenicol, often considered by clinicians to be a valuable drug in severe purulent chest infections, has been usefully defined in a group of patients with advanced disease. Chloramphenicol given by injection (500 mg. 8 hourly) for 2 days followed by oral treatment (500 mg. 6 hourly) for 12 days gave significantly better results than ampicillin (500 mg. by injection 8 hourly for 2 days followed by 1 g. 6 hourly by mouth for 12 days) in severely ill patients with purulent exacerbations of bronchitis (Pines *et al.*, 1972b). For moderately ill patients chloramphenicol was compared with tetracycline, both given orally, and were found equally effective, although chloramphenicol was the better tolerated (Pines *et al.*, 1972c). Another point emerging from this last trial was the outstanding superiority of either antibiotic over the placebo. The value of antibiotics in bronchitis is often held in doubt, which may be justified of mild virus-induced exacerbations treated at home; but the results of these and other trials leave no doubt of the importance of bacterial infection in exacerbations bad enough to lead to hospital admission.

The same group of workers (Pines *et al.*, 1970) have also

studied methods of treating patients severely ill with chronic bronchitis or bronchiectasis who have a profuse growth of *Ps. aeruginosa* in their sputum. Colistin alone, gentamicin alone and moderate doses of carbenicillin alone were ineffective, but carbenicillin combined with gentamicin, or carbenicillin intravenously in doses up to 18 g. daily, gave good, albeit temporary, improvement in many patients.

Bronchiectasis

Treatment follows the same principles as in purulent chronic bronchitis, especially as *H. influenzae* may be a dominant pathogen and treatment should be directed against this organism. In other cases the sputum contains a mixed flora which includes anaerobes, and antibiotic sensitivity tests should be used to guide treatment.

Staphylococcal infection in children with cystic fibrosis poses a difficult and long-term problem since antibiotic-resistant strains are commonly present. Oral cloxacillin, to which flucloxacillin is now preferred, has been given for very long periods starting from the time of diagnosis, and Wright and Harper (1970) have obtained good results with the combination of fusidic acid and lincomycin. Superinfection by *Ps. aeruginosa* is very common, especially as the patient begins to deteriorate, and evidence of infection by *H. influenzae* is also commonly found.

REFERENCES

ADDY, M. G., ELLIS, P. D. M. & TURK, D. C. (1972). *Brit. med. J.* **1**, 40.
ANDERSON, R., BAUMAN, M. & AUSTRIAN, R. (1968). *Amer. Rev. Resp. Dis.* **97**,
BASS, J. W., KLENK, E. L., KOTHEIMER, J. B., LINNEMANN, C. C. & SMITH,
914.
    M. H. D. (1969). *J. Pediat.* **75**, 768.
BASS, J. W., STEELE, R. W., WIEBE, R. A. & DIERDORFF, E. P. (1971). *Pediatrics* **48**. 417.
BASS, J. W., COHEN, S. H., CORLESS, J. D. & MAMURES, P. (1967). *J. Amer. med. Ass.* **202**, 697.
BATH, J. C. J. L., BOISSARD, G. P. B., CALDER, M. A. & MOFFAT, M. A. J. (1964). *Brit. J. Dis. Chest* **58**, 1.
CALDER, M. A., LUTZ, W. & SCHONELL, M. E. (1968). *Brit. J. Dis. Chest* **62**, 93.
COFFEY, J. D. (1968). *J. Pediat.* **72**, 693.
DAVIS, S. D. & WEDGEWOOD, R. G. (1965). *Amer. J. Dis. Child.* **109**, 544.
FIALA, M. (1969). *Amer. J. med. Sci.* **257**, 44.
FRY, J. (1958). *Brit. med. J.* **2**, 883.
HOWE, J. G. & WILSON, T. S. (1972). *Lancet* **2**, 184.
HOWIE, V. M., PLOUSSARD, J. H. & LESTER, R. L. (1970). *Pediatrics* **45**, 29.
HUGHES, D. T. D. (1969). *Brit. med. J.* **4**, 470.
HUMPHREY, J. H., JOULES, H. & VAN DER WALT, E. D. (1948). *Thorax* **3**, 112.

JOHNSTON, R. N., McNEILL, R. S., SMITH, D. H., DEMPSTER, M. B., NAIRN, J. R., PURVIS, M. S., WATSON, J. M. & WARD, F. G. (1969). *Brit. med. J.* 4, 265.

KAMME, C., LUNDGREN, K. & RUNDCRANTZ, H. (1969). *Scand. J. infect. Dis.* 1, 77.

KAMME, C. (1970). *Scand. J. Inf. Dis.* 2, 117.

KINGSTON, J. R. & nine others (1961). *J. Amer. med. Ass.* 176, 118.

LAL, S., BHALLA, K. K. (1969). *Postgrad. med. J.*, 45, Suppl. p. 91.

LAMBERT, H. P. & STERN, H. (1972). *Brit. med. J.* 3, 323.

LAXDAL, O. E., MERIDA, J. & JONES, R. H. T. (1970). *Canad. med. Ass. J.* 102, 263.

McCLOSKEY, R. V., ELLER, J. J., GREEN, M., MAUNEY, C. U. & RICHARDS, S. E. M. (1971). *Ann. intern. Med.* 75, 495.

McKERROW, C. B., OLDHAM, P. D. & THOMSON, S. (1961). *Lancet* 1, 185.

MALONE, D. N., GOULD, J. C. & GRANT, I. W. B. (1968). *Lancet* 2, 594.

MEDICAL RESEARCH COUNCIL (1951). *Brit. med. J.* 2, 1361.

MEDICAL RESEARCH COUNCIL (1953). *Lancet* 1, 1109.

MEDICAL RESEARCH COUNCIL (1966). *Brit. med. J.* 1, 1317.

NILSON, B. W., POLAND, R. L., THOMPSON, R. S., MOREHEAD, D., BAGHDAS-SARIAN, A. & CARVER, D. H. (1969). *Pediatrics* 43, 351.

NYLEN, O., JEPPSSON, P-H., BRANEFORS-HELANDER, P. (1972). *Scand. J. infect. Dis.* 4, 43.

PINES, A., RAAFAT, H., GREENFIELD, J. S. B., SIDDIQUI, G., LENOX-SMITH, I. & LINSELL, W. D. (1972a). *Practitioner* 208, 265.

PINES, A., GREENFIELD, J. S. B., RAAFAT, H., SIDDIQUI, G. (1972b). *Brit. J. Dis. Chest* 66, 116.

PINES, A., RAAFAT, H., GREENFIELD, J. S. B., LINSELL, W. D. & SOLARI, M. E. (1972c). *Brit. J. Dis. Chest* 66, 107.

PINES, A., RAAFAT, H., GREENFIELD, J. S. B., MARSHALL, M. J. & SOLARI, M. (1971). *Brit. J. Dis. Chest* 65, 91.

PINES, A., RAAFAT, H., PLUCINSKI, K., GREENFIELD, J. S. B., LINSELL, W. D. & SOLARI, M. E. (1968) *Brit. J. Dis. Chest* 62, 19.

PINES, A., RAAFAT, H., SIDDIQUI, G. & GREENFIELD, J. S. B. (1970). *Brit. med. J.* 1, 663.

RITCHIE, J. M. (1958). *Lancet* 1, 618.

ROSS, P. W., CHISTY, S. M. K. & KNOX, J. D. E. (1971). *Brit. med. J.* 2, 624.

SHAMES, J. M., GEORGE, R. B., HOLLIDAY, W. B., RASCH, J. R. & MOGABGAB, N. J. (1970). *Arch. intern. Med.* 125, 680.

STRANGERT, K. (1969). *Scand. J. infect. Dis.* 1, 67.

STENHOUSE, A. C. (1967). *Brit. med. J.* 3, 461.

STILLERMAN, M., ISENBERG, H. D. & MOODY, M. (1972). *Amer. J. Dis. Child.* 123, 457.

STUART-HARRIS, C. H. (1968). *Abstr. Wld Med.* 42, 649.

TAYLOR, R. B., PUGLIESE, W. M., WIERSUM, J., MESCHES, D. N. & HENRIQUEZ, C. (1969). *Amer. J. Dis. Child.* 117, 139.

TILLOTSON, J. R. & LERNER, A. M. (1968). *Medicine* 45, 65.

TRAKAS, J. C. & LIND, H. E. (1966). *Antimicrob. Agents & Chemother.* (1965), p. 717.

WRIGHT, G. L. T. & HARPER, J. (1970). *Lancet* 1, 9.

Chapter 23

ANTIBIOTICS IN OBSTETRICS

Prolonged Labour

Although the amniotic fluid, placenta, and foetus are normally sterile, the vagina and cervical canal contain a variable bacterial flora which frequently includes potential pathogens (Morris and Morris, 1967).

These organisms are barred from ascent to the uterus by the membranes and provided these remain intact, intrauterine infection is uncommon. The membrane barrier can be involved by vaginal inflammatory disease and breached by premature (including surgical) rupture.

There is no conclusive proof that inflammatory conditions of the lower genital tract allow these organisms to gain access to the foetal membranes but the circumstantial evidence is considerable. Infections of the lower genital tract increase the prematurity rate (Hawkinson and Schulman, 1966) and sometimes reach the foetus from infected amniotic fluid entering the foetal respiratory tract. Such infection may be present without inducing symptoms in the mother.

Ascent of vaginal organisms is facilitated by repeated vaginal examination. The total duration of prolonged labour is less important in determining the risk of infection than the interval between rupture of the membranes and onset of labour.

Both foetus and mother may suffer the consequences of ascending infection and there is a sharp rise in perinatal mortality and maternal morbidity when the membranes have been ruptured for more than 24 hours (Still and Adamson, 1967). Uterine sepsis may develop insidiously, with no evidence of infection beyond a foul or foetid vaginal discharge for as long as 48 hours. The result of untreated sepsis may be a foul-smelling still-birth and, in the mother, bacteraemia with a 30-60 per cent incidence of septic shock.

With such potentially serious consequences, it generally continues to be the practice in premature rupture of the membranes to protect the foetus, as far as possible, by maternal antibacterial prophylaxis. So far, however, convincing evidence is lacking that either systemic treatment of the mother, or the instillation of topical antibacterial agents into the genital tract, significantly reduces the incidence of infections in the amnion or foetus (Brelje and Kaltreider, 1966; Hawkinson and Schulman, 1966).

There is no such doubt about the need and efficacy of antibiotic protection of the mother. The only fatality from streptococcal infection in the puerperium recorded in Britain for some years occurred in a patient in whom this precaution was omitted, in spite of prolonged labour and manual removal of the placenta. A policy for management commonly practised in obstetric units and outlined by MacVicar (1970) is to start antibiotic treatment if the baby is not delivered within 24 hours of membrane rupture, either naturally or by surgical intervention. Antibiotics are not, however, given after premature rupture of membranes in women not in labour unless signs of infection develop.

Choice of Agent

In selecting the appropriate antibiotic its antibacterial spectrum and its capacity to pass into the liquor amnii and into the foetal circulation must be borne in mind. The organisms principally concerned are *Escherichia,* other enterobacteria, staphylococci, and streptococci, including some anaerobic strains. *Listeria monocytogenes* is frequently mentioned amongst more exotic organisms likely to infect the foetus, but while its role is indisputable, it does not appear to be an important cause of foetal loss (Ansbacher *et al.,* 1966). Only negligible amounts of streptomycin, the tetracyclines and chloramphenicol reach the liquor amnii, whereas with penicillins and cephalosporins high and prolonged levels result from excretion by the foetal kidneys. Benzyl penicillin has been found to produce levels up to 32 times those in the blood and Blecher *et al.* (1966) have shown that after three 500 mg. doses of ampicillin to the mother, the liquor amnii usually contains 2·5 μg. per ml. or more. Barr and Graham (1967) found that doses of 1 g.

of cephaloridine produced levels of 1-8 μg./ml. in both the amnion and the cord serum of the majority of babies, but in 5-10 per cent, the levels were less than 1 μg./ml.

A number of studies comparing antibiotic concentrations in maternal and umbilical blood have shown that penicillin, streptomycin and the tetracyclines administered to the mother all reach the foetal circulation within about half an hour but the concentrations are substantially lower than those found in maternal blood. Chloramphenicol reaches the foetal circulation rather less readily. It appears therefore that the best protection against ascending vaginal organisms is likely to be afforded by agents which besides being active against the main incriminated pathogens are concentrated in the liquor.

Cervical swabs should be taken and examined bacteriologically, but while waiting for a report it appears that cover will probably be provided by ampicillin, or cephaloridine, but they are not likely to produce adequate foetal blood levels unless large doses are given.

PUERPERAL PYREXIA

Slight fever in the puerperium without clinical signs should be observed and not treated with antibiotics in the absence of positive findings. Observation should include examination of the urine and high vaginal or cervical swabs. If haemolytic streptococci of Lancefield groups A, C or G are found in vaginal or cervical swabs antibiotic treatment must always be given and penicillin is the drug of choice. The presence of other organisms in the vagina, even those commonly associated with puerperal infection, does not necessarily indicate antibiotic treatment, in the absence of clinical evidence of infection.

Puerperal Infection of the Genital Tract

Patients with severe pyrexia of more than 24 hours' duration or with clinical signs of genital tract infection should always be given antibiotic treatment. Infection is still the most important cause of maternal death (Stevenson, 1969). The bacteriological investigation of puerperal infection of the genital tract is not very satisfactory. In most hospitals reliance is placed on the high vaginal swab, which is perfectly adequate if the infecting agent is *Str. pyogenes* but in other cases may give misleading results, either because the infecting agent is not isolated or because the organism isolated is so frequently present in the vagina of apparently healthy women in the puerperium that its pathogenic significance is doubtful.

These cases arise in the same way as the ascending infection which may complicate premature rupture of the membranes. Cervical swabs and blood cultures should be obtained and treatment instituted with ampicillin or cephaloridine along the lines suggested on page 394. Amongst possible infecting organisms *Staph. aureus* is likely to be resistant to ampicillin, and bacteroides to cephaloridine (some strains are sensitive to ampicillin). As it happens, both of these possibilities can be covered by adding clindamycin to either agent for the first day or two until the nature of the infection is established. The problems of concomitant shock are mentioned on page 308. Other organisms of uncertain significance in puerperal pyrexia are the genital mycoplasmas. *M. hominis* has been associated with a few cases of post-partum septicaemia (Tully and Smith, 1968) and puerperal sepsis associated with the isolation of a T-strain mycoplasma from blood, urine and vagina has also been reported (Sompolinski *et al.*, 1971).

Puerperal Bacteriaemia in Patients with Heart Disease

It has been claimed that bacteriaemia can be demonstrated in up to 5 per cent of women during delivery and that there is a corresponding risk of endocarditis in those with heart disease. Baker and Hubbell (1967) found the incidence to be only a tenth of this, with no bacteriaemia after the first 24 hours. They doubt the necessity of giving prophylactic antibiotics during the uncomplicated delivery of women with heart disease.

SEPTIC ABORTION

Infection is liable to occur in cases of incomplete abortion, where all or part of the placenta is retained, or in cases where abortion is illegally performed by the inexpert use of unsterile instruments. Smith *et al.* (1970) grew the following organisms from blood cultures in patients with septic abortion; anaerobic streptococci from 13 patients, *Bacteroides* 7, *Cl. welchii* 3, beta-haemolytic streptococci (not Groups A or D) 3, and enterococci from 2 patients. After instrumental abortion, particularly if the uterus is ruptured, gas gangrene may occur. More than half of all maternal deaths result from septic abortion.The mortality rate is variously reported as 0·29-3·25 per cent and is especially high in those with septic shock. Moritz and Thompson (1966) emphasize that these patients often appear deceptively well for some time and then suddenly deteriorate. The clinical picture of *Cl. welchii* abortal sepsis, which has a mortality of 53-85 per cent, is described by Decker and Hall (1966).

The antibiotic therapy of septic abortion cannot be separated from other parts of the treatment which are also of great importance but which cannot be discussed in detail here; this applies especially to the treatment of septic shock, many aspects of which are still controversial. As regards antibiotic treatment, large doses of benzyl penicillin should be given if gas gangrene is suspected. In other cases the common problem arises of providing broad cover for a wide range of organisms which include both gram-positive and gram-negative aerobes and a variety of anaerobes. In all cases cervical swabs and blood cultures should be taken for bacteriological examination.

Ampicillin with cloxacillin, or cephaloridine alone, have been widely used in recent years, but the increased incidence of drug resistance in gram-negative flora suggests that, in seriously ill patients, wider cover should be provided by adding gentamicin or kanamycin to the scheme of treatment. Thus a suitable scheme for very ill patients would be cephaloridine or cephalothin, with gentamicin or kanamycin. Few clinical trials have been undertaken in septic abortion but Ostergaard (1970), in a series of 28 patients, made a random allocation between penicillin with chloramphenicol, and cephalothin with kanamycin, finding no difference in the clinical course between the two methods. He evacuated the uterus 12 to 24 hours after beginning antibiotic treatment. Freel *et al.* (1969) advocate delaying curettage until intensive antibiotic treatment has rendered the patient afebrile for at least 24 hours, while others (Decker and Hall, 1966) curette the infected uterus at the earliest opportunity.

Trichomoniasis in Pregnancy

Trichomonas infection is usually reported to occur in 10-20 per cent of pregnant patients although figures as high as 50 per cent have been given (Sands, 1966). Despite the efficacy of oral metronidazole in trichomoniasis (p. 468), there has been reluctance to prescribe it for pregnant patients for fear of foetal toxicity. Rodin and Hass (1966) review the previously published results of treatment during pregnancy and add 78 patients of their own, including 10 treated during the first 8 weeks with the conventional dose of 200 mg. metronidazole 8-hourly for 7 days. In no instance was any congenital malformation attributable to the drug. This is supported by Sands (1966) who gave 750 mg. metronidazole daily for only three days. Only 2/113 patients failed to respond. There was no foetal abnormality and no maternal disturbance other than a rash in one patient and vomiting in another. He suggests that metronidazole treatment of trichomoniasis in pregnancy is not only safe but necessary because of evidence that inflammatory conditions of the cervix and vagina significantly increase the prematurity rate Hawkinson and Schulman, 1966).

Vaginal Candidiasis

This is common in pregnancy and readily transferred to the infant during birth producing oral thrush. It may be controlled by vaginal tablets containing 100,000 units of nystatin inserted once, or in severe cases, twice a day. Csonka (1967) cured 9/11 pregnant and all 18 non-pregnant patients with 15 days' treatment, and found that amphotericin B pessaries were no better. Other polyene antibiotics have also been used. Using vaginal tablets containing pimaricin, Don (1967) cured 9/17 pregnant and 29/40 non-pregnant patients. Cameron (1969) claims excellent results without side effects from preparations containing 0·3 per cent candicidin.

BREAST ABSCESS

Breast abscess in the puerperium is invariably due to *Staph. aureus* and the general principles of chemotherapy are the same as those outlined for staphylococcal infection generally in Chapter 18. Treatment should be started with cloxacillin or flucloxacillin pending a bacteriological report, since penicillin resistance is common among staphylococci in and out of hospital. It is impossible to say how often surgery is avoided by the use of antibiotics in incipient breast abscess, but Goodman and Benson (1970) found no evidence of benefit from their use once surgery had become necessary. In their series 59 of 115 abscesses arising in hospital were caused by penicillin-sensitive strains of staphlyococci, as were 5 of 9 developing after home delivery.

NEONATAL INFECTIONS

Babies born to mothers receiving chemoprophylaxis because of premature rupture of the membranes should continue on treatment especially if the membranes have been ruptured for some time or if the mother's temperature has risen during labour. It is also generally felt that because of the high risk and danger of respiratory infection, prophylactic antibiotics should also be given to babies asphyxiated at birth or with the respiratory distress syndrome, or those requiring tracheal intubation or assisted respiration.

Generalised Infection

If an infant is seriously ill with no obvious cause, cultures of blood and urine and swabs from any local lesions, nose, throat and umbilicus should be examined bacteriologically: a lumbar puncture may also be indicated.

Difficulty of localizing infection and rapid deterioration of the new-born not infrequently demand the institution of treatment before the nature of infection is fully established. Choice of antibiotics in these circumstances is difficult, since it must provide cover for a variety of enterobacteria, *Pseudomonas,* streptococci of various types, and staphylococci; some guidance may be obtained by the local prevalence of strains of known resistance pattern, or the known presence of a nursery outbreak caused by a particular organism. Combinations of ampicillin and cloxacillin, or cephaloridine alone, have been widely used for generalized neonatal infection of uncertain cause, but neither method is suitable if *Pseudomonas* infection is likely, and a number of other enterobacteria are now resistant to these drugs. Gentamicin has now been used quite extensively in neonates (Klein *et al.*, 1971) and dose limits for this age group well defined. A combination of gentamicin with a penicillin or a cephalosporin provides cover against most gram-negative pathogens as well as against streptococci and penicillin–resistant staphylococci. Septicaemia in neonates is often accompanied by meningitis, and further discussion of this topic will be found on p. 356. Once the identity of the invading organism is known, other drugs than those used to initiate treatment may prove more suitable.

Thrush

This is usually confined to the mouth and can be treated by local application of gentian violet or nystatin. The lesions sometimes extend down the alimentary tract, in which case nystatin should be given orally in a dose of 100,000 units every six hours. If the infant is having a broad spectrum antibiotic, this should be stopped.

REFERENCES

ANSBACHER, R., BORCHARDT, K. A., HANNEGAN, M. W. & BOYSON, W. A. (1966). *Amer. J. Obstet. Gynec.* **94**, 386.
BAKER, T. H. & HUBBELL, R. (1967). *Amer. J. Obstet. Gynec.* **97**, 575.
BARR, W. & GRAHAM, R. (1967). *Postgrad. med. J.* **43** (Suppl. Aug.), 101.
BLECHER, T. E., EDGAR, W. M., MELVILLE, H. A. H. & PEEL, K. R. (1966). *Brit. med. J.* **1**, 137.
BRELJE, M. C. & KALTREIDER, D. F. (1966). *Amer. J. Obstet. Gynec.* **94**, 889.
CAMERON, P. F. (1969). *Practitioner* **202**, 695.
CSONKA, G. W. (1967). *Brit. J. vener. Dis.* **43**, 210.
DECKER, W. H. & HALL, W. (1966). *Amer. J. Obstet. Gynec.* **95**, 394.
DON, R. A. (1967). *Med. J. Aust.* **1**, 382.
FREEL, J. H., GARDNER, W. M. & GEITTMANN, W. F. (1969). *Amer. J. Obstet. Gynec.* **104**, 651.
GOODMAN, M. A. & BENSON, E. A. (1970). *Med. J. Aust.* **1**, 1034.
HAWKINSON, J. A. & SCHULMAN, H. (1966). *Amer. J. Obstet. Gynec.* **94**, 898.
KLEIN, J. O., HERSCHEL, M., THERAKAN, R. M. & INGALL, D. (1971). *J. infect. Dis.* **124**, Suppl. p. 224.
MACVICAR, J. (1970). *Clin. Obstet. Gynec.* **13**, 272.
MORITZ, C. R. & THOMPSON, N. J. (1966). *Amer. J. Obstet. Gynec.* **95**, 46.
MORRIS, C. A. & MORRIS, D. F. (1967). *J. clin. Path.* **20**, 636.
OSTERGARD, D. R. (1970). *Obstet. Gynec. N.Y.* **36**, 473.
RODIN, P. & HASS, G. (1966). *Brit. J. vener. Dis.* **42**, 210.
SANDS, R. X. (1966). *Amer. J. Obstet. Gynec.* **94**, 350.
SMITH, J. W., SOUTHERN, P. M. & LEHMANN, J. D. (1970). *Obstet. Gynec. N.Y.* **35**, 704.
SOMPOLINSKY, D., SOLOMON, F., LEIBA, H., CASPI, E., LEWINSOHN, G. & ALMOG, C. (1971). *Israel J. med. Sci.* **7**, 745.
STEVENSON. C. S. (1969). *Amer. J. Obstet. Gynec.* **104**, 699.
STILL, R. M. & ADAMSON, H. S. (1967). *J. Obstet. Gynaec. Brit. Cwlth.* **74**, 412.
TULLY, J. G. & SMITH, L. G. (1968). *J. Amer. med. Ass.* **204**, 827.

CHAPTER 24

URINARY TRACT INFECTIONS

ABOUT 80 per cent of acute urinary tract infections are caused by *E. coli* (Mond *et al.*, 1965; McGeachie, 1966); *Proteus* species (almost all *Pr. mirabilis*) account for another 8-12 per cent. The remainder are *Staph. albus, Str. faecalis,* and other enterobacteria. In chronic infections, *Escherichia* are much less common and various other enterobacteria, notably *Proteus Klebsiella,* and *Ps. aeruginosa* are found (Brumfitt, 1972). The most important feature shared by these organisms is their resistance to antibacterial agents.

Another important difference is that acute infection is almost always caused by a single bacterial species. In chronic infection, particularly in patients with gross structural or functional abnormalities of the urinary tract, more than one kind of organism is frequently present.

Diagnosis

The presence of urinary infection and the efficacy of its treatment cannot be established without bacteriological examination of the urine. Many infections, particularly the later infections of a series, are asymptomatic and can only be recognized by laborious bacteriological follow-up. Conversely, sometimes in the child (Stephens *et al.*, 1966) and frequently in the adult, typical symptoms, notably frequency and dysuria, are unaccompanied by infected urine. About half the symptomatic women seen in general practice fall into this category (Gallagher *et al.*, 1965) and are said to be suffering from the ' urethral syndrome ' (Editorial, 1968).

This is almost certainly a complex of disorders of which one major variety is associated with subsequent urinary infection and may be very clearly related to sexual activity. In a minority of persistently symptomatic patients some underlying gynaecological, intestinal or other disorder can be demonstrated which may respond to appropriate measures (O'Grady,

Charlton *et al.*, 1973). The treatment of the remainder is generally very satisfactory. Some patients respond to treatment as for urinary infection, to local antibacterial or other applications, to a single dose of an antibacterial agent taken prior to intercourse, or to repeated urethral dilatation.

Acute Infection

The treatment of patients with acute urinary infection is now reasonably well defined but is not universally successful. Most infections are due to *Escherichia* sensitive to a great variety of agents excreted in the urine (Table 40) all of which have been successfully used for treatment as reported in a great and growing literature. Most commonly used have been sulphonamides, usually in the form of sulphadimidine or sulphafurazole (2 g. initial plus 1 g. 6-hourly), but longer-acting sulphonamides such as sulphamethoxazole (2 g. initially plus 1 g. 12-hrly), sulphamethoxypyridazine or sulphamethoxydiazine (1 g. initially plus 500 mg. daily) and even sulfadoxine (page 26) given as a single 1 g. dose, have been successfully employed. Also widely used are nitrofurantoin (100 mg. 6-hrly) ampicillin (500 mg. 6-hrly) and, in some centres cycloserine (250 mg. 8-hrly). Increasing use is being made of cephalexin (250 mg. 6-hrly), nalidixic acid (1 g. 6-hrly) and co-trimoxazole (2 tablets 12-hrly). In more resistant infections use must be made of the agents lower in Table 40 amongst which the aminoglycosides have the advantage that they will frequently eradicate sensitive organisms from the urine within 24 hours.

So far, the evidence accumulated from the copious use of all these agents has failed to establish with any certainty the optimum dosage and duration of therapy. A substantial number of acute infections resolve spontaneously (Brumfitt, 1972) or respond to minimum treatment. For example, of the cases described by Fairley *et al.* (1967) a number were cured by rinsing out the bladder with a single dose of neomycin. Brumfitt *et al.* (1970) cured a proportion of their patients with a single dose of cephaloridine and Williams and Smith (1970) a proportion of theirs with a single dose of streptomycin. About 80 per cent of patients respond to most regimens and it is probable that a week's treatment is sufficient to achieve this result although two weeks' treatment has commonly been employed. No better results are obtained by increasing the duration of therapy to six weeks (Kincaid-Smith and Fairley, 1969).

As far as the agents are concerned, it appears that there is little to choose between them providing the organism is sensitive *in vitro* (Brumfitt and Pursell, 1972; Slade and Crowther, 1972). Claims that patients commonly respond to agents to which the infecting organism is said by the laboratory to be resistant may be due to several things : sensitivity tests on organisms recovered from poorly collected specimens and having no relation to the patient's condition; spontaneous resolution of infection, or to an erroneous sensitivity report. False reports of *Escherichia* resistant to sulphonamides or *Proteus* resistant to ampicillin are prominent amongst errors made in routine sensitivity tests (Report, 1965).

Very similar results from treatment with agents which have very different modes of antibacterial action, and very different pharmacokinetic properties could, of course, mean not that they have strikingly similar effects but that they have little or no effect beyond that exerted by the natural clearance mechanisms.

Intrinsic Clearance Mechanisms

In women, organisms derived from the bowel (Grüneberg, 1969) cancolonize the introitus (O'Grady *et al.*, 1970) and gain access to the urine during micturition (Hinman, 1966). In the male, the anatomical arrangement makes such access much less likely and it is generally supposed that this accounts in large part for the different prevalence of urinary infection in the two sexes: about 26 per 1000 married women, but only 1·8 per 1000 men per annum in general practice in Britain (Mond *et al.*, 1965).

In the urine enterobacteria are able to grow freely but are normally soon eliminated by dilution with incoming ureteric urine and discharge at the next voiding—a process which is enhanced by the frequent micturition naturally excited by urinary infection (O'Grady and Cattell, 1966). Organisms which remain in the normally very small volume of residual urine (Hinman and Cox, 1967; Shand *et al.*, 1968) will be disposed of by cellular or humoral mechanisms (Norden *et al.*, 1968; Stamey *et al.*, 1968). During the overnight period, the rate of ureteric urine flow naturally falls and there is a long period without micturition during which organisms have a special opportunity to establish themselves. In the same way, where bladder emptying is impaired infection is particularly likely to occur and especially difficult to treat. Shand *et al.* (1970) showed that patients in whom the residual volume was increased by only a few ml. were more difficult to treat and more liable to recurrent infection than patients whose bladder emptying was completely normal.

Treatment Regimen

This suggests that optimum results will be obtained if antibacterial therapy is used to support the natural clearance mechanisms by encouraging patients to drink copiously, and to empty the bladder completely (if necessary by double or triple micturition) at frequent intervals. The last of the daily doses of antibacterial agent should be taken immediately before retiring to bed, having emptied the bladder completely, in order to control the re-growth of bladder bacteria overnight.

It may be objected that fluid loading will exert a detrimental effect on antibacterial therapy by diluting the agent in the urine. In fact, agents used for the treatment of urinary infection normally appear in the urine in very high concentrations (Table 40) and the degree of dilution which can be achieved by increased drinking still leaves a concentration greatly in excess of that required to inhibit sensitive organisms.

Moreover, many antibacterial agents exert much less effect on the high concentrations of bacteria found in infected urine than they do on the very much smaller numbers used as inocula in conventional determinations of minimum inhibitory concentrations. Direct comparison of the effect of a single dose of an antibiotic with and without fluid loading on the concentration of organisms in the urine (Cattell *et al.,* 1968) showed that the beneficial effect of diluting the culture greatly outweighed any detrimental effect of diluting the agent.

Failure of Initial Therapy

In a proportion of patients infection is not controlled or promptly returns on cessation of therapy, and more intensive treatment is necessary. Fluid loading and frequent complete micturition should be continued and the patient given a two-week course of a second agent chosen on the basis of *in vitro* sensitivity tests. Amongst adult women, failure to respond to initial or re-treatment is the simplest way of identifying those who require more complex management and investigation.

Relapse and Re-infection

In some patients whose infections rapidly reappear after re-treatment the organisms prove (even on the closest study of their antigenic structure) to be identical with those responsible for the original infection. It is reasonable to conclude in such cases that therapy succeeded only in suppressing growth of the organisms which somehow hid in the urinary tract and quickly re-established infection when treatment was withdrawn. Such recrudescence of the original infection is described as *relapse*. In other patients, and typically after a longer interval, bacteriuria reappears but is shown to be due to *re-infection* with a different organism. In practice, it is not always easy to distinguish relapse from re-infection in the individual patient.

Localization of Infection

Much has been made of the distinction between relapse and re-infection because of the belief that relapse commonly indicates persistence of infection within the kidney, with the attendant dangers of progressive renal damage and ultimate failure, while re-infection indicates simply susceptibility to bladder infection which is easily treated and carries little risk to the upper urinary tract. Various ways by which the differentiation of relapse from re-infection may be attempted are reviewed by Reeves and Brumfitt (1968).

Indirect indications of renal involvement such as high levels of circulating antibodies to the infecting organism or impaired urinary concentrating ability, have received a good deal of attention. A recent study (Cattell *et al.*, 1973) by the method—ureteric catheterization—which shows with the least equivocation whether or not bacteria are present in the upper tract-confirmed that a greater proportion of patients whose disease involved the upper tract relapsed and a greater proportion of those whose disease involved the lower tract became re-infected, but the differences were not great. It was concluded that while localization studies may have much to contribute towards elucidating the pathogenesis and natural history of intractable infection, they have little or no part to play in the management of the individual patient.

TABLE 40

Sensitivity to Drugs of Bacteria causing Urinary Infections

Drug	Concentration attained in urine (μg./ml.)	Minimum Inhibitory Concentration (μg./ml.)					
		Esch. coli	Proteus mira-bilis	Kl. aero-genes	Ps. aeru-ginosa	Staph. aureus	Str. faecalis
Sulphonamides	1000	8	8	R	50	4-16	R
Nitrofurantoin	125	16	200	100	R	4	25
Ampicillin	250+	8	4	R	R	0·04	2
Cycloserine	250	64	250	64	128	16	128
Cephalexin	500+	4	4	32	R	4	128
Nalidixic acid	250+	4	4	16	R	64	R
Trimethoprim	100	0·5	2	2	R	0·5	0·5
Penicillin	250+	20->100	8	R	R	0·02	4
Carbenicillin	2000	5	2·5	250	50	0·5-50	25
Cephaloridine	300	4	4	4-R	R	0·1-5	16
Streptomycin	1000	5	50	5	50	10	100
Kanamycin	300	2	4	2	64	0·5	64
Gentamicin	50	1-4	2-8	1-2	1-8	0·1-1	8-16
Tetracyclines	300	5	R	100	10	200	0·5
Polymyxin	50	1	R	1	1	R	1

R = resistant to concentrations attainable.

Mechanism of Relapse

The re-appearance of sensitive strains after what should have been adequate courses of therapy is usually explained either by failure of antibacterial agent to reach the site of infection, or by indifference of the organism to its action, even though it appears sensitive on conventional *in vitro* testing. Such evidence as we have does not support the idea that deficient overall tissue concentrations are a common cause of failure.

Tissue Concentrations

The measurement of concentrations of antibacterial agents in the interstitium of the kidney presents considerable technical difficulties. Apart from the fact that important concentration differences may exist in the vicinity of different micro-anatomical structures, homogenates of kidney cannot be used to determine 'tissue concentrations' because they contain varying quantities of blood and, more important, of urine, the presence of which usually results in grossly high false values.

An elegant method of determining tissue fluid levels is described by Cockett et al. (1965) who found that in a proportion of dogs the surface lymphatics arising from the cortex and medulla of the kidney can be separately cannulated. Chisholm et al. (1968), who discuss the technical difficulties, found renal lymph levels of nitrofurantoin to be about twice those of the plasma in three of five dogs but similar in the other two. The levels of gentamicin in the renal lymph (2·5-6 μg./ml.) were slightly lower than those in the plasma.

Even when 'tissue' levels are adequate, however, it does not follow that the agent is appropriately distributed. It is likely that it is precisely in those areas where function is deranged by infection that the adequate levels demonstrable in adjoining normal tissue are not reached. Gross examples of this may be found where the ureteric urine is sterilized on the side where renal function has been moderately preserved, but not on the other side, where renal function is grossly deficient.

One example of metabolic indifference of organisms to an agent to which they are sensitive on conventional testing is the production of L-forms (Gutman et al., 1967). Treatment with agents which interrupt cell-wall synthesis can result in the production of spheroplasts which are excreted in the urine where their integrity is preserved by the high osmolality. When no longer exposed to the agent, cell-wall is re-synthesized and infection re-appears. L-forms of enterobacteria, unlike the parent organism, may be sensitive to erythromycin, and Proteus infection has been eradicated by successive treatment with ampicillin and erythromycin (Gutman et al., 1967).

While this example has the benefit of a demonstrable mechanism, the importance of L-forms in chronic renal infection is arguable (Guinan et al., 1972) and the persistence of organisms in the presence of high concentrations of agents to which they are ' sensitive ' on conventional testing is not restricted to agents which interrupt cell-wall synthesis. It occurs with many (perhaps all) agents when large bacterial inocula are used, presumably because some of the organisms at the time of exposure to the antibiotic are in a ' dormant' state (Greenwood and O'Grady, 1969).

Treatment of Persistent Relapse

It must first be established that failure is not due to the emergence of a resistant mutant. This is a very uncommon cause of failure except with streptomycin and, in some series, nalidixic acid.

In patients who relapse after re-treatment, there is a high chance that radiology will show some abnormality of the urinary tract which may be surgically correctable, and uroradiology is essential at this stage. The most important example of renal infection uncontrollable before and controlled after surgery is that associated with stones.

Persistence in the form of spheroplasts is most likely to be a feature of infection with *Proteus* in which eradication may be achieved by sequential treatment with a cell-wall-inhibiting agent, such as ampicillin or cephalexin, followed by a spheroplast inhibitor such as erythromycin (Gutman *et al.,* 1967). We have confirmed the success of this regimen, but it is much less likely to be useful in relapsing infection due to *Escherichia* since only the minority of its survivors from exposure to cell-wall-inhibiting agents are in the form of spheroplasts (Greenwood and O'Grady, 1969).

It might reasonably be hoped that failure to achieve adequate agent concentration at the site of infection following oral treatment would be overcome by intensive parenteral therapy. This certainly sometimes succeeds but must obviously be done in hospital using agents chosen on the basis of *in vitro* sensitivity tests. Suitable agents are ampicillin, cephaloridine or cephalothin, streptomycin or kanamycin (1·5 g. per day for three days). Dosage should be given frequently, preferably by rapid intravenous infusion. The effect of the penicillins or cephalosporins should be enhanced by probenecid and that of aminoglycosides by alkalinization of the urine. This can be achieved with sodium bicarbonate, or more rapidly with acetazolamide. Administration of the antibiotic should not be started until the pH of the first specimen passed on waking is at least 7·0, and it should be verified daily that this reaction is being maintained. If surgery is undertaken (for example for the removal of renal stones) intensive therapy should begin at the time of operation. Patients who fail to respond to these measures require long-term suppressive therapy (see below).

Treatment of Re-infection

Irrespective of the ease with which infection is eradicated some patients become re-infected with a new organism. The management of patients subject to such re-infection depends on the frequency with which infections occur. If new infections occur infrequently (not more than 2 or 3 a year) and respond readily to treatment, each episode is probably best treated as a first infection as described on page 401. If, on the other hand, attacks occur frequently, or if infection, once established, is difficult to eradicate, then such patients are probably better managed on long-term prophylaxis. Infection should be eradicated, if necessary by intensive therapy, and chemoprophylaxis instituted as soon as the initial treatment has been shown to be successful, in order to prevent the establishment of fresh exogenous infection.

As with patients who repeatedly relapse, full uro-radiological examination of patients who suffer frequent re-infection may reveal correctable abnormalities.

Long-Term Therapy

Much disagreement about the place and efficacy of long-term therapy results from failure to recognize that such treatment may be used for three distinct purposes: (1) cure, (2) suppression (3) prophylaxis. Patients who relapse even after extended or intensive therapy may benefit from prolonged treatment which keeps the urine ' sterile ' as long as sufficient antibacterial agent is present. Such suppressive treatment may provide symptomatic relief and prevent fresh acute attacks but since it is not curative there is a possibility that resolution of symptoms may conceal the progression of urinary tract disease. There are undoubtedly, however, a significant number of patients in whom therapy may be discontinued after six months or more without infection re-appearing (Kaye *et al.*, 1968; O'Grady, Fry *et al.*, 1973). Successful long-term therapy has been described with a number of agents, including mandelamine, cycloserine, sulphonamides, nitrofurantoin and co-trimoxazole. Once control has been established patients can often be maintained on a single nightly dose. In the case of co-trimoxazole, adults with persistently relapsing infection or with frequent re-infections have been successfully maintained for years (O'Grady, Fry *et al.*, 1973) on a dosage which was halved at fortnightly intervals (from 12-hourly to nightly, alternate nightly) as long as control was maintained.

Long-term therapy has two main foreseeable disadvantages: toxicity and superinfection with resistant organisms. These hazards may be minimized by choosing the least toxic agent and progressively reducing the dose to the effective minimum; and by accepting only the most compelling reasons for bringing patients into hospital where the most undesirable organisms live. Long-term toxic effects on these regimens must, of course, be constantly watched for, and only time will tell whether such protracted medication is completely safe.

Special Groups

Particular problems arise when infection occurs in children, in men, in pregnancy, in obstructive uropathy or in the presence of calculi or renal failure.

In children, the danger of renal damage is very real (Smellie, 1970). In the very young the still developing defence mechanisms often fail to localize infection and where this involves the urinary tract there may be grave damage to the kidney. In the older child, urinary infection, especially if repeated, can lead to the distortion and scarring of the kidney identified radiologically as ' chronic pyelonephritis ', and to ultimate loss of renal function.

It follows that in the child infection must be recognized early, treated promptly with a demonstrably effective agent and pursued for signs of recurrence (which may be asymptomatic) into adolescence. This means that bacteriological control of treatment and subsequent bacteriological surveillance are essential. Treatment should be along the lines already discussed : short term initial therapy, repeated if necessary, followed where this fails by more intensive or prolonged treatment. Just as in the adult, if infection cannot be eradicated or there is frequent re-infection, surgically remediable abnormalities may be demonstrable and long-term therapy may be required. The most important lesion likely to be revealed by uroradiology in childhood is vesico-ureteric reflux (Rolleston *et al.*, 1970). Considerable success has been claimed in some centres for anti-reflux operations but effective long-term therapy is generally all that is required except in a minority of children in whom infection cannot be controlled or in whom, despite anti-bacterially effective treatment, fresh renal scarring occurs (Govan and Palmer, 1969; Smellie, 1970). Elaborate schemes for prolonged or combined initial therapy followed by rotating administration of different antibiotics have been proposed but there is no evidence that such complex therapy is necessary or desirable.

Smellie and Normand (1968) have shown on prolonged follow-up of a large group of children with recurrent infection (including many with pyelonephritic scarring and reflux) that kidney growth which is halted by infection can commonly be restored. Most of the children were treated with sulphadimidine or sulphafurazole (less than 1 year of age: 0·25 g. daily; 1-5 years: 0·5 g. daily; more than 5 years 1 g. daily). Nitrofurantoin (2·4 mg. per kg. per day) or ampicillin were used in a few children.

Infection in the Adult Male

Spontaneous uncomplicated infection occurs in the adult male but it is a very rare condition compared with that seen in the adult female. Underlying abnormalities of the urinary tract are common in the infected male and early recourse to investigation is necessary. Recurrent infection in the absence of other abnormalities is commonly associated with prostatitis and Stamey and his colleagues have described how the diagnosis can be made and its bacterial aetiology established (Meares and Stamey, 1972).

Failure to eradicate prostatic organisms may result from the fact that the concentration of most agents active against Gram-negative organisms is considerably less in the prostate than it is in the plasma. Winningham *et al.* (1968) argue that to be concentrated in the acid secretion of the prostate, a drug must be basic and lipid-soluble. Amongst commonly used antibiotics only the macrolides fulfil these criteria and they are predominantly active against Gram-positive organisms. Reeves and

Ghilchik (1970) show that trimethoprim, a basic, lipid-soluble compound (p. 29), achieves peak concentrations in the prostatic fluid of the dog 2 to 3 times higher than those of the blood. However, sulphamethoxazole, the other component of co-trimoxazole (p. 25), behaves quite differently in that its concentration in the prostate is only about a third of that in the blood. The antibacterial spectrum of co-trimoxazole makes it very suitable for the treatment of bacterial prostatitis but this difference in the pharmacokinetic behaviour of the two components must be taken into account.

Bacteriuria in Pregnancy

E. H. Kass has been responsible for drawing attention to the frequency with which pregnant women develop symptomless urinary infection (Norden and Kass, 1968). The usual prevalence found has been about 4-6 per cent although both lower and higher figures have been quoted, partly perhaps because of the influence of age and social class (G. L. Williams et al., 1969). The condition is important because about a quarter or a third of the patients develop clinical pyelonephritis and a number of studies have shown that bacteriuric patients are more likely to suffer abortion or premature labour and to deliver small or dead babies.

Kass showed that treatment of asymptomatic bacteriuria would prevent the development of pyelonephritis and this has been generally confirmed. On the other hand a good deal of controversy has raged about the claims that uncontrolled urinary infection in pregnancy exerts detrimental effects on the foetus which can be prevented by adequate antibacterial therapy (Williams et al., 1973). Whether or not entirely satisfactory statistical evidence for these claims can be produced it may still be argued that both mother and foetus must be better off if continuing maternal infection can be eradicated. The issue (rather like that of the treatment of trichomonas vaginitis in pregnancy: p. 397) turns largely on whether the foetus is likely to suffer more from the drug used in treatment than from maternal infection.

Tetracycline should certainly not be given in pregnancy (p. 157) and various disadvantages have been postulated for most of the other agents used for treatment. However, J. D. Williams et *al.* (1969) treated a number of patients in various stages of pregnancy with co-trimoxazole without mishap and Grüneberg *et al.* (1969) safely used sulphonamides (usually sulphadimidine or sulphafurazole for 8 days) with which they cured 75 per cent of patients after the first course and a further 16 per cent after the second.

Nitrofurantoin reaches the foetus with such difficulty (p. 45) that it is hard to see how conventional doses could be injurious.

It is evident that as in the non-pregnant patient there is a variety of urinary tract infection which responds comparatively readily to treatment, and a variety which is very resistant. In a proportion of these very resistant patients—but by no means all—radiological abnormalities of the renal tract are demonstrable (Gower *et al.*, 1968). In Australia, Kincaid-Smith and Bullen (1965) found that in a third of their patients significant bacteriuria was still present 6 months after delivery. Over half their patients had abnormal pyelograms and it appears that pregnancy may effectively advertise the existence of long-standing renal disease.

Since some patients respond readily to treatment it seems reasonable to give them the chance to do so, thereby avoiding the disadvantages of prolonged medication. Patients who fail to respond may require suppressive therapy throughout pregnancy, and should undergo urological investigation post-partum. Safe and successful therapy throughout pregnancy has been described with a variety of agents including sulphamethoxydiazine (0·5 g. per day) changing after the 13th week to sulphadimidine (1 g. 8-hourly); sulphamethoxypyridazine (0·5 g. per day); ampicillin (500 mg., 8-hourly) and nitrofurantoin (100 mg. nightly: Bailey, 1970).

Infection in the Grossly Abnormal Urinary Tract

Urinary infections in patients with grossly impaired bladder emptying or with obstructive uropathy are frequently distinguished from those in patients with radiologically normal tracts by being caused by more than one bacterial species, often including resistant organisms such as *Pr. vulgaris, Klebsiella,* and particularly *Ps. aeruginosa,* or by resistant strains of otherwise sensitive species such as *E. coli.* By using selective media it is often possible to show, even when infection appears to be with only one organism, that other species are present in small numbers (Slade and Linton, 1965). These minor members of the bacterial population inevitably come to predominate if they are resistant to an agent effective in suppressing initially more numerous organisms. Better results of treatment are sometimes obtained if these minor species are isolated and an agent chosen for therapy which is active also against them or if suitable combined therapy is instituted.

In many such patients instrumentation in hospital for diagnostic or therapeutic purposes is unhappily responsible for the introduction of resistant organisms. The importance of avoiding such infections, which enormously increase the difficulty of managing these patients, is obvious.

Therapeutically, these patients present a series of difficulties which tend to compound one another. The abnormalities of their urinary tracts greatly impair both natural resolution and response to treatment. The resulting need for repeated therapy (plus instrumentation) facilitates the emergence of organisms sensitive only to a few agents, the more potent of which are toxic—the kidney itself being one of the organs affected. Impaired kidney function results both in poor concentrations of administered agents in the renal tract, and where dosage is not scrupulously regulated, to their accumulation in the blood with increased remote toxic effects and perhaps further impairment of renal excretion.

Because of the extreme resistance of some of the organisms and the need to monitor dosage, these patients cannot be managed without full bacteriological surveillance. As much as possible should be done to rectify anatomical and functional abnormalities. Patients with large residual volumes should be encouraged to empty their bladders at frequent and regular intervals, practising double or, if necessary, triple micturition (MacGregor and Williams, 1966). Systemic antibacterial therapy in such patients is seldom successful and should be avoided (particularly if the organisms prove to be sensitive only to toxic agents) unless there is evidence of systemic upset. Control may sometimes be established by washing out the bladder two or three times a day and instilling 50 ml. of a 0·1 per cent solution of an appropriate antibiotic (for example polymyxin or neomycin) or antiseptic (for example chlorhexidine or noxytiolin) which is allowed to remain until the bladder refills. Once the urinary bacterial count has been substantially reduced, recurrent symptoms and even re-emergence of high counts of urinary bacteria can sometimes be prevented by long-term suppressive therapy.

In patients with renal calculi, short-term therapy even if intensive is seldom successful but a proportion of patients can be controlled by long-term suppressive therapy (O'Grady, Fry et al., 1973). Eradication of infection is very unlikely unless the stones are removed. Once this has been achieved it is important to maintain the patient on long-term low dose prophylaxis in order to prevent re-accumulation of calculi.

Instrumental Infection

Where there is obstructive uropathy or bladder emptying is expected or known to be impaired: for example in obstetric patients or in prostatic obstruction—especially where the natural male anatomical advantage is set aside by catheterization—the importance of avoiding infection is obvious. Short-term catheterization can be successfully ' covered ' by giving the patient nitrofurantoin, or washing out the bladder with neomycin, plus polymyxin if pseudomonas infection is at large (Cox et al., 1967). Over the long-term, with the use of indwelling catheters, the inevitable result of continuous medication—as with other forms of prolonged prophylaxis for endogenously acquired infections—is superinfection with resistant organisms.

Several authors have emphasized the importance of aspects of the management other than the use of antibacterial agents, and Gillespie and his colleagues (1967) have drawn particular attention to the importance of closed drainage. There have been several kinds of approach to the problem of preventing urinary infection after prostatectomy. Although it is clear that substantial reductions in infection rate can be achieved (Marshall, 1967), many urologists still seem to take infection for granted, and minimize its importance. The patients themselves, over-joyed at having cleared the most dangerous hurdle in later male life, make light of discomfort and accept it as a natural consequence of what they have gone through. They would surely be better off if their urine could be kept sterile.

Renal Failure

A special problem is presented by the need to treat patients—especially with streptomycin and its relatives or with polymyxins—when the capacity to excrete these agents is impaired. Conventional dosage will cause the drug to accumulate with neurological sequelae and possible further kidney damage without achieving therapeutically effective concentrations in the urine. The toxic effects are discussed under the individual agents. Suitable adjustment of dosage can be so successful that renal function improves while the patient is treated with a potentially nephrotoxic agent because of the beneficial effect of controlling infection. Guidance to suitable dosage in relation to the level of renal function is given on page 293.

REFERENCES

BAILEY, R. R. (1970). *N.Z. med. J.* **71**, 216.
BRUMFITT, W. (1972). *J. roy. Coll Physcns. Lond.* **6**, 194.
BRUMFITT, W., FAIERS, M. C. & FRANKLIN, I. N. S. (1970). *Postgrad. med. J.* **46** (Suppl. Oct.), 65.
BRUMFITT, W. & PURSELL, R. (1972). *Brit. med. J.* **2**, 673.
CATTELL, W. R., CHARLTON, C. A. C., FRY, I. K., McSHERRY, M. A. & O'GRADY, F. (1973). *Urinary Tract Infection II*. Ed. Brumfitt, W. & Asscher, A. W., Oxford, *in press.*
CATTELL, W. R., SARDESON, J. M., SUTCLIFFE, M. B. & O'GRADY, F. (1968). In *Urinary Tract Infection*, p. 212, ed. O'Grady, F. and Brumfitt, W. London, Oxford University Press.
CHISHOLM, G. D., CALNAN, J. S. & WATERWORTH, P. M. (1968). In *Urinary Tract Infection*, p. 194, ed. O'Grady, F. and Brumfitt, W. London, Oxford University Press.
COCKETT, A. T. K., MOORE, R. S. & KADO, R. T. (1965). *Brit. J. Urol.* **37**, 650.
COX, F., SMITH, R. F., ELLIOTT, J. P. & QUINN, E. L. (1967). *Antimicrob. Agents Chemother.* 1966, 165.
EDITORIAL (1968). *Brit. med. J.* **2**, 192.
FAIRLEY, K. F., BOND, A. G., BROWN, B. & HABERSBERGER, P. (1967). *Lancet* **2**, 427.
GALLAGHER, D. J. A., MONTGOMERIE, J. Z. & NORTH, J. D. K. (1965). *Brit. med. J.* **1**, 622.
GILLESPIE, W. A., LENNON, G. G., LINTON, K. B. & PHIPPEN, G. A. (1967). *Brit. med. J.* **2**, 90.
GREENWOOD, D. & O'GRADY, F. (1969). *J. med. Microbiol.* **2**, 435.
GOVAN, D. E. & PALMER, J. M. (1969). *Pediatrics,* **44**, 677.
GOWER, P. E., HASWELL, B., SIDAWAY, M. E. & DE WARDENER, H. E. (1968). *Lancet* **1**, 990.
GRÜNEBERG, R. N. (1969). *Lancet* **2**, 766.
GRÜNEBERG, R. N., LEIGH, D. A. & BRUMFITT, W. (1969). *Lancet* **2**, 1.
GUINAN, P. D., NETER, E. & MURPHY, G. P. (1972). *J. Urol.* **108**, 50.
GUTMAN, L., SCHALLER, J. & WEDGWOOD, R. J. (1967). *Lancet* **1**, 464.
HINMAN, F. JR. (1966). *J. Urol.* **96**, 546.
HINMAN, F. JR. & COX, C. E. (1967). *J. Urol.* **97**, 641.
KAYE, D., VIANNA, N. J., McGOVERN, J. H., SHINEFIELD, H. R. & ROSH, M. (1968). *Amer. J. Dis. Child.* **116**, 166.

KINCAID-SMITH, P. & BULLEN, M. (1965). *Lancet*, **1**, 395.
KINCAID-SMITH, P. & FAIRLEY, K. F. (1969). *Brit. med. J.* **2**, 145.
MCGEACHIE, J. (1966). *Brit. J. Urol.* **38**, 294.
MACGREGOR, M. E. & WILLIAMS, C. J. E. W. (1966). *Lancet* **1**, 893.
MARSHALL, A. (1967). *Brit. J. Urol.* **39**, 307.
MEARES. E. M. JR. & STAMEY, T. A. (1972). *Brit. J. Urol.* **44**, 175.
MOND, N. C., PERCIVAL, A., WILLIAMS, J. D. & BRUMFITT, W. (1965). *Lancet* **1**, 514.
NORDEN, C. W., GREEN, G. M. & KASS, E. H. (1968). *J. clin. Invest.* **47**, 2689.
NORDEN, C. W. & KASS, E. H. (1968). *Ann. Rev. Med.* **19**, 431.
O'GRADY, F. & CATTELL, W. R. (1966). *Brit. J. Urol.* **38**, 149.
O'GRADY, F., CHARLTON. C. A. C., FRY, I. K., MCSHERRY, A. & CATTELL, W. R. (1973). *Urinary Tract Infection II*. Ed. W. Brumfitt & A. W. Asscher, Oxford, *in press.*
O'GRADY, F., FRY, I. K., MCSHERRY, A. & CATTELL, W. R. (1973). *J. infect. Dis. in press.*
O'GRADY, F. W., RICHARDS, B., MCSHERRY, M. A., O'FARRELL, S. M. & CATTELL, W. R. (1970). *Lancet* **2**, 1208.
REEVES, D. S. & BRUMFITT. W. (1968). In *Urinary Tract Infection*, p. 53, ed. O'Grady, F. and Brumfitt, W. London, Oxford University Press.
REEVES, D. S. & GHILCHIK, M. (1970). *Brit. J. Urol.* **42**, 66.
REPORT (1965). *J. clin. Path.* **18**, 1.
ROLLESTON, G. L., SHANNON, F. T. & UTLEY, W. L. F. (1970). *Brit. med. J.* **1**, 460.
SHAND, D. G., O'GRADY, F., NIMMON, C. C. & CATTELL, W. R. (1970). *Lancet* **1**, 1305.
SHAND, D. G., MACKENZIE, J. C., CATTELL, W. R. & CATO, J. (1968). *Brit. J. Urol.* **40**, 196.
SLADE, N. & CROWTHER, S. T. (1972). *Brit. J. Urol.* **44**, 105.
SLADE, N. & LINTON. K. B., (1965). *Brit J. Urol.* **37**, 73.
SMELLIE, J. M. & NORMAND, I. C. S. (1968). In *Urinary Tract Infection*, p. 123, ed. O'Grady. F. and Brumfitt. W. London, Oxford University Press.
SMELLIE, J. M. (1970) *Brit. med. J.* **4**, 97.
STAMEY, T. A., FAIR, W. R., TIMOTHY, M. M. & CHUNG, H. K. (1968). *Nature* **218**, 444.
STEPHENS, F. D., WHITAKER, J. & HEWSTONE, A. S. (1966). *Med. J. Aust.* **2**, 840.
WILLIAMS, G L., CAMPBELL, H. & DAVIES, K. J. (1969). *J. Obst. Gynaec. Brit. Cwlth* **76**, 229.
WILLIAMS, J. D.. BRUMFITT, W., CONDIE, A. P. & REEVES, D. S. (1969). *Postgrad. med. J.* **45** (Suppl. Nov.), 71.
WILLIAMS, J. D. & SMITH. E. K. (1970). *Brit. med. J.* **4**, 651.
WILLIAMS, J. D. (1973). *Urinary Tract Infection II*. Ed. W. Brumfitt & A. W. Asscher, Oxford, *in press.*
WINNINGHAM, D. G., NEMOY, N. J. & STAMEY. T. A. (1968). *Nature* (*Lond.*) **219**, 139.

CHAPTER 25

INFECTIONS OF THE EYE

THE treatment of serious ocular infections is a highly special-
ised task, and a full account of it would be out of place in a
work of this kind. The following is no more than an outline
of the underlying principles and of the more important
methods employed.

Superficial infections respond readily to various forms of
local treatment, and few of them present any problems. Those
involving the interior of the eye do present a special problem,
that of penetration of the affected area by anti-bacterial drugs.
Since adequate concentrations may only be obtainable there
by the method of sub-conjunctival injection of a substantial
dose in a small volume, the choice is limited by two considerations, solubility and local tolerance. Antibiotics easily
administered for their systemic effect may be excluded from
this special use on one or other of these grounds.

Intra-ocular Concentrations after Systemic Administration

Systemic administration is seldom used in the treatment of
intra-ocular infection but some anti-bacterial drugs diffuse into
the aqueous humour in therapeutic concentrations after administration by the ordinary route: the levels attained in the
vitreous are much lower and often undetectable. This penetration has been studied extensively in both animals and man,
employing a variety of doses including some very large ones.
This and other variables discourage any too concise and quantitative expression of the results. Simmons and O'Rourke (1968)
point out that with the uveal blood flow of about 0·2 ml. per
min. it takes a week for the blood volume to perfuse the eye.
Hence prolonged rather than transiently high blood levels are
necessary if systemic treatment is to be used to control intra-
ocular infection.

SULPHONAMIDES. The concentration of sulphadimidine attained in the aqueous is about 30 per cent of that in the blood

in the rat, and about 60 per cent in the rabbit, 30 minutes after the intravenous administration of a large dose. Experimentally, sulphonamides will control intra-ocular infections due to a fully sensitive organism such as *Str. pyogenes*. No other drugs penetrate with this facility.

PENICILLIN. Benzyl penicillin is useful, despite poor penetration, because of the large doses which can be given and its great intrinsic activity. An intramuscular dose of 1,000,000 units (0·6 g.) produces a concentration in the aqueous of about 0·5 unit per ml.

AMPICILLIN. Kurose *et al.* (1965) found single doses of 250 mg. gave maximum concentrations in the aqueous of 0·16 μg. per ml. after 4 hours. Single doses of 1 or 2 g. gave maximum aqueous concentrations after 6 hours of 0·96 μg. per ml. and 1·6 μg. per ml. respectively. One hour after the last of six hourly doses of 250 mg., the aqueous concentration was 0·12 μg. per ml., and after similar doses eight hourly, 0·18 μg. per ml. They conclude that unless the drug is given 4- to 6-hourly, or in very large doses, intra-ocular concentrations adequate for the treatment of any other than the most sensitive organisms are unlikely to be achieved. Furgiuele (1964) failed to detect ampicillin in the aqueous after 10-20 mg. per kg. body weight when the serum concentration was 0·025 to 1·0 μg. per ml.

METHICILLIN. After 20 or 40 mg. per kg. intra-muscularly, Green and Leopold (1965) found 0·2 or 0·8 μg. per ml. in the aqueous of the normal rabbit eye. In the presence of an intense keratitis produced by 0·2 N. HCl. the concentration was considerably increased : after 40 mg. per kg. to 5·7 μg. per ml. Furgiuele (1964) found that oxacillin and nafcillin failed to penetrate the eye after doses of 5 to 10 mg. per kg.

CEPHALOSPORINS. In patients about to undergo cataract operations who were given 1 g. cephalothin by rapid intravenous infusion, Records (1968) found concentrations in the aqueous of 0-2·5 μg./ml. at 15 min. and 0-1·0 μg./ml. after 30 min., the corresponding serum levels being 22-100 and 10-14 μg./ml. Cephaloridine, given in the same way and in the same dose produced considerably higher levels between 1 and 2 hours which persisted to give 2·5-17 µg./ml. after 8 hours (Records, 1969).

ERYTHROMYCIN. The estolate (p. 171) gave levels in the aqueous of rabbits' eyes of 0·09-0·6 and 0·39-1·62 µg. per ml. after oral doses of 44 and 500 mg. per kg. respectively (Shorr *et al.*, 1969).

FUCIDIN. In 18 patients about to undergo cataract extractions, and treated for three days preoperatively with 500 mg. fucidin three times daily, Chadwick and Jackson (1969) found aqueous levels of 0·8-2·0 µg./ml. with corresponding serum levels of 10-200 µg./ml. On the same regimen and with the last dose given 12 hours before operation, Williamson *et al.* (1970) found aqueous levels around 1·2 µg./ml. with serum levels of 52-72 µg./ml. After only two days' preoperative treatment, the aqueous and serum levels were 1·2 and 18-64 µg./ml., and after one day's treatment, 0·1-0·84 and 4-36 µg./ml. Fucidin was present in the vitreous of three patients whose eyes were enucleated. In two the levels were 2 to 3 times as high as those in the aqueous. In one patient presumably as the result of prolonged inflammation, the vitreous level was 28·8 (aqueous 12·8) µg./ml. and in another patient the vitreous level was still 0·32 (aqueous 0·1) µg./ml. 4 days after the last dose of fucidin.

SULPHOMETHYL COLISTIN. By intra-arterial infusion in dogs with experimental endophthalmitis, Simmons and O'Rourke (1968) produced levels of sulphomethyl colistin in the aqueous of 5-20 µg./ml. and in the vitreous of 0-0·6 µg./ml. when the serum levels were 40-80 µg./ml.

AMPHOTERICIN B. Green *et al.* (1965) were unable to demonstrate amphotericin B in the normal eyes of systemically treated rabbits, but found that in the presence of albumen-induced uveitis, levels of 0·16 to 0·18 µg. per ml. were obtained 6 hours after intravenous doses of 1 mg. per kg. Significantly, the drug penetrated less well when given sub-conjunctivally.

OTHER ANTIBIOTICS. The evidence with regard to streptomycin and chloramphenicol is somewhat conflicting, but it seems that by giving exceptionally large doses concentrations of either antibiotic of the order of 10 µg. per ml. or more can be attained in the aqueous and lower ones in the vitreous. The

TABLE 41

*Dosage for Injections in the Eye**

	Sub-conjunctival	Intra-ocular
Benzyl penicillin	0·5-1 mega unit	1,000-4,000 units
Methicillin	150 mg.	1 mg.
Neomycin	100-500 mg.	2·5 mg.
Streptomycin	50 mg.	—
Kanamycin	10-20 mg.	—
Polymyxin B (or Colistin) sulphate	0·1 mega unit	1,000 units
Bacitracin	10,000 units	500-1,000 units
Chloramphenicol	1 mg.	1-2 mg.
Tetracycline	2·5-5 mg.	—
Erythromycin	2·5-50 mg.	1-2 mg.

* LEOPOLD, I. H. (1964). *Invest. Ophthal.* **3,** 504.

TABLE 42

Concentrations of Various Agents Achieved in Normal Rabbits' Eyes after Systemic Injection

Agent	Dose	Route	Interval after Last Dose	Concentration, µg. per ml.		
				Aqueous	Vitreous	Serum
Chlor- amphenicol	50 mg./kg.	i/v	15 min	12	≦6	48
Erythro- mycin	6·5 mg./kg. 8 hrly × 4	i/v	2½ hr	0·1	0	0·36
Tetracycline	20 mg./kg. 12 hrly × 3	i/v	2½ hr	0·5	0	2-4
Kanamycin	50 mg./kg.	i/v	1 hr	8-16	0	128-256
	50 mg./kg. hrly × 2	i/m	15 min	1·6	0	26
Ampicillin	1 g. 2 g.	Oral	6 hr	0·96 1·6	0	—
	250 mg. 8 hrly	Oral	1 hr	0·08	0	—
Methicillin	20 mg./kg. 40 mg./kg.	i/m	1 hr	0·8 0·2	0	—
Vancomycin	45 mg./kg. 12 hrly × 3	i/v	2½ hr	1·5	0	23

Furgiuele, F. P., *et al.* (1960). *Amer. J. Ophthal.* **50,** 614. Furgiuele (1964). Green and Leopold (1965). Kurose, *et al.* (1965).

concentrations obtained by treatment with various agents are shown in Table 42. Furgiuele (1964) found that the intra-ocular concentrations of the agents which he studied were not affected by giving acetazolamide intravenously (7·2 mg. per kg.)

Sub-conjunctival Injection

There are several ways of introducing anti-bacterial substances locally, apart from application to the lids or conjunctiva. Injection into the orbit gives poor penetration, and direct injections into the chambers of the eye are not often indicated. The method of choice is sub-conjunctival injection, a fine

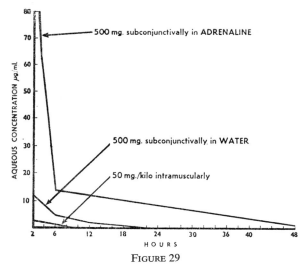

FIGURE 29

Aqueous levels of streptomycin after subconjunctival injection in water or adrenaline contrasted with the low level obtained by intramuscular injection of a large dose (Sorsby, A. and Ungar, J., 1960: *Antibiotics and Sulphonamides in Ophthalmology,* Oxford University Press).

needle being inserted between the conjunctiva and the sclera usually below the cornea since the injections are often painful and the patient tends to roll the eyeball up. Up to 1 ml. of solution can be injected. Trapped in this situation, the substance diffuses into the cornea and the chambers of the eye, where concentrations are attained far higher than any to be achieved by systemic administration, and maintained above the therapeutic minimum for as long as 48 hours. It should not be forgotten that antibiotics will be absorbed from this site and there is the possibility of remote toxic effects with such agents as neomycin—which can be given by this route in substantial doses—especially in patients with impaired renal function. The addition of adrenaline to the solution prolongs the effect. The concentrations of streptomycin attainable in the aqueous, contrasted with those obtained by systemic administration are shown in Figure 29.

Antibiotics suitable for administration by this route are :

PENICILLIN is in this situation as in most others the best tolerated: 1,000,000 units (0·6 g.) is often the dose given. Because of possible sensitization (but see p. 304) and the

TABLE 43

Concentrations of Various Agents Achieved in Normal Rabbits' Eyes after Subconjunctival Injection

Agent	Dose	Interval after Injection	Concentration μg. (or units) per ml.	
			Aqueous	Vitreous
Penicillin	50,000 units	1 hr.	>32 units	17 units
Methicillin	20 mg.	1 hr.	13	0
	40 mg.		20	
Streptomycin	10 mg.	3 hr.	8-20	—
Kanamycin	10 mg.	1 hr.	8	0-4
	20 mg.		10	0
Neomycin	500 mg.	4 hr.	240	33
Polymyxin E	250,000 units	1-3 hr.	10-200 units	20-200 units
Sulphomethyl-polymyxin B	500,000 units	45-120 min.	95-750 units	—

Sorsby, A. & Ungar, J. (1947). *Brit. J. Ophthal.* **31**, 517.
Gardiner, P. A., *et al.* (1948). *Brit. J. Ophthal.* **32**, 449.
Ainslie, D. & Smith, C. (1952). *Brit. J. Ophthal.* **36**, 352.
Furgiuele, *et al.* (1960). Ainslie, D. (1965). *Brit. J. Ophthal.* **49**, 98. Green and Leopold (1965).

inactivity of penicillin against the majority of enterobacteria, treatment is most commonly initiated with neomycin or, where *Pseudomonas* infection is feared, with a polymyxin or gentamicin. Methicillin is much less well tolerated, even considerably smaller amounts being liable to cause chemosis, a fact of some consequence to the treatment of penicillin-resistant staphylococcal infections. Cloxacillin is damaging to the eye and should not be used for this purpose nor as ophthalmic drops.

AMINOGLYCOSIDES. Neomycin is well tolerated in a dose of up to 0·5 g., and produces high and well sustained intra-ocular concentrations. There is clinical confirmation of its efficacy. Framycetin has been used in the same way with naturally corresponding results. Streptomycin and kanamycin behave similarly but smaller doses have generally been recommended (Table 41). Furgiuele (1970) gave 10 mg. gentamicin in 0·25 ml. by subconjunctival injection before cataract extraction and found aqueous levels of 0-4 μg./ml. after 30 minutes and 1·2-9·0 μg./ml. at 1-2$\frac{1}{2}$ hours.

POLYMYXIN. This antibiotic, invaluable for the treatment of one of the most dangerous of eye infections, that due to *Ps. aeruginosa,* is unfortunately much less well tolerated. The assessment of results with it is complicated by the use of two different polymyxins, B. and E (colistin), and of two different salts, the sulphate and the methane sulphonate, of which the latter evidently causes much less local reaction, in the eye as elsewhere (p. 185).

Doses recommended for sub-conjunctival and intra-ocular injection are given in Table 41. The intra-ocular concentrations of various agents achieved by the sub-conjunctival route are shown in Table 43.

The Treatment of Superficial Infections

Cant (1969) emphasizes the simple measures such as removal of a lash or encrusted exudate, and expression of pus from a blocked tear duct, which are essential to success and may be the only therapy necessary. The possibility that continuing or recrudescent inflammation is a reaction to locally applied antibacterial agent must be considered.

Superficial application may take the form of drops or ointment. The former may need very frequent application. Ointments, which obscure vision, are convenient for application last thing at night. Among the sulphonamides, sulphacetamide, as 10 per cent drops or 2·5-6 per cent ointment, has been chiefly used in this way because of its high solubility: it is doubtful whether there is any purpose for which an antibiotic is not more effective. Penicillin is also used in the form of drops containing up to 10,000 units (6 mg.) per ml. The validity of the commonly expressed fear of allergic reactions to such local applications of penicillin is discussed on page 304.

In ointments the antibiotic can be incorporated in the base in solid form, which ensures stability, and a slow process of solution in the lachrymal secretion gives a persistent effect. Penicillin can be used in this way in almost any desired concentration, and an ointment containing 50,000 units (30 mg.) per g. even gives some penetration into the interior of the eye. Ointments containing streptomycin, neomycin, tetracyclines or chloramphenicol are usually made up to contain one per cent. Ointment containing 10,000 and 4,000 units of polymyxin and bacitracin respectively per g. has been found satisfactory for a variety of purposes. Magnuson and Suie (1970) have confirmed their previous finding that gentamicin (0.3 per cent) ophthalmic drops and ointment are highly effective in the treatment of conjunctivitis, blepharitis or meibomiantis. In a double-blind, bacteriologically monitored comparison, Gordon (1970) found gentamicin at least as effective as a mixture of neomycin, bacitracin and polymyxin.

The minutiae of the treatment of various conditions of the eyelids and conjunctiva and of the lachrymal system, which include measures other than the application of anti-bacterial agents, are outside the scope of this book. Apart from the fact that staphylococci, which are responsible for most infections involving the eyelids, may be resistant to penicillin or tetracyclines, the organisms concerned are sensitive to most of the antibiotics mentioned. Even the two Gram-negative species causing conjunctivitis, the Koch-Weeks bacillus (a *Haemophilus*) and the Morax-Axenfeld bacillus, are sensitive to penicillin, as well as to other antibiotics more usually thought of in connection with Gram-negative infections.

Gonococcal ophthalmia in the infant is best treated by the instillation of penicillin solution at intervals at first of only one minute, but gradually extended. Systemic treatment may be advisable in addition, and is said to be invariably indicated in the adult.

Pseudomonas Ophthalmia. This dangerous condition has received publicity through outbreaks traced to contamination of solutions used for ophthalmic medication. The danger of contamination of eye medicaments and the importance of avoiding multi-dose containers for this reason has several times been emphasized. In a controlled trial of various treatments for experimental pseudomonas keratitis, Hessburg *et al.*, (1966) found that colistin sulphate irrigation (1mg. per ml.) was effective, and that the addition of sulphacetamide (1mg. per ml.) did not significantly improve the results. Furgiuele *et al.*, (1965) successfully controlled the condition with local applications of 1 per cent gentamicin drops.

Treatment with daily subconjunctival injections of gentamicin or a polymyxin-neomycin mixture for seven days is also effective (Furgiuele, 1968) but has the disadvantage that some of the potentially toxic agent will be absorbed. To overcome the need to make frequent instillations of drops in human infections, Hessburg (1966) describes a method of continuous corneal lavage. He used lavage, at 6-8 drops per minute, with 0·05 per cent colistin and 0·05 per cent sulphacetamide. He suggests that treatment should be continued for about 14 days, followed by 1 per cent colistin ointment hourly during the day and several times during the night for 3 weeks, followed again by 10 or 15 per cent sulphacetamide eye drops hourly during the day for 3 further weeks.

Fungus Infections of the Eye

In recent years there has been considerable interest in these infections and in the role of broad-spectrum antibiotics and corticosteroids in encouraging their emergence. A great variety of fungi have been identified (sometimes only on morphological grounds) in mycotic keratitis and endophthalmitis. They include both organisms normally regarded as saprophytic, such as cephalosporium and mucor, and some which are conceded more general pathogenic roles such as sporotrichum, aspergillus and candida (Jones *et al.*, 1969). It appears to be the consensus of opinion on both experimental and clinical grounds (Rheins *et al.*, 1966) that broad spectrum antibiotics do not predispose to fungus infections of the eye but corticosteroids do, and numerous warnings have been issued against the indiscriminate use of corticosteroids in the eye. Fungus infection should be suspected wherever purulent corneal ulceration cannot be explained by bacterial infection. Most authors believe that any applications of corticosteroid must be stopped (even though this may result in initial apparent deterioration), but that antibiotics should be continued in order to limit, as far as possible, secondary bacterial invasion.

Until recently, the only agents of proven value were the polyene antibiotics (p. 229). Nystatin is irritating but reasonably safe as ointment (100,000 units per g.). Amphotericin is more effective and can be given as drops containing up to 3 mg. per ml. of the colloidal suspension for injection, in distilled water (not saline) which can be supplemented by subconjunctival injections of 125 μg. Local treatment with amphotericin B is unpleasant and irritating, has often to be supplemented with debridement and must be continued for months. Newmark *et al.*, (1970) obtained good visual results in 7 patients suffering from cephalosporium or fusarium keratitis treated with pimaricin. At hourly intervals, they instilled alternately a 5 per cent suspension of pimaricin and 1 per cent potassium iodide drops. They originally used potassium iodide in the belief that it exerted an antifungal effect but suggest that the benefit is due to the potassium which helps to maintain the physiological state of the cornea and reduce the chance of intraocular sequelae. Treatment was continued for 2 to 4 weeks. The pimaricin suspension was non-irritant and sufficiently viscous to remain in the cul-de-sac for long periods.

The results of treatment of fungal endophthalmitis with polyenes are very unsatisfactory. There is little intraocular penetration of nystatin or amphotericin from subconjunctival injection, and intraocular injections are not well tolerated so that the final visual result even if the fungus is eliminated is likely to be poor.

Intra-ocular levels of amphotericin are obtained by systemic therapy, but the dangers of this (p. 419) are such that the treatment should only be undertaken in proven cases of fungal infection. Intra-ocular injections of amphotericin are exceedingly irritating but doses of 35-40 μg. in 0·05 ml. distilled water are tolerated. Injections of 200 units nystatin directly into the

aqueous or vitreous are tolerated, but produce inhibitory levels
(6-12 μg. per ml.) for only 24 hours. Larger or repeated injections cause vitreous degeneration. Encouraging results were
obtained by Richards *et al.*, (1969) who saved the sight of a
candida-infected eye by combining topical and oral treatment
with 5-fluorocytosine (150 mg./kg., later raised to 200 mg./kg.).

Trachoma

Inclusion conjunctivitis, inclusion blenorrhoea and trachoma are caused by the TRIC agent which belongs to the group
of *Chlamydia* (p. 486). It has also been suggested that in the
trachoma-infected eye, commensal bacteria may function as
opportunist pathogens and partly determine the severity of the
lesions (Arm and Woolridge, 1966). In keeping with the sensitivity of the causal organism and the possible role of bacterial
super-infection, trachoma was held to respond either to prolonged systemic sulphonamide treatment or to the local application of ointment containing tetracycline. Subsequent
experience was, however, much less encouraging. In 475 cases
randomized into three groups: untreated, treated with sulphamethoxypyridazine, or treated with local tetracycline, Foster,
Powers and Thygeson (1966) were unable to demonstrate any
difference in the cure rates when patients were re-examined
after one year. It did not appear that this apparent decline
in responsiveness was associated with increased resistance to
the antimicrobial agents (Shiao *et al.*, 1967). Grayston (1967)
discussed possible reasons for long-term poor results (including
re-infection) and suggested that therapy was of value in limiting spread of the disease even if it was not curative. Tarizzo
(1972) takes a much less gloomy view and warns that ' a
hypercritical approach may hinder positive action '. He believes
that currently available treatment, while not wholly effective,
can do much to control the disease and sees the possibility of
further improvement with the introduction of new agents such
as the rifamycins (p. 219).

Herpes Simplex Keratitis. This condition, which resolves
spontaneously in about 10 per cent of patients, can respond
well to idoxuridine (0·1 per cent drops) one-hourly by day and
two-hourly by night. Birge (1963) was successful in treating
75/76 of his patients. Idoxuridine (p. 482) has, however, two

disadvantages: the effective dose is very close to the maximum permissible so that severe reactions may occur, and resistance develops to it relatively easily. In a general review of the prospects for treating viral infections of the eye, Jones (1967) concludes that idoxuridine offers no advantage over cauterization in the treatment of dendritic ulcers. He suggests that its principal use may be in controlling deleterious effects of steroids on amoeboid ulcers and deep keratitis. Cytarabine (page 483) has been successfully used for the treatment of various herpes infections (Hryniuk *et al*, 1972) and a number of other synthetic agents have been tried experimentally (Maichik, 1971).

Post-operative Endophthalmitis

PRE-OPERATIVE PROPHYLAXIS. Opinions differ on the advisability of performing cultures before such operations as cataract extraction when there is no sign of infection. Even when secretion is obtained, as it should be, with a loop from the depths of the lower conjunctival sac, a few *Staph. albus* from the lid may be cultivated, and *C. xerosis* is a normal inhabitant. If a pathogenic organism such as *Staph. aureus* is found, preoperative treatment with antibiotic drops is indicated. Ointments may enter the eye during operation and are contraindicated.

POST-OPERATIVE PROPHYLAXIS. The majority view appears to be against routine antibiotic administration, whether systemic or subconjunctival, after clean operations. In 8 cases of post-operative infection reported by Aronstam (1964), 4 had had post-operative sub-conjunctival injections of penicillin plus streptomycin and 4 had not. This treatment delayed both the development and recognition of infection, and the ultimate visual result was poorer in the treated group. In contrast, Kolker *et al.* (1967), who gave alternate patients 100,000 units of penicillin and 66 mg. streptomycin subconjunctivally at the conclusion of operation, found one infection in 480 treated patients and 7 in 494 untreated. Over the next two years, all patients were treated and 2 out of 1480 developed endophthalmitis. McCoy *et al.* (1968) irrigated the anterior chamber after lens delivery with a solution containing 5 mg neomycin and 1 mg. polymyxin B per ml. and had no infection in 200 operations and no untoward effects. However, it must be pointed out that the infection rate in the untreated patients described by Kolker *et al.* (1967) is high compared with some other series in which patients receiving no prophylaxis have had very low infection rates (Rollins, 1965). The position is different after removal of an intra-ocular foreign body: the infection which may follow this is usually staphylococcal, and subconjunctival neomycin or cephaloridine is indicated.

TREATMENT OF ESTABLISHED INFECTION. Bacterial endophthalmitis after clean surgery is an unusual and serious complication occurring in most series in about 0·1 to 0·3 per cent of cases. In the series reported by Rollins (1965) there was loss of useful vision in 71 per cent of affected patients. The principal organisms are now *Staph. aureus* and *Pseudomonas aeruginosa* followed by *Klebsiella, Proteus* and *Escherichia.* The classical causes of eye infection, pneumococci and streptococci, appear now to be of much less importance. A bacteriological diagnosis is urgent in such a case. Conjunctival swabs can be misleading by yielding organisms other than those responsible for intra-ocular infection, and several pleas have been made for early anterior chamber aspiration. Gram-stained smears of this material may offer the most valuable guide to therapy since even where organisms are seen they may prove impossible to cultivate.

TABLE 44

Minimum Inhibitory Concentrations (μg./ml.) of Antibiotics Administrable by Subconjunctival Injection for Bacterial Species causing Ocular Infections

	Penicillin	Gentamicin	Neomycin	Polymyxin
Staph. aureus	0·03-R	0·12-1	1	R
Str. pyogenes	0·015	16	R	R
Str. pneumoniae	0·015	16-32	128	R
Ps. aeruginosa	R	1-8	50	0·12
Proteus spp.	5-R	1-8	5-50	R
Klebsiella spp.	R	0·5-4	2	0·25
Escherichia	R	1-4	8	0·25

The choice of an antibiotic for subconjunctival injection must take account of the properties of the four principal antibiotics available as stated in Table 44. Penicillin is clearly indicated for pneumococcal and streptococcal infection, but staphylococci responsible for hospital-acquired infection are almost certain to be resistant. Polymyxin is active, and to a high degree, against *Ps. aeruginosa, Klebsiella,* and *Escherichia;* but not against *Proteus* or the Gram-positive cocci. Neomycin and gentamicin on the other hand, have satisfactory activity against all these problem organisms: staphylococci, whether penicillin-resistant or not, and both *Ps. aeruginosa* and *Proteus.*

Kanski (1970) successfully treated 13 out of 20 patients with subconjunctival injections of a mixture of gentamicin, framycetin and methicillin.

REFERENCES

ARM, H. G. & WOOLRIDGE, R. L. (1966). *Med. J. Aust.* **2,** 351.
ARONSTAM, R. H. (1964). *Amer. J. Ophthal.* **57,** 312.
BIRGE, H. L. (1963). *Amer. J. med. Sci.* **246,** 239.
CANT, J. S. (1969). *Practitioner* **202,** 787.
CHADWICK, A. J. & JACKSON, B. (1969). *Brit. J. Ophthal.* **53,** 26.
FOSTER, S. O., POWERS, D. K. & THYGESON, P. (1966). *Amer. J. Ophthal.* **61,** 451.
FURGIUELE, F. P. (1964). *Amer. J. Ophthal.* **58,** 443.
FURGIUELE, F. P. (1968). *Amer. J. Ophthal.* **66,** 276.
FURGIUELE, F. P. (1970). *Amer. J. Ophthal.* **69,** 481.
FURGIUELE, F. P., KIESEL, R. & MARTYN, L. (1965). *Amer. J. Ophthal.* **60,** 818.
GORDON, D. M. (1970). *Amer. J. Ophthal.* **62,** 300.
GRAYSTON, J. T. (1967). *Amer. J. Ophthal.* **63,** 1583.
KUROSE, Y., LEVY, P. M. & LEOPOLD, I. H. (1965). *Arch. Ophthal.* (N.Y.) **73,** 769.
GREEN, W. R. & LEOPOLD, I. H. (1965). *Amer. J. Ophthal.* **60,** 800.
HESSBURG, P. C. (1966). *Amer. J. Ophthal.* **61,** 896.
HESSBURG, P. C., TRUANT, J. P. & PENN, W. P. (1966). *Amer. J. Ophthal.* **61,** 49.
HRYNIUK, W., FOERSTER, J., SHOJANIA, M. & CHOW, A. (1972). *J. Amer. med. Ass.* **219,** 715.
JONES, B. R. (1967). *Trans. ophthal. Soc. U.K.* **87,** 437.
JONES, B. R., RICHARDS, A. B. & MORGAN, G. (1969). *Trans. Ophthal. Soc. U.K.* **89,** 727.
KANSKI, J. J. (1970). *Brit. J. Ophthal.* **54,** 316.
KOLKER, A. E., FREEMAN, M. I. & PETTIT, T. H. (1967). *Amer. J. Ophthal.* **63,** 434.
KUROSE, Y., LEVY, P. M. & LEOPOLD, I. H. (1965). *Arch. Ophthal. (Chicago)* **73,** 366.
MAGNUSON, R. & SUIE, T. (1970). *Amer. J. Ophthal.* **70,** 734.
MAICHUK, Y. F. (1971). *Invest. Ophthal.* **10,** 408.
McCOY, D. A., McINTYRE, M. W. & TURNBULL, D. C. (1968). *Arch. Ophthal.* (N.Y.) **79,** 506.
NEWMARK, E., ELLISON, A. C. & KAUFMAN, H. E. (1970). *Amer. J. Ophthal.* **69,** 458.
RECORDS, R. E. (1968). *Amer. J. Ophthal.* **66,** 441.
RECORDS, R. E. (1969). *Arch. Ophthal.* (N.Y.) **81,** 331.
RHEINS, M. S., SUIE, T., VAN WINKLE, M. G. & HAVENER, W. H. (1966). *Brit. J. Ophthal.* **50,** 533.

RICHARDS, A. B., JONES, B. R., WHITWELL, J. & CLAYTON, Y. M. (1969). *Trans. Ophthal. Soc. U.K.* **89,** 867.

ROLLINS, H. J. (1965). *Sth. med. J.* **58,** 353.

SHIAO, L.-C., WANG, S.-P. & GRAYSTON, J. T. (1967). *Amer. J. Ophthal.* **63,** 1558.

SHORR, N., MACK, L. W. JR. & SMITH, J. L. (1969). *Brit. J. Ophthal.* **53,** 331.

SIMMONS, R. E. & O'ROURKE, J. (1968). *Amer. J. Ophthal.* **66,** 295.

TARIZZO, M. L. (1972). *W.H.O. Chronicle* **26,** 99.

WILLIAMSON, J., RUSSELL, F., DOIG, W. M. & PATERSON, R. W. W. (1970). *Brit. J. Ophthal.* **54,** 126.

CHAPTER 26

TUBERCULOSIS

CHEMOTHERAPY has radically transformed the outlook in this disease. A mortality rate which had been falling by only 3 per cent per annum from 1900 to 1948, fell thereafter by 15 per cent per annum (Fig. 30) and this reduction was even steeper in the lower age groups. The significance of the year 1948 is that it marks the general introduction of streptomycin for treating the disease: since then many other antibiotics and synthetic drugs have followed, the introduction of isoniazid in 1952 being of particular importance. Deaths from tuberculosis in England in 1970 were 1465, the lowest ever recorded, but even this is an overestimate, since nearly one third of death certificates carrying the diagnosis of tuberculosis relate to deaths from respiratory failure long after the infection has healed.

It is our purpose to describe the properties of these drugs, and to give a general account of the chief methods of treatment. Needless to say, the treatment of tuberculosis is a speciality, and should be directed only by those experienced in it.

STANDARD DRUGS

The three standard drugs used in the treatment of tuberculosis are, in order of their discovery, streptomycin, para-aminosalicylic acid and isoniazid. Although they still form the main basis of antituberculous chemotherapy, the distinction between the three standard drugs and the drugs of second choice is less sharp than formerly. This follows the introduction of several compounds which are acceptable substitutes for PAS as companion drugs to the major antituberculous agents. The general properties of streptomycin are described in Chapter 6 and those of para-aminosalicylic acid and isoniazid are summarized below.

Para-Aminosalicylic Acid (PAS)

The anti-tuberculous activity of PAS was discovered in Sweden in 1946 in the course of a systematic study of analogues of salicylic acid and benzoic acid. Of 50 derivatives prepared, *p*-aminosalicylic acid was the most active and caused 50-75 per cent inhibition of the BCG bovine strain of tubercle bacillus in a concentration of 1 in 650,000 (Lehmann, 1946).

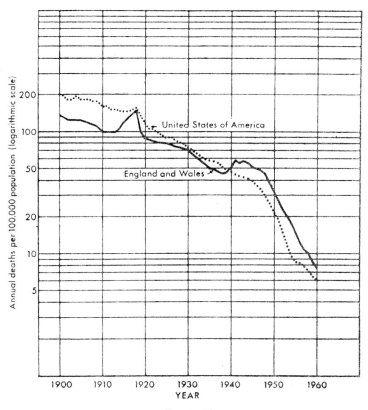

FIGURE 30

Annual deaths from tuberculosis per 100,000 population in England and Wales, and the United States of America 1900-1960. (In 1970 there were 3·2 deaths per 100,000 in England and Wales, and 2·7 in the U.S.A.)

COMPARATIVE MERITS. In comparison with most other anti-tuberculous drugs the activity of PAS is not very great and it is bacteristatic and not bactericidal. Its rôle is mainly that of preventing the development of resistance to the major compounds given at the same time. It is well absorbed from the gastro-intestinal tract, but large daily doses, 10-12 g., have to be given. It has the advantages, however, that it is absorbed from the intestinal tract and although not free from side effects these are rarely of sufficient severity to interfere with treatment.

SIDE EFFECTS. Gastric discomfort and nausea, with or without diarrhoea, occur in nearly all patients treated with large doses of the drug. These effects often subside in the first weeks of treatment, but an appreciable proportion of patients are unable or unwilling to continue taking PAS. Many preparations have now been evolved with the aim of reducing gastro-intestinal side-effects and, by combining PAS with isoniazid, ensuring that the patient receives either appropriate combined chemotherapy or none at all.

Allergic reactions in the form of rashes with or without fever are unfortunately common and may be severe. Other reactions such as hepatitis, a syndrome resembling infectious mono-nucleosis, and rarely an encephalitis-like syndrome may occur. These reactions are usually dealt with by replacing PAS with another drug, but desensitization can be achieved, at least after the milder reactions. An initial dose of 0·5 g. is given, and this is increased by 0·5 g. daily. Severe reactions are treated by corticosteroids.

PAS causes slight interference in the metabolism of iodine in the thyroid gland and after six months or more of treatment some patients may develop a goitre and occasionally signs of myxoedema. These symptoms can be relieved by giving thyroid, without stopping PAS.

Isoniazid

Isoniazid or 1-isonicotinyl hydrazide was synthesized as long ago as 1912 (Meyer and Mally, 1912) but its anti-tuberculous properties were first announced in the American press in February, 1952. A series of papers indicating the activity of the drug against *Myco. tuberculosis in vitro,* in experimental infection in laboratory animals and in human infection quickly followed (Grunberg and Schnitzer, 1952; Grunberg *et al.*, 1952; Robitzek *et al.*, 1952) and in March, 1952, the Medical Research Council launched a large controlled clinical trial, which established the value of isoniazid in the treatment of tuberculosis (Report, 1952).

COMPARATIVE MERITS. Isoniazid has an active bactericidal action on *Myco. tuberculosis* and inhibits the growth of most pre-treatment strains in a concentration as low as 0·2 μg./ml. It has the advantage over streptomycin that it is readily absorbed from the intestinal tract, diffuses well into the body tissues and fluids, including the cerebro-spinal fluid, and penetrates into macrophages, so that it is effective against intracellular tubercle bacilli. It is effective clinically in small doses (e.g. 200-300 mg. daily) and with this dosage toxicity is very low. It has the disadvantage that tubercle bacilli very readily develop resistance to it. Isoniazid-resistant bacilli are of diminished virulence for guinea-pigs (Mitchison, 1954), but the clinical significance of this is not clear. Resistance affects only some of the cells in the population, and the drug may therefore still have a useful therapeutic effect by its action on the remainder.

METABOLISM. Metabolism of isoniazid in the body has been shown to vary very greatly in different individuals. Broadly speaking people can be divided into one of two groups usually referred to as rapid and slow inactivators of isoniazid. Six hours after a dose of 10 mg. per kg. body weight the latter group usually have blood levels of 3-6 μg./ml. whereas with the former group the blood level is less than 2·5 μg./ml. The speed of isoniazid inactivation is genetically controlled, rapid inactivation being the dominant character. Isoniazid inactivation status has an important effect on the results of intermittent chemotherapy for tuberculosis (p. 444).

EXCRETION. Isoniazid is excreted in the urine in three forms, free drug, its acetyl derivative and hydrazones. The proportion in the latter form is constant: that in the free form is higher in slow inactivators, and that in the form of acetyl isoniazid is higher in rapid inactivators. A determination of this ratio is an alternative to blood assay for distinguishing between the two groups (Short, 1962).

SIDE EFFECTS. Toxic effects are not common with the usual dosage of 200-300 mg. but are significantly more frequent among slow inactivators when larger doses are used. The most common side effects are restlessness, insomnia, muscle twitching and difficulty in starting micturition. More serious effects are peripheral neuritis and psychotic upsets. The incidence of toxic symptoms is reduced by the simultaneous administration of pyridoxine.

Resistance to Standard Drugs

Primary resistance to these drugs (i.e. resistance in newly diagnosed patients who have had no treatment) has fortunately remained very uncommon in advanced countries. In surveys in Great Britain, Canada and the United States, the percentage of strains resistant to streptomycin has varied from 2·0-3·1, to isoniazid from 1·5-4, and to PAS from 0·7-4·6. In developing countries resistance is much more common, although some so-called primary resistance is no doubt attributable to inadequate or self-administered treatment. The proportion of resistant strains is between 20 and 25 per cent in parts of India, Africa and Korea, and is even higher in Vietnam (Editorial, 1970). France occupies an intermediate position, with an overall primary resistance rate of 9·8 per cent (Canetti *et al.*, 1972) to one or more of the three standard drugs.

OTHER ANTITUBERCULOUS DRUGS

These include both antibiotics and synthetic compounds.

Rifampicin

Earlier derivatives of rifamycin had little success in the treatment of this disease, but rifampicin (see also p. 220) represents an enormous advance on them in two directions. It can be administered orally, attaining high and well sustained blood levels, and it has greatly enhanced antibacterial activity. Apparent activity against *Myco. tuberculosis* varies with the medium used, but in a Tween-albumin medium Hobby, Lenert and Maier-Engallena (1969) found the mean M.I.C. for 20 strains to be only 0·018 μg./ml. As with all rifamycin derivatives, bacterial populations contain a minute proportion of resistant cells which grow out unless this is prevented by the presence of another active drug.

Of now numerous experimental studies the most comprehensive are those of Grumbach, Canetti and Le Lirzin (1969) who treated mice with various combinations of rifampicin and other drugs and different systems of dosage, judging results by quantitative cultures of liver and spleen after 3 and 6 months. The most effective combination was rifampicin plus isoniazid: daily treatment sterilized the organs of all mice at 6 months. Rifampicin plus ethambutol given daily was almost as effective, but less so when the latter part of the course was intermittent. Isoniazid plus ethambutol was inferior to either of the foregoing. Although the addition of streptomycin to a regime of rifampicin plus isoniazid had little effect, that of an initial one month of rifampicin to a course of isoniazid plus streptomycin had a pronounced effect, particularly on the organ counts at 5 months, i.e. long after rifampicin had been discontinued. These authors predict that the use of rifampicin may enable the usual period of clinical treatment to be shortened and there is now evidence to support this contention (see p. 446).

Needless to say, rifampicin must always be used in combination with one or more other drugs to which the patient's organisms are susceptible. Resistant strains emerge rapidly if it is used alone. The use of rifampicin in antituberculous treatment is discussed below (p. 446); widespread use is at present limited by its high cost.

Disturbance of liver function tests is commonly detected during rifampicin treatment, but the changes are often transient. Clinically significant adverse reactions are less frequent but transient rashes are not uncommon and occasionally patients develop violent sensitivity reactions leading to discontinuation of treatment. Girling and Fox (1971) have described a number of symptom complexes associated with rifampicin treatment, and outlined a procedure for their management. Thrombocytopenic purpura is an uncommon but potentially important adverse effect, and is associated with rifampicin-dependent antibodies in the serum (Poole *et al.*, 1971). Adverse reactions from rifampicin appear to be more frequent when the regimen also includes isoniazid (Lees *et al.*, 1971), and a high incidence of unwanted effects has been recorded in a twice weekly regimen including a high dose of rifampicin (Poole *et al.*, 1971).

Ethambutol

This is the dextrorotatory isomer of 2.2'-(ethylenediimino)-di-1-butanol. The compound inhibits the growth of human and bovine strains of *Myco. tuberculosis* in a concentration of 1-5 μg./ml. and is effective in the treatment of experimental infection in mice and guinea-pigs (Thomas *et al.*, 1961; Karlson, 1961a and b). It is well absorbed after oral administration in man, and has been found effective both alone and in various combinations.

The use of ethambutol has until recently been restricted because it can cause impairment of vision, due to a retrobulbar neuritis, of which the first signs are blurred vision and inability to distinguish colours. Recovery from this seems to have been invariable, and according to the authors cited and to Leibold (1966) it can be prevented by regulating the dose: 25 mg. per kg. for 60 days should then be reduced to 15 mg. This scheme of dosage has now become widely accepted and ocular toxicity is now rare. For example, only one of 72 patients treated with this dose by Lees *et al.* (1971) developed optic neuritis. Routine tests of colour vision and of the visual fields should precede treatment and patients should be warned to stop treatment if they have visual symptoms. Routine eye tests are not, however, useful in anticipating toxic effects (Citron, 1969).

Thiacetazone (Conteben: TBI)

Thiosemicarbazones were used for the treatment of tuberculosis in Germany as long ago as 1946. They were introduced by Domagk and his colleagues at the Farbenfabriken Bayer Laboratories at Elberfeld, where the antibacterial activity of the sulphonamides had been discovered (Domagk *et al.*, 1946). The most active was 4-acetylaminobenzaldehyde thiosemicarbazone which was given the name thiacetazone; *in vitro* and in experimental infection in laboratory animals, thiacetazone in large doses appears to have an activity greater than that of *p*-aminosalicylic acid and similar or slightly inferior to that of streptomycin.

Thiacetazone is a reliable companion drug, and excellent results have been reported from its use with isoniazid, especially when treatment is initiated with a phase of additional daily streptomycin (E. African/British MRC, 1970). Its value is somewhat limited by adverse reactions, especially by rashes: other side-effects include nausea, vomiting and dizziness. An international investigation showed that 16·1 and 17·6 per cent of patients on two thiacetazone-containing regimens developed rashes, 20 per cent of which were severe. By comparison, 7·7 per cent of patients receiving streptomycin and isoniazid developed rashes, and of them, only 6 per cent were severe (Ferguson et al., 1971). The incidence of rashes varies greatly in different areas. In E. Africa adverse effects are not so common as to outweigh the advantages, including cheapness, of thiacetazone-containing schemes of treatment. In Chinese patients in Hong Kong, and in all the three racial groups in Singapore, the incidence of rashes is unacceptably high, and thiacetazone-containing regimens cannot be generally used. (Singapore Tuberculosis Services, 1971).

Ethionamide

This compound, like isoniazid, is a derivative of isonicotinic acid, with the full chemical name, alpha-ethylthioisonicotin-amide.

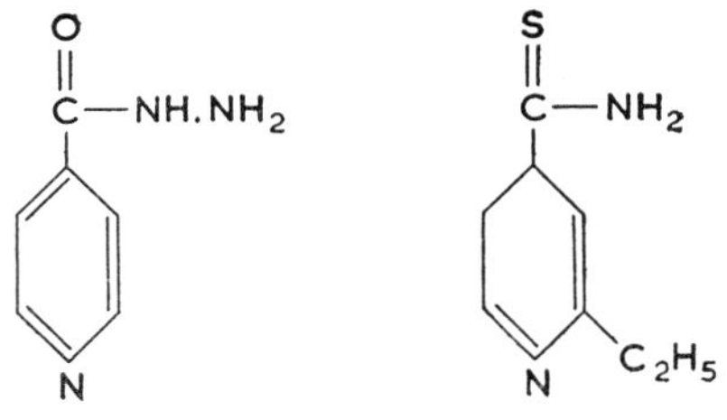

ISONIAZID   ETHIONAMIDE

In spite of the structural similarity between isoniazid and ethionamide, tubercle bacilli do not show cross-resistance and ethionamide is fully active against isoniazid-resistant tubercle bacilli. The activity of ethionamide *in vitro* and in experi-

15

mental infection is about twice that of streptomycin but inferior to that of isoniazid. Like streptomycin and isoniazid the action of ethionamide on tubercle bacilli is bactericidal (Rist *et al.*, 1959). As with isoniazid, ethionamide-resistant tubercle bacilli emerge rapidly, and there is cross-resistance between thioacetazone and ethionamide (Rist *et al.*, 1959).

The full dose, a total of 1 g. daily, is liable to cause nausea and anorexia, and may on that account have to be somewhat reduced: neurotoxic effects may also occur (Brouet *et al.*, 1959). Prothionamide is somewhat less likely to provoke severe gastro-intestinal symptoms, at least in males, and may therefore be preferred to ethionamide, with which there is complete cross-resistance.

Pyrazinamide

Following the discovery of the anti-tuberculous activity of nicotinamide a number of nicotinic acid derivatives were synthesized, of which pyrazinamide was the most active (Kushner *et al.*, 1952). Although *in vitro* and in experimental infections in mice and guinea-pigs the activity of pyrazinamide was only moderate, trials in man showed apparently greater activity (Yeager *et al.*, 1952). Moreover, combined treatment with isoniazid and pyrazinamide in experimental infections of mice freed the animals from tubercle bacilli more completely than did any of the standard drugs used singly or together, and early clinical trial suggested that this combination gave better bacteriological and radiographic results than did combinations of any of the three standard drugs (Schwartz and Moyer, 1953; McDermott *et al.*, 1955). Equally good results are not, however, obtained in all cases. This may be partly explained by the fact that a proportion of pre-treatment strains of tubercle bacilli are resistant to pyrazinamide (Riddell *et al.*, 1960).

The disadvantage of pyrazinamide is hepatotoxicity. This was caused in earlier studies mainly by rather large doses, and it seems from the observations of Velu *et al.* (1961) and subsequent experience that a dose limited to 1·5 g. daily is reasonably safe. This dose, divided into three of 0·5 g., was found by Ellard (1969) in a thorough pharmacological study to maintain a blood level about 5 μg./ml. almost continuously. Patients should be under frequent observation, and blood transaminase estimations should be done regularly.

Capreomycin

Capreomycin is a peptide derived from *Streptomyces capreolus* and is available as the sulphate. It has little action on species other than mycobacteria. Streptomycin-resistant tubercle bacilli are sensitive to it, but there is some cross-resistance with viomycin and kanamycin. It is an alternative to these two antibiotics, and possibly less toxic than either, although damage both to the eighth nerve (usually auditory) and to the kidney may be caused: reports of the frequency of these effects differ. Hesling (1969) described adverse reactions in 34 patients treated with 1 g. daily, 14 of whom completed two years' treatment. The drug was stopped because of renal damage in 8 patients, because of hearing loss in 3, and because of an allergic reaction in one

Viomycin

This is another antibiotic isolated from a species of *Streptomyces* and similar in many ways to streptomycin, both in its anti-bacterial activity and in its toxicity to the eighth cranial nerve. It also has to be given by intramuscular injection. Unfortunately its anti-bacterial activity is lower than that of streptomycin and its toxicity is higher. With daily treatment for long periods giddiness, deafness and renal damage are frequent, but the incidence of side effects is greatly reduced by giving the drug on only two days of the week, and 1 g. twice a day on each of the two days is the usually recommended dose. There is cross-resistance between viomycin and both streptomycin and kanamycin, but once again it is usually one-way, so that strains which have become resistant to streptomycin and kanamycin are often still sensitive to viomycin, but viomycin-resistant strains are usually resistant to both the other two.

Cycloserine

This is a broad spectrum antibiotic, sometimes used for other purposes than this (see Chapter 12). It has a relatively weak action on the tubercle bacillus *in vitro*, but is effective *in vivo*, with the double advantage that resistance to it develops only slowly and that its inclusion in combinations strongly deters the development of resistance to other drugs. The aim should be to administer 0·5 g. twice daily, but the peculiar neurotoxic effects liable to be caused may necessitate reduction of this dose. Confusion, excitability, hallucinations and depression have all been reported, and treatment should be stopped promptly if any mental or neurological signs develop.

Kanamycin

This is described fully in Chapter 7. It belongs to the same group as streptomycin and has a similar *in vitro* action on *Myco. tuberculosis*. Strains resistant to streptomycin are sensitive to it, although the reverse does not obtain. Its only drawback is ototoxicity, the frequency of which varies greatly in different reports. A good account of the use of kanamycin is given by Kreis (1966) who prefers it to viomycin both for its greater activity and because should resistance to kanamycin develop, viomycin sensitivity is retained: the converse is not true.

Thiocarbanilides

Many substituted thioureas have been shown to have therapeutic activity in mice and guinea-pigs, but there is very little correlation between activity *in vitro* and *in vivo*. Clinical trials with one of the most effective compounds in animals, 4-isobutoxy-4'-(2-pyridyl) thiocarbanilide, were disappointing and it was thought that the compound was poorly absorbed from the human intestinal tract. More recently another carbanilide, 4-4'-diisoamyloxythiocarbanilide (isoxyl) has been introduced, and some success was claimed from a combination of this drug in a dose of 500 mg. daily with streptomycin, but recently it has been little used.

Tetracyclines

These antibiotics have a very weak action against tubercle bacilli, but when given in large doses (2 g. twice a day) in combnation with streptomycin or isoniazid appear to prevent the emergence of tubercle bacilli resistant to the two latter. Similarly the tetracyclines in the same dose reduce the incidence of viomycin-resistant organisms when given with viomycin. Administration of tetracyclines does not appear to delay the emergence of strains resistant to pyrazinamide or ethionamide (Crofton, 1960).

STANDARD TREATMENT

Both standard treatment and that with ' second-line ' drugs are well described by Crofton and Douglas (1969), and only an outline will be given here. The necessity for giving at least two, often three, and sometimes even more than three drugs together has long been recognized, and the evidence that bacillary resistance is thus prevented or at least long delayed is now familiar. Originally furnished by studies with streptomycin and PAS in Great Britain over twenty years ago, it has since been extended to many other combinations. Perhaps the principal change in management during recent years has been the recognition that sanatorium treatment is unnecessary for the average patient: provided that drug administration is feasible he can remain at home.

Initial Treatment

The treatment of active pulmonary disease is usually started with a combination of all three of the standard drugs, streptomycin, isoniazid and PAS (Report, 1962a). The dose for young adults is streptomycin 1 g. daily by intramuscular injection, together with isoniazid and PAS. The two oral drugs are normally given together in one of a number of combined preparations designed to give a daily dose of 300 mg. isoniazid with 12 g. PAS. For patients over 40 years the amount of streptomycin should be reduced to 1 g. on three days a week because of the greater risk of vestibular damage in older people (Crofton, 1960).

Continued Treatment

Provided sensitivity tests on the original isolates show that the infecting bacilli are fully sensitive to all three drugs, treatment can then be continued with oral isoniazid and PAS alone. In practice this means that most patients receive an initial intensive phase of daily streptomycin, isoniazid and PAS for two to three months, but this phase may be longer in patients with extensive disease. The development of additional ' second line ' drugs has made physicians less inclined to persist with PAS or to attempt desensitization in patients intolerant or allergic to this drug, a sizeable problem since 24 per cent of patients are unable to go on taking PAS (Stradling and Poole, 1970). Now that its dosage in relationship to efficacy and toxicity has been well established (p. 438), ethambutol is commonly administered as the companion drug with streptomycin and isoniazid. Treatment must be continued for at least 18 months, and for two years in patients with extensive disease (Report, 1962). Rifampicin and isoniazid have also been used with success in previously untreated patients (Lees *et al.*, 1972).

INTERMITTENT CHEMOTHERAPY

Although standard regimens of antituberculous chemotherapy achieve excellent results under the closely supervised conditions of a clinical trial, their results are far from ideal under conditions which normally prevail during treatment, and this is found both in wealthy and in developing countries. A number of schemes of intermittent chemotherapy have now been tried and shown to be at least as good, and sometimes better, than standard chemotherapy. These methods, which are of great theoretical interest, have important practical advantages because they can be closely supervised and because, in some cases, the incidence of adverse drug reactions is less than that encountered with daily chemotherapy. The first step towards intermittent chemotherapy followed an investigation in Madras (Gangadharam *et al.*, 1961) which showed that a dose of 400 mg. of isoniazid administered once a day (as part of a standard scheme of combined treatment) was more effective than 200 mg. given twice daily, although the latter scheme produced continuous levels of isoniazid in the plasma while the former did not. Since then a number of trials have been completed in which standard chemotherapy has been compared with various schemes of intermittent treatment. Of patients with severe cavitated pulmonary tuberculosis 94 per cent achieved quiescence after one year of treatment with twice weekly streptomycin and high dose isoniazid (15 mg./kg.), while 84 per cent achieved quiescence on conventional treatment with daily PAS and low dose isoniazid.

Remarkable results were achieved in a closely supervised trial in which schemes of standard or intermittent treatment followed an intensive phase in which all patients received three months' treatment with daily streptomycin, PAS and isoniazid. All 233 patients on twice-weekly streptomycin and high-dose isoniazid achieved quiescence, as did 163 of the 165 patients receiving conventional daily PAS and low dose isoniazid (Czech/WHO/MRC, 1971). It would clearly be of great advantage if treatment could be given even less often than twice weekly, but the individual dose of isoniazid cannot be much increased over about 15 mg./kg. because of the risk of acute toxic effects. Trials of once-weekly streptomycin and high dose isoniazid have given clearly inferior results to the twice weekly schemes, but when these findings are analysed in relation to isoniazid inactivator status, it emerges that the disadvantages of this form of treatment is confined to the rapid inactivators. The poor results of once weekly chemotherapy for rapid inactivators of isoniazid can be overcome neither by the addition of pyrazinamide nor by an initial intensive phase of one month's daily treatment with streptomycin and isoniazid. A preparation of isoniazid is needed which, by its delayed absorption, would enable a fast inactivator of isoniazid to maintain effective levels of the drug for as long as a slow inactivator does with ordinary isoniazid. Several slow release preparations have been devised and one of them, given in a dose of 30 mg./kg., may be suitable for a once weekly scheme (Ellard et al., 1972). Intermittent chemotherapy would be much easier to apply if injections of streptomycin could be avoided. Schemes involving only drugs administered by mouth have now been successfully used, following an initial intensive phase of treatment including daily streptomycin. Lahlou (1970), in N. Africa, gave ethionamide and isoniazid twice weekly, while in Madras, patients have been given 10 g. PAS and 15 mg./kg. isoniazid twice weekly (Fox, 1971). Both schemes gave good results which might have been even better with a longer initial intensive phase. The value of rifampicin in intermittent chemotherapy is still being assessed, since some authors (Poole et *al.*, 1971), have encountered a high incidence of toxic effects when large doses of this drug are given twice weekly. The theoretical basis and practical results of intermittent chemotherapy have been reviewed by Fox (1971).

SHORT COURSE CHEMOTHERAPY

Effective standard chemotherapy leads to rapid radiological and clinical improvement, and to the disappearance of cultivable tubercle bacilli from the sputum, but a long total period of chemotherapy, at least 18 months, is essential to ensure a low risk of relapse after treatment is discontinued. The introduction of new and powerful antituberculous drugs raises the possibility that shorter regimens of chemotherapy might be devised which would nevertheless be followed by an acceptably low relapse rate. This hope would apply particularly to rifampicin-containing schemes in view of the remarkable bactericidal efficacy of this drug, especially in combination with isoniazid (Grumbach *et al.*, 1969; Batten, 1969).

A trial has now been completed in East Africa comparing four six-month regimens with one of the standard 18-month schemes (E. African/British MRC, 1972). All the methods gave immediately favourable results, but significant differences between them emerged in the six months after chemotherapy was completed. Daily streptomycin, isoniazid and rifampicin, and daily streptomycin, isoniazid and pyrazinamide were followed by low rates of relapse, 4 per cent and 6 per cent respectively. The other two methods, daily streptomycin, isoniazid and thiacetazone, and daily streptomycin and isoniazid only, were followed by high relapse rates, 21 per cent and 18 per cent. The standard 18-month scheme of daily isoniazid and thiacetazone, with daily streptomycin in addition during the first 8 weeks of treatment, had a relapse rate of 2 per cent. It is notable that the rate at which cultures became negative during the first 3 months of treatment was more rapid in the rifampicin- and the pyrazinamide-containing regimens, and that all bacilli cultivated during relapses were fully drug-sensitive.

Although any regimen involving daily injections of streptomycin for six months, as all these schemes do, must be of limited value in countries with restricted health services, successful short-course chemotherapy is potentially of great practical importance as well as much theoretical interest.

Meningitis

In cases of tuberculous meningitis all three of the standard drugs should be given. Initially the dose should be strepto-mycin 1 g. daily, or 40 mg./kg. for infants and small children, by intramuscular injection, PAS 10-15 g. daily by mouth; and isoniazid at least 300 mg. daily or 10 mg./kg. by mouth. Treatment should be continued for at least a year. A good case could be made for using ethionamide instead of PAS as the third drug, since it passes into the CSF fairly readily even in the absence of meningitis (Hughes *et al.*, 1962). Ethambutol too achieves modest concentrations in the CSF in tuberculous meningitis, although it does not do so in normal subjects (Place *et al.*, 1969; Pilheu *et al.*, 1971). The efficacy of rifampicin as an antituberculous drug makes this also a possible addition to the treatment of tuberculous meningitis, since it shows some ability to penetrate into the CSF (D'Oliveira, 1972). Large scale trials of newer methods have yet to be published, but the continuing severity of the disease in areas of high tuberculosis prevalence can be gauged by the report of Freiman and Geefhuysen (1970) who treated 131 African children with tuberculous meningitis. Two thirds of them were unconscious on admission, 40 per cent had died within a year, and half the survivors showed serious sequelae.

Whether intrathecal treatment should be given or not is still in dispute; reports from many centres suggest that intra-thecal injections of any kind are now unnecessary and possibly undesirable because of their irritant effect (Anderson *et al.*, 1953; Bulkeley, 1953; Report, 1954). A more cautious view is expressed by Lorber (1960) who suggests that intrathecal injec-tions of streptomycin should not be wholly abandoned. He re-commends a course of 10 injections and more if the clinical condition or cerebro-spinal fluid findings are unsatisfactory at any subsequent date. The intrathecal dose should not exceed 100 mg. or 25–50 mg. in children.

Additional treatment with corticosteroids may be helpful in severe cases. Lorber (1960) recommends this for patients unconscious on admission or for children under one year of age. The dose must be adequate and the duration rarely needs to exceed one month. If intrathecal injections of hydrocortisone are contemplated, special precautions must be taken to prevent secondary infection. Freidman and Geefhuysen, whose experience is quoted above, believe that their results have been improved by the addition of intrathecal streptomycin and hydrocortisone.

Surgical Tuberculosis

The treatment of this differs in no way in principle, and very little in practice, from that of pulmonary disease. For genito-urinary tuberculosis there is now general agreement that treatment should be continued for two years. The two drugs mainly to be relied on are PAS and isoniazid : since the organism is sometimes of the bovine type and 17 per cent of these are PAS-resistant (Wallace and Webber, 1956), verification of sensitivity is desirable. Some authors have obtained satisfactory results with this combination alone (e.g. Band and Murray, 1958): others favour the addition of streptomycin, at least for the first few months (Halkier and Meyer, 1959). In patients with extensive renal disease who are given streptomycin, blood levels should be determined and the dose reduced if these are found to be unduly high. Surgery is now rarely necessary for disease of either the kidney or the epididymis, and lesions of the bladder which formerly led to severe disability now resolve with good restoration of function.

Initial surgical treatment is often still advisable in tuberculosis of bone : chemotherapy follows the same lines as in other forms of the disease.

TREATMENT FOR PATIENTS WITH DRUG-RESISTANT INFECTION

The choice of treatment in such patients is a matter for the expert and can only be briefly discussed here. Careful preliminary sensitivity tests and assessment of their likely results in the light of the patient's previous history of drug administration are very important; these and other factors of importance in establishing a suitable scheme of treatment have been reviewed by Crofton (1971). At least three drugs and sometimes four are advocated for strains resistant to the standard drugs and a combination of ethionamide, pyrazinamide and cycloserine has been widely used. The introduction of new drugs has widened the effective choices for these difficult problems, and, although most authors still favour the use of at least three drugs, good results have been achieved in drug-resistant tuberculosis with daily ethambutol and rifampicin (Lees *et al.*, 1971; Somner *et al.*, 1971).

Hypersensitivity to a standard drug presents the same problem as resistance to it, except that de-sensitization by initially very small and frequently repeated doses may be possible.

Chemoprophylaxis

Recent contacts should in the first place have a tuberculin test and a chest X-ray. Those with positive tuberculin tests and X-ray changes should be investigated and treated on the usual principles as presumed cases of tuberculosis. Child contacts with normal X-ray but positive tuberculin tests should be treated for one year. The upper age limit for prophylactic chemotherapy of contacts with a positive tuberculin test will vary with the prevalence of infection in the community. Treatment should be given to any child contact under the age of three years, and the age limit for treatment will rise as the prevalence of tuberculous infection in the community declines. The use of chemoprophylaxis on a larger scale is discussed below. A special case among contacts is the infant of a tuberculous mother. If the disease has been diagnosed and adequately treated during pregnancy, so that it is quiescent at term, the infant is vaccinated with BCG at birth and need not be separated from the mother. A serious problem arises if the disease is diagnosed late in pregnancy, or even after delivery. If the infant is vaccinated with BCG segregation is necessary until the tuberculin test has converted, but in many communities this is impracticable and itself dangerous to the infant. In these circumstances the infant should be given oral isoniazid for a year, and then vaccinated with BCG. The production of immunity by BCG is impaired by simultaneous administration of isoniazid, but chemoprophylaxis and vaccination can be combined by using an isoniazid-resistant strain of BCG, as suggested by Canetti (1956) and used successfully by Gaisford and Griffiths (1961). If this preparation is available, vaccination need not then be delayed until after the period of isoniazid prophylaxis.

Apart from the use of chemoprophylaxis in infant and child contacts of patients with tuberculosis, isoniazid has also been used on a much larger scale in attempting to prevent infection and to lessen the incidence of tuberculous disease in infected subjects.

The U.S. Public Health Service has carried out extensive controlled trials in children with asymptomatic primary tuberculosis, in household contacts, among Alaskan villages in which ' the disease was so widespread that for all practical purposes everyone could be regarded as a close contact of an active case of tuberculosis ', in patients in mental institutions and in people with inactive lesions compatible with healed tuberculosis. These and other controlled trials have been extensively reviewed by Ferebee (1969). The degree of protection afforded by one year's treatment with isoniazid varied greatly with the different trials. At its best, among the good pill takers in the trial of household contacts, the tuberculosis morbidity was reduced by 88 per cent during the treatment year. Of great interest is the finding that these beneficial effects are maintained in lesser degree during the following years, suggesting that chemoprophylaxis has a long term effect on the risks of endogenous breakdown. In the trial quoted, morbidity was reduced by 60 per cent in the post-treatment phase, with a follow-up of 5-10 years.

Adverse reactions do not present a serious problem with the dose used, 5 mg./kg./day, but 1·9 per cent of contacts, and 6 per cent of those with inactive lesions, discontinued treatment because of reactions, mainly gastro-intestinal upsets and rash. Unwanted effects are more common in older patients, and in a prospective study in the U.S. Army (Byrd, Nelson and Elliott, 1972) 16 of 160 men were unable to complete one year of chemoprophylaxis.

Enthusiasm for the results of controlled trials has led to discussion of even more widespread use of these schemes, which might in theory be extended to the whole tuberculin-positive section of the population. The logistics of schemes for chemoprophylaxis have been examined by Katz and Kunofsky (1971), who confirm that a useful reduction of tuberculosis morbidity can be expected by treating special groups, namely patients with inactive tuberculosis who have received inadequate or no chemotherapy in the past, certain patients at special risk, contacts of cases, and known recent tuberculin converters. By contrast, the use of isoniazid in large groups such as all positive tuberculin reactors at school entry, or in adolescence, would require enormous numbers to be treated for a very low yield of cases prevented. The useful limits of programmes of chemoprophylaxis will, of course, vary with the tuberculosis morbidity of the population concerned.

LEPROSY

If the treatment of tuberculosis is a speciality, that of leprosy is even more narrowly so, and can only briefly be discussed here. Its study has been facilitated by two discoveries which circumvent to some extent the grave handicap imposed by the non-cultivability of *Myco. leprae* and thus the unavailability of the usual methods of testing chemotherapeutic activity in the laboratory.

One of these discoveries is of a method for producing a transmissible infection by the human bacillus in animals. Shepard (1962), inspired by some earlier observations on other mycobacteria by Fenner, inoculated the footpads of CFW mice intradermally with suspensions of bacilli from human lesions. Slow multiplication followed (50-1000 fold in up to 10 months) and serial transmission succeeded. The mouse foot pad technique has now been widely applied in studying the effects of different treatments, and has been used to evaluate the incidence and significance of bacillary resistance to anti-leprosy drugs. The second observation is that bacilli showing irregular staining by Ziehl-Neelsen are probably dead, corresponding as they do with bacilli showing degenerative changes on electron microscopy (Rees and Valentine, 1962). Estimation of the proportion of bacilli in skin biopsies showing irregular staining (morphological index) is now in general use as a method of assessing the results of treatment.

For many years diaminodiphenylsulphone (dapsone) has been the mainstay of treatment. Experimental results with the mouse foot pad method have shown that the minimal inhibitory dose of dapsone is extremely small. This finding has led to considerable reduction in the dose of dapsone, and standard treatment now begins with 25 mg. weekly, increasing slowly to a maximum of 100-200 mg. weekly. Treatment is continued for a period of years, the duration varying with the type of leprosy. The difficulties of achieving regular treatment for a long time, so important in the management of tuberculosis, are also found in leprosy, and have stimulated the development of long-acting preparations. 4-4-Diacetyldiamino-diphenylsulphone (DADDS) has been given by intramuscular injection in a dose of 225 mg. every 77 days (Shepard *et al.*, 1968) and shown to be as active as dapsone in its effects on the number of bacilli (bacteriological index) and on the morphological index. The existence of drug resistance can now be established by inoculating mouse foot pads with bacilli from the patient, and measuring the dose of dapsone necessary to prevent multiplication. Resistance is probably rare overall but was convincingly demonstrated by Rees (1967) in about half of a group of selected relapsed patients; resistance to thiambutosine was also shown by the same method.

Of the many other drugs used in leprosy, two recent additions have proved important. The rapid and bactericidal action of rifampicin on *Myco. tuberculosis* naturally led to its evaluation in leprosy, with highly encouraging results in a preliminary study by Rees, Pearson and Waters (1970). Even the smallest dose given to mice (0·0025 per cent in the diet) prevented bacillary multiplication in the foot pad. In the lesions of treated patients the morphological index (proportion of bacilli staining normally) fell to *nil* in four weeks: a comparable reduction from dapsone required 18 weeks. Moreover the infectivity of lesion material for mice was reduced within 3 to 24 days, whereas during dapsone treatment this change occurs only after 69 days. As the authors point out, this is evidence of a bactericidal effect not exerted by other anti-leprotic drugs.

The second important addition is clofazimine (Lamprene, B663). This orally administered drug is a fat soluble phenazine dye, with activity in experimental systems against a number of mycobacteria (Vischer, 1969). Its efficacy in leprosy has been recorded in many uncontrolled studies, and in a controlled clinical trial appears to be of the same order as that of dapsone (Karat *et al.*, 1971). The remarkable feature of clofazimine is that it possesses anti-inflammatory as well as antibacterial properties. Patients who receive it appear to develop erythema nodosum leprosum less often than do patients on dapsone, and trials have shown it to be more effective than prednisone (Karat *et al.*, 1970) and more effective than a placebo (Helmy, Pearson and Waters, 1972) in controlling lepra reactions. The dose needed to control ENL is larger (300 mg. daily), than that needed for basic treatment (100 mg. twice a week), so that the dose of the drug is actually raised when lepra reactions develop. A disadvantage of clofazimine is the red-brown pigmentation produced in the skin and conjunctivae, and the darkening of the lesions themselves. Apart from this, the only adverse effects have been, in a few patients, abdominal discomfort and mild diarrhoea. Clofazimine appears, incidentally, to provide effective treatment for tropical ulcers caused by infection by *Myco. ulcerans* (Lunn and Rees, 1964). Thiambutosine (4-butoxy-4-dimethyl-amino-diphenylthiourea, Ciba 1906) is slightly less effective than dapsone but also less toxic, and has been used in patients intolerant of dapsone. The dose is gradually increased to 2 g. daily in divided doses and a parenteral compound has been formulated, suitable for once weekly administration. Thiambutosine resistance tends to develop after about two years' treatment.

Other drugs used in leprosy include ditophal (diethodithiol iso-phthalate, Etisul), a disadvantage of which is its nauseating smell, and long acting sulphonamides such as sulphadoxine (formerly called sulphormethoxine, Fanasil), which are, however, more expensive than dapsone without being less toxic or more effective.

The possibility of preventing leprosy has attracted much attention in recent years. As well as trials of BCG vaccine, which have given widely variable results, other workers have used chemoprophylaxis by dapsone or by repository dapsone (DADDS) in epidemic areas (Sloan *et al.*, 1971). Results so far suggest that leprosy can be prevented by treatment of contacts, but the effect of long-term low-dose dapsone on the incidence of drug resistance has yet to be assessed.

PHARMACEUTICAL PREPARATIONS

CAPREOMYCIN SULPHATE (*Dista Products*) vials containing 1 g. of base for solution for intramuscular injection. Usual dose 1 g. daily.

CLOFAZIMINE (' Lamprene ' Geigy) 100 mg. capsules 3 weekly.

DAPSONE (' Avlosulfon ', *I.C.I.*)
    Tablets of 50 and 100 mg. Also as powder, suspension, and solution for injection. Usual dose 100-150 mg. once or twice weekly.

DITOPHAL (' Etisul ', *I.C.I.*)
    Application for inunction. Dose 5 g. three times a week.

ETHAMBUTOL HYDROCHLORIDE (' Myambutol ', *Lederle*)
    Tablets of 100 and 400 mg. Usual dose (combined with other drugs) 25 mg. per kg. for 60 days, then 15 mg. per kg.

ETHIONAMIDE (' Trescazide ', *May & Baker*)
    Tablets of 125 mg. Usual dose 125 mg. four times a day.

ISONIAZID
    Tablets of 100 mg. Usual dose up to 300 mg. daily. Also as injection, syrup, and in many combinations with PAS.

KANAMYCIN. See page 130.

PAS (' Para-aminosalicylic Acid ')
    Tablets of 500 mg. Usual dose 10-16 g. daily. Also available as sodium or calcium salt in sachets, and in numerous combinations with isonizid.

PYRAZINAMIDE
    Tablets of 500 mg. Usual dose 500 mg. three times a day.

RIFAMPICIN. See page 222. 450-600 mg. daily.

STREPTOMYCIN. See page 113.

THIAMBUTOSINE (' Ciba ' 1906, *Ciba*)
    Tablets of 500 mg. Dose 500 mg. increasing to 2 g. daily.

THIOACETAZONE (' Thioparamizone ', *Smith & Nephew*)
    Tablets of 25, 50 and 75 mg. Dose up to 150 mg. daily.

VIOMYCIN SULPHATE
    Vials containing equivalent of 1 g. of the base for solution for intramuscular injection. Usual dose 1 g. twice in the day on 2 days of the week.

REFERENCES

ANDERSON, T., KERR, M. R. & LANDSMAN, J. B. (1953). *Lancet* **2**, 691.
BATTEN, J. C. (1969). *Tubercle* **50**, 294.
BAND, D. & MURRAY, W. A. (1958). *Practitioner* **181**, 279.
BROUET, G., MARCHE, J., RIST, N., CHEVALLIER, J. & LeMEUR, G. (1959). *Amer. Rev. Tuberc.* **79**, 6.
BULKELEY, W. C. M. (1953). *Brit. med. J.* **2**, 1127.
BYRD, R. B., NELSON, R. & ELLIOTT, R. C. (1972). *J. Amer. med. Ass.* **220**, 1471.
CANETTI, G. (1956). *Amer. Rev. Tuberc.* **74**, Suppl. p. 13.
CANETTI, G., GAY, PH. & LE LIRZIN, M. (1972). *Tubercle,* **53**, 57.
CITRON, K. M. (1969). *Tubercle* **50**, Suppl. p. 32.
CROFTON, J. (1960). *Brit. med. J.* **2**, 370, 449.
CROFTON, J. & DOUGLAS, D. (1969). *Respiratory Diseases.* Oxford: Blackwell.
CROFTON, J. (1971). *Postgrad. med. J.* **47**, 748.
Czechoslovakian Tuberculosis Service/WHO/British MRC Cooperative Investigation (1971). *Bull. WHO.*
D'OLIVIERA, J. J. G. (1972). *Amer. Rev. resp. Dis.* **106**, 432.

DOMAGK, G., BENISCH, R., MIETZSCH, F. & SCHMIDT, H. (1946). *Naturwissenschaften* **33**, 315.

East African/British MRC (1970). *Tubercle*, **51**, 353.

East African/British MRC (1972). *Lancet* **1**, 1079.

EDITORIAL (1970). *J. Amer. med. Ass.* **212**, 2113.

ELLARD, G. A. (1969). *Tubercle* **50**, 144.

ELLARD, G. A. and 7 others (1972). *Lancet* **1**, 340.

FEREBEE, S. H. (1970). *Adv. Tuberc. Res.* **17**, 28.

FREIMAN, I. & FEEFHUYSEN, J. (1970). *J. Pediat.* **76**, 895.

FERGUSON, G. C., NUNN, A. J., FOX, W., MILLER, A. B., ROBINSON, D. K. & TALL, R. (1971). *Tubercle* **52**, 166.

FOX, W. (1971). *Postgrad. med. J.* **47**, 729.

GAISFORD, W. & GRIFFITHS, M. I. (1961). *Brit. med. J.* **1**, 1500.

GANGADHARAM, P. R. J., DEVADATTA, S., FOX, W., NAIR, C. N. & SELKON, J. B. (1961). *Bull. WHO* **25**, 793.

GIRLING, D. J. & FOX, W. (1971). *Brit. med. J.* **4**, 231.

GRUMBACH, F., CANETTI, G. & LE LIRZIN, M. (1969). *Tubercle* **50**, 280.

GRUNBERG, E., LEIWANT, B., D'ASCENSIO, I. L. & SCHNITZER, R. J. (1952). *Dis. Chest* **21**, 369.

GRUNBERG, E. & SCHNITZER, R. J. (1952). *Quart. Bull. Sea View Hosp.* **13**, 3.

HALKIER, E. & MEYER, J. (1959). *Danish med. Bull.* **6**, 97.

HELMY, S. H., PEARSON, J. M. H. & WATERS, M. F. R. (1972). *Lepr. Rev.* **42**, 167.

HESLING, C. M. (1969). *Tubercle* **50**, Suppl. p. 39.

HOBBY, G. L., LENERT, T. F. & MAIER-ENGALLENA, J. (1969). *Proc. Soc. Exp. Biol. (N.Y.)* **131**, 323.

HUGHES, I. E., SMITH, H. & KANE, P. O. (1962). *Lancet* **1**, 616.

KARLSON, A. G. (1961a & b). *Amer. Rev. resp. Dis.* **84**, 902, 905.

KARAT, A. B. A., JEEVARATNAM, A., KARAT, S. & RAO, P. S. S. (1970). *Brit. med. J.* **1**, 198.

KARAT, A. B. A., JEEVARATNAM, A., KARAT, S. & RAO, P. S. S. (1971). *Brit. med. J.* **4**, 514.

KATZ, J., KUNOFSKY, S. (1971). *Chest* **59**, 600.

KREIS, B. (1966). *Ann. New York Acad. Sci.* **132**, Art. 2, 912.

KUSHNER, S., DALATIAN, H., SANJWZJO, J. L., BACH, F. L. JR., SAFIR, S. R., SMITH, V. K. JR., & WILLIAMS, J. H. (1952). *Med. Chem. Sect., Amer. chem. Soc.*, Milwaukee, Wisconsin, April 1st.

LAHLOU, M. (1970). *Bull. Un. int. Tuberc.* **43**, 289.

LEES, A. W., ALLAN, G. W., SMITH, J., TYRRELL, W. F. & FALLON, R. J. (1971). *Tubercle* **52**, 182.

LEES, A. W., ALLAN, G. W., SMITH, J., TYRRELL, W. F. & FALLON, R. J. (1972). *Amer. Rev. resp. Dis.* **105**, 132.

LEHMANN, J. (1946). *Lancet* **1**, 15.

LEIBOLD, J. E. (1966). *Ann. New York Acad. Sci.* **135**, Art 2, 904.

LORBER, J. (1960). *Brit. med. J.* **1**, 1309.

LUNN, H. F. & REES, R. J. W. (1964). *Lancet* **1**, 247.

McDERMOTT, W., ORMOND, L., MUSCHENHEIM, C. & DEUTSCHLE, K. (1955). *13th Conf. Chemother. Tuberc.*, p. 170. Washington: Veterans Administration.

MEYER, H. & MALLY, J. (1912). *Mschr. Chem.* **33**, 393.

MITCHISON, D. A. (1954). *Brit. med. J.* **1**, 128.

POOLE, G., STRADLING, P., WORLLEDGE, S. (1971). *Brit. med. J.* **3**, 343.

PILHEU, J. A., MAGLIO, F., CETRANGOLO, R. & PLEUS, A. D. (1971). *Tubercle* **52**, 117.

PLACE, V. A., PYLE, M. M. & DE LA HUERGA, J. (1969). *Amer. Rev. resp. Dis.* **99**, 783.

REES, R. J. W. (1967). *Int. J. Lepr.* **35**, 625.

REES, R. J. W., PEARSON, J. M. H. & WATERS, M. F. R. (1970). *Brit. med. J.* **1**, 89.

REES, R. J. W. & VALENTINE, R. C. (1962). *Int. J. Lep.* **30**, 1.

REPORT, MEDICAL RESEARCH COUNCIL (1952). *Brit. med. J.* **2,** 735.

REPORT, MEDICAL RESEARCH COUNCIL (1962). *Tubercle (Lond.)* **43,** 201.

REPORT, VETERANS ADMINISTRATION (1954). *Trans. 13th Conf. Chemother. Tuberc.,* p. 191. Washington.

RIDDELL, R. W., STEWART, S. M. & SOMNER, A. R. (1960). *Brit. med. J.* **2,** 1207.

RIST, N., GRUMBACH, F. & LIBERMANN, D. (1959). *Amer. Rev. Tuberc.* **79,** 1.

ROBITZEK, E. H., SELIKOFF, I. J. & ORNSTEIN, G. G. (1952). *Quart. Bull. Sea View Hosp.* **13,** 27.

SCHWARTZ, W. S. & MOYER, R. E. (1953). *12th Conf. Chemother. Tuberc.,* p. 296. Washington: Veterans Administration.

SHEPARD, C. C. (1962). *Int. J. Lep.* **30,** 291.

SHEPARD, C. C., TOLENTINO, J. G. & MCRAE, D. H. (1968). *Amer. J. trop. Med. Hyg.* **17,** 192.

SHORT, E. I. (1962). *Tubercle (Lond.)* **43,** 33.

Singapore Tuberculosis Services/Brompton Hospital/British MRC Investigation (1971). *Tubercle* **52,** 88.

SLOAN, N. R., WORTH, R. M., JANO, B., FASAL, P. & SHEPARD, C. C. (1971). *Lancet* **2,** 525.

SOMNER, A. R., SELKON, J. B., WALTON, M. & WHITE, A. B. (1971). *Tubercle* **52,** 266.

STRADLING, P. & POOLE, G. W. (1970). *Tubercle* **51,** 44.

THOMAS, J. P., BAUGHN, C. O., WILKINSON, R. G. & SHEPHERD, R. G. (1961). *Amer. Rev. resp. Dis.* **83,** 891.

VELU, S., ANDREWS, R. H., ANGEL, J. H., DEVADATTA, S., FOX, W., JACOB, P. G., NAIR, C. N. & RAMAKRISHNAN, C. V. (1961). *Tubercle (Lond.)* **42,** 136.

VISCHER, W. A. (1969). *Lepr. Rev.* **40,** 107.

WALLACE, A. T. & WEBBER, W. J. (1956). *Tubercle* **37,** 358.

YEAGER, R. L., MUNROE, W. G. C. & DESAU, F. I. (1952). *Trans. 11th Conf. Chemother. Tuberc.* Washington Veterans Administration.

CHAPTER 27

VENEREAL DISEASES AND NON-VENEREAL SPIROCHAETOSES

IT is a remarkable fact that the most sensitive of all micro-organisms to penicillin are those causing the two principal forms of venereal disease. Their treatment is now within the capacity of anyone, but because clinical skill and special laboratory facilities are necessary to verify cure and some-times even to make a diagnosis, the subject must remain a speciality.

Syphilis

THE degree of sensitivity of *Treponema pallidum* to anti-bacterial agents cannot be measured in the ordinary way *in vitro* since the organism cannot be cultured artificially, but the results of curative tests in rabbits are highly significant. Early experiments showed that four days after the intratesticular or intracutaneous inoculation of rabbits a very small dose of peni-cillin sufficed to abort the infection, even though administered in a long-acting form giving very low blood levels. At two weeks a dose about seven times larger was required to produce the same effect. These findings indicated the possibility of aborting the disease in man by a single dose of a long-acting preparation administered at an early stage.

The object in treating established syphilis is to maintain a therapeutic level in the blood continuously for a period varying somewhat with the stage of the disease. The most certain way of doing this is to give daily injections of 600,000 units of a suspension of procaine penicillin: such a course should ideally be uninterrupted, even on Sundays, although it is common practice to give 1·2 mega units on Saturday to cover the week-end. Because penicillin therapy may be interrupted by patients defaulting or by the development of allergy, some prefer to give an initial dose of 2·4 mega units of a long-acting penicillin which will itself render the patient non-infectious and may even be curative. Preparations containing benethamine or benzathine penicillin give much more prolonged action, but the levels produced, particularly by benzathine penicillin, are lower and inconstant, the rate of absorption varying with the site of injection and still more with degree of muscular activity. Such treatment appears to be indicated only for those unable to attend for a full course of daily injections. Treatment with procaine penicillin is given daily for 10 days in primary and secondary syphilis, but continued for as long as 15 days in late syphilis. In pregnancy too treatment is continued for 10-15 days. Congenital syphilis is treated by daily procaine penicillin to a total dose of 0·5 mega units per kg. body wt. over 10 days, or by a single injection of benzathine penicillin 50,000 units per kg. The current recommendations of the United States Public Health Service for the treatment of syphilis are summarized in an extensive review by Sparling (1971). It is generally recommended that in her first pregnancy after treatment a woman should receive a further 10-day course although there is no good evidence that this is necessary (King, 1965). Established congenital syphilis is treated with 0·5 mega units per kg. body weight over 10 days, but such delayed treatment may not prevent later development of interstitial keratitis or nerve deafness.

JARISCH-HERXHEIMER REACTION. Within a few hours of starting penicillin treatment, over half the patients with early syphilis develop fever, sweating, malaise and headache, often with exacerbation of their symptoms or signs. Putkonen et al. (1966) found a rise in axillary temperature to at least 37·6°C. in 95 per cent of patients with secondary or sero-positive primary syphilis. The incidence falls with increasing duration of the disease. Similar reactions are described in other spirochaetal infections (p. 472).

The classical explanation has been that the reaction is due to the liberation of toxic products from the massive destruction of treponemes, and this is in keeping with the reaction occurring most frequently in the primary and early part of the secondary stages when organisms are most numerous. It is, however, an all-or-none response independent of the dose of penicillin, and this and other evidence has led to the suggestion that the reaction has an allergic basis.

The reaction is harmless in the primary and secondary stages, but the focal reaction can be dangerous in certain cases of gummatous, cardiovascular, or neurosyphilis. It has been traditional to try to avoid the reactions in late syphilis by beginning treatment with bismuth. The efficacy of this has long been doubted, and it has been agreed that this regimen will not suppress the reaction in general paralysis. Knudsen and Aastrup (1965), in a direct comparison of 149 patients treated with penicillin with 184 patients treated with bismuth and organic arsenicals, found no difference in the course or frequency of Jarisch-Herxheimer reactions in the two groups. De Graciansky and Grupper (1961) reduced the frequency and severity of the reaction by simultaneous treatment with corticosteroids, and C. S. Nicol (personal communication) has been successful for some years with prednisolone 5 mg. 8 hourly for 2 days before and after the first injection. It has been felt wise to treat active general paralysis in hospital under barbiturate sedation in the hope of avoiding the occasional psychosis and epileptiform seizures which may follow the first dose of penicillin.

PERSISTENCE OF TREPONEMES IN TREATED SYPHILIS. Several investigators have claimed that treponemes are recoverable from the tissues of some penicillin-treated patients long after the disease was believed to have been eradicated (Collart *et al.*, 1962). It has been suggested that these surviving organisms may be avirulent but antigenic and responsible for the persistence of a positive T.P.I. reaction after adequate treatment. The possibility of recrudescent infection from these organisms, particularly in patients treated with steroids, has aroused considerable interest. In patients believed to have been adequately treated, Rice *et al.* (1970) demonstrated by darkground and immunofluorescent microscopy the persistence in the aqueous humour and C.S.F. of forms at least some of which were *Treponema pallidum*. It is generally felt, however, that as the clinical results of treatment are excellent and only the moist early lesions are infectious, there is no reason to modify the present treatment regimens.

PENICILLIN ALLERGY. Concern has several times been expressed that the growing frequency of allergic reactions to penicillin is seriously interfering with venereal disease control.

Willcox (1964) reviews the reactions to penicillin and ways of preventing them. Amongst more than 74,000 patients receiving a single dose of penicillin, the incidence of reaction was less than 1 per cent. Amongst those receiving multiple injections for the treatment of syphilis, the incidence was 6·6 to 10·2 per cent (less in negroes). On the other hand fatalities were very uncommon.

So far, there has been very little trouble in mass campaigns for the control of treponematoses and the principal threat is in the treatment of adult syphilis in urban communities. In his own series, Willcox (1964) found that a history of allergy contraindicated the use of penicillin in less than 4 per cent. In the course of multiple injections, 7·5 per cent developed reactions, but by then all but 22 per cent of these had received curative doses.

Patients so highly sensitized as to prohibit treatment with penicillin have been successfully treated with tetracycline (750 mg. 6 hourly for 15 days) or erythromycin (500 mg. 6 hourly for 10 days: Fernando, 1969). Many venereologists repeat the course of tetracycline or erythromycin after an interval of six months. South et al. (1964) reported the birth of an infant with congenital syphilis to a pregnant girl treated with erythromycin two months before delivery, but she had received a total dose of only 15 g.

Galla et al. (1965) found cephaloridine as effective as penicillin against rabbit syphilis and superior to tetracycline, chloramphenicol, novobiocin, or streptomycin. Cephaloridine has been used in primary and secondary syphilis in doses ranging from 0·5-2·0 g. daily and for periods ranging from a few days to several weeks; it is probable that daily injections of 0·5 or 1·0 g. for 10 days provide adequate treatment (Sparling, 1971). Cephaloridine is best avoided in any patient with a well documented history of a severe penicillin reaction, but some patients known to be hypersensitive to penicillin show no signs of reaction.

Other Treponematoses

Late yaws is now seen relatively commonly in immigrants to this country and bejel may be occasionally encountered (Wray, 1966).

BEJEL (and PINTA) are reported to respond well to a single large dose of a repository penicillin preparation.

YAWS. *T. pertenue* is also highly penicillin-sensitive, and this disease has commonly been treated with a single dose of PAM (procaine penicillin in oil with 2 per cent aluminium monostearate), the dose being 0·6 and 1·2 mega unit in children and adults respectively. Fry and Rodin (1966) emphasize the importance of recognizing the occasional case of infectious yaws, and successfully treated a child from St. Vincent with 0·3 mega units aqueous procaine penicillin daily for 14 days. For adults with palmar and plantar hyperkeratosis and those with late lesions, Gentle (1965) recommends 4-6 mega units aqueous procaine penicillin spread over a period of several weeks. Contacts and latent cases can be treated with 0·6 mega unit benzathine penicillin and active cases with 1·2 mega units benzathine penicillin (children under 10 should receive half these amounts). Nicol (1962) emphasizes the difficulty of distinguishing with certainty between yaws and syphilis and recommends that where there is any doubt treatment should be with procaine penicillin 0·6 mega units intramuscularly daily for 10 days. Reports on yaws eradication campaigns emphasize the necessity for treating the entire population of an area, and not merely overt cases, since others may be latent or in the stage of incubation.

Gonorrhoea

The treatment of gonorrhoea has been transformed twice in the past 30 years. The first success, that of sulphonamides, was relatively short-lived, resistant strains of gonococci becoming common within a few years. That of penicillin has been both more dramatic and more prolonged, but is now failing from the same cause.

The gonococcus is the most sensitive to penicillin of all ordinary bacteria. It disappears from the exudate within two hours of a moderate dose being given, and that single dose is usually curative. This rapid destructive action, leaving the organism no time to adapt itself, was believed to be the reason why no resistant strains appeared, although it was very early shown that by careful training resistance could be increased *in vitro* several thousand-fold.

The first unequivocal evidence of the existence of resistant strains was obtained in 1958, when it was evident that treatment failures were becoming rather more frequent. Of 1,984 strains examined in nine centres in England (Report, 1961) 262 (13·2 per cent) were inhibited only by concentrations of 0·125 to 1·0 unit per ml., the normal inhibitory concentration being <0·01 unit per ml. Moreover, it was clearly shown that these strains of higher resistance are associated with treatment failure. During the exclusive use of penicillin for treating gonorrhoea, gonococci have largely reverted to sulphonamide sensitivity. Resistance to streptomycin is so readily developed and of such a degree that it was soon apparent that extensive use could not succeed for long.

Substantial increase in the incidence of gonorrhoea and in the female to male ratio continues (British Co-operative Clinical Group, 1970). In this country there has been no marked increase in penicillin resistance but elsewhere great changes have occurred, and in South East Asia increase in both the incidence and degree of resistance has reached a crisis (Willcox, 1970).

No other infectious disease has been the subject of so many therapeutic trials but despite the ready (and increasing) availability of patients, and the relatively large numbers treated in centres designed for this purpose, the design and conduct of the trials have not always been as impeccable as might be hoped.

Where less sensitive strains have become common, the recommended dose of penicillin has been progressively raised from a single intramuscular injection of 1·2 mega units aqueous procaine penicillin for acute uncomplicated gonorrhoea in the male (repeated the next day for the female) to 4·8 mega units. The size of the injection precludes increase beyond this point but even so there have been 5 per cent or more of failures. Willcox (1970) reviews the reasons for failure which include not only infection with less-sensitive gonococci, but misdiagnosis, re-infection, and failure of the anti-bacterial agent to reach adequate levels either in the blood or at the site of infection.

Despondency engendered by decreasing penicillin sensitivity amongst gonococci is likely to lead to insistence on more exacting schedules for all patients. There is copious evidence that therapeutic success is directly related to the *in vitro* sensitivity of the strain, and where sensitive strains predominate, as they currently do in this country, treatment with modest doses of penicillin can still be expected to be curative. At the same time it must be acknowledged that the successful control of gonorrhoea involves other considerations than the sensitivity of the organism. In a more perfectly regulated society (where gonorrhoea might in any case be less common) it would be reasonable to use modest doses for initial treatment and to re-treat the failures. This would, however, permit the spread of less sensitive strains on re-exposure during the interval before re-treatment and there arises a natural demand for near-100 per cent success rates on initial treatment.

This ideal may be approached in two ways: by magnified penicillin therapy or by the use of other agents. The high incidence of defaulters after a first attendance is another important factor which influences methods of treatment, and there is a strong tendency to favour regimens which are completed at one visit. The desire for instant success and the problem of defaulters in treatment also makes it highly desirable that this effect should be achieved by a single injection or at least by treatment of a very limited duration.

MAGNIFIED PENICILLIN THERAPY. The peak penicillin level may be improved by giving benzyl penicillin in addition to procaine penicillin, by giving more frequent doses, and giving probenecid and thus prolonging treatment. This last method has gained favour in recent years, since Holmes *et al* (1967) obtained improved results by giving 1 g. probenecid by mouth one hour before an intramuscular injection of 2.4 mega units of fortified procaine penicillin. Probenecid may also be given in conjunction with benzyl penicillin. Olsen and Lumholt (1969) cured 99 per cent of 832 patients with 5 mega units benzyl penicillin and 1 g. probenicid, and Niordson and Ullmann (1971) also obtained excellent results with this method, with 97 per cent of primary cases in 428 out-patients.

OTHER AGENTS. Numerous other agents have been tried. Oral treatments which need to be continued for several days are at a disadvantage because of defaulting by an appreciable proportion of patients, and several one-dose oral treatments have shown a high failure rate. On the other hand, several oral drugs have proved effective when given as two doses at an interval of five hours. These methods have been reviewed by Willcox (1971); it is hoped that a higher proportion of patients might be relied upon to take one additional dose of a drug a few hours after leaving the clinic than could be expected to complete a five or seven day course. There is also the problem that a proportion of strains more resistant to penicillin are also more resistant to other agents, possibly as the result of previous alternative treatment (Reyn and Bentzon, 1969, Phillips et al., 1970).

Parenteral Agents. Because of resistance, streptomycin is no longer suitable for treatment and parenteral tetracycline, because of relatively low blood levels, gives poor results unless supplemented by oral therapy (Willcox, 1970). Spectinomycin (p. 223) has had several very favourable reports. Given as a single dose of 2 g. to 108 males and 28 females, it gave 100 per cent cure in the hands of Cornelius and Domescik (1970) who describe it as one of the most effective agents for gonorrhoea. It is not at present commercially available and has not been tested against the most intractable strains. Kanamycin, as a single intramuscular injection of 2 g., continues to give consistent results with failure rates around 5 per cent (Fishnaller et al., 1968; Farrell, 1969). Intramuscular cephaloridine in a 2 g. dose supplemented by 1 g. the following day was successful in 93·6 per cent of females treated by Jouhar and Fowler (1968) while Shapiro and Lentz (1970) obtained 94·3 per cent of cures, also in female patients, after a single dose of 2 g.

Oral Agents. Most attention has been given to the possible use of ampicillin, tetracyclines and drug combinations. Successful two dose treatment has been applied with ampicillin, tetracyclines and cephalexin. Groth and Hallqvist (1970) treated 311 patients, males and females infected with penicillin-sensitive strains, with two oral doses of 1 g. ampicillin separated by 5 hours. After exclusion of probable reinfections, the failure rate was less than 1 per cent. Good results have also been obtained by a single dose of 2 g ampicillin given with 1 g probenecid (Gundersen et al., 1969).

It is worth noting that gonococcal strains show a narrower range of sensitivity to ampicillin than to benzyl penicillin. Although the M.I.C. of ampicillin for sensitive strains is higher than that of benzyl penicillin, penicillin-resistant strains are more sensitive to ampicillin than to benzyl penicillin (Johnson et al., 1970). Two doses of 1·2 g. demethylchlortetracycline were associated with a failure rate of 4·3 per cent (Willcox, 1969), and two doses of cephalexin (2 g.) with a failure rate of 14·6 per cent (Willcox and Woodcock, 1970). Of the newer tetracyclines, minocycline has been used in attempting satisfactory single dose treatment, but even with a dose of 400 mg. the failure rate was about 25 per cent (Duncan et al., 1971). Rifampicin as a single dose of 900 mg. was given by Panduro (1971) in two groups of 62 and 36 patients, with cure rates of 87 and 91 per cent.

Several attempts have been made to improve results by using combinations of agents. Garrod and Waterworth (1967) examined the in vitro effects on the gonococcus of three such combinations. Kanamycin and penicillin were indifferent or no more than additive (p. 283). Kanamycin and sulphafurazole were usually additive so that simultaneous treatment with sulphafurazole might allow the dose of kanamycin to be reduced. Trimethoprim and sulphonamide were strongly synergic (p. 283). This combination was very successfully used by Csonka and Knight (1967) and by Carroll and Nicol (1970) who gave four tablets (each 80 mg. trimethoprim plus 200 mg. sulphamethoxazole) as one dose daily for 5 days. Arya et al. (1970) gave four tablets 12-hourly and found that 65 per cent of the patients were cured after two doses and 96 per cent after three or four. Short course treatment with cotrimoxazole was also used by Ullman et al., (1971) who gave two doses at an eight-hour interval to 144 patients, with a 98 per cent cure rate. In contrast, Wright and Grimble (1970) found that the drug given 6-hourly for five days failed to cure 38 per cent of 97 men, all but one of whom responded to 0·9 mega unit procaine penicillin daily for three days. Their poor results with cotrimoxazole were associated with an asymptomatic carrier state, shown by routine examination of urethral smears in 15 of the 33 failures in the main group of their study. The possibility that superior results might be obtained in gonor-

rhoea by the use of a different ratio of trimethoprim to sulphonamide is discussed on page 30.

Concern has often been expressed that the use of other
agents or the increased dose of penicillin necessary to treat
less sensitive gonococci will mask the development of concurrent syphilis. It goes without saying that every patient
treated for gonorrhoea should undergo serological tests for
syphilis six months later. Provided that this is done, cannot
the possible effect on incubating syphilis be disregarded? The
ordinary dose of penicillin might only be suppressive: larger
doses might well be curative of syphilis at that stage. Tetracyclines and erythromycin are also active against *T. pallidum*:
streptomycin and kanamycin are not, and this is claimed as an
advantage in their use.

RE-TREATMENT OF FAILURES. There is nothing in the clinical
status of patients which helps to identify the potential failures,
except that more prolonged infections are less likely to respond
(Wray, 1965). Previously treated patients in Evans' (1966)
series showed no special liability to relapse. The most important single factor in failure is reduced sensitivity of the gonococcus to penicillin. In patients infected with gonococci sensitive to 0·1 unit per ml. or less Rantsalo *et al.* (1964) found
a failure rate of 5·4 per cent. Amongst those infected with more
resistant organisms the failure rate was 4 times as high. Borring
(1965) shows a systematic decline in success rate with decreasing
sensitivity of the infecting organism. There is also evidence that
organisms with reduced sensitivity both to penicillin and to
streptomycin are particularly resistant to penicillin treatment
(Rantsalo *et al.*, 1964; Evans, 1966). In heterosexual gonorrhoea the chance is about 90 per cent that treatment which has
already failed in the partner will be unsuccessful (Evans, 1966).

In the male, relapse usually occurs in the first week after
treatment without the urine having cleared completely. In
streptomycin-treated patients, Evans (1966) found that relapse
occurred immediately on cessation of treatment but in penicillin-treated patients there was a delay of 2-7 days. In the
female, relapse is frequently not detectable without bacteriological examination.

The drugs other than penicillin discussed in the preceding

pages are used for re-treatment, including two-dose oral regimens with demethylchlortetracycline and ampicillin, and injection methods with one or two doses of cephaloridine or kanamycin.

COMPLICATED INFECTIONS. Proctitis is more resistant to treatment than urethritis, as shown by Evans' (1966) finding that in homosexual partners similar doses of procaine penicillin cured urethritis in the active partner but not proctitis in the passive. Proctitis should respond to procaine penicillin 1·2 mega units daily for 3-5 days. Tubal infections require still more active treatment: benzyl penicillin, 1 mega unit 6-hourly for 10 days is recommended. Rees and Annels (1969) begin treatment with penicillin and three days later, when the sensitivity of the gonococcus is known, change the treatment if necessary. Acute gonococcal arthritis usually responds rapidly to penicillin treatment (Cooke *et al.*, 1971). Septic gonococcal dermatitis, now not uncommon in Britain, is cured by penicillin, the fever and joint symptoms being relieved within two to seven days of starting treatment (Barr and Danielsson, 1971).

Non-gonococcal Urethritis

The cause of this disease (if there is a single cause) still eludes final demonstration and this, combined with its spontaneous remissions and recurrences, make the assessment of treatment difficult. Recent contenders as the cause of non-specific urethritis are TRIC (trachoma-inclusion conjunctivitis) agents (Dunlop *et al.*, 1965) and T-strain mycoplasma (Csonka and Corse 1970). Chlamydia have been grown in tissue culture using material from non-specific urethritis by Gordon *et al.* (1969). Both chlamydia and mycoplasma have the attraction of being sensitive *in vitro* to tetracyclines to which the disease commonly responds. It has also several times been suggested that the condition is an allergic reaction to an unidentified antigen (Weston, 1965). The immediate benefits of tetracycline are not maintained to the same degree as follow-up is continued, partly because of the accumulation of defaulting and re-infected patients (Csonka, 1965). Fowler (1970), using tetracycline 1 g. daily for four days, found 72 per cent of his patients were free of urethritis, compared with 37 per cent of the placebo group. Many relapses then occurred in the following four weeks, so that after ten weeks the cure rate fell to 55 per cent for the tetracycline group and 34 per cent for the placebo group. By three months tetracycline had only benefited 10 per cent more patients than the placebo.

Morton and Wray (1966) treated 50 patients with methacycline (150 mg. 6-hourly for 4 days) and obtained cures in almost 80 per cent. Wright (1969) was less successful. He found the results no better than those obtained with other tetracyclines, and Andrew et al. (1969) say the same for clomocycline.

Results with streptomycin and sulphonamides (short, medium and long-acting), alone and in combination, have been conflicting (Csonka, 1965). Alergant (1964) found that a single dose of streptomycin (0·5 g.) plus sulphamethoxydiazine (1 g.) was slightly more effective than the same dose of streptomycin plus sulphadimidine (1 g., 6-hourly for 5 days). The two regimens had failure rates at 7-14 days of 10·8 and 12·3 per cent, and at 14-28 days of 23·7 and 27·8 per cent. Almost identical results were obtained by Willcox (1968) in 106 patients using erythromycin stearate 250 mg. 6-hourly for 6 days. Csonka and Spitzer (1969) treated 51 patients with oral lincomycin 500 mg. 6-hourly for 5 days and cured only a quarter of the patients—a result equivalent to that obtained with a placebo. Retreatment with erythromycin cured 68 per cent. They argue that this supports the aetiological role of T-strain mycoplasma since this, unlike *Mycoplasma hominis,* is sensitive to erythromycin but resistant to lincomycin (Csonka and Corse, 1970). Trimethoprim-sulphamethoxazole was so unsuccessful in a dozen patients treated by Carroll and Nicol (1970) that they abandoned the trial.

Trichomoniasis

Trichomonas vaginalis was found in 513/1,355 (38 per cent) cases of sexually transmitted infection in the female (Wisdom and Dunlop, 1965). On treatment with metronidazole (Flagyl: 200 mg., 8-hourly by mouth for 7 days) 98 per cent of 284 cases were clear immediately after cessation of treatment and 72 per cent of 144 cases three weeks later. Conventional seven day treatment has been compared with single dose treatment by Csonka (1971); the former cured 94 per cent of 54 patients, while a single dose of 2 g cured 82 per cent of 58 patients, an insignificant difference. The propriety of using the drug early in pregnancy is discussed on page 97. There is no evidence that increased resistance of *Trichomonas* to metronidazole is a cause of failure, or that the presence in the vagina of numerous bacteria which inactivate metronidazole significantly affects the response to treatment (MacFadzean *et al.*, 1969). There have been a number of disputed claims that metronidazole treatment can precipitate vaginal candidiasis. Oller (1969) discusses the factors influencing this complication and shows that it can be controlled by the use of amphotericin pessaries (50 mg. nightly ×7). Since symptomatic superinfection is generally infrequent, he suggests that such combined treatment should be reserved for high risk patients: in pregnancy, diabetes, or following recent vaginal candidiasis.

Nifuratel, a nitrofuran marketed under the name *Magmilor* has been used for vaginal trichomoniasis when given by combined oral (200 mg. 3 times daily for 7 days) and local (250 mg. pessaries nightly × 10) administration but has been shown as less effective than metronidazole in a comparative trial by Evans and Catterall (1970). Nimorazole, a nitrimidazole derivative formerly known as nitrimidazine, has also been compared with metronidazole and found less effective (Evans and Catterall, 1971), with cure rates of 68 per cent and 89 per cent respectively, although results as good as those with metronidazole were reported by Moffett *et al.* (1971) and by Cohen (1971). Metronidazole emerges as superior to the newer contenders in the treatment of trichonosoniasis. Its continued efficacy in circumstances in which treatment can be rigidly controlled has been established by Keighley (1971) who cured 488 of 496 female prisoners (98·3 per cent) with one seven-day course. Nevertheless, occasional patients are seen who will be cured by, or will be more tolerant of, one of the newer drugs. A complication of the use of nitrofuratel is the broad antibacterial spectrum which it shares with other nitrofurans (it is also active against candida). Churcher and Evans (1969) point out that before instituting treatment it is important to exclude gonorrhoea which is otherwise likely to be masked by the local antibacterial effect. Trichomonas was found in 93/1,646 (5·6 per cent) cases of non-gonococcal urethritis in the male and was cleared by

the same regimen as that used in women from all 71 cases
seen immediately after treatment and from 93 per cent of the
41 cases who returned for follow-up 90 days later. Similar success rates are reported by Schapira (1965) who holds to the view
that male infection constitutes the main source of the female
disease. Difficulty in persuading male consorts to undergo treatment is increased by the fact that only about 10 per cent of male
infections produce symptoms. Some observers claim that the
male disease is commonly self-limiting if re-infection is prevented
by treatment of the female. The organism may nevertheless
underly some chronic infections in the male, and Catterall
(1965) successfully managed 27/38 cases of prostatitis, believed to be of trichomonal origin, with metronidazole.

Chancroid

Haemophilus ducreyi has similar sensitivities to other
species in this genus, and there is therefore a considerable
choice of suitable drugs. Willcox (1965) recommends streptomycin 1-3 g. daily in divided doses for 5 days or tetracycline or
chloramphenicol 250-500 mg. 6-hourly for 4-5 days. McDaniel
(1964) continues tetracycline therapy for 12 days if the nodes
have suppurated. Some prefer sulphonamides (4 g. daily until
healing) or streptomycin to tetracyclines because they eliminate
the risk of masking syphilis, and on the ground of lesser cost.
Among American troops in Saigon, Kerber *et al.* (1969)
obtained good results with sulfisoxazole (sulphafurazole) 4 g.
daily and with this drug together with tetracycline, but very
poor results with tetracycline alone. They postulate that drug
resistance may have emerged because of the large amount of
' bootleg ' antibiotics consumed by prostitutes in Vietnam.

Lymphogranuloma Venereum

The nomenclature of this and the following disease is confused : the above is now the accepted name for the undoubtedly
venereal disease having a trivial primary lesion and followed by secondary suppurative lymphadenitis going on to
fibrosis involving inguinal glands in the male and pelvic in
the female. The cause is an agent related to that of psittacosis and susceptible to various chemotherapeutic agents.
When ' aureomycin ' was first introduced this disease was

claimed to be one of its triumphs: even secondary rectal strictures in the female were said to relax. Some of the effects observed may have been due to an action on secondary bacterial infection. Tetracycline (250 mg. 6-hourly) is given for different periods at various stages of the disease by McDaniel (1964): 2 weeks for the acute inguinal disease, 3 weeks for the acute rectal disease, and 6 weeks or more for chronic disease. Willcox (1965) uses larger doses: up to 500 mg. 6-hourly in the male and more in the female. The prognosis is poor in the most chronic cases. It has been claimed that sulphonamides are as effective as tetracyclines and more so than chloramphenicol. Incision of fluctuant nodes is contraindicated but aspiration may hasten resolution (Abrams, 1968). The treatment of chlamydial infections is further discussed on p. 486.

Granuloma Inguinale

This doubtfully venereal disease is due to *Donovania granulomatis*. Most authors are agreed that the choice lies between streptomycin (1 g. 6-hourly for 5 days) or tetracycline (500 mg. 6-hourly for 10-15 days). Goldberg and Bernstein (1964) describe two cases, one on each of these regimens, which resolved within six weeks. Davis (1970) describes 14 cases, all negroes, 7 of whom also had evidence of syphilis; 8 of the 10 males were homosexuals. With one exception, all responded to tetracycline 2 g. per day given until the lesions were completely healed (1-4 weeks). Two patients treated over several weeks with ampicillin (up to 4 g. per day) failed to respond and were subsequently successfully treated with tetracycline.

OTHER SPIROCHAETOSES

RELAPSING FEVER. *Borrelia recurrentis* (reviewed by Southern and Sanford, 1969) is sensitive to arsenicals and to various antibiotics. Penicillin, which originally replaced arsenicals, is now generally considered inferior to tetracyclines. Only a short course is necessary, but the dose recommended varies from 1 to 3 g. daily and the duration from three to six days. In fact, very much less tetracycline is effective. Bryceson *et al.* (1970) found that 250 mg. tetracycline given

16

intravenously over 2 to 3 minutes cleared the blood of spirochaetes within $2\frac{1}{2}$ hours. Two intramuscular injections of 150 mg. at an interval of 6 hours were also effective. There was no relapse in 18 patients so treated, nor in 45 patients given a total dose of 4·3-5·5 g. over 4 to 5 days. All patients given an effective dose developed a characteristic Jarisch-Herxheimer-like reaction showing the prodromal, chill and flush phases of endotoxic fever. Cardiorespiratory disturbance in the flush phase may be so severe that patients die. Correction of extracellular fluid depletion, cardiac failure and hypoxia may prevent fatalities, but large doses of hydrocortisone did not influence the reaction (Warrell *et al.*, 1970). In patients in whom vigorous reactions might be dangerous (one was pregnant), Bryceson *et al.* (1970) substituted an injection of 20,000 units of benzylpenicillin plus 60,000 units of procaine penicillin for the initial dose of tetracycline. Penicillin is, however, poor at eradicating spirochaetes from the brain, some strains of *Borrelia* are resistant, and relapse on penicillin treatment is common. They recommend therefore that the initial dose of penicillin be followed the next day by 250 mg. tetracycline.

RAT-BITE FEVER. Roughgarden (1965) describes the clinical manifestations, diagnosis and laboratory investigation of the acute illnesses caused by *Streptobacillus moniliformis* and *Spirillum minus*. Penicillin is the drug of choice for both infections, which respond to as little as 0·6 mega units daily. Treatment should be given for not less than 7 days. Streptomycin and tetracycline are also effective, but sulphonamides have uniformly failed. McGill *et al.* (1966) successfully treated two patients in this country with penicillin (0·5 mega units, 6-hourly) plus streptomycin (0·5-1 g., 12-hourly). Bacterial endocarditis due to either organism is said to require 12-15 mega units penicillin per day for three to four weeks.

Leptospirosis

This infection is in a different category, in regard both to the causative organism and to its response to treatment. Arsenicals are without effect, but *Leptospira* spp. are susceptible in varying degrees to most of the major antibiotics. Nevertheless the evalution of their effect presents unusual difficulties in all three spheres, *in vitro,* in the experimental animal and in the clinical field, and their place in the treatment of this disease is still the subject of a controversy which breaks out in print from time to time.

In vitro studies are complicated by the fact that different degrees of anti-leptospiral activity are exerted by antibiotics over a very wide range of concentrations, and any quantitative result depends on the criterion adopted. Very low concentrations of penicillin, of the order of 0·1 unit per ml., will inhibit the normally slow growth of the organism, but motility is retained, and very much higher concentrations fail to sterilize a culture. The effective concentrations determined by various authors, using different methods, are therefore not comparable or worth quoting.

Animal studies meet another difficulty: the guinea-pig and hamster, although suitably susceptible to the infection, are also uniquely susceptible to a ' toxic ' effect not only of penicillin (see p. 61) but of tetracyclines and macrolides, and are liable to succumb to this when adequate doses are given. These drug deaths have interfered with animal studies of the treatment of *L. icterohaemorrhagiae* infection, but several workers have nevertheless satisfied themselves of a curative effect, superior to that of penicillin, from large doses of erythromycin or oleandomycin and of curative effects from streptomycin and tetracyclines. Stalheim (1966) believes that in previous animal studies demonstration of leptospiral survival was attempted too soon after cessation of treatment. In his own studies penicillin, chloramphenicol and erythromycin were ineffective in doses corresponding with those generally used in man: chlortetracycline destroyed most of the renal population of leptospira, but dihydrostreptomycin (and hence presumably streptomycin) was the most effective agent.

The clinical value of antibiotic treatment is difficult to assess (Heath, *et al.,* 1965). It is clearly necessary to distinguish the severe infection caused by *L. icterohaemorrhagiae,* occurring sporadically, the diagnosis of which is often delayed, from those due to other serotypes, which are not only milder, but often because epidemic or endemic are recognized earlier.

Examples of such mild infections, almost never fatal and rarely even causing jaundice, are those caused by *L. australis* in Queensland and *L. bataviae* in Malaya. These appear to respond regularly to about 4 mega units of penicillin daily, which causes a characteristic Jarisch-Herxheimer-type reaction, followed by rapid recovery. Kocen (1962) and others working in Malaya, report a shortened duration of fever from treatment with oxytetracycline and penicillin respectively. The infection caused by *L. canicola* is also comparatively mild, and the review by Pertzelan and Pruzanski (1963) concludes in favour of its treatment with tetracycline.

The proper treatment for *L. icterohaemorrhagiae* infections cannot be so confidently defined. The view has been taken that no antibiotics are of any value, but this may well be, as suggested by several authors, because too little is given too late. It certainly seems that by the time the diagnosis is made in a sporadic case of severe leptospirosis, renal damage may already have reached its maximum, and a curative effect is not necessarily to be expected, whatever the anti-leptospiral activity of the drug. The choice appears to lie between full doses of tetracycline, given at first intravenously, and large doses of penicillin. Some authors give streptomycin in addition to penicillin, but this is probably best avoided without better evidence of benefit since renal failure is so common a feature of severe leptospirosis. Sarasin *et al.* (1963) gave 40 mega units of penicillin daily by intravenous infusion and 1 g. streptomycin twice daily to a patient with laboratory-acquired infection, who became afebrile within 24 hours, but early treatment evidently contributed to this happy result.

REFERENCES

ABRAMS, A. J. (1968). *J. Amer. med. Ass.* **205,** 199.
ALERGANT, C. D. (1964). *Brit. J. vener. Dis.* **40,** 266.
ANDREW, G. S., EDWARDS, J. C. & OLLER, L. Z. (1969). *Brit. J. vener. Dis.* **45,** 154.
ARYA, O. P., PEARSON, C. H., RAO, S. K. & BLOWERS, R. (1970). *Brit. J. vener. Dis.* **46,** 214.
BARR, J. & DANIELSSON, D. (1971). *Brit. med. J.* **1,** 482.
BORRING, J. (1965). *Brit. J. vener. Dis.* **41,** 193.
BRITISH CO-OPERATIVE CLINICAL GROUP (1970). *Brit. J. vener. Dis.* **46,** 62.
BRYCESON, A. D. M., PARRY, E. H. O., PERINE, P. L., WARRELL, D. A., VUKOTICH, D. & LEITHEAD, C. S. (1970). *Quart. J. Med.* **39,** 129.
CATTERALL, R. D. (1965). *Brit. J. vener. Dis.* **41,** 302.
CARROLL, B. R. T. & NICOL, C. S. (1970). *Brit. J. vener. Dis.* **46,** 31.
CHURCHER, G. M. & EVANS, A. J. (1969). *Brit. J. vener. Dis.* **45,** 149.
COHEN, L. (1971). *Brit. J. vener. Dis.* **47,** 177.
COLLART, P., BOREL, L. J. & DUREL, P. (1962). *Ann. Inst. Pasteur* **103,** 953.

COOKE, C. L., OWEN, D. S., IRBY, R. & TOONE, E. (1971). *J. Amer. med. Ass.* **217,** 204.
CORNELIUS, C. E., III, & DOMESCIK, G. (1970). *Brit. J. vener. Dis.* **46,** 212.
CSONKA, G. W. (1965). *Brit. J. vener. Dis.* **41,** 1.
CSONKA, G. W. (1971). *Brit. J. vener. Dis.* **47,** 456.
CSONKA, G. & CORSE, J. (1970). *Brit. J. vener. Dis.* **46,** 203.
CSONKA, G. W. & KNIGHT, G. J. (1967). *Brit. J. vener. Dis.* **43,** 161.
CSONKA, G. W. & SPITZER, R. J. (1969). *Brit. J. vener. Dis.* **45,** 52.
DAVIS, C. M. (1970). *J. Amer. med. Ass.* **211,** 632.
DE GRACIANSKY, P. & GRUPPER, C. (1961). *Brit. J. vener. Dis.* **37,** 247.
DUNCAN, W. C., GLICKSMAN, J. M., KNOX, J. M. & HOLDER, W. R. (1971). *Brit. J. vener. Dis.* **47,** 364.
DUNLOP, E. M. C., AL-HUSSAINI, M. K., GARLAND, J., TREHARNE, J. D., HARPER, I. A. & JONES, B. R. (1965). *Lancet* **1,** 1125.
EVANS, A. J. (1966). *Brit. J. vener. Dis.* **42,** 251.
EVANS, B. A. & CATTERALL, R. D. (1970). *Brit. med. J.* **2,** 335.
EVANS, B. A. & CATTERALL, R. D. (1971). *Brit. med. J.* **4,** 146.
FARRELL, L. (1969). *Brit. J. vener. Dis.* **45,** 232.
FERNANDO, W. L. (1969). *Brit. J. vener. Dis.* **45,** 200.
FISCHNALLER, J. E., PEDERSEN, A. H. B., RONALD, A. R., BONIN, P. & TRONCA, E. L. (1968). *J. Amer. med. Ass.* **203,** 909.
FOWLER, W. (1970). *Brit. J. vener. Dis.* **46,** 464.
FRY, L. & RODIN, P. (1966). *Brit. J. vener. Dis.* **42,** 28.
GALLA, F., PAGNES, P. & FERRARI, M. (1965). *Chemotherapia (Basel)* **10,** 2·.
GARROD, L. P. & WATERWORTH, P. M. (1968). *Brit. J. vener. Dis.* **44,** 75.
GENTLE, G. H. K. (1965). *Brit. J. vener. Dis.* **41,** 155.
GOLDBERG, J. & BERNSTEIN, R. (1964). *Brit. J. vener. Dis.* **40,** 137.
GORDON, F. B., HARPER, I. A., QUAN, A. L., TREHARNE, J. D., DWYER, R. ST. C. & GARLAND, J. A. (1969). *J. infect. Dis.* **120,** 451.
GROTH, O. & HALLQVIST, L. (1970). *Brit. J. vener. Dis.* **46,** 21.
GUNDERSEN, T., ÖDEGAARD, K. & GJESSING, H. C. (1969). *Brit. J. vener. Dis.* **45,** 235.
HEATH, C. W., ALEXANDER, A. D. & GALTON, M. M. (1965). *New Engl. J. Med.* **273,** 857, 915.
HOLMES, K. K., JOHNSON, D. W. & FLOYD, T. M. (1967). *J. Amer. med. Ass.* **202,** 461.
JOUHAR, A. J. & FOWLER, W. (1968). *Brit. J. vener. Dis.* **44,** 223.
JOHNSON, D. W., KVALE, P. A., AFABLE, V. L., STEWART, S. S., HALVERSON, C. W. & HOLMES, K. K. (1970). *New Engl. J. Med.* **283,** 1.
KERBER, R. E., ROWE, C. E. & GILBERT, K. R. (1969). *Arch. Dermatol.* **100,** 604.
KEIGHLEY, E. E. (1971). *Brit. med. J.* **1,** 207.
KING, A. J. (1965). *Practitioner* **195,** 589.
KNUDSEN, E. A. & AASTRUP, B. (1965). *Brit. J. vener. Dis.* **41,** 177.
KOCEN, R. S. (1962). *Brit. med. J.* **1,** 1181.
MCDANIEL, W. E. (1964). *J. Kentucky med. Ass.* **62,** 281.
MCFADZEAN, J. A., PUGH, I. M., SQUIRES, S. L. & WHELAN, J. P. F. (1969). *Brit. J. vener. Dis.* **45,** 161.
MCGILL, R. C., MARTIN, A. M. & EDMUNDS, P. N. (1966). *Brit. med. J.* **1,** 1213.
MOFFETT, M., MCGILL, M. I., SCHOFIELD, C. B. S. & MASTERTON, G. (1971). *Brit. J. vener. Dis.* **47,** 173.
MORTON, R. S. & WRAY, P. M. (1966). *Brit. J. vener. Dis.* **42,** 195.
NICOL, C. S. (1962). *Practitioner* **189,** 491.
NIORDSON, A-M., & ULLMAN, S. (1971). *Acta Derm-vener. (Stockh.)* **51,** 311.
OLLER, L. Z. (1969). *Brit. J. vener. Dis.* **45,** 163.
OLSEN, G. A. & LOMHOLT, G. (1969). *Brit. J. vener. Dis.* **45,** 144.
PANDURO, J. (1971). *Brit. J. vener. Dis.* **47,** 440.
PERTZELAN, A. & PRUZANSKI, W. (1963). *Amer. J. trop. Med. Hyg.* **12,** 75.

PHILLIPS, I., RIMMER, D., RIDLEY, M., LYNN, R. & WARREN, C. (1970). *Lancet* **1**, 263.
PUTKONEN, T., SALO, O. P. & MUSTAKALLIO, K. K. (1966). *Brit. J. vener. Dis.* **42**, 181.
RANTASALO, I., SALO, O. P. & WALLENIUS, J. O. (1964). *Brit. J. vener. Dis.* **40**, 273.
REES, E. & ANNELS, E. H. (1969). *Brit. J. vener. Dis.* **45**, 205.
REPORT (1961). *Lancet* **2**, 226.
REYN, A. & BENTZON, M. W. (1969). *Brit. J. vener. Dis.* **45**, 223.
RICE, N. S. C., DUNLOP, E. M. C., JONES, B. R., HARE, M. J., KING, A. J., RODIN, P., MUSHIN, A. & WILKINSON, A. E. (1970). *Brit. J. vener. Dis.* **46**, 1.
ROUGHGARDEN, J. W. (1965). *Arch. intern. Med.* **116**, 39.
SARASIN, G., TUCKER, D. N. & AREAN, V. M. (1963). *Amer. J. clin. Path.* **40**, 146.
SCHAPIRA, H. E. (1965). *J. Urol.* **93**, 303.
SHAPIRO, L. & LENTZ, J. W. (1970) *Amer. J. Obst. Gynec.* **108**, 471.
SOUTH, M. A., SHORT, D. H. & KNOX, J. M. (1964). *J. Amer. med. Ass.* **190**, 70.
SOUTHERN, P. M. & SANFORD, J. P. (1969). *Medicine (Baltimore)* **48**, 129.
SPARLING, P. F. (1971). *New Engl. J. Med.* **284**, 642.
STALHEIM, O. H. V. (1966). *Amer. J. vet. Res.* **27**, 803.
ULLMAN, S., NIORDSON, A-M. & ZACHARIAE, H. (1971). *Acta Dermvener. (Stockh.)* **51**, 394.
WARRELL, D. A., POPE, H. M., PARRY, E. H. O., PERINE, P. L. & BRYCESON, A. D. M. (1970). *Clin. Sci.* **39**, 123.
WESTON, T. E. T. (1965). *Brit. J. vener. Dis.* **41**, 107.
WILLCOX, R. R. (1964). *Brit. J. vener. Dis.* **40**, 200.
WILLCOX, R. R. (1965). *Curr. Med. Drugs* **6** (2), 14.
WILLCOX, R. R. (1968). *Brit. J. vener. Dis.* **44**, 157.
WILLCOX, R. R. (1969). *Acta Dermvener. (Stockh.)* **49**, 103.
WILLCOX, R. R. (1970). *Brit. J. vener. Dis.* **46**, 217.
WILLCOX, R. R. (1971). *Brit. J. vener. Dis.* **47**, 31.
WILLCOX, R. R. & WOODCOCK, K. S. (1970). *Postgrad. med. J.* **46**, Suppl. Oct. 103.
WISDOM, A. R. & DUNLOP, E. M. C. (1965). *Brit. J. vener. Dis.* **41**, 90.
WRAY, P. M. (1965). *Brit. J. vener. Dis.* **41**, 117.
WRAY, P. M. (1966). *Brit. J. vener. Dis.* **42**, 25.
WRIGHT, D. J. M. (1969). *Brit. J. vener. Dis.* **45**, 167.
WRIGHT, D. J. M. & GRIMBLE, A. S. (1970). *Brit. J. vener. Dis.* **46**, 34.

CHAPTER 28

VIRAL AND CHLAMYDIAL INFECTIONS

UNTIL very recently it was held that viruses are not susceptible to any of the agents used for the treatment of bacterial diseases. It now appears that some antibacterial agents, albeit in concentrations very much greater than those required to inhibit the growth of sensitive bacteria, exert some antiviral effects. Rifampicin in a concentration about 1,000 times that effective against sensitive bacteria has been shown to inhibit the growth of several poxviruses and an adenovirus. It acts, both in bacteria and viruses, by inhibiting DNA-dependent RNA-polymerase, and resistant variants of vaccinia virus arise quickly in experimental systems (Heller *et al.*, 1969; Subak-Sharp *et al.*, 1969). Fusidic acid and cephalosporin P$_1$ (p. 87) in concentrations of 25-50 μg. per ml. inhibit rhinoviruses and coxsackievirus A 21 (Acornley *et al.*, 1967). These are encouraging signs that viruses are perhaps not quite so insusceptible to attack as was once feared, but the very high plasma concentrations of these agents which would be required for treatment makes it unlikely that these findings will have any immediate clinical benefit. The *Chlamydia*, which were at one time included amongst the viruses but differ from them fundamentally (p. 486) are sensitive to tetracyclines and some other agents.

The present striking contrast between bacteria and viruses in the availability of effective antimicrobial therapy arises from a number of special difficulties. The metabolism of bacterial pathogens is often sufficiently different from that of the host to make them susceptible to agents which have little or no effect on the host's metabolism. Viral replication, on the other hand, occurs by distortion of normal cellular processes causing the cell to synthesize viral nucleic acids and proteins in place of normal cellular components. This intimate relationship between normal and infected cell processes means that compounds capable of interrupting viral replication will have to show an extraordinary degree of selective toxicity if they are not at the same time to

477

inhibit similar processes crucial to the metabolic needs of normal cells. Nevertheless, any enzymic capacity possessed by the virus itself, for example the RNA-polymerase of the pox viruses (Kates and McAuslan, 1967), or even host enzymes sufficiently modified to subserve the parasite's needs, may well show (just as bacterial enzymes do) different susceptibility to inhibitors from that of the corresponding mammalian enzyme.

One serious therapeutic difficulty is that the signs and symptoms of virus disease often appear after peak viral growth is over, the clinical manifestations being due to inflammatory and other processes. It may be, therefore, that symptomatic control of such infections is more likely to be obtained with compounds which interfere with the host response than with those which interfere with viral growth. It follows that substances which inhibit viral replication are more likely to be of use in prophylaxis than in treatment.

Large and growing numbers of compounds have been shown to exert anti-viral activity both *in vitro* and against experimental infections in animals (Thompson, 1964; Tyrrell, 1969). Amongst those of current interest are benzimidazole derivatives active against poliovirus and certain coxsackie, echo and adeno viruses (O'Sullivan *et al.*, 1969). Whether these antiviral effects can be put to any clinical use remains to be seen. A number of compounds have already risen to trials in man; two, idoxuridine and methisazone have established a place in current therapeutics, and two others, amantadine and cytarabine, have also shown promising results.

Interferons

First described by Isaacs and Lindemann (1957), interferons are a family of closely related proteins liberated by cells which are actively synthesizing virus and which act on other cells reducing their susceptibility to viral infection (Finter, 1966). With some exceptions, interferons will protect only the cells of the animal species in which they were manufactured, or those of closely related species. On the other hand, the protection afforded includes not only the inducing virus but a wide variety of unrelated viruses. Interferon production is blocked by actinomycin D which inhibits the synthesis of messenger-RNA and it appears that viral infection of the cell may induce (or de-repress) the production of a messenger-RNA which codes the ribosome to produce interferon (Ho, 1964; Baron and Levy, 1966). They are proteins of molecular weight variously calculated to be between 19,000 and 160,000. They are destroyed by proteolytic but not by other enzymes and are otherwise remarkably stable. Some preparations are said to withstand 72°C. for 1 hour but human interferon is considerably less heat-stable (Glasgow, 1965). They are active against a wide variety of both DNA and RNA viruses but viral sensitivity differs considerably. Their potency is at least comparable with that of antibacterial antibiotics: partially purified preparations inhibit viral growth in concentrations of about 1 or 2 μg. per ml. Interferons are apparently of low toxicity and very poor antigens. Unlike neutralizing antibody, interferon has no effect on extra-cellular virus and does not prevent virus from penetrating cells. It appears to exert its effect very soon after the virus has entered the cell, interfering with the earliest stages of viral replication. Since they have generally little activity in species unrelated to the one in which they were produced, only human or possibly primate interferon is likely to be of any use for therapy in man. Human placenta or leucocytes are possible rich sources of interferon but the danger of transmitting serum hepatitis with such products must obviously be circumvented. Considerable technical difficulties remain over the purification, potency and standardization of interferon.

Monkey interferon has been shown to prevent smallpox vaccination from 'taking' if it is injected at the site 24 hours previously (M.R.C., 1962) but it failed to influence the course of experimental respiratory virus infections in volunteers (M.R.C., 1965). Jones *et al.* (1962) successfully treated 5 patients suffering from vaccinial keratitis with topical monkey interferon.

Interferon Inducers. Of considerable interest is the possibility of treating systemic infections by stimulating endogenous interferon production. Petralli *et al.* (1965) showed that injection of a virulent measles virus might be used to stimulate endogenous interferon production in a patient suffering from another virus disease (since interferon is non-specific in its anti-viral activity) but the development of antibody against the stimulating virus would soon render this procedure ineffective.

An assortment of substances has been found to excite the production or release of preformed interferons. It appears that the anti-viral effects of the fungal products helenine (derived from *Penicillium funiculosum*) and statolon (derived from *Penicillium stoloniferum*) are exerted in this way (Rytel *et al.*, 1966) and the mechanism of these effects is of great theoretical interest. Lampson *et al.* (1967) showed that the interferon inducer in helenine is double-stranded-RNA. Double- and multiple-stranded RNA is produced in cells infected with RNA viruses and this suggests that the origin of the interferon inducer in statolon and helenine is fungal virus and that the inducer is polystranded RNA (Banks *et al.*, 1968; Kleinschmidt *et al.*, 1968). This raises the possibility of using extracted polystranded RNA or synthetic analogues for therapeutic purposes. Some multi-stranded complexes of synthetic polyisosinic and polycytidinic acids are active inducers of interferons (Field *et al.*, 1967). Experimental keratitis in rabbits has been treated successfully by these compounds (Park and Baron, 1968), but Nesburn and Ziniti (1971) found the suppressive effect was only temporary. In man, the effect of an interferon inducer, administered intranasally, on the course of experimental rhinovirus and influenza virus infection has been assessed (Hill *et al.*, 1972). Only minimal amounts of nasal interferon were stimulated and the results were unimpressive. Interferon induction has also been attempted in herpes simplex encephalitis (Bellanti *et al.*, 1971), and in subacute sclerosing panencephalitis (Leavitt *et al.*, 1971), One of three patients to whom a pyran copolymer was administered in an attempt to influence the course of S.S.P.E. developed a haemolytic uraemic syndrome. More information will doubtless be forthcoming about the properties and potential toxicity of these interesting compounds.

Amantadines

These drugs have been fairly extensively investigated and are believed to act by blocking entry of adsorbed virus into the cell (Dickinson *et al.*, 1967). *In vitro* they inhibit influenza A and C and rubella viruses. The effect is not profound and cell-to-cell spread of some strains of virus is prevented only if the infecting dose of virus is small. Some viral strains appear to contain relatively high proportions of more resistant particles, and in one study viral susceptibility was lost after a single passage in the presence of the drug (Sabin, 1967).

Experimental influenza A infection in volunteers was prevented by prophylactic use of the drug in some studies (Togo *et al.,* 1968) but not in others (Tyrrell *et al.,* 1965). Similarly discordant results have been obtained in the prophylaxis of natural infection. Galbraith *et al.* (1969a) found that early prophylactic treatment of the household contacts of index cases reduced the incidence of clinical influenza to less than a quarter of that in placebo-treated contacts, and also significantly reduced the frequency of serological evidence of infection. Yet in a similar trial (Galbraith *et al.,* 1969b), they failed to find any protection against the Hong Kong strain. They suggest that the difference may be accounted for by the greater level of immunity in the first population studied. This is in keeping with Quilligan *et al.* (1966) who found that they could suppress clinical and subclinical influenza A2 infection in children providing they had some pre-existing immunity from previous infection or vaccination. Oker-Blom *et al.* (1970), in a controlled field trial among Finnish students, recorded a modest degree of protection against natural infection with influenza A2/Hong Kong. Serological evidence of infection was obtained in 27 of 192 amantadine-treated students, and in 57 of 199 in the placebo group, a protection rate of 52 per cent.

In terms of the prospects for antiviral chemotherapy, there have been several very encouraging reports of the therapeutic use of amantadines. In natural outbreaks of influenza A2, there was more rapid defervescence of illness in patients treated within about 20 hours of the onset of symptoms with amantadine than in those treated with placebo (Hornick *et al.,* 1969; Togo *et al.,* 1970). The results in naturally occurring influenza A2/Hong Kong in Britain were somewhat disappointing (Galbraith *et al.,* 1971). The mean duration of fever was significantly reduced in the treated group, but the duration of a variety of symptoms was no different in the two groups. No effect was demonstrated on rubella in the 1964 outbreak (Sabin, 1967) and Dickinson *et al.* (1967), using 1-adamantanamine-HCl (Symmetrel) and α-methyl-1-adamantanemethyl-amine-HCl (Rimatadine) confirmed previous reports that these agents are inactive against influenza B. They also failed to demonstrate any effect on the clinical or immunological response of children having live measles vaccine. Adverse effects have not been a problem. Amantadine hydrochloride has been used for the treatment of Parkinson's disease (Parkes et al., 1970).

Idoxuridine

This compound (2'-deoxy-5-iodouridine) synthesized by Prusoff (1959) is a white crystalline odourless powder with a molecular weight of 354·1. It is sparingly soluble in water (1 in 500) and alcohol (1 in 400) and even less soluble in chloroform and ether. A 0·1 per cent aqueous solution has a pH of about 6. It is stable when stored dry and the 0·1 per cent ophthalmic solution is said to retain its potency for a year at room temperature but this has been disputed and refrigeration is recommended. The solution is sensitive to light and should be stored in amber bottles. About half the potency is lost on autoclaving at 120°C. for 20 minutes.

Idoxuridine and the corresponding 2'-deoxy-5-bromouridine are thymidine analogues which inhibit the utilization of thymidine in the rapid synthesis of DNA which normally occurs in herpes-infected cells. The possibility of a similar effect in uninfected cells and the rapid dehalogenation of these compounds in the body makes them unpromising for systemic use although some success has been claimed in the treatment of herpes encephalitis. Viral resistance to idoxuridine is said to develop relatively easily. It has been used principally for the treatment of herpes keratitis and cutaneous herpes. The beneficial result claimed in both conditions has been disputed.

HERPES KERATITIS. This has usually been treated with 0·1 per cent idoxuridine drops, hourly by day and 2-hourly by night. Several authors reporting large series of cases have been satisfied with the results (Maxwell, 1965) but Jones (1967) takes the view that the results are no better than cauterization in the treatment of dendritic ulcer (p. 427).

CUTANEOUS HERPES. The failure of some workers to enjoy the same success as others in the treatment of recurrent cutaneous herpes may be the result of poor contact between the agent and the infected cells. Juel-Jensen and MacCallum (1965) who had previously failed to influence the disease by local applications of idoxuridine ointment, reduced the average duration of lesions from 8·9 to 5·5 days, by injecting 0·1 per cent idoxuridine into the affected skin with a spray-gun.

HERPES ZOSTER. Juel Jensen *et al.* (1970) conducted a controlled trial in 20 patients with herpes zoster. The treated group received idoxuridine in the form of a 40 per cent solution in dimethylsulphoxide, continuously applied to the affected area. No new lesions appeared after idoxuridine treatment was started, and pain abated much more quickly than in the controls.

HERPES SIMPLEX ENCEPHALITIS. This form of encephalitis carries a poor prognosis, with a high risk of death or of residual neurological damage. Idoxuridine has been used in the form of daily intravenous infusions, and occasionally by intra-carotid infusion, in an attempt to mitigate the results of the infection. Although the disease is serious, the course varies greatly and unpredictably in individual patients and, as in other forms of brain damage, the effects of a particular form of treatment are difficult to assess; nor is the condition common enough to make a controlled trial possible. A number of favourable individual reports have been published and a larger series was reported by Nolan, Carruthers and Lerner (1970). They described 13 patients with herpes simplex encephalitis, of whom six were treated with idoxuridine. They claimed their results could not be matched by previous descriptions of the course of herpes encephalitis without specific treatment, and that the potentially toxic treatment was thus justified. Other authors have been less sanguine, and have observed equally favourable results by careful non-specific treatment of coma combined with dexamethasone to reduce cerebral oedema (Upton *et al.*, 1971). The use of steroids in this form of encephalitis without apparent detriment is of interest since herpetic keratitis provides one clear-cut example of the possible detrimental effects of corticosteroids in active viral infection. Cytarabine (v.i.) has also been used in herpes simplex encephalitis.

Cytarabine

Cytosine arabinoside (1-β-D-arabinofuranosyl-cytosine hydrochloride), like the halogenated nucleosides, acts by inhibition of nucleic acid synthesis. It appears to act by depressing the formation of phosphorylated derivatives of deoxycytidine from their ribose-containing precursors. It is active against herpes group viruses and has been used in patients with severe varicella-zoster arising in the course of leukaemia and other malignant diseases, in zoster without underlying malignancy, and in severe herpes simplex infections. Its use in 25 patients including eight of their own, is summarized by Chow *et al.* (1971), who noted dramatic clinical improvement in several instances. Most authors used a dose of 100 mg./sq.m./day intravenously but in a later report Hryniuk *et al.* (1972) claim that a response can be achieved with a lesser risk of toxic effects by lower doses, ranging from 10-100 mg. per sq.m per day for $1\frac{1}{2}$ to 7 days. On the other hand varicella arising in the course of a malignant condition is not necessarily fatal or even severe, and a final judgment must wait upon the results of carefully controlled trials.

Another interesting possible application for cytarabine has been propounded by Kraybill *et al.* (1972) who administered the drug to two infants with congenital cytomegalovirus infection. Infection was not suppressed in either but the dose used was small.

Methisazone

This compound (N-methylisatin β-thiosemicarbazone) was shown by Bauer *et al.* (1962) to be active against variola following a number of observations over the years that various thiosemicarbazones would inhibit pox viruses in mice and chick embryos. It is a fine orange-yellow powder almost insoluble in water but soluble in acetone (1 in 25) and sparingly in chloroform (1 in 800). Brief exposure to light causes a reversible change, but prolonged exposure causes decomposition and it must be suitably protected. Methisazone is believed to affect a late stage of virus maturation (Easterbrook, 1962).

Anorexia, nausea and vomiting are common in those treated with the drug, occurring in 95 per cent of Landsman and Grist's (1964) cases and 66 per cent of the cases of do Valle *et al.* (1965) despite the use of cyclizine or chlorpromazine. Diarrhoea, rashes and thinning of the hair have also been described. Alcohol may exacerbate the side-effects and it is currently recommended that the drug should not be given to pregnant women or to those with liver or kidney disease.

VARIOLA. By the time lesions have appeared viral multiplication is rapidly declining, and methisazone has no effect on the course of smallpox. The principal use of these compounds has been in the contact prophylaxis of small-pox. Several successful trials have been reported in variola major. Bauer (1965) reported 6 cases with two deaths amongst 2,297 close contacts treated with methisazone and 114 cases with 20 deaths amongst 2,842 similar untreated contacts. Similar success has been described in the prophylaxis of variola minor (do Valle et al., 1965). Subsequent trials in West Pakistan in contacts of variola major have given much less favourable results (Heiner et al., 1971) and it appears that methisazone is less valuable in prophylaxis that at first appeared. Using a related compound, M & B 7714 for the prophylaxis of variola major, Rao et al. (1966) were successful, finding 40 cases with 7 deaths amongst 196 treated contacts and 80 cases with 12 deaths amongst 201 untreated contacts.

VACCINIA. Methisazone given at the time of vaccination depresses the local reaction but also possibly impairs the antibody response (Landsman and Grist, 1964). In an uncontrolled trial, Jaroszynska-Weinberger and Mészáros (1966) vaccinated children with a history of eczema without any developing eczema vaccinatum. In a later report (Jaroszynska-Weinberger, 1970) good results were claimed in 16 patients with ectopic vaccinial lesions, in four with eczema vaccinatum, and two with vaccinia gangrenosa. Established eczema vaccinatum was favourably influenced by methisazone treatment in 14/24 of Adels' and Oppé's (1966) patients, some of whom also received antivaccinial gamma globulin. Progressive vaccinia (vaccinia gangrenosa) which without treatment is almost invariably fatal has been treated by a number of authors (usually together with anti-vaccinial gamma globulin) and half have recovered (Connolly, 1966).

Methisazone should not be used as a substitute for vaccination, which currently remains the best prophylactic, and treatment should not begin before vaccination lest it interfere with the development of immunity.

Isoquinolines

Larin *et al.* (1968) showed that two isoquinoline derivatives inactivated the infectivity of influenza A and B, parainfluenza and measles viruses, but appeared not to affect viral multiplication. With rhino- and echoviruses there was a suppressive effect on replication but not on infectivity; with rubella both processes were affected and respiratory syncytial virus was suppressed but the mode of action was obscure. Beare *et al.* (1968) compared one of these compounds (UK 2371) with a placebo in volunteers challenged intranasally with influenza B virus. A week's treatment begun the day before challenge halved the incidence of clinical and subclinical infection, but similar activity was not shown in a further trial using the Hong Kong strain of influenza A2 (Reed *et al.*, 1970). In a review of the properties of UK 2054 (' famotine ') and UK 2371 (' memotine ') Williamson and Jackson (1969) found the evidence for their activity in man inconclusive. In a well-designed and controlled trial, Stark *et al.* (1970) found that prophylactic use of the drug failed to influence the incidence of respiratory viral infection, including influenza, amongst students in a hall of residence during the mild winter outbreak of 1969.

CHLAMYDIA

The organisms responsible for trachoma, inclusion conjunctivitis and inclusion blenorrhoea (TRIC agents), lymphogranuloma venereum and psittacosis have many properties in common and are now grouped together under the name *Chlamydia* (Moulder, 1966). Like the viruses, they are obligate intra-cellular parasites of small size, but unlike viruses and like bacteria they multiply by binary fission, they have cell walls resembling those of Gram-negative bacteria, they have ribosomal structures with the susceptibility to antibiotics characteristic of bacterial ribosomes, and those which are sulphonamide-sensitive synthesize folate. Their obligate intra-cellular nature (and perhaps their small size) may be accounted for by their complete, or almost complete, lack of mechanisms for the production of metabolic energy.

There are two groups. The first group, including those

causing trachoma and lymphogranuloma venereum, produce compact cytoplasmic inclusions and are sensitive to sulphonamides and cycloserine. The other group, including the psittacosis agent, produce diffuse cytoplasmic inclusions and are resistant to sulphonamides and cycloserine (Moulder, 1966).

It has been the general view for a long time that the diseases caused by *Chlamydia* respond to tetracyclines, but more recent, perhaps more critical, study indicates that the results are far from perfect (Jawetz, 1969). The efficacy of tetracyclines (and sulphonamides) in trachoma has been seriously questioned (p. 427) and there is evidence, both in this country (Watson and Gairdner, 1968) and in America, that the effects of neonatal inclusion conjunctivitis are by no means as benign as once thought, and that the tetracycline treatment used to date is, in some cases at least, inadequate (Forster *et al.*, 1970). It is of interest that rifampicin in low concentrations shows activity against the trachoma agent in infected cell lines and in embryonated eggs (Becker & Zakay-Rones, 1969). The results of tetracycline treatment of psittacosis are similarly imperfect (Anderson and Bridgwater, 1968) and, as with other chlamydial infections, adequate information is especially lacking about the correct duration of treatment. The treatment of lymphogranuloma venerum is discussed on p. 470). Increasing availability of improved diagnostic methods will no doubt result in more frequent recognition of these diseases and the opportunity to undertake the review of their treatment which is evidently now required.

PHARMACEUTICAL PREPARATIONS AND DOSAGE

IDOXURIDINE (IDU; 5 IDUR)

Ophthalmic solution 0·1 per cent. (Dendrid, *Alcon Laboratories, Vestric Ltd;* ' Kerecid ' and ' Stoxil ', *Smith, Kline and French*) 1 drop hourly by day and 2 hourly by night. Ophthalmic ointment 0·25 per cent. in sterile eye ointment base, B.P.

METHISAZONE (' Marboran ', *Burroughs Wellcome*)

Capsules 1·5 g. Optimum dosage schedules not yet established. Cyclizine or chlorpromazine may assist in controlling nausea and vomiting. Connolly (1966) recommends: *Prevention of variola* 3 g.+3 g. 12 hours later. *Prevention of complications of vaccinia* on fourth day after vaccination 100 mg./kg./day followed by 50 mg./kg./day for 3–6 days. *Treatment of eczema vaccinatum or progressive vaccinia* 200 mg./kg. followed by 200 mg./kg./day in divided doses for 2 days.

REFERENCES

ACORNLEY, J. E., BESSELL, C. H., BYNOE, M. L., GOTFREDSEN, W. O. & KNOYLE, J. M. (1967). *Brit. J. Pharmacol.* **31**, 210.

ADELS, B. R. & OPPÉ, T. E. (1966). *Lancet* **1**, 18

ANDERSON, J. P. & BRIDGWATER, F. A. J. (1968). *Brit. J. Dis. Chest* **62**, 155.

BANKS, G. T., BUCK, K. W., CHAIN, E. B., HIMMELWEIT, F., MARKS, J. E., TYLER, J. M., HOLLINGS, M., LAST, F. T. & STONE, O. M. (1968). *Nature (Lond.)* **218**, 542.

BARON, S. & LEVY, H. B. (1966). *Ann. Rev. Microbiol.* **20**, 291.

BAUER, D. J. (1965). *Ann. N.Y. Acad. Sci.* **130**, 110.

BAUER, D. J., DUMBELL, K. R., FOX-HULME, P. & SADLER, P. W. (1962). *Bull Wld Hlth Org.* **26**, 727.

BEARE, A. S., BYNOE, M. L. & TYRRELL, D. A. J. (1968). *Lancet* **1**, 843.

BECKER, Y. & ZAKAY-RONES, Z. (1969). *Nature* **222**, 851.

BELLANTINI, J. A., CATALANO, L. W. JR. & CHAMBERS, R. W. (1971). *J. Pediat.* **78**, 136.

CHOW, A. W., FOERSTER, J., HRYNIUK, W. (1971). *Antimicrob. Agents Chemother.*—1970, p. 214.

CONNOLLY, J. H. (1966). *Practitioner* **197**, 373.

DICKINSON, P. C. T., CHANG, T-W. & WEINSTEIN, L. (1967). *Antimicrob. Agents Chemother.*, 1966, 521.

DO VALLE, L. A. R., DE MELO, P. R., DE SALLES GOMES, L. F. & PROENCA, L. M. (1965). *Lancet* **2**, 976.

EASTERBROOK, K. B. (1962). *Virology* **17**, 245.

FIELD, A. K., TYTELL, A. A., LAMPSON, G. P. & HILLEMAN, M. R. (1967). *Proc. Nat. Acad. Sci. (Wash.)* **58**, 1004.

FINTER, N. B. (Ed.) (1966). *Interferons.* Philadelphia, Saunders.

FORSTER, R. K., DAWSON, C. R. & SCHACHTER, J. (1970). *Amer. J. Ophthal.* **69**, 467.

GALBRAITH, A. W., OXFORD, J. S., SCHILD, G. C. & WATSON, G. I. (1969a). *Lancet* **2**, 1026.

GALBRAITH, A. W., OXFORD, J. S., SCHILD, G. C. & WATSON, G. I. (1969b). *Bull. Wld Hlth Org.* **41**, 677.

GALBRAITH, A. W., OXFORD, J. S., SCHILD, G. C., POTTER, C. W. & WATSON, G. I. (1971). *Lancet* **2**, 113.

GLASGOW, L. A. (1965). *J. Pediat.* **67**, 104.

HELLER, E., ARGAMAN, M., LEVY, H. & GOLDBLUM, N. (1969). *Nature (Lond.)* **222**, 273.

HEINER, G. G. & 11 others. (1971). *Amer. J. Epidem.* **94**, 435.

HILL, D. A. & 7 others. (1972). *J. Amer. med. Ass.* **219**, 1179.

HO, M. (1964). *Bact. Rev.* **28**, 367.

HORNICK, R. B., TOGO, Y., MAHLER, S. & IEZZONI, D. (1969). *Bull. Wld Hlth Org.* **41**, 671.

HRYNIUK, W., FOERSTER, J., SHOJANIA, M. & CHOW, A. (1972). *J. Amer. med. Ass.* **219**, 715.

ISAACS, A. & LINDEMANN, J. (1957). *Proc. roy. Soc. B.* **147**, 258.

JAROSZYŃSKA-WEINBERGER, B. & MÉSZÁROS, B. (1966). *Lancet* **1**, 948.

JAROSZYNSKA-WEINBERGER, B. (1970). *Arch. Dis. Child.* **45**, 573.

JAWETZ, E. (1969). *Adv. Pharmacol. Chemother.* **7**, 253.

JONES, B. R. (1967). *Trans. Ophthal. Soc., U.K.* **87**, 537.

JONES, B. R., GALBRAITH, J. E. K., & AL-HUSSAINI, M. K. (1962). *Lancet* **2**, 875.

JUEL-JENSEN, B. E. & MACCALLUM, F. O. (1965). *Brit. med. J.* **1**, 901.

JUEL-JENSEN, B. E., MACCALLUM, F. O., MACKENZIE, A. M. R. & PIKE, M. C. (1970). *Brit. med. J.* **4**, 776.

KATES, J. R. & MCAUSLAN, B. R. (1967). *Proc. Nat. Acad. Sci. (Wash.)* **58**, 134.

KLEINSCHMIDT, W. J., ELLIS, L. F., VAN FRANK, R. M. & MURPHY, E. B. (1968). *Nature (Lond.)* **220**, 167.

KRAYBILL, E. N., SEVER, J. L., AVERY, G. B. & MOVASSAGHI, N. (1972). *J. Pediat.* **80**, 485.

LAMPSON, G. P., TYTELL, A. A., FIELD, A. K., NEMES, M. M. & HILLEMAN, M. R. (1967). *Proc. Nat. Acad. Sci. (Wash.)* **58**, 782.

LANDSMAN, J. B. & GRIST, N. R. (1964). *Lancet* **1**, 330.

LARIN, N. M., BEARE, A. S., COPPING, M. P., McDONALD, C. R., McDOUGALL, J. K., ROBERTS, B. & SMITH, J. B. (1968). *Antimicrob. Agents Chemother.* —1967, p. 646.

LEAVITT, T. J., MERIGAN, T. C. & FREEMAN, J. M. (1971). *Amer. J. Dis. Child.* **121**, 43.

MAXWELL, E. (1965). *Amer. J. Ophthal.* **59**, 42.

MEDICAL RESEARCH COUNCIL SCIENTIFIC COMMITTEE ON INTERFERON (1962). *Lancet* **1**, 873.

MEDICAL RESEARCH COUNCIL SCIENTIFIC COMMITTEE ON INTERFERON (1965). *Lancet* **1**, 505.

MOULDER, J. W. (1966). *Ann. Rev. Microbiol.* **20**, 107.

NESBURN, A. B. & ZINITI, P. J. (1971). *Amer. J. Ophthal.* **72**, 821.

NOLAN, D. C., CARRUTHERS, M. M. & LERNER, A. M. (1970). *New Engl. J. Med.* **282**, 10.

OKER-BLOM, N., HOVI, T., LEINIKKI, P., PALOSUO, T., PETTERSSON, R. & SUNI, J. (1970). *Brit. med. J.* **3**, 676.

O'SULLIVAN, D. G., PANTIC, D., DANE, D. S. & BRIGGS, M. (1969). *Lancet* **1**, 446.

PARK, J. H. & BARON, S. (1968). *Science, N.Y.* **162**, 811.

PARKES, J. D., ZILKHA, K. J., MARSDEN, P., BAXTER, R. C. H. & KNILL-JONES, R. P. (1970). *Lancet* **1**, 1130.

PETRALLI, J. K., MERIGAN, T. C. & WILBUR, J. R. (1965). *Lancet* **2**, 401.

PRUSOFF, W. H. (1959). *Biochem. biophys. Acta* **32**, 295.

QUILLIGAN, J. J., JR., HIRAYAMA, M. & BAERNSTEIN, H. D., JR. (1966). *J. Pediat.* **69**, 572.

RAO, A. R., McFADZEAN, J. A. & KAMALASHKI, K. (1966). *Lancet* **1**, 1068.

REED, S. E., BEARE, A. S., BYNOE, M. L. & TYRRELL, D. A. J. (1970). *Ann. N.Y. Acad. Sci.* **173**, Art. 1, 760.

RYTEL, M. W., SHOPE, R. E. & KILBOURNE, E. D. (1966). *J. exp. Med.* **123**, 577.

SABIN, A. B. (1967). *J. Amer. med. Ass.* **200**, 943.

STARK, J. E., HEATH, R. B., OSWALD, N. C., BOOTH, V., TALL, R., FOX, W., MOYNAGH, K. D. & INGLIS, J. M. (1970). *Thorax.* **25**, 649.

SUBAK-SHARPE, J. H., TIMBURY, M. C. & WILLIAMS, J. F. (1969). *Nature (Lond.)* **222**, 341.

THOMPSON, R. L. (1964). *Adv. Chemother.* **1**, 85.

TOGO, Y., HORNICK, R. B. & DAWKINS, A. T. (1968). *J. Amer. med. Ass.* **203**, 1089.

TOGO, Y., HORNICK, R. B., FELITTI, V. J., KAUFMAN, M. L., DAWKINS, A. T., KILPE, V. E. & CLAGHORN, J. L. (1970). *J. Amer. med. Ass.* **211**, 1149.

TYRRELL, D. A. J. (1969). *The Scientific Basis of Medicine Annual Reviews,* 1969, p. 294.

TYRRELL, D. A. J., BYNOE, M. L. & HOORN, B. (1965). *Brit. J. exp. Path.* **46**, 370.

UPTON, A. R. M., BARWICK, D. D. & FOSTER, J. B. (1971). *Lancet* **1**, 290.

WATSON, P. G. & GAIRDNER, D. (1968). *Brit. med. J.* **3**, 527.

WILLIAMSON, G. M. & JACKSON, D. (1969). *Bull. Wld Hlth Org.* **41**, 665.

CHAPTER 29

LABORATORY CONTROL

EXCEPT in a few diseases with a single bacterial cause always sensitive to the drug of first choice, ' chemotherapy without bacteriology is guesswork' (Howie, 1962). The first task of the laboratory is to make a bacteriological diagnosis, and skill and experience in identifying the cause of an infection are even more important to-day than they were in the past. Many of the taunts directed at the proceedings about to be described, because patients have responded to treatment with an antibiotic to which their organisms have been reported resistant, are a reflection not on the method but on its user, who has seen nothing in his cultures but commensals.

No more need usually be done if the organism found is, for instance, a Group A streptococcus or a pneumococcus, which may safely be assumed to be sensitive to penicillin. Such species are unfortunately the exception: most others commonly found, particularly in the kinds of non-specific infection of the air passages, urinary tract, wounds etc., which make up the bulk of infective disease in temperate climates, cannot be depended on to be fully sensitive to a given drug. Hence most bacteriological examinations now include determinations of bacterial sensitivity, at least to certain antibiotics.

The vast number of these tests which must now be carried out in all routine laboratories demand a quick reliable method which will indicate whether the infection is likely to respond to treatment with a given drug rather than the precise amount of the drug required to inhibit growth. Some form of diffusion test is generally used for this purpose, and various methods with innumerable modifications have been used. In recent years a considerable effort has been made to standardize these tests and the Report of the International Collaborative Study, which spent eight years investigating the disc test, has now appeared (Ericsson and Sherris, 1971). We understand that the method recommended in this Report (I.C.S., see p 498) is in use

490

throughout Scandinavia and some attempt is being made to have it adopted in various countries in Europe. The Kirby-Bauer method (Bauer *et al.*, 1966, see p. 498), with some modifications, has now been made the official F.D.A. method in the United States (Federal Register 1972). The main alternative to the I.C.S. method is to continue to use plates of ordinary size and lower content discs and to interpret zone size by comparison with that in a culture of a control organism on a plate of the same medium. Proposals for standardizing such a method (and for a few particular tests for which neither it nor the I.C.S. method is applicable), including consideration of media, disc content, and limitation of the number of drugs against which common bacterial species need to be tested, are made by Garrod and Waterworth (1971) and Stokes and Waterworth (1972).

A comparative study of the various methods is in progress in Great Britain and it is hoped that it will be possible to make recommendations based on this and also on the results of Quality Control trials currently being carried out in hospital and Public Health Laboratories.

It may be that it is not possible, or even desirable, to have a single method adopted universally, and the desired effect might more easily be achieved by greater standardization of media and discs, increased availability of reference strains and more general participation in quality control.

DIFFUSION TESTS OF BACTERIAL SENSITIVITY

In these tests the antibiotic diffuses from a focus through a solid medium, inhibiting the growth of an organism on or in it to a distance depending, *inter alia*, on the sensitivity of the organism. This focus is usually a blotting paper disc on which a known amount of antibiotic has been dried, but blotting paper strips can be used with advantage when multiple strains are tested against a single drug (Fig. 32). Whichever the method used, its results will be affected by certain basic factors which therefore require control.

Factors Affecting Results of Diffusion Tests

MEDIUM. Some constituents of laboratory media affect certain antibiotics; the addition of blood will reduce the inhibition zone of antibiotics heavily protein-bound (e.g. fucidin, novobiocin). Electrolytes affect many antibiotics: the activity of the aminoglycosides is depressed but others may be enhanced (e.g. bacitracin, fucidin and novobiocin, and penicillins against *Proteus* spp.). The M.I.C. of gentamicin varies with the magnesium content of the medium (Garrod and Waterworth, 1969). The addition of a sugar enlarges zones of inhibition produced by nitrofurantoin (Report, 1965) and ampicillin and penicillin (Garrod and Waterworth, 1971) against some organisms. This is seen only in a diffusion test; M.I.C. are not altered.

The agar used for solidifying medium can affect not only the diffusion of some drugs (polymyxin; Bechtle and Scherr, 1958); polymyxin and the aminoglycosides (Kunin and Edmondson, 1968), but may also affect the M.I.C. of gentamicin (Garrod and Waterworth, 1969, see p. 124 and Fig. 34) and of neomycin, kanamycin and polymyxin (Hanus, Sands, and Bennett, 1967).

There is no doubt that more consistent and reliable results are obtained if a specially formulated sensitivity test medium is used. Mueller-Hinton agar is recommended for both the I.C.S. and Kirby-Bauer methods, but Garrod and Waterworth (1971) reported considerable variation between different manufacturers' products. These variations can be accounted for by variations in the constituents of the medium: Bovallius and Zacharias (1971) found very considerable differences in the cation content of commercial media from different sources and even between different batches from a single source.

Whatever the medium used, plates must be flat-bottomed and poured on a level surface (some laboratory benches do not qualify for this description) and the medium must be of uniform depth. The medium used must support free growth of the organism to be tested, blood being added if required. Selective media should not be used.

pH OF MEDIUM. Streptomycin is about 500 times more active at pH 8·5 than at 5·5: kanamycin, gentamicin and tobramycin are affected similarly to a lesser degree. The macrolides are also favoured by alkalinity. Tetracyclines and some other antibiotics are more active in an acid medium (see Table 45). The pH of the medium should not be altered to favour an antibiotic, but it should be remembered that circumstances which do alter it may affect the result. Thus incubation in CO_2 which lowers the pH, may make an organism which is partially resistant to tetracycline appear sensitive. Growth of most species raises the pH of nutrient agar in the surrounding area, and if the antibiotic is favoured by acidity (*e.g.* fucidin) the change may be sufficient to permit growth on an otherwise inhibitory concentration. 'Satellitism' may have a similar explanation. If the antibiotic is favoured by alkalinity (*e.g.* erythromycin) the same effect can be produced by adding glucose to the medium. Any organism which ferments this will lower the pH of the surrounding medium (P. M. Waterworth, unpublished observations).

TABLE 45

Effect of pH on Antibiotics

Little Affected	Less Active in Acid Medium	Less Active in Alkaline Medium
Penicillin Chloramphenicol Polymyxins Vancomycin	Aminoglycosides Lincomycin Erythromycin group Cephaloridine	Tetracyclines Methicillin Cloxacillin Fucidin

INOCULUM. The activity of many antibiotics is little affected by the number of bacteria present, but nevertheless all zones of inhibition are reduced if the inoculum increases (Fig. 35). The probable explanation of this contradiction is that visible growth appears more quickly if the inoculum is heavy, thus allowing less time for the diffusion of the antibiotic. It should be such as will produce 'dense but not confluent growth' (Fig. 36) and it is also essential that it be uniformly distributed. The best results are obtained by flooding with a suspension of the organism, but the preparation of dilutions is time-consuming and this method is not without risk to the operator and should not be used with highly pathogenic organisms. Whole plates cannot be adequately spread with a wire loop. Photographs are often published showing zones which are much wider on one side of the disc than on the other, due to the reduction of the inoculum when spreading with a loop. The Kirby-Bauer method inoculates plates with a swab dipped in diluted culture, but this too is dependent on careful standardization and dilution. Barry, Garcia & Thrupp (1970) recommend inoculating plates by adding a 0·001 ml. calibrated loopful of culture to 8 ml. of a melted and cooled 1·5 per cent aqueous solution of agar which was mixed well and poured over the surface of a 15 cm plate of Mueller Hinton agar. On the other hand, highly satisfactory results can be achieved without any dilutions if a small loopful of fully grown culture is spread with a sterile dry swab (Felmingham and Stokes, 1972). Such a culture is illustrated in Fig. 37.

INOCULATION OF PLATES. (a) *By flooding*. Overnight broth cultures require diluting approximately 1/100 for streptococci, 1/1000 for staphylococci and 1/5000 for coliforms. Suitable dilutions can be prepared by adding a 2 mm. loopful to 1 ml. saline (streptococci) to 4 ml. saline (staphylococci) and to 10 ml. saline (coliforms), the loop being held vertically. Using a sterile pasteur pipette, flood the plate with a well shaken suspension diluted as described, drain the excess to the side by tilting and remove with the same pipette. If only plate cultures are available, suspend portions of 5-10 colonies in a small volume of broth to give a similar density to an overnight broth culture and proceed as above.

(b) *Spreading with a swab*. A 5 mm. loopful, the loop held vertically, of well-grown broth culture is transferred to the plate and spread with a dry swab, closely and evenly, over the area to be covered. The precise size of the loop does not matter greatly, presumably because a large proportion of the cells adheres to the swab. In the absence of a broth culture, a suspension can be made in a small volume of broth.

DISCS. There is still no general agreement on the ideal content of discs; indeed in a survey carried out in 645 laboratories in Great Britain in 1970, it was found that as many as 9 different disc contents were being used for penicillin and tetracycline (Castle and Elstub, 1971). The choice of disc content must be governed by the method of interpretation being used. The I.C.S. method uses high content discs throughout as does the Kirby-Bauer method for most drugs. On the other hand, if results are being interpreted by other methods, particularly without adequate controls, it must be remembered that the *concentration per ml.* of the drug in the immediately surrounding medium will exceed the stated disc *content*; thus discs containing 30 μg. kanamycin may give a 12 mm. zone with an organism having an M.I.C. of 64 μg./ml. The exclusive use of discs of high content may mask small but clinically significant increases in resistance and may also give a zone of inhibition with a clinically insensitive organism (e.g. *E. coli* with erythromycin).

Suitable discs for use with the methods advocated on pp. 496 and 504 together with those used in the I.C.S. and Kirby-Bauer methods are given in Table 46.

STORAGE OF DISCS. Discs must be stored in the cold and kept dry. On removal from the refrigerator they should be allowed to attain room temperature before being opened, to avoid condensation. Only sufficient for the day's use should be removed and any left over should be discarded. When applying individual discs each must be pressed firmly in position—diffusion cannot take place unless the disc is in close contact with the medium.

TABLE 46

Suitable disc contents (μg.)

	Low	High	ICS	Kirby-Bauer (F.D.A.)
*Ampicillin	10	25	10	10
*Carbenicillin	10	100	100	50
*Cephalosporins	—	30	30	30
Chloramphenicol	10	30	30	30
Clindamycin	2	—	—	2
Colistin	50	50	30	10
Erythromycin	5	—	30	15
Fucidin	10	—	50	—
Gentamicin	10	10	30	10
Kanamycin	30	30	30	30
Lincomycin	2	—	15	—
Methicillin	10	—	10	5
Nalidixic acid	—	30	30	—
Nitrofurantoin	—	200	30	—
Novobiocin	5	—	—	30
Penicillin	2†	10†	10	10†
Polymyxin B sulphate	300†	300†		300†
Streptomycin	10	25	30	10
Sulphonamide	100	100	250	—
Tetracycline	10	30	30	30
Trimethoprim	1·25	1·25	—	—

*High content discs can be used to test coliform bacilli from specimens other than urine, but the fully sensitive control must be used to make it clear that such infections will respond only to high doses (see p. 498).

† units

PREDIFFUSION. Ericsson (1960), who has studied the whole of this subject with admirable thoroughness, makes a strong plea for a three-hour period of pre-diffusion as giving more significant results. Satisfactory results are obtained without it, and in clinical work the difficulties involved would seem to outweigh any possible advantage.

LENGTH OF INCUBATION. This should be the minimum required for the normal growth of the test organism. If it is prolonged, loss of activity of the drug may permit growth of sensitive organisms which were inhibited though not killed. This method is suitable only for organisms of a rapid rate of growth. It should be remembered that anything which reduces the speed of growth (*e.g.* poor or selective medium or lower temperature of incubation) will enlarge the inhibition zones.

Control Cultures

All these sources of error can be eliminated or at least the error recognized by the correct use of control cultures, which are also necessary for the proper interpretation of the test. The method described on page 504 is ideal in this respect as it controls every disc. This is not possible if whole plates are used for the specimen and it is then essential that control tests are set up every day for every drug and medium that has been used. Time can be saved and the risk of contamination is greatly reduced if control plates are inoculated with swabs impregnated in bulk with diluted culture (Felmingham and Stokes, 1972).

Add about 15 drops overnight broth culture of the Oxford *Staph. aureus* to 20 ml. nutrient broth. (For *E. coli* NCTC 10418 and *Ps. aeruginosa* 10662, about 7 drops of culture is usually sufficient.) Shake well and pour into a jar containing sterile 3 in. Q-tip swabs* (the quantity of broth is sufficient to impregnate about 90 swabs). Store in a screw cap glass or plastic jar at 4°C and use one swab per plate. They should keep at least one week.

Three organisms are necessary, *Staph. aureus* (*e.g.* N.C.T.C. 6571), *E. coli* (*e.g.* N.C.T.C. 10418) and *Ps. aeruginosa* (*e.g.* N.C.T.C. 10662). Their correct use is discussed on page 497.

Control cultures should be maintained at room temperature on agar slopes and sub-cultivated once a month. Broth cultures should be made from these once a week and either kept in the refrigerator or sub-cultivated daily in broth.

Interpretation of Results

1. COMPARISON WITH A CONTROL. The most usual method of interpreting disc sensitivity tests in routine diagnostic work in

* Available from Chesebrough-Ponds, Victoria Road, London N.W.10.

Great Britain, is to use low content discs and compare the zone produced with the unknown organism to that given by a control. The control should be an organism known to respond to treatment with normal doses of the drug concerned, and the Oxford staphylococcus (N.C.T.C. 6571) can be used for all the common drugs except polymyxins, when *E. coli* (*e.g.* N.C.T.C. 10418) should be used. If a drug is excreted by the kidneys more resistant infections can be treated in the urinary tract. A more resistant control should then be used, but again it must be one known to respond to treatment, *E. coli* (*e.g.* N.C.T.C. 10418) serves well: higher strength discs may also be used. Suitable discs for use with this method are given in Table 46.

In either case results are reported as sensitive, moderately resistant or resistant and the generally accepted definition of these terms is:

' *Sensitive* '—zone equal to or larger than that of the control, inferring that the infection should respond to treatment with normal doses.

' *Resistant* '—no zone or one of not more than 2 mm. radius, inferring that clinical response to treatment is unlikely.

'*Moderately Resistant* '—zone radius over 3 mm. smaller than that of the control (the inocula must be comparable and both measurements made by the same operator). This may signify:

a. Resistance in a normally sensitive species insufficient to justify the term ' resistant '. Whether the drug should be used will depend on other factors.

b. Usual sensitivity of a species which is more resistant than the control organism but may still respond to treatment with normal dosage (*e.g. H. influenzae* and ampicillin and *Ps. aeruginosa* with gentamicin and carbenicillin) or to high dosage (*e.g. Str. faecalis* and penicillin). This should be made clear in the report by describing it either as normally sensitive for the species or as sensitive to high doses. Abnormal resistance of these organisms is difficult to detect and is of particular importance with *Ps. aeruginosa* where any increase in resistance may jeopardize treatment with either gentamicin or carbenicillin. This difficulty can be overcome by using a sensitive strain of the same species as a control (*e.g.* N.C.T.C. 10662); equal sized zones then infer sensitivity normal *for the species,* and a reduced zone moderate resistance (see Fig. 38 B).

With this exception it must be emphasized that the choice of the control depends on the concentration of the drug at the site of the infection and not the species being tested. Urinary pathogens isolated from other parts of the body must be compared to the fully sensitive control and not to the *E. coli*: this is particularly important if high content discs are used and is illustrated in Fig. 38 A.

It must always be remembered that other factors besides the activity of the drug affect the result (*e.g.* diffusibility). The activity of different drugs cannot be directly compared by this method even if the discs contain the same amount.

2. THE ZONE OR NO ZONE METHOD employs both high and low content discs for each drug. Zones are not measured; any inhibition round the low content disc indicates sensitivity, a zone round the high disc only, infers moderate sensitivity and no zone round either indicates resistance. Very misleading results are obtained if only high content discs are used.

3. THE KIRBY-BAUER METHOD (Bauer *et al.*, 1966), defines 3 degrees of sensitivity according to zone diameter. For example, using a 30 μg. tetracycline disc zones of >19 mm. = sensitive. 15-18 mm. = intermediate and <15 mm. = resistant. The breakpoints for each drug can be obtained from published tables, which have been worked out taking into consideration both the corresponding M.I.C. of the organism and the blood levels attainable with normal dosage, and the distribution of zone sizes among species of known clinical responsiveness. The method uses mainly high content discs. Mueller-Hinton agar in plates 5-6 mm. deep, and carefully standardized inocula applied with a cotton wool swab, giving confluent growth. It must be stressed that the tables are only applicable if the method is followed *exactly;* full details are given by Anderson (1970).

4. THE I.C.S. METHOD is based on that devised by Ericsson (1960) and depends on the fact that for most antibiotics there is a linear relationship between the diameter of the zone of inhibition and the log of the M.I.C. A regression line is prepared by plotting the M.I.C. of at least 100 organisms of widely varying sensitivity against the diameter of the zone

produced by a high content disc, both tests being run simultaneously under similar controlled conditions. A regression line prepared by one of us for the International Working Party is illustrated in Figure 31. The zone given by an unknown organism tested in similar conditions can be converted

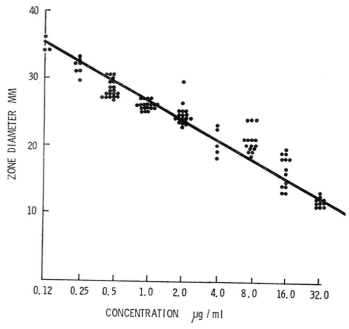

FIGURE 31

Regression line for kanamycin prepared by plotting the M.I.C. of 100 organisms against the diameter of the zone of inhibition produced by a 30 μg. disc.
(The organisms with an M.I.C. of 8 μg./ml. giving points consistently above the line, were Gram-positive cocci isolated from environmental studies. These usually grow more slowly than most pathogens and therefore produce larger zones of inhibition.)

into M.I.C. by reference to this line; M.I.C. are not reported but are translated into 4 categories of susceptibility which are based on M.I.C. and drug levels attainable *in vivo*. In practice regression lines are not referred to, zone diameters are measured with calipers which are then applied to scales which translate directly into the appropriate category.

Both the last two methods require a high degree of standardization if published break-points are to be applicable and it may be questioned whether this is attainable in the average diagnostic laboratory. There is no doubt that many laboratories find the preparation of the required dilutions of culture too time consuming to be acceptable. Unless both the size and distribution of the inoculum can be guaranteed, we feel that these methods may give a false sense of security. The break-points must also, to some extent, be a matter of individual opinion. A further difficulty is the availability of regression lines. These (or scales based on them) are required for every drug tested, and although the I.C.S. Report recommended their use, it did not provide them.

Common Sources of Error

PENICILLINASE-PRODUCING STAPHYLOCOCCI are resistant to penicillin by virtue of their ability to destroy the drug, but they may show quite large inhibition zones round a penicillin disc. These organisms can be identified by their appearance at the edge of the inhibition zone. Colonies are full-sized, giving a heaped-up edge (Fig. 36) in contrast to the smooth edge produced by colonies of diminishing size in the control culture. The same effect is seen with ampicillin. Such organisms should be reported as penicillinase-producing or resistant.

Tube dilution tests with these organisms are much affected by the size of the inoculum. The literature contains hundreds of reports to the effect that strains of resistant staphylococci were inhibited by certain concentrations of penicillin, often without specifying the size of the inoculum: without this information the concentration figure is meaningless.

METHICILLIN-RESISTANT STAPHYLOCOCCI. Cultures of most of these organisms contain only a small proportion of cells capable of appearing resistant if grown on normal medium and incubated at 37°C. for 18 hours, and resistance is often not obvious unless a heavy inoculum is used and incubation continued for 48 hours. It was shown by Barber (1964) that the addition of 5 per cent NaCl enabled the entire population of such cultures to grow on higher concentrations of methicillin. Disc tests on this medium usually give satisfactory results, though Hewitt,

Coe and Parker (1969) found some batches relatively inhibitory to resistant strains. A method using salt agar and requiring only 4 hours' incubation is given on p. 505.

Annear (1968) reported that enhanced and nearly uniform resistance was seen with ordinary medium if cultures were incubated at 30°C. for 18 hours, though this made little or no difference to sensitive strains (see Fig. 32). Hewitt, Coe and Parker (1969), who investigated this problem most thoroughly, concluded that this was the most dependable method and that practically all resistant strains will grow to within 1 mm. of a 10 μg. methicillin disc on nutrient agar, with or without blood, if incubated at 30°C. for 18 hours. It has recently been reported that the Kirby-Bauer method (see p. 498) gives reliable results when cultures are incubated at 35°C. (Drew et al., 1972). As there are no recognized contra-indications to maintaining diagnostic laboratory incubators at this temperature, it would seem that this is the easiest way of overcoming the problem of detecting methicillin resistance. It is essential that the temperature is adequately controlled and does not rise above 35°C., and that the inoculum is heavy.

Only methicillin should be tested. Although there is cross-resistance between methicillin, cloxacillin and flucloxacillin, both clinically and when tests are done by a dilution method, diffusion tests with cloxacillin and flucloxacillin do not always reveal resistance and should not be relied upon (Fig. 33). This phenomenon has recently been explained by Drew et al. (1972). They found that although the concentration of cloxacillin required totally to inhibit growth was similar to that of methicillin, nafcillin and oxacillin, the proportion of cells in the culture capable of surviving the intermediate concentrations was very much lower, 99·99 per cent being inhibited by 1·6 μg./ml. cloxacillin.

These authors also draw attention to the instability of methicillin discs, emphasizing the need for storing these in a refrigerator with a desiccant. They recommend the use of oxacillin in discs as this is more stable than methicillin and gives equally reliable results.

CEPHALORIDINE RESISTANCE in staphylococci is of a similar nature but the problem of detecting it is even greater. Although

cephaloridine is much more resistant to staphylococcal penicillinase than benzyl penicillin, some strains of staphylococci
can partially inactivate it, and if tested with a heavy inoculum
will appear resistant because of this. There is always cross-
resistance between methicillin, cloxacillin and the cephalosporins, and staphylococci proved to be resistant to methicillin
may be assumed to be resistant to the cephalosporins.

PROTEUS spp. Much confusion arises from the ability of some
strains to swarm into inhibition zones. Organisms taken from
inside the zone and re-tested are no more resistant than the
parent culture and as long as there is a clear edge to the zone,
measurements may be taken from this and swarming disregarded. See Figure 41.

CYCLOSERINE activity is depressed by D-alanine (see p. 198).
Results will therefore be affected by the content of this amino
acid in the medium and the M.I.C. may be high. In an
experiment using a commercial dehydrated medium, M.I.C.'s
ranged from 32 μg. per ml. for *Staph. aureus* and *E. coli* to
256-512 μg. per ml. for *Proteus* spp. and *Ps. aeruginosa*. The
drug is very unstable and solutions must be freshly prepared.

POLYMYXINS diffuse very poorly and though growth up to the
disc can safely be taken to indicate resistance, a zone of inhibition is only a very rough indication of sensitivity. Determinations of M.I.C. by tube dilution methods are much affected by
the medium; we have found that the most consistent results
are obtained using either nutrient agar or peptone water.

SULPHONAMIDES AND TRIMETHOPRIM are much affected by
the composition of the medium. Harper and Cawston (1945)
showed that many laboratory media contain substances which
inhibit the action of sulphonamides and that these could be
neutralized by the addition of lysed horse blood. Trimethoprim
is similarly affected and Koch and Burchall (1971) have shown
that this is due to the presence of thymidine or end-products
of folate metabolism, which enable bacteria to by-pass the
action of these drugs. Such media permit growth throughout
the zone of inhibition, colonies varying from very small to full
size. Oxoid Sensitest agar and Wellcome Wellcotest agar are
suitable for use with these drugs but Mueller-Hinton agar varies

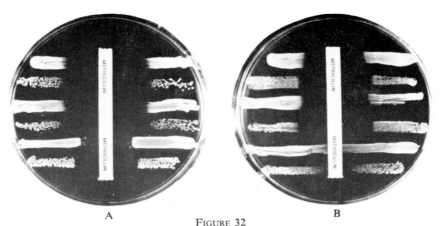

A   B

FIGURE 32

The use of blotting paper strips for testing sensitivity to methicillin.
Organisms (top to bottom)—Oxford staphylococcus, penicillinase-producing
Staph. aureus and a methicillin-resistant *Staph. aureus*, with a heavy and
light inoculum of each. Strips contain 100μg. methicillin.

A. Incubated overnight at 37°C. When the inoculum is heavy the zone of
the resistant strain is reduced and contains resistant colonies, but when the
inoculum is light there is a large zone of inhibition.

B. Incubated overnight at 30° C. The resistant strain grows up to the strip
from both heavy and light inocula.

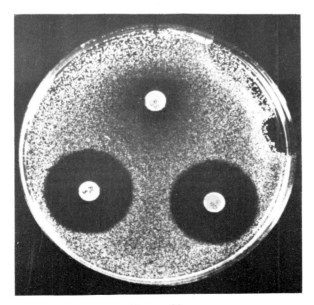

FIGURE 33

Disc sensitivity on a methicillin-resistant strain of *Staph. aureus* incubated
at 30° C. Discs contain: (top) methicillin 10 μg., (lower left) flucloxacillin
5 μg., (lower right) cloxacillin 5 μg. (See page 501) (Garrod and Waterworth,
1971).

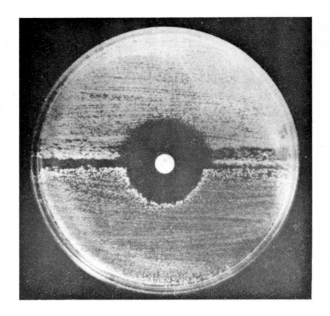

A

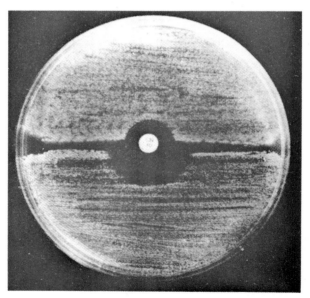

B

FIGURE 34

Effect of agar on the relative sensitivity of *Ps. aeruginosa* (top half of plate) and *E. coli* (lower half of plate) to gentamicin. Discs contain 10 μg.

A. Oxoid nutrient broth No. 2 solidified with Oxoid agar No. 1.
B. Oxoid nutrient broth No. 2 solidified with Oxoid agar No. 3.

Both the broth itself and agar No. 1 have a very low magnesium content so that *Ps. aeruginosa* appears highly sensitive to gentamicin. Agar No. 3 contains a considerable amount of magnesium and other minerals and its addition to the broth reduces the sensitivity of *Ps. aeruginosa* although that of *E. coli* is unaffected (see page 124). (Garrod and Waterworth, 1969).

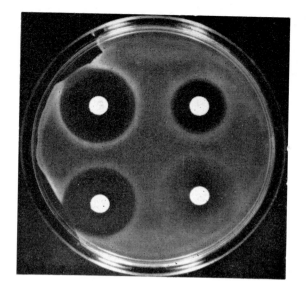

A

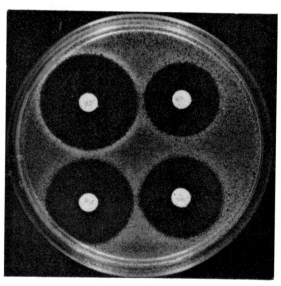

B

FIGURE 35

Effect of the size of inoculum on disc sensitivity tests. Discs contain: (top left) ampicillin 25 μg., (top right) kanamycin 30 μg., (lower left) tetracycline 30 μg., (lower right) sulphafurazole 100 μg.

A. Plate flooded with overnight broth culture of *E. coli*.
B. Plate flooded with the same culture of *E. coli* diluted 1 in 5000.

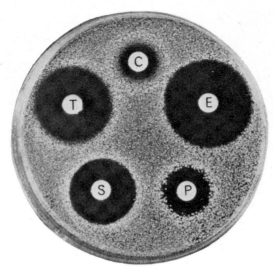

FIGURE 36

Disc sensitivity test on a strain of *Staph. aureus* inoculated to give 'dense but not confluent growth'. Colonies at the edge of the zone round the penicillin disc (P) are full-size, making an irregular edge and indicating that the strain produces penicillinase.

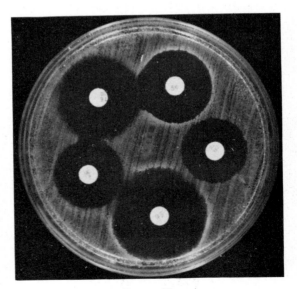

FIGURE 37

Plate inoculated with one loopful of an overnight broth culture of *E. coli* and spread with a dry swab.

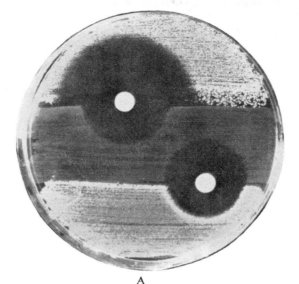

A

FIGURE 38A

The choice of control for disc tests on organisms of intermediate sensitivity.
A. Sensitivity of *Str. faecalis* (centre) to ampicillin. When isolated from the
urine it should be compared to the *Esch. coli* control (bottom), when it will
appear fully sensitive and the infection is likely to respond to normal doses.
If isolated from other parts of the body it should be compared with the
fully sensitive staphylococcal control (top) when it will be seen to be only
moderately sensitive and higher dosage will be required.
Discs—ampicillin 25 μg. (Waterworth, 1969b).

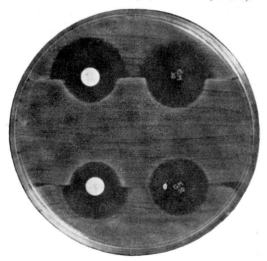

FIGURE 38B

B. Sensitivity of *Ps. aeruginosa* (centre) to carbenicillin and gentamicin. If
compared to the control *Esch. coli* (top) it appears moderately resistant to
both drugs, but when a standard strain of the same species (bottom) is used
as a control, the test strain is seen to have *normal sensitivity* to gentamicin
but increased resistance to carbenicillin.
Discs—Left—carbenicillin 100 μg. Right—gentamicin 30 μg.

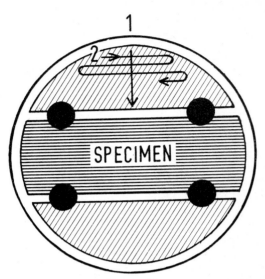

FIGURE 39

Diagram showing the preparation of a sensitivity test on a primary culture by the Stokes method.

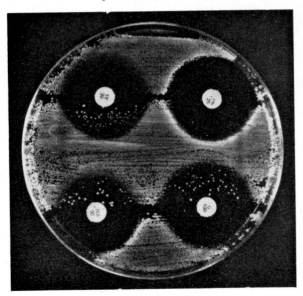

FIGURE 40

Sensitivity test on a primary culture of a specimen of urine. Growth consists mainly of *E. coli* but includes a smaller number of *Str. faecalis*, which are easily seen because of their resistance to three of the drugs tested. Discs contain: (top left) tetracycline 30 μg., (top right) ampicillin 25 μg., (lower left) nalidixic acid 30 μg., (lower right) sulphafurazole 100 μg.

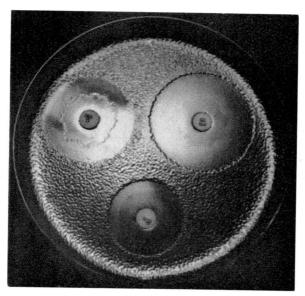

FIGURE 41

Sensitivity test on *P. mirabilis.* Discs contain: (top left) sulphafurazole 100 μg., (top right) ampicillin 25 μg., (bottom) kanamycin 30 μg. Note swarming into the zones. So long as there is a clear shoulder to the zone, swarming within it can be disregarded (see page 502).

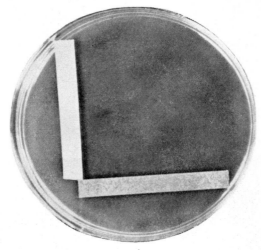

A

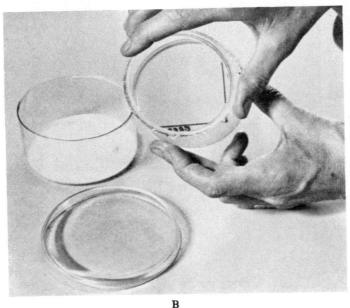

B

FIGURE 42 A and B

The cellophane transfer method.

A. Blotting paper strips containing antibiotic applied to nutrient agar and the antibiotic allowed to diffuse out.

B. Sterile tambour applied to the plate after the strips have been removed.

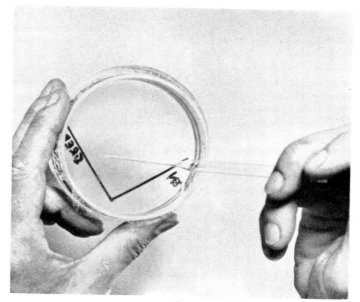

C

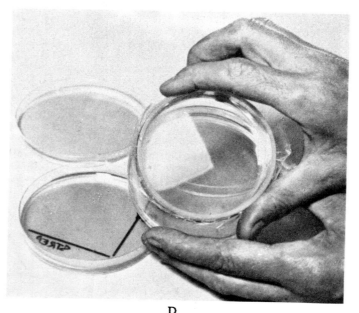

D

FIGURE 42 C and D

C. The inside of the tambour is flooded with bacterial suspension.
D. After incubation the tambour is transferred to antibiotic-free
medium. Note that the growth is on the cellophane, the plate to
which it had been applied remaining sterile.

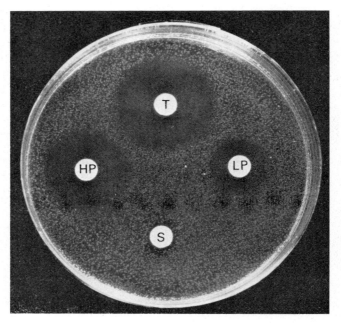

FIGURE 43 A

Fig. 43 A-D. Disc tests and tests by the cellophane transfer method on a strain of *Str. faecalis* isolated from a patient (G. F.) with bacterial endocarditis.

A. Disc test showing high bacteristatic sensitivity to tetracycline (T), moderate resistance to penicillin (P, LP=1·5 units, HP=5 units) and resistance to streptomycin (S).

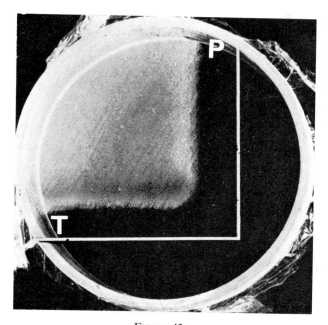

FIGURE 43 B

B. Tambour after overnight incubation on a plate into which penicillin and tetracycline had been pre-diffused from blotting paper strips. This shows bacteristatic sensitivity.

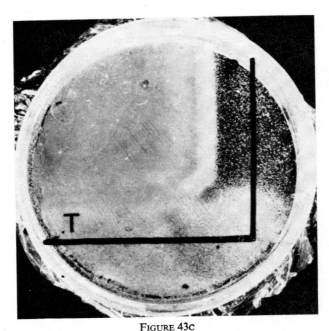

FIGURE 43c

C. The same tambour after a further 24 hours' incubation on antibiotic-free medium. Tetracycline alone was purely bacteristatic. Penicillin alone killed most of the inoculum but left some survivors. Where both drugs are present in the area round the angle formed by the strips, the tetracycline has eliminated the bactericidal effect of the penicillin (antagonism).

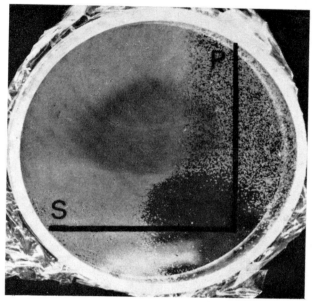

FIGURE 43D

D. Tambour after incubation on antibiotic-free medium following exposure to penicillin and streptomycin. Penicillin alone left survivors, streptomycin alone was barely inhibitory. The presence of both drugs sterilized the inoculum (synergy).

This patient, a man of 71, had been ill for 9 months and had received many courses of antibiotics, always relapsing after treatment was stopped. As a result of these tests he made a complete recovery following treatment with penicillin and streptomycin. A re-infection with the same organism 9 months later was again successfully treated with this combination and the patient remained free from infection until his death 9 years later.

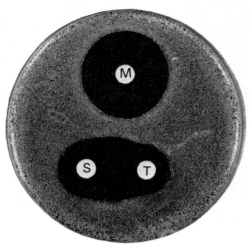

FIGURE 44

Bacteristatic synergy between trimethoprim and sulphonamide against a strain of *Pr. morgani*. Discs contain: T—trimethoprim 2·5 μg. S—sulphafurazole 50 μg. M—the same amount of both.

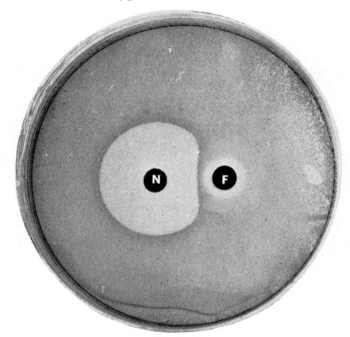

FIGURE 45

Bacteristatic antagonism between nitrofurantoin (F) and nalidixic acid (N) against *Pr. rettgeri*.

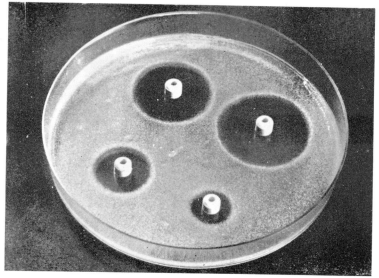

FIGURE 46

' Fish-spines ' containing antibiotic solutions on an agar plate seeded with
S. lutea.

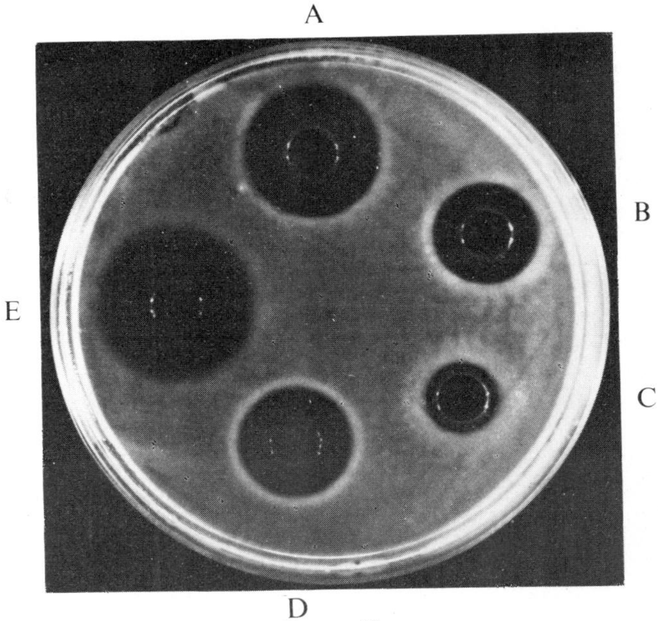

A

E

B

C

D
FIGURE 47

Five hour gentamicin assay using a fast-growing *Klebsiella*. Cups A, B and C contain gentamicin standards in serum (10, 2 and 0·4 μg./ml.). Cups D and E contain sera from patients receiving gentamicin and the specimens were collected immediately before the next dose was due. The zone round E is larger than that given by the 10 μg./ml. standard and the appearance of the zone edge is different from those round the other cups. This patient was said not to be receiving any other drugs, but enquiry revealed that treatment had now been changed to co-trimoxazole, and the first dose had been given 1½ hours before the blood was collected.

considerably (Garrod and Waterworth, 1971) and requires the addition of 4 per cent lysed horse blood. This addition is also necessary with Oxoid D.S.T. agar.

Sulphonamides are inactivated by *p*-aminobenzoic acid and sensitivity tests are invalidated by a heavy inoculum (which contains enough *p*-aminobenzoic acid to inactivate the drug). Zones are not just reduced; they disappear completely (Fig. 35). If these tests are over-inoculated resistance cannot be assumed; the test must be repeated. Among the more active sulphonamides, it matters very little which is used : results obtained with one apply with little difference to others, with the possible exception of some strains of *Ps. aeruginosa*, against which sulphadiazine has greater activity than other sulphonamides. As a result some strains may give a zone of inhibition round a 300 μg. sulphatriad disc (which contains sulphadiazine) though appearing resistant to sulphafurazole and cotrimoxazole. We do not believe this difference to be clinically significant.

The M.I.C. of trimethoprim for a number of organisms known to respond to treatment covers an unusually wide range and this presents some technical problems. *E. coli,* normally used for the more resistant urinary control, is one of the most sensitive species (M.I.C. 0·12 μg./ml.) : thus not only are very large zones produced with this organism, but also many potentially treatable organisms (*e.g. Proteus,* M.I.C. 1-2 μg./ml.) must appear significantly more resistant than the control. This can only be overcome either by using a special control for this drug (*e.g. Pr. morgani* or *Klebsiella* with an M.I.C. of 1 μg./ml.), or by modifying the interpretation of the test.

Synergy between trimethoprim and sulphonamide can be demonstrated either by placing discs containing each drug singly about 15 mm. apart, when the zones may coalesce by extension, or by showing that a zone produced by a disc containing both drugs is larger than that given by the same amount of each singly (Fig. 44). It cannot be shown using only one disc containing both drugs. The practical value of such tests is questionable. Synergy will only be seen if the drugs are present in the ratio appropriate for the organism being tested; therefore failure to demonstrate it does not mean that it will not occur. It is preferable to test both drugs separately. An

17

organism should only be reported as sensitive to cotrimoxazole when there is at least a small zone round *each* disc.

Further information concerning the *in vitro* activity of tri-methoprim can be found in the following papers: Bushby and Hitchings (1968), Darrell, Garrod and Waterworth (1968), Bushby (1969), Waterworth (1969a).

ANTI-FUNGAL DRUGS. As an increasing number of these drugs becomes available there is a greater demand for sensitivity tests. These can best be done by the dilution method and glucose-peptone broth or agar is satisfactory for all except 5-fluorocytosine. This is neutralized by the constituents of ordinary media but tests can be done in yeast nitrogen base (Difco) with 0·15 per cent asparagine and 1 per cent dextrose added and the pH brought to 7·4 (Shadomy, 1969). A sensitive strain of *C. albicans* can be used as a control for tests of most of these drugs except griseofulvin.

SENSITIVITY TESTS IN PRIMARY CULTURES

Diffusion tests can be incorporated in primary culture. These tests have advantages, of which the foremost are speed and simplicity; they also reveal the presence of small numbers of resistant organisms (Fig. 40); and often facilitate the identification of organisms present in mixed cultures because of the selective action on different species.

The method is particularly suitable for swabs of pus, and for urine specimens which have been shown by direct microscopy, or other methods (Thomas and Baldwin, 1971), to be infected. If anaerobes are expected, sensitivity tests should also be carried out anaerobically. The method given below (Stokes, 1968, Fig. 39) has the advantage that each disc has a control, making direct comparison easy and the results more reliable. Figure 40 illustrates such a culture.

If the specimen is a swab inoculate a broad area across the middle of the plate with this as evenly as possible. If it is urine, transfer 1 loopful to the plate and spread this with a dry sterile swab. The inoculum will usually be too heavy if the swab is dipped in the urine. Spread a loopful of control culture over each of the remaining areas with a dry swab, or alternatively, use a pre-inoculated swab (see p. 496) leaving not more than 5 mm. between control and test areas of inoculation. Place 4 discs in these gaps between the 2 inocula, each about 1 cm. from the edge of the plate: inhibition zones will then be formed in both control and test cultures.

If whole plates are used for the specimen, zones must be compared with those given by the control organism on a separate plate inoculated in the same way.

The main objection is the difficulty of controlling the size of the inoculum and whilst a number of tests will have to be repeated because the inoculum was too heavy or too light, allowance can be made for small variations and a surprisingly large proportion can be reported the day after receipt of the specimen.

It must be borne in mind that penicillinase-producing staphylococci destroy penicillin and may thus make a sensitive organism also present in a mixed culture appear resistant. Similarly, chloramphenicol may be inactivated by organisms which are resistant to it and other organisms present may then grow on a concentration which is normally inhibitory (Waterworth, 1966). In such cases the test should be repeated on a pure culture.

Suitable drugs for testing are given in Table 47.

Rapid Methods on Pure Cultures

To obtain a pure suspension takes at least one day, but the test itself can be made to occupy less time by employing a colour indicator of early growth. In a tube dilution test this may simply be a pH indicator in a medium containing glucose, or methylene blue, resazurin or a tetrazolium salt. Gillissen and Becher (1957) favour the last-named, and define conditions for its use. An alternative is to place antibiotic discs on an inoculated layer of blood agar and cover this with plain agar: growth reduces the haemoglobin except in the zones of inhibition. Fust and Böhni (1961) read the results of such a test after six hours: Davis (1959) claims for his modification of it that a two-hour reading may be possible. In view of the problems of testing for methicillin resistance (p. 500), the method recently devised by Kensit and Simmons (1973) for use with this drug is particularly interesting. Triphenyltetrazolium chloride (TTC) is added to salt agar with a very heavy inoculum and the result can be read in about 4 hours.

The method can be used for other antibiotics if the salt is omitted from the medium.

THE CHOICE OF DRUGS TO BE TESTED

The increasing array of chemotherapeutic agents available makes it impossible to test them all and it is better to test a few suitable ones well than to report many unreliably. It must be remembered that hospital use of antibiotics is greatly influenced by laboratory reports and the unnecessary use of potentially toxic drugs should not be encouraged by indiscriminate reporting of sensitivity to them. If primary sensitivity tests are done it is usually sufficient to test 4 as in the Stokes method, further tests being done if the organism is resistant to more than 2. In emergencies 8 or more may be included on the primary culture. The 4 drugs to be tested should be agreed with the clinicians and can be varied to suit individual preferences. Suitable drugs for different types of specimens and bacterial species are given in Table 47.

The number of tests required can be cut down by testing only one representative of the following closely related groups, within which there is almost always cross-resistance: tetracyclines (tetracycline), sulphonamides (sulphafurazole), polymyxins (polymyxin B sulphate), cephalosporins (cephaloridine), penicillinase-resistant penicillins (methicillin), rifamycins (rifamide). There are some minor exceptions to these rules: e.g. ampicillin-resistant enterobacteria, may sometimes be resistant to cephaloridine and cephalothin but sensitive to cephalexin (Waterworth, 1971). If gentamicin is preferred to kanamycin clinically, there seems little point in testing the latter except for local treatment: kanamycin should then be tested in preference to neomycin, which gives less reliable results with staphylococci (Waterworth, 1966). Drugs inapplicable to the specimen (*e.g.* nitrofurantoin for organisms for any source but urine) or unsuited to the method should not be tested. It was pointed out by Waterworth (1962) that laboratory sensitivity tests with methenamine mandelate (Mandelamine) are misleading, because its anti-bacterial activity is dependent on the liberation of formaldehyde, which only occurs in an acid environment. Solutions of methenamine mandelate from which discs are prepared are highly acid, so that disc tests only show the sensitivity of organisms to formalin. Waterworth (1962) found that in such tests, strains of *Proteus*

Choice of Drugs for Sensitivity Tests

	Penicillin	Methicillin	Ampicillin	Carbenicillin	Cephaloridine	Erythromycin	Lincomycin Clindamycin	Fucidin	Tetracycline	Chloramphenicol	Streptomycin	Kanamycin	Gentamicin	Polymyxin	Sulphonamide	Trimethoprim	Nitrofurantoin*	Nalidixic Acid*
Primary Cultures																		
Pus	1					1	1		1				1					
Sputum			1			2	2		1	2					1	1		
Urine			1						2	3	2	2	2		1	1	1	1
Sub-culture																		
Staphylococcus	1	1			2	1	1	2	1		2	2	2		2	2		
Streptococcus	1					1	1		1						1	1		
Haemophilus			1		1	2	2		1	2								
Bacteroides						1	1		1	2								
Escherichia			1		2				1	2	2	2	1	2	1	1	1	1
Klebsiella					1				2			1	1	2	1	1	1	1
Proteus				1	1						2	2	2		1	1	1	1
Salmonella			1							2	1	2	2		1	1		
Shigella			1							1	1	2	2		1	1		
Pseudomonas				1							1		1	1				

* Applicable only to organisms from the urine. Figures indicate order of priority.

species were among the most sensitive organisms, whereas infections of the urinary tract due to *Proteus* are among the least susceptible to the drug because of the high alkalinity they produce in the urine.

DILUTION METHODS

These methods are too time-consuming for general use. Indications for them are:

1. When dosage is to be based on determination of the minimum inhibitory (or bactericidal) concentration, as in the treatment of bacterial endocarditis.

2. For tests of slowly growing organisms, notably *Myco. tuberculosis* and *Actinomyces israeli*.

3. For demonstrating small degrees of acquired bacterial resistance.

Tube Dilution Test

With the exception of tests with *Myco. tuberculosis* (see below) these tests are usually performed with fluid medium, and as with diffusion tests, results will be affected by both its composition and pH. The size of the inoculum is less critical but should be comparable to that used in diffusion tests and about 10^5 organisms per ml is satisfactory (*i.e.* 1 drop of a $1/100$ dilution of an overnight broth culture) to 1 ml. volumes.

DETERMINATION OF M.I.C. Prepare 2 sets of two-fold dilutions of the antibiotic in broth (5% serum may be added if necessary for the growth of the organism). Inoculate one set with 1 drop of an overnight broth culture of the test organism diluted $1/100$ (if growth is sparse the dilution should be reduced). Inoculate the second set of tubes with a similar number of a suitable control organism. Incubate overnight.

Assuming that the control is inhibited by the correct concentration, the M.I.C. of the test organism is taken as the lowest concentration showing no visible growth.

The same method can be used for determining the minimum bactericidal concentration (M.B.C.). In this case the inoculum should be heavier than for the determination of the MIC and 1 drop of a $1/10$ dilution of an overnight broth culture is usually satisfactory.

DETERMINATION OF M.B.C. Dilutions are prepared as for M.I.C. but in this case the control tube containing no antibiotic is subcultivated immediately after inoculaton by spreading a loopful as evenly as possible over ¼ of a plate of suitable medium. The test is then incubated overnight and any tubes showing no growth are sub-cultivated in the same way and any growth compared to that given by the control before incubation.

Sub-cultures may show : —

1. Growth similar to that from the control before incubation —bacteristatic action only.

2. Small number of colonies—incomplete bactericidal action.

3. Sterility—total bactericidal action.

Agar Dilution Method

If many strains are to be tested, dilutions can be prepared in agar plates, when a number of strains can be tested on each. A solid medium also has the advantage that it reveals whether the whole inoculum has grown or only a few cells.

Prepare a range of double-dilutions of the drug in water, twenty times the final strengths required in agar. Place 1 ml. of each in previously labelled Petri dishes. Add to each 19 ml. melted agar (cooled to about 60°C.) and mix well. Allow to set and dry well at 37°C. with the lids tipped. Inoculate with a loop or multiple replicator with broth culture diluted approximately 1/100.

Preparation of Stock Solutions

Tablets and capsules should not be used to prepare solutions: they contain binding materials, ' fillers ' and other materials as well as the antibiotic. The pure substance must be obtained, and is available for many antibiotics in preparations supplied for injection. Many antibiotics are highly soluble: for those which are not there are special preparations for injection and these are suitable for laboratory purposes with the following exceptions : —

CHLORAMPHENICOL. Chloramphenicol succinate has little activity *in vitro*. Chloramphenicol powder is available and should be used but has a solubility of only 2·5 mg./ml. in water. Pure chloramphenicol powder can be dissolved to give 10 mg. per ml. in ethyl alcohol.

FUCIDIN AND CYCLOSERINE are not available as injection preparations. The pure substances should be obtained from the manufacturers : both are freely soluble in water.

ERYTHROMYCIN LACTOBIONATE (injection preparation) may be used but if erythromycin base is used this must first be dissolved to give 10 mg. per ml. in ethyl alcohol, after which it may be diluted in water.

NYSTATIN is insoluble in water, but owing to its very fine particle size it can be used as a suspension. It is very unstable and must be freshly prepared.

SULPHONAMIDES, NITROFURANTOIN AND NALIDIXIC ACID all have a low solubility in water but can be brought into solution by raising the pH. The drug should be suspended in the appropriate volume of water and 10N NaOH added a drop at a time until the solution is clear. Sodium nitrofurantoin, which is freely soluble in water, can be obtained for laboratory use from Eaton Laboratories.

TRIMETHOPRIM is available from the manufacturers. The lactate is soluble in water and the base can be brought into solution by lowering the pH with lactic acid.

POLYMYXINS. The sulphomethyl form of both polymyxin B and colistin (polymyxin E) is unsuitable for sensitivity testing (see p. 185): the sulphate should be used.

RIFAMPICIN has a low solubility in water but dissolves readily in N/100 HCl.

AUTOMATED METHODS

The simplest form of automation is that practised by the group of hospitals included in the Department of Medical Microbiology in the University of Toronto. One or two concentrations of each drug are added to agar and plates poured in bulk: these may be stored for at least 1 week at 4°C. without loss of activity (Ryan *et al.*, 1970). These, together with plates of any media required for the identification of species are inoculated with a multiple replicator from broth cultures made from primary cultures earlier in the day. Any number of concentrations can, of course, be used, and the method has the advantage that it is much less affected by the size of the inoculum than are diffusion methods

In the United States there is currently much interest in fully mechanized procedures, both for testing single concentrations of multiple drugs in broth and for the determination of M.I.C. in broth by microtitre methods. In the latter, using as little as 50 μl. volumes in wells in plastic trays, results are read in the usual way. In the former, when pre-seeded broth is automatically distributed in wells either containing antibiotic, or to which a disc is added, results are read automatically after only short incubation. Some of these machines are now undergoing trials in the United States, meanwhile an excellent account of the present position is given by Schoenknecht and Sherris (1973).

SENSITIVITY TESTS FOR MYCO. TUBERCULOSIS

So many drugs are now available for the treatment of tuberculosis that most laboratories either use the ready-made sensitivity sets commercially available or send their cultures to special centres.

Tests are done by the tube dilution method, usually with double dilutions in Löwenstein-Jensen medium. The inoculum must be carefully standardized and a duplicate set of slopes inoculated similarly with H37Rv. Cultures are incubated for 14 days or until a control slope containing no drug shows good growth.

INOCULUM. Standardization of the size of the inoculum is important. About 2 cu. mm. (judged by eye) representative growth from a primary diagnostic Löwenstein-Jensen slope, is transferred with a wire loop to 0·5 ml. sterile distilled water in a ¼ oz. screw-capped bottle containing 6 (3 mm.) glass beads. A suspension is prepared by shaking for 1 minute and a full 3 mm. loopful is then spread over the surface of each slope.

This procedure should only be carried out by trained personnel in a suitably ventilated cabinet. Tests must be done not more than 2 weeks after the culture has become positive and subcultures of H37Rv must not be more than 4 weeks old.

The M.I.C. is taken as the lowest concentration yielding <20 colonies and the result reported as the resistance ratio, obtained by dividing the M.I.C. for the test organism by that for the H37Rv. A ratio of 8:1 indicates resistance; if 4:1 the test should be repeated and i fthe result is confirmed it should be reported as resistant.

Some drugs are unstable. Clark (1967) found that ethionamide lost activity even when stored at 4° C, and at 18° C isoniazid and cycloserine also deteriorated. All drug-containing media should therefore be supplied marked with an expiry date and it is essential not only that this be observed but also that all tubes used for both test and control bear the same date.

In the Proportion Method, viable counts of a culture of the test organism are done on both drug-containing and drug-free media and the proportion of the culture found to be resistant reported. This method is not recommended for routine laboratories; full details of both this and the resistance ratio method can be found in the paper by Canetti *et al.* (1963).

TESTS OF COMBINED ACTION

These are chiefly of interest for the purpose of identifying a synergic combination for treating a difficult and serious infection, such as an endocarditis due to a streptococcus relatively resistant to penicillin. Total bactericidal effect must be the aim in such treatment: anything short of this may fail, and merely bacteristatic action, in however low a concentration, is notoriously incapable of eliminating the infection. Sensitivity tests must therefore reveal whether the organism has been killed or merely prevented from growing.

Tests in Liquid Medium with Subculture

Tubes of liquid medium containing each antibiotic alone and in all combinations are heavily inoculated, incubated overnight and sub-cultivated on suitable solid medium to determine whether the inoculum has been killed. The result of the test is much affected by the size of the inoculum: if it is very large nothing will sterilize it, but if too small results will be unduly optimistic. The final test mixtures should contain about 10^6 organisms per ml.

TESTS OF COMBINED ACTION. Each antibiotic is added to broth singly and in all possible combinations, using a single concentration of each attainable in the blood (conveniently 10 μg. per ml.). If a number of drugs are to be tested, tubes can conveniently be arranged in the form of a 'half chess board' (Fig. 48). Prepare solutions of each antibiotic containing 100 μg. per ml. and pipette 0·5 ml. of each into the appropriate rows of tubes. Add 4 ml. broth pre-inoculated to contain 10^6 organisms per ml. (i.e. about 5 drops of undiluted overnight broth culture to 100 ml. broth) to each tube containing 2 antibiotics and 4·5 ml. to those with only one. Shake well. Subcultivate a control tube containing no antibiotic on suitable solid medium. After overnight incubation subcultivate any tubes showing no growth; incubate overnight.

Bulger and Nielson (1968) studied the bactericidal action of antibiotic combinations in both Mueller-Hinton broth and human serum with almost identical results. They recommend sub-cultivating the test mixtures by preparing a pour-plate from 0·001 ml. delivered by a calibrated loop, after only 4 hours' incubation.

Sub-cultures are interpreted as in determinations of M.B.C. (page 509). The disadvantages of the method are:

1. Only one concentration of each drug is tested. 2. Only a minute proportion of the original inoculum is sub-cultivated. 3. If the organism is highly sensitive, growth of surviving cells may be inhibited by carry-over of antibiotic on sub-culture. This can be partially overcome by placing a loopful of each mixture on a marked area of a plate and allowing the fluid to be absorbed before thoroughly spreading over a wider area. Colonies may then surround a sterile area.

Velvet Pad Replica Plate

In this method, devised by Elek and Hilson (1954), a wooden block cut to fit into a Petri dish is covered with sterile velvet. The pad so formed is first pressed firmly onto an ordinary disc sensitivity test which has been incubated overnight, and then on to a plate of fresh medium. This is incubated overnight and any colonies appearing within the inhibition zones represent survivors from the original inoculum· Combined action can be studied either by placing discs side by side or by using blotting paper strips set at right angles to each other. The disadvantage of the method is that the velvet pad transfers only about 0·5 per cent of the cells present.

Cellophane Transfer Method

This method, originally described by Chabbert and his colleagues and fully described by Garrod and Waterworth (1962) and Chabbert and Waterworth (1965) requires special apparatus and some practice for its proper execution, but its results are remarkably revealing. A cellophane tambour, inoculated on the inside with the test organism, is placed on a plate into which antibiotics have been pre-diffused from blotting paper strips placed at right angles. Nutrients and antibiotics diffuse through the cellophane to permit growth on the inside of the tambour, the plate remaining sterile. After a period of incubation the tambour is transferred to a plate of normal medium and any bacteria surviving in the inhibition zones will then grow. The final culture will show the bactericidal effect of each drug alone at the ends of each strip and their combined action in the area surrounding the angle where the strips meet.

TECHNIQUE. Immerse 0·5 × 5 cm. strips of sterile blotting paper in antibiotic solution (Table 48), remove excess fluid by lightly blotting on sterile blotting paper and place at right angles on a plate of suitable medium (Fig. 42A). Allow to diffuse at 37°C. for 5 hours or overnight at 4°C.

Tambours are prepared by stretching cellophane PT 300 (commercially available as jam pot covers) across a pyrex glass ring 8 cm. in diameter and 2·5 cm. high* and securing it with a strong rubber band. The cellophane should first be softened to permit stretching; with the present day material it is usually sufficient to wet it in cold water, but if necessary this can be brought to the boil. Tambours must not be allowed to dry before use; they should be placed in glass pots with the cellophane resting on moist filter paper and sterilized by autoclaving for 10 min. at 121°C.

Remove the strips from the plate and apply the tambour to the surface, taking care to avoid trapping any air between the medium and the cellophane. Flood the inside of the tambour with a suspension of the organism containing about 10^7 organisms per ml., removing any surplus with a Pasteur pipette. Place the culture in the incubator with the lid tipped until the surface of the cellophane is dry, then remove the lid and continue incubation overnight with the culture inverted over clean blotting paper (see Figs. 42A-D).

Transfer the tambour to a well-dried plate of suitable medium containing no antibiotic and incubate a further 24 hours.

Some antibiotics, particularly those heavily protein-bound, are carried over by the cellophane and if the concentration in the medium is too high, sufficient may be carried over to prevent growth of the surviving organisms. Suitable solutions for preparing the strips are given in Table 48.

Choice of Antibiotics

The tests are made unnecessarily laborious if unsuitable drugs are tested. Table 49 gives the antibiotics most likely to have bactericidal activity against most of the common infections. The bactericidal action of penicillins is always antagonized by the presence of a bacteristatic antibiotic and even if the organism has been shown to be highly sensitive to tetracycline or chloramphenicol, it is a waste of time to include either in bactericidal tests with penicillins. On the other hand, penicillin and streptomycin, gentamicin or kanamycin may act

* Obtainable from Stanmore Surgical Company, 62 Lamorna Grove, Stanmore, Middlesex

synergically against streptococci even though the strain is relatively resistant to any or all of them (see p. 105). These combinations should always be included when testing streptococci (see Fig. 43). Penicillin-resistant streptococci other than enterococci may be sensitive to cephaloridine (Tozer, Boutflower and Gillespie, 1966), and this should be included in tests of such organisms.

It is generally agreed that rifampicin should not be used indiscriminately because of the risk of unknowingly producing

TABLE 48

Solutions recommended for preparation of blotting paper strips (μg. per ml.)

*Ampicillin	50	Kanamycin	1000
Carbenicillin	1000	Lincomycin	200
*Cephaloridine	50	Methicillin	1000
Chloramphenicol	1000	*Penicillin	50
Clindamycin	200	Rifamide	50
Cloxacillin	200	Streptomycin	1000
Erythromycin	200	Tetracycline	200
Fucidin	50	Vancomycin	1000
Gentamicin	100		

* Use 500 μg. per ml. if testing enterococci and Gram-negative bacilli.

N.B. Closely related drugs vary and it should not be assumed that the same concentrations will apply.

Based on Chabbert & Waterworth (1965).

resistance in tubercle bacilli. Nevertheless, as Peard *et al.* (1970) have shown, it can be invaluable in life-endangering staphylococcal infection where other treatment has failed. Resistant cells are present in most cultures of staphylococci and if bactericidal tests are done in fluid media, tubes must be sub-cultivated after 4 or 6 hours as growth of resistant organisms may occur later. Either rifamide or rifampicin can be used for *in vitro* tests; the former is preferable as it is readily soluble in water and less carried over by cellophane.

Fucidin and methicillin or cloxacillin are commonly antagonistic (see p. 201). Polymyxin is very heavily carried over by cellophane and must be tested by the tube dilution method.

Interpretation of Results

Combined bactericidal tests can show any of three results:

1. Indifference—the action of the two drugs together is no greater than that of the more active alone.

2. Antagonism—the bactericidal effect of one is reduced by the presence of the other.

3. Synergy—neither drug alone is completely bactericidal but the two together sterilize the inoculum.

TABLE 49

COMBINATIONS OF DRUGS LIKELY TO SHOW
BACTERICIDAL SYNERGY

Streptococci		
penicillin, cephalosporins or erythromycin	+	streptomycin, kanamycin or gentamicin
Staphylococci		
methicillin or a cephalosporin	+	streptomycin, gentamicin or kanamycin
streptomycin, gentamicin or kanamycin	+	erythromycin or clindamycin
rifamide	+	erythromycin or fucidin
Gram-negative bacilli		
ampicillin, carbenicillin or a cephalosporin	+	streptomycin gentamicin or kanamycin

Antagonism between penicillin and tetracycline and synergy between penicillin and streptomycin against *Str. faecalis* are demonstrated by the cellophane transfer method in Figure 43. Similar results obtained by the broth dilution method are given in the ' half chess board ' illustrated in Figure 48.

Ideally the drugs recommended for the treatment of endocarditis will have been shown to be totally bactericidal *in vitro*. If this has not been achieved other combinations should be tried before finally choosing that which shows the smallest number of survivors.

The cellophane transfer method is a severer test of performance than the broth dilution test, and it is not uncommon for sub-cultures from the latter to be sterile although there are survivors from the same drug on the tambour. This is probably due mainly to the small amount of the inoculum sub-cultivated from the fluid cultures.

	Penicillin	Streptomycin	Tetracycline	Erythromycin	Kanamycin
Penicillin	+	−	+ +	+	−
Streptomycin		+ + +	+ +	+	+ +
Tetracycline			+ +	+	+ +
Erythromycin				+	+
Kanamycin					+ +

FIGURE 48

'Half Chess Board' bactericidal sensitivity test. Tubes containing each drug singly and in all combinations are arranged as above and results of sub-cultures recorded as follows. Broth itself turbid ' + + + '. Numbers of colonies approximately equal to the original inoculum ' + + '. Marked reduction in the number of colonies '+'; '−' = no growth.

Tests of Combined Bacteristatic Action

The combined effects described above cannot be demonstrated by discs containing mixtures of antibiotics, since these reflect only the activity of the more active or more diffusible.

The modern practice of testing many discs on a single plate has revealed a number of bacteristatic interactions between drugs placed next to each other. The best known are the synergy between polymyxin and sulphonamides or trimethoprim against *Proteus* spp. and the antagonism between nitrofurantoin and nalidixic acid against various organisms (see p. 283). The synergy between trimethoprim and sulphonamides is of much greater importance and is discussed on page 503 (see Fig. 44). Bacteristatic antagonism is shown in Figs 15 and 45.

ANTIBIOTIC ASSAYS IN BODY FLUIDS

These are perhaps less often performed than they should be, and can be useful for two main purposes, apart from studying the absorption, distribution and excretion of a new drug.

1. To verify that adequate concentrations are being attained, as in the blood when absorption from the alimentary tract may be defective, or in the cerebro-spinal fluid during the treatment of meningitis.

2. To guard against excessive blood levels, particularly of antibiotics liable to damage the eighth nerve (streptomycin, gentamicin, kanamycin, vancomycin) in patients with any impairment of renal function.

The interval between the collection of the blood and the last dose is important and should be stated. If the level is being determined for the second reason, blood should be taken immediately before the next dose is due. Peak levels vary greatly and when high do not necessarily indicate delayed excretion as does a significant level at the end of the interval between doses (Line, Poole and Waterworth, 1970). It is obviously essential to know whether any other antibiotic is being given, but this information is only too often omitted. It should also be remembered that blood from a patient with impaired renal function may still contain an antibiotic given a week or more earlier.

Assays may be done by tube dilution or diffusion methods. A variety of organisms recommended for different antibiotics are listed in Table 50. Spore suspensions are particularly satisfactory for plate diffusion methods. They can be produced in bulk, standardized and stored in small volumes at 4°C.; they keep indefinitely and are always ready for use. A single suspension of *B. subtilis* can be used for penicillins (except carbenicillin), cephalosporins, all aminoglycosides, erythromycin, lincomycins, and vancomycin. In an emergency any antibiotic can be assayed against either the *Staph. aureus* or *E. coli* used as sensitivity test controls.

PREPARATION OF SPORE SUSPENSIONS. Grow cultures on agar, preferably in Roux Bottles, for 1 week at 37°C. (30°C. for *B. cereus*). Suspend the growth in sterile distilled water and heat for 30 minutes at 65°C. Wash the spores in water and resuspend in water. Suspensions will keep at 4°C. indefinitely.

SUSPENSIONS OF VEGETATIVE ORGANISMS can be prepared from broth cultures (if not granular) or by suspending growth from solid medium in broth. They will keep at 4°C. for up to 4 weeks or may be stored indefinitely at −70°C. or in liquid nitrogen.

TABLE 50

Appropriate Organisms for Assaying Antibacterial Drugs

Drug	Organism	NCTC Number	Optimum pH
Penicillins Cephaloridine	*Staph. aureus* *S. lutea* *B. subtilis*	6571 8340 8236	6·8
* Carbenicillin	*Ps. aeruginosa*	10490	
Streptomycin	*Staph. aureus* *Kl. pneumoniae* *B. subtilis*	6571 7242 8236	7·8
Kanamycin Gentamicin	*Staph. aureus* *B. subtilis*	6571 8236	
Tetracycline	*B. cereus* *Staph. aureus*	10320 6571	6·6
Chloramphenicol	*Esch. coli* *S. lutea*	10418 8340	
Erythromycin Lincomycin	*Staph. aureus* *B. subtilis*	6571 8236	7·8 7·8
Fucidin	*C. xerosis*	9755	6·6
Vancomycin	*Staph. aureus* *B. subtilis*	6571 8236	7·8
Polymyxins	*Bord. bronchiseptica* *Esch. coli*	8344 10418	7·3
Anti-fungal	*Sacch. cerevisiae* *C. albicans*	10716	7·3
Trimethoprim	*B. pumilis*	8241	7·3

* Usually contains traces of benzylpenicillin and must therefore be assayed against an organism resistant to this.

18

Stock solutions may be prepared in water but standards used for assaying serum must be prepared in serum. Ideally pooled human serum should be used, but that collected from blood sent for serological examination is not suitable, as some of the patients concerned may be receiving antibiotics. If human serum of known origin is not available, horse serum should be used. If the specimen is plasma, standards should also be in plasma (Sabath *et al.*, 1970).

When assaying urine, the pH of the specimen must first be brought to the optimum for the drug concerned (Table 50). The standard solutions and any dilutions of the unknown should be prepared in buffer of the same pH.

The aminoglycosides, vancomycin and chloramphenicol are all very stable and solutions can be kept frozen for several months: other antibiotics must be freshly prepared.

Plate Diffusion Methods

In these methods the size of the inhibition zones produced by the unknown fluid is compared with a graph of the sizes of inhibition zones produced by known concentrations of the antibiotic. There is a linear relationship between the diameter of the zone and the log of the concentration so that 3 standards are usually sufficient; suitable concentrations for some common drugs are given in Table 51. The standards and the unknown, diluted when necessary, are applied to seeded agar plates; any of various methods of application can be used. Zones from the standards are measured and plotted against concentration on semi-log paper. The resulting line should be straight; when assays are done by inexperienced workers, it is advisable to use more standards with smaller differences between them. The zone produced by the unknown is measured and the concentration can then be read off the standard line.

What dilutions of the unknown should be tested depends on the probable antibiotic content. If this is likely to be high as in urine or in serum from patients receiving high dosage penicillin or with gross renal insufficiency, the specimen must be diluted until it falls within the range of the standard curve. With penicillin serum levels, two or three 1 in 5 dilutions may be necessary.

Plates can be inoculated either by pre-seeding the melted agar or by surface flooding. It is not generally necessary to prepare a special assay medium; that used for sensitivity tests will suffice. The sensitivity of the assay is increased if the pH is brought to the optimum for the drug concerned (Table 50) but in practice this is seldom strictly necessary except with streptomycin. It is essential that all the plates used in any assay are prepared from a single batch of medium and identically inoculated at one time.

The depth of the medium affects the size of the zones in any test in which the antibiotic is applied to the surface of the medium unless it is more than 8 mm. deep. The thinner the layer of medium, the more sensitive the test. If very thin plates are used for any method, care must be taken to prevent their drying up during incubation. Results will be affected by the size of the inoculum and the sensitivity of the test will be reduced if it is too heavy. It will be increased by allowing a period of pre-diffusion and by incubating cultures at 30°C.

The original diffusion method described by Heatley (1944) for the assay of penicillin employed porcelain cylinders. These have the advantage that the material for assay need not be sterile but considerable skill is required for their use. Cylinders must be heated just sufficiently to form a seal of agar when placed on the plate: if heating is inadequate or excessive they will either leak when filled or sink too far into the medium and interfere with diffusion. They also require a considerable depth of medium, making the test less sensitive and necessitating some means of preventing the lid of the petri dish resting on them. Stainless steel cylinders do not require heating but slide very easily and have been reported to inactivate some antibiotics (Snell and Lewis, 1959).

The method employing fish spine electrical insulating beads (Fig. 46) given below was described by Lightbown and Sulitzeanu (1957). This has the advantage that beads are filled and placed in position in one operation, they are light and do not move easily and can be used on very thin agar plates.

Holes punched in agar plates are being increasingly used. These can be as little as 4·5 mm. in diameter in plates only 2·5 mm. deep, thus requiring little serum. The surrounding medium must not be lifted when the plug of agar is removed. According to Bennett et al. (1966), who give an excellent description of this method, cups must be completely filled, slight overflow not affecting the results. An alternative is to place a measured volume in each. If rather larger holes (8-9 mm.) are used, smaller amounts of antibiotic can be detected by this method than by any other.

TABLE 51

Suitable standard solutions, in serum, for serum assays

Drug	Test organism	μg./ml.
*Streptomycin Kanamycin Gentamicin Tobramycin	B. subtilis Staph. aureus Klebsiella	75, 15, 3 50, 10, 2 10, 2, 0·4 10, 2, 0·4
Vancomycin	B. subtilis Staph. aureus	50, 10, 2
Penicillin	Staph. aureus B. subtilis	1, 0·5, 0·25, 0·12 10, 2, 0·4
Carbenicillin	Ps. aeruginosa NCTC 10490	50, 25, 12-5, 6·2

* pH of medium must be raised to 7·8.

Blotting paper discs require little serum and can be used with a thin layer of agar. Measured volumes of standards and unknown are pipetted on to discs (which must be large enough to absorb all the fluid completely), before they are applied to the seeded medium. Some types of paper may bind a considerable proportion of many antibiotics and zones will then be smaller than expected and the resulting line may not be straight.

Fish Spine Diffusion Assay

PREPARATION OF FISH SPINES (obtainable from Griffin & George Ltd., Cat. No. L96-320/015).

Boil in 5NHCl. Wash with water until the washings are free from chloride when tested with silver nitrate. Dry at 100°C. overnight. Heat in a muffle furnace at 500°C. for 30 minutes (or roast on asbestos gauze).

PREPARATION OF PLATES. Melt nutrient agar and cool to 48°C. Inoculate to give about 10^5 organisms per ml. Mix well and pipette 10 ml. amounts into flat 9 cm. Petri dishes on a level surface, bursting any bubbles with a hot wire. Allow to dry at room temperature for 1 hour. Alternatively, dry plates containing 10 ml. agar at 37°C. for 30 min. and inoculate by flooding with a suspension of the test organism containing about 10^6 organisms per ml. Drain any excess to the side and remove with a Pasteur pipette. Allow to dry at room temperature.

Prepare standards in serum and if high levels are likely in the specimen, dilute in normal serum. Place all dilutions in shallow wells, as in a suitable blood grouping tile. Fish spines fill by capillarity. Using curved forceps, pick one up as near the top as possible, allow the open end to come in contact with the fluid, lift without tilting and gently place in position on the agar plate without piercing the medium. A ring of fluid appears at the base of the fish spine and does not indicate leakage.

All tests must be done in triplicate.

Incubate overnight, measure zones of inhibition and average the results.

Plot a standard curve and read the concentration corresponding to the diameter of the unknown from this.

Vertical Diffusion Method

The vertical diffusion method devised by Mitchison and Spicer (1949) for the assay of streptomycin can be used for any aminoglycoside and for vancomycin. Standard solutions and unknown are pipetted into narrow tubes containing a column of agar seeded with *Staph. aureus.* The antibiotic diffuses downwards and the edge of the zone of inhibition is marked by a band of large colonies making it possible to measure the zone microscopically, using a micrometer eye piece and the vernier on the moving stage.

Other antibiotics do not give this band of large colonies; the edge of the zone is ill-defined and impossible to measure microscopically (Fig. 49). This has the advantage that it is at once apparent if a second antibiotic is present, even if this was not suspected.

The method was modified by Fujii, Grossman and Ticknor (1961) who added blood to the medium, used *Str. pyogenes* as the test organism and measured the inhibition of haemolysis in the same way. This method can be used for any antibiotic active against *Str. pyogenes.*

Whilst these tubes take longer to read than plate diffusion methods, they are admirable for routine laboratories where few assays are done, being both quick and easy to set up. The material for assay need not be sterile and very small specimens will suffice. In a recent study on neonates (Davies *et al.,* 1970), kanamycin, penicillin and polymyxin were each assayed separately in specimens of <1 ml. blood by using 3 modifications of the method.

TECHNIQUE. Assay medium. Nutrient agar diluted with an equal amount of 1 per cent peptone in water and brought to pH 7·8. Tube in 19 ml. amounts.

Melt the agar and cool to 48°C. Dilute an overnight broth culture of the Oxford *Staph. aureus* 1 in 100, *shake well* to break up clumps and add 1 ml. to the cooled medium. Mix well. Pipette seeded agar into tubes having an internal diameter of 3 mm. to give a column 2-3 cm. deep. Allow to set at least 5 min. Pipette standards and unknown into at least 3 tubes each: the size of the zone is unaffected by the volume as long as the layer is at least 1 mm. deep. Incubate at 37° C. overnight.

To measure zones lay a tube on a slide and fix in position with plasticine. Place on a microscope with a micrometer eye-piece and using the ⅔ objective and reduced light, move the slide until the line in the eye piece falls across the bottom of the meniscus between the serum and the agar. Record the

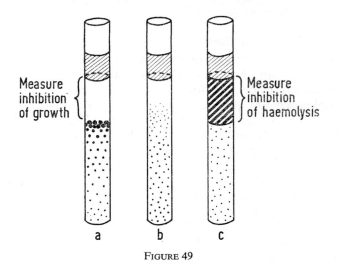

FIGURE 49

Diagrammatic illustration of vertical diffusion assays.
a. Streptomycin over assay agar inoculated with *Staph. aureus*. A band of large colonies gives a clear edge to the zone of inhibition.
b. Penicillin over assay agar inoculated with *Staph. aureus*. Colonies gradually increase in size giving no clear definition to the inhibition zone.
c. Penicillin over blood agar inoculated with *Str. pyogenes*. Haemolysis is inhibited through a well-defined zone, the width of which can be measured accurately.

figure on the vernier on the moving stage. Move the slide across until the large colonies forming the bottom of the zone reach the line; read this measurement and obtain the depth of the zone by subtracting one from the other. The readings for each set of tubes are averaged and a graph constructed from the standards by plotting the log of the concentration against the zone squared (for vancomycin the zone need not be squared). The zone given by the unknown can then be interpreted from this.

BLOOD AGAR MODIFICATION. Melt 17 ml. nutrient agar and cool to 48°C.
Add 2 ml. warmed blood and 1 ml. well shaken overnight culture of *Str. pyogenes* diluted to contain about 10^6 organisms per ml. Mix well and pipette into narrow tubes. Allow to set at least 5 min. Pipette standards and unknown onto at least 3 tubes each and incubate overnight. Measure the zones of inhibition of haemolysis microscopically as in the foregoing method and average the results.

The same standards are used as for other diffusion methods and a straight line is usually obtained by plotting the depth of the zone against the log of the concentration.

Tube Dilution Test

This method is simple to perform and has the advantage that no advance preparations are required, as all drugs can be assayed against either the Oxford staphylococcus or the standard *E. coli* (N.C.T.C. 10418), but the dilutions are widely spaced and results are often inexplicably erratic. When serum is assayed it must first be inactivated by heating to 56°C for 20 minutes.

MEDIUM. Aminoglycosides are considerably affected by the composition of the medium. We have determined the M.I.C. of streptomycin for the Oxford staphylococcus in 6 commercially available nutrient broths and peptone water, all containing 10 per cent of serum. It was found to vary from 8 μg./ml. in tryptone-soya broth to 1 μg./ml. in peptone water (2 brands of peptone gave similar results) and there were similar differences with gentamicin and kanamycin. Aminoglycosides should therefore not be assayed in nutrient broth unless that in use is known not to depress their activity. The peptone water usually available is quite adequate for assaying most drugs, but the addition of 0·5 per cent dextrose and an indicator facilitates reading the results. At least 10 per cent serum should be added and if the drug is heavily protein-bound this should be increased to 50 per cent.

TECHNIQUE. Prepare serial two-fold dilutions in serum peptone-water, in volumes of 1 ml. If blow-out pipettes are used, 2 or 3 two-fold dilutions may be made with the same pipette so long as it is rinsed several times in each. Prepare a control series of dilutions in the same medium from a known solution of the antibiotic. Inoculate both sets of tubes with a standard drop of a suspension of the test organism containing about 10^5 organisms per ml.

The amount of antibiotic in the patient's serum is calculated by multiplying the concentration inhibiting growth in the control series by the dilution of the patient's serum inhibiting growth.

Rapid Assays

When assays are required to monitor treatment with aminoglycosides during renal failure, they are of greater value if the result is available on the same day. The method described by Noone *et al.* (1971) based on the change of pH produced by *Proteus* species in a urea medium requires only 2 hours' incubation, and has the advantage that the presence of most other antibiotics does not interfere with the test. On the other hand, it is laborious to do and requires a pH meter such as is not often available in diagnostic laboratories.

A radio-active assay method based on an R-factor mediated enzyme that adenylates gentamicin and kanamycin (see p. 264) has recently been described by Smith et al. (1972). This is claimed to be more accurate than most microbiological methods, to provide an answer within 1 hour and to require only 0·05 ml. serum. This method can be used to assay gentamicin, kanamycin and tobramycin and is not interfered with by other antibiotics but is only likely to be of interest to departments already doing radio-active assays.

A much simpler procedure is to use a heavy inoculum of a fast-growing test organism with the plate diffusion method; zones can be measured after from 3-5 hours' incubation. Sabath et al. (1970) recommended B. subtilis, pre-seeded plates being prepared in bulk and stored in plastic bags at 4°C. for 2 or more weeks. Warren et al. (1972) recommend Staph. aureus, adding 2 ml. fully grown culture to 100 ml. agar. Neither of these organisms can be used if a second drug is present unless this can first be inactivated (see p. 527) but this problem seldom arises if the Klebsiella (NCTC 10896) recommended on p. 528 is used as test organism. Reeves (1972) recommends the storage of aliquots of a suspension of a Klebsiella containing 5×10^7 organisms per ml. in liquid nitrogen. This is diluted 1 in 50 when required and plates are surface seeded by flooding. If well-dried, thin plates containing a measured volume of agar, and the standard antibiotic solutions in serum are kept prepared at 4°C., these tests can be set up within a few minutes of receiving the specimen. Very little serum is required. This method needs rather longer incubation than those mentioned above, about 4 hours, but it seems to us that in patients with delayed excretion, so long as the result is obtained on the same day, the difference of 2–3 hours is immaterial. The simplicity of this method commends it for general use..

Polymyxin Assays

Polymyxins diffuse poorly through agar but satisfactory results can be obtained with both plate and vertical diffusion methods using *Bord. bronchiseptica* and a medium consisting of tryptone-soya broth + 1 per cent polysorbate 80 (Tween 80), and 1·2 per cent agar, and incubating at 27°C.

If they are assayed by the dilution methods, results can be much affected by the medium and the most consistent results are obtained using serum-peptone water and a small inoculum (10^5 organisms per ml.). The complications of assaying sulphomethyl polymyxins are discussed on page 185.

Trimethoprim Assays

Trimethoprim is always administered with sulphamethoxazole and whilst it is possible to determine the dilution of the serum which will inhibit growth, this cannot be converted into μg./ml. of the mixture. The trimethoprim content can be assayed by inactivating the sulphonamide with *p*-aminobenzoic acid. In either case a thymidine-free medium must be used (see p. 502) together with 0·005 per cent *p*-aminobenzoic acid if required. A spore suspension of *B. pumilis* is generally used for plate diffusion assays but *E coli* is satisfactory: the inoculum should be light.

Anti-fungal Drugs

The majority of these can be assayed by the plate diffusion method using glucose-peptone agar with *Sacch. cerevisiae* or *C. albicans* as test organism, or, if the levels are high enough, by the tube dilution method with glucose-peptone broth. 5-fluorocytosine is inactivated by these media and that described

Assays During Combined Treatment

on page 504 should be used for this drug.

It is often necessary to perform assays on the serum of patients receiving more than one antibiotic. In some cases levels of both drugs may be required (*e.g.* penicillin and streptomycin during the treatment of endocarditis), but more commonly only the aminoglycoside level is required, usually in patients with poor renal function.

If a penicillin or cephalosporin is present, these can be inactivated by the addition of a suitable β-lactamase. Commercial ' penicillinases ' vary greatly in their capacity to inactivate the penicillinase-resistant penicillins and cephalosporins (Newsom,

1967, Newsom and Walsingham, 1973), largely because of the instability of β-lactamase II, the enzyme responsible. The freeze-dried preparation of zinc-stabilized enzymes described by Sabath and Abraham (1966) (Whatman Biochemicals Ltd) which is guaranteed to contain both β-lactamases I and II is of great value to clinical microbiologists. If reconstituted to give 1000 units/ml. and 1 part added to 5 parts serum before assay this will immediately inactivate all penicillins and cephalosporins now in therapeutic use at levels in excess of those encountered in clinical practice. The result of the assay must then be corrected for this dilution. Alternatively, if the vertical diffusion method is used for assay (p. 523) 0·2 ml. of enzyme can be added to 10 ml. agar : this is particularly useful when only small amounts of serum are available.

In the absence of such an enzyme, or when any other antibiotic is present, distinction between these and the aminoglycoside is usually based on their selective bacteristatic activity. A strain of *Klebsiella* is now available (NCTC 10896) which is resistant to most of the common anti-bacterial drugs and can be used for the assay of gentamicin, tobramycin or kanamycin despite the presence of any of those shown in Table 52. This strain was a clinical isolate and it must be remembered that resistance in a normally sensitive species, whether acquired *in vivo* or from *in vitro* training, is not necessarily stable and may be lost during storage. It is important that stock cultures of such organisms be either freeze-dried or stored at $-70°C$. or in liquid nitrogen, and the resistance of subcultures should be checked regularly. Methods for assaying aminoglycosides in the presence of other antibiotics is given in Table 52.

Isoniazid, PAS, ethionamide, ethambutol, pyrazinamide and thiacetazone do not interfere with the assay of aminoglycosides.

Sulphonamides are inactivated by the addition of 0·005 per cent of p-aminobenzoic acid but this has no action on trimethoprim. Both drugs are neutralized by thymidine : 4 $\mu g.$/ml. should be added to the medium.

The unsuspected presence of a second drug may sometimes be detected by careful observation of the zone edge, as is illustrated in Fig. 47. The value of the vertical diffusion method in this respect is described on page 523.

The greater diffusibility of penicillin and the relative resistance of *Str. pyogenes* to aminoglycosides make it possible to assay penicillin by the blood agar vertical diffusion method despite the presence of streptomycin or kanamycin.

Polymyxins can be assayed in the presence of an aminoglycoside if the pH of the medium is lowered to 6·0. This can be achieved by adding 1 per cent KH_2PO_4 to the medium recommended on page 526.

TABLE 52

Methods for assaying gentamicin, tobramycin or kanamycin in the presence of other drugs.

Penicillins Ampicillins Carbenicillin Cloxacillins Methicillin Cephalosporins	Inactivate with suitable β-lactamase or	
Chloramphenicol Clindamycin Lincomycin Fucidin Macrolides Tetracycline		Use *Klebsiella* (NCTC 10896) as test organism
Trimethoprim Sulphonamides	Add thymidine to medium or	
Polymyxins	Use *Staph. aureus* as test organism	
Rifampicin	Use resistant *Staph. aureus* as test organism*	

* A suitable strain can readily be obtained if broth containing about 2 μg./ml. rifampicin or rifamide is heavily inoculated with any *Staph. aureus* which is sensitive to the aminoglycoside to be assayed (including streptomycin).

Assays of Bactericidal Activity

The tube dilution method can be used for estimating the bactericidal activity of the patient's serum during treatment, a proceeding chiefly of interest in cases of bacterial endocarditis.

A series of two-fold dilutions are made in suitable medium and heavily inoculated with the organism isolated from the patient's blood. As with bactericidal sensitivity tests, the result is greatly influenced by the size of the inoculum: 10^6 organisms per ml. is recommended. Any tubes showing no growth after overnight incubation are subcultivated on suitable solid medium and any growth compared with that from the control tube plated before incubation. The greatest dilution giving no growth (or less than 10 colonies in the convention of some laboratories) is reported, and serum bactericidal in a dilution of 1 in 4 is considered satisfactory. This test is based on that described by Jawetz (1962) who also discusses its interpretation and value.

REFERENCES

ANDERSON, T. G. (1970). In *Manual of Clinical Microbiology*, p. 299. Ed. Blair, J. E., Lenette, E. H. & Truant, J. P. Bethesda, Md., *American Society for Microbiology*, p. 299.
ANNEAR, D. I. (1968). *Med. J. Aust.* **1**, 444.
BARBER, M. (1964). *J. gen. Microbiol.* **35**, 183.
BARRY, A. L., GARCIA, F. & THRUPP, L. D. (1970). *Amer. J. clin. Path.* **53**, 149.
BAUER, A. W., KIRBY, W. M. M., SHERRIS, J. C. & TURCK, M. (1966). *Amer. J. clin. Path.*, **45**, 493.
BECHTLE, R. M. & SCHERR, G. H. (1958). *Antibiot. & Chemother.* **8**, 599.
BENNETT, J. V., BRODIE, J. L., BENNER, E. J. & KIRBY, W. M. M. (1966). *Appl. Microbiol.* **14**, 170.
BOVALLIUS, A. & ZACHARIAS, B. (1971). *Appl. Microbiol.* **22**, 260.
BULGER, R. J. & NIELSON, K. (1968). *Appl. Microbiol.* **16**, 890.
BUSHBY, S. R. M. (1969). *Postgrad. med. J.* **45** (Suppl. Nov.) 10.
BUSHBY, S. R. M. & HITCHINGS, G. H. (1968). *Brit. J. Pharmacol.* **33**, 72.
CANETTI, G. & 9 others (1963). *Bull. Wld Hlth Org.* **29**, 565.
CASTLE, A. R. & ELSTUB, J. (1971). *J. clin. Path.* **24**, 773.
CHABBERT, Y. A. & WATERWORTH, P. M. (1965). *J. clin. Path.* **18**, 314.
CLARK, J. (1967). *J. med. Lab. Technol.* **24**, 212.
DARRELL, J. H., GARROD, L. P. & WATERWORTH, P. M. (1968). *J. clin. Path.* **21**, 202.
DAVIES, P. A., DARRELL, J. H., CHANDRAN, K. R. & WATERWORTH, P. M. (1970). In *The Control of Chemotherapy*, p. 49. Ed. Watt, P. J. Edinburgh: Livingstone.
DREW, W. L., BARRY, A. L., O'TOOLE, R. & SHERRIS, J. C. (1972). *Appl. Microbiol.* **24**, 240.
ELEK, S. D. & HILSON, G. R. F. (1954). *J. clin. Path.* **7**, 37.
ERICSSON, H. M. (1960). *Scand. J. clin. Lab. Invest.* **12**, Suppl. 50.
ERICSSON, H. M. & SHERRIS, J. C. (1971). *Acta path. microbiol. scand.* Section B Suppl. 217.
FEDERAL, REGISTER (1972). **37**, 20525.
FELMINGHAM, D. & STOKES, E. J. (1972). *Med. Lab. Technol.* **29**, 198.
FUJII, R., GROSSMAN, M. & TICKNOR. W. (1961). *Pediatrics* **28**, 662.
GARROD, L. P. & WATERWORTH, P. M. (1962). *J. clin. Path.* **15**, 328.
GARROD, L. P. & WATERWORTH, P. M. (1969). *J. clin. Path.* **22**, 534.
GARROD, L. P. & WATERWORTH, P. M. (1971). *J. clin. Path.* **24**, 779.
HANUS, F. J., SANDS, J. G. & BENNETT, E. O. (1967). *Appl. Microbiol.* **15**, 31.
HARPER, G. J. & CAWSTON. W. C. (1945). *J. Path. Bact.* **57**, 59.
HEATLEY, N. G. (1944). *Biochem. J.* **38**, 61.
HEWITT, J. H., COE, A. W. & PARKER, M. T. (1969). *J. med. Microbiol.* **2**, 443.
HOWIE, J. W. (1962). *Lancet* **i**, 1137.
JAWETZ, E. (1962). *Amer. J. Dis. Child.* **103**, 81.
KENSIT, J. G. & SIMMONS, N. A. (1973). *Brit. med. J.* **1**, 230.
KOCH, A. E. & BURCHALL, J. J. (1971). *Appl. Microbiol.* **22**, 812.
KUNIN, C. M. & EDMONDSON, W. P. (1968). *Proc. Soc. Exp. Biol. (N.Y.)* **129**, 118.
LIGHTBOWN, J. W. & SULITZEANU, D. (1957). *Bull. Wld Hlth Org.* **17**, 553.
LINE, D. H., POOLE, G. W. & WATERWORTH, P. M. (1970). *Tubercle* **51**, 76.
MITCHISON, D. A. & SPICER, C. C. (1949). *J. gen. Microbiol.* **3**, 184.
NEWSOM, S. W. B. (1967). *Brit. med. J.* **3**, 678.
NEWSOM, S. W. B. & WALSINGHAM, B. M. (1973). *J. med. Microbiol.* **6**, 59.

NOONE, P., PATTISON, J. R. & SAMSON, D. (1971). *Lancet* **2**, 16.
PEARD, M. C., FLECK, D. G., GARROD, L. P. & WATERWORTH, P. M. (1970). *Brit. med. J.* **4**, 410.
REEVES, D. S. (1972). *Lancet* **2**, 1369.
REPORT (1965). 'Report on the antibiotic sensitivity test trial organized by the Bacteriology Committee of the Association of Clinical Pathologists. *J. clin. Path.* **18**, 1.
RYAN. K. J., NEEDHAM, G. M., DUNSMOOR, C. L. & SHERRIS, J. C. (1970). *Appl. Microbiol.* **20**, 447.
SABATH, L. D. & ABRAHAM, E. P. (1966). *Biochem. J.* **98**, 11c.
SABATH, L. D., LODER, P. B., GERSTEIN, D. A. & FINLAND, M. (1968). *Appl. Microbiol.* **16**, 877.
SABATH, L. D., CASEY, J. I., RUCH, P. A., STUMPF, L. L. & FINLAND, M. (1971). *Antimicrob. Agents and Chemother.*—1970. p. 83.
SCHOENKNECHT, F. D. & SHERRIS, J. C. (1973). In *Recent Advances in Clinical Pathology,* Series 6. Ed. Dyke, S. C. Edinburgh: Churchill Livingstone. p. 275.
SHADOMY, S. (1969). *Appl. Microbiol.* **17**, 871.
SMITH, D. H., VAN OTTO, B. & SMITH, A. L. (1972). *New Engl. J. Med.* **286**, 583.
SNELL, N. S. & LEWIS, J. C. (1959). *Antibiot. Chemother.* **6**, 609.
STOKES, E. J. (1968). *Clinical Bacteriology,* Third Edition. London: Arnold. p. 179.
STOKES, E. J. & WATERWORTH, P. M. (1972). Association of Clinical Pathologists Broadsheet No. 55 (Revised).
THOMAS, M. & BALDWIN, G. (1971). *J. clin. Path.* **24**, 320.
TOZER, R. A., BOUTFLOWER, S. & GILLESPIE, W. A. (1966). *Lancet* **1**, 686.
WARREN, E. SNYDER, R. J. & WASHINGTON, J. A. II (1972). *Antimicrob. Agents and Chemother.* **1**, 46.
WATERWORTH, P. M. (1962). *J. med. Lab. Technol.* **19**, 163.
WATERWORTH, P. M. (1966). *J. med. Lab. Technol.* **23**, 96.
WATERWORTH, P. M. (1969a). *Postgrad. med. J.* **45** (Suppl. Nov.), 21.
WATERWORTH, P. M. (1969b). *J. med. Lab. Technol.* **26**, 106.
WATERWORTH, P. M. (1971). *Postgrad. med. J.* **47** (Suppl. Feb.), 25

INDEX

The Central Press (Aberdeen) Ltd